Ophthalmic Care

Ophthalmic Care

Edited by,

JANET MARSDEN MSc, BSc, RGN, OND
Manchester Metropolitan University,
Chair of Royal College of Nursing,
Ophthalmic Nursing Forum

WILEY

Other Wiley Editorial Offices

John Wiley & Sons Inc., 111 River Street, Hoboken, NJ 07030, USA

Jossey-Bass, 989 Market Street, San Francisco, CA 94103-1741, USA

Wiley-VCH Verlag GmbH, Boschstr. 12, D-69469 Weinheim, Germany

John Wiley & Sons Australia Ltd, 42 McDougall Street, Milton, Queensland 4064, Australia

John Wiley & Sons (Asia) Pte Ltd, 2 Clementi Loop #02-01, Jin Xing Distripark, Singapore
129809

John Wiley & Sons Canada Ltd, 22 Worcester Road, Etobicoke, Ontario, Canada
M9W 1L1

Wiley also publishes its books in a variety of electronic formats. Some content that appears in
print may not be available in electronic books.

A catalogue record for this book is available from the British Library

ISBN -13   978-1-86156-488-7 (PB)

Printed and bound in Great Britain by TJ International Ltd, Padstow, Cornwall

This book is printed on acid-free paper responsibly manufactured from sustainable forestry
in which at least two trees are planted for each one used for paper production.

Contents

Foreword

To paraphrase Bill Clinton's celebrated campaign slogan, the adage - "it's the patient, stupid"- would seem to sum up perfectly the essential message of this new treatise on eye care written for and by ophthalmic professionals. As the book's editor Janet Marsden herself points out whilst discussing emergency service provision ..... "It is irrelevant who cares for the patient, as long as the clinician who does so is competent to undertake the role, understands the parameters of the role, is able and willing to refer when necessary to more appropriate care and that the care of the patient as well as his presenting problem is paramount." This role statement differs in no material respect from the essence of the Royal College of Ophthalmologist's description of what an ophthalmologist can and should be doing. Yet this book is being published at a time when the Royal Colleges in the UK (and especially the surgical Colleges) are in disarray over the extent to which, and the circumstances under which, care that they perceive to be the primary prerogative of medical school-trained practitioners should be undertaken by others, and not least by nurses. It is fully acknowledged that the depth of understanding, the mastery of surgical techniques and the experience required of medical specialists (who are ultimately responsible for the patients' care) will exceed that of other members of the multidisciplinary team in certain areas of practice. However, it is also arguably the case that the need for a book of this nature signals a current failure to put the patient's needs squarely at the centre of the training agenda for the variety of health professionals with whom the patient may have contact. That is not to say that 'one-size-fits-all' educational material would be appropriate, but rather that 'fit-for-purpose' is the basic aspiration for training of a range of practitioners whose contributions should overlap wherever possible if eye care is to be other than an exercise in passing the parcel.

The management needs of the majority of ophthalmic patients, including drug prescribing and technical procedures, can be met by appropriately trained individuals who have not had recourse to a dozen or more years of progressively specialized medical and surgical training. Admittedly, high standards of practical expertise can only be acquired through on-the-job experience and guidance, but this manual by an international panel of contributors will underpin in-service development, and its concise readability will surely help to encourage enthusiasm for our subject. Happily, generic caring skills and attitudes are entirely transferable to the small world of ophthalmology and, once its vocabulary has been addressed if not mastered, learning to provide expert care for those with eye afflictions can be intensely rewarding, a sentiment that this book subliminally conveys throughout.

The pre-qualification training of health professionals in 'ophthalmics' is universally disproportionate (ie inversely proportionate) to the frequency with which patients present themselves with their wide array of eye- and vision-related problems. Fortunately, obtaining a good history remains the key to successful diagnosis and management notwithstanding the extraordinary brevity accorded to history-taking and recording by the majority of ophthalmologists. Eliciting an accurate history contributes enormously to the safety of telephone triage and advice, a key role often undertaken by nurses in our modern-day eye service. Indeed, one of the great attractions of our specialty is the considerable extent to which the professional-of-first-encounter with the patient can come to an accurate conclusion about the clinical problem without recourse to extensive laboratory tests and distressing, expensive or time-consuming investigations (making it all the more surprising that general medical practitioners have largely abdicated from this particular area of patient care). This presumes, of course, that the individual involved has the necessary examination skills and is secure in his/her knowledge of eye anatomy, physiology and pathology. Fostering the acquisition of such comprehensive and fundamental knowledge in nurses, while maintaining an emphasis on the holistic approach and on clarity over professional roles and responsibilities, is both the challenge and success of this book.

David McLeod
Professor of Ophthalmology and Honorary Consultant
Ophthalmic Surgeon, Manchester Royal Eye Hospital.

May 2005

Preface

The concept of this book arose out of a recognition by ophthalmic nurses that, in general, existing text books for nurses working in the speciality did not have the depth of content to inform and evidence their practice. This book is designed therefore, to meet the needs of ophthalmic professionals and most especially, ophthalmic nurses, whose practice has expanded exponentially over the past few years, into areas we would never have dreamed possible. This expansion though has often been accompanied by a lack of accessible evidence to underpin it and this is the gap the book aims to bridge.

It has been written by an international team of ophthalmic practitioners, all experts in their fields who have given up a large amount of time, immensely willingly, to develop the dream into the reality because of their passion for and dedication to their area of practice.

It is hoped that the book, while combining depth and breadth of content, does this in an accessible manner which enables it to be used as a comprehensive resource not just for ophthalmic professionals, but for any health care professional who ever cares for a patient with an eye problem, thus enabling them to develop the knowledge and skills to incorporate consideration of their patients' eye problems into their practice.

The book is divided into three parts. The first section considers some general aspects relating to the understanding of the function and structure of the eye. The first two chapters cover the physiology of vision including embryology (in order to give an overview of how we see), and basic optics as applied to the eye. This section goes on to consider how drugs affect the eye and the main categories of ophthalmic drugs and delivery systems as well as some of the adverse effects of systemic and ophthalmic drugs. It concludes with a section about drugs and the nurse, considering both legal aspects prescription, supply and administration of drugs by nurses in the UK. The eye examination chapter considers the requirements for effective assessment of the patient including, physical surroundings, taking a history and obtaining accurate visual acuity. It stresses the need for systematic eye examination and considers both the structures that may be examined and what the examiner should be looking for. It goes on to consider the use of more sophisticated ophthalmic equipment.

The second section of the book considers issues surrounding patient care. It begins by considering visual impairment, its effects on the patient and strategies that may be used both by the patient, and carers and health professionals in order to maximise autonomy and independence. Patient education is considered, both in general terms and for this particular client group and the chapter entitled "Work and the eye" considers some work related issues and some of the UK legislation pertaining to eye care and visual standards. Care of the patient in the ophthalmic setting makes up the next five chapters considering, in turn, care of the patient undergoing day surgery and inpatient care, care of the child in the ophthalmic setting and care of the ophthalmic patient in the theatre area. The chapter entitled "care of patients presenting with acute problems" discusses triage and telephone triage both in general terms and relating to the speciality. It goes onto discuss the diagnosis, care and treatment of patients presenting with ophthalmic trauma and with acute, non traumatic 'red eyes'. This section concludes with a chapter which considers some of the challenges facing those working in eye health settings in developing countries.

The third section takes a systematic approach to the care of patients with ophthalmic problems. The work of all ophthalmic health professionals are very closely intertwined and this is reflected in the structure of these chapters. Following the theme developed in the discussion of systematic eye examination and working from the front to the back of the eye, each chapter considers the anatomy and physiology of a structure (e.g. lens, cornea) or group of structures (The eyelids and lacrimal drainage system) and follows this with discussion of some of the common disorders of these structures. This includes, the causes, presentation, special tests, diagnosis and treatment of these disorders integrated with the care of the patient presenting with this problem. The final chapter considers the ocular manifestations of a number of the more common systemic diseases which may be encountered by health professionals.

After the ocular systems related chapters, there follows an appendix which gives useful addresses and the contact details of many organisations and sources of support to health care professionals and patients. Ophthalmology has a language of its own which can be confusing for people new to the speciality, those outside it and even some very experienced practitioners on occasion. The book therefore concludes with a glossary.

It must be remembered that the legal aspects of practice discussed here are of necessity, UK based and the reader should consider recommendation in the light of their national legal framework as well as local policies.

I hope the reality of the book, enables the dream of effective, evidence based, informed and thinking practice for all those with eye problems, via those who care for them.

Janet Marsden

May 2005

Contributors

Sharon Andrew MRPharmS, NHS Liaison Executive (formerly Directorate Pharmacist, Surgery, Manchester Royal Infirmary), Alcon Laboratories UK (Ltd)

Jilly Bradshaw RGN, RSCN, Paediatric Nurse, Bournemouth Eye Unit, Bournemouth

Olga HL Brochner RGON PgDip, Staff Nurse and Research Co-ordinator, Ophthalmology Department, Auckland Hospital

Gayle Catt BHSc, Staff Nurse, Ophthalmology Department, Auckland Hospital

Ingrid Cox RGN, KRN, COA, ENB 176, Training Advisor for Mid-Level Eye Care, Christian Blind Mission International, Central and East Africa

Helen Davies MSc, RGN, ONC, Dip PP, Lead Nurse, HM Stanley Hospital, St Asaph, Denbighshire, Wales

Patricia Evans PGCE, BSc (Hons), ENB 346, RGN, Lecturer Practitioner (Ophthalmology), Moorfields Eye Hospital NHS Foundation Trust, London and St Bartholomew School of Nursing and Midwifery, City University, London

Dorothy E Field PhD, RGN, OND, BSc(Hons), PGCE(A), MA, EdD, Bournemouth Eye Unit, Royal Bournemouth General Hospital

Margaret Gurney RN, OND, BSc(Hons), MSc, Consultant Nurse, Maidstone and Tunbridge Wells Trust

Bradley Kirkwood MA, BN, ONC, Ophthalmic Nurse Practitioner, Flinders Medical Centre, Adelaide, South Australia

Agnes Lee MPhil, BSc(Hons), DipN, RGN, SCM, OND, Lecturer Practitioner, Manchester Royal Eye Hospital, Manchester

Janet Marsden MSc, BSc, RGN, OND, Senior Lecturer Manchester Metropolitan University and Chair of the RCN Ophthalmic Nursing Forum

Les McQueen RGN, OND, Dip HE, Ophthalmic Charge Nurse, North Glasgow University Hospitals Division, Stobhill Hospital, Glasgow

Yvonne Needham MA, BSc, RGN, OND, Director of Pre-Registration Nursing and Midwifery, Faculty of Health and Social Care, University of Hull

Andrew R Potter MBE, MA, MRCGP, MRCOphth, DTM&H, Ophthalmologist, Christian Blind Mission International, Republic of Benin, West Africa

Susanne Raynel MA, RGON, ADN, BHSc, OND, Manager, Ophthalmology Department, Auckland Hospital, Auckland

Allyson Ryder DBO(D), Orthoptic Clinical Specialist, Wrightington, Wigan and Leigh NHS Trust

Ramesh Seewoodhary BSc(Hons), RGN, OND(Hons), RCNT, RNT, CertEd, Senior Lecturer, Ophthalmic Nursing Programme, Thames Valley University

Mary E Shaw MSc, BA, RN, RNT, RCNT, OND, Cert Ed, Senior Nurse/ Lecturer Practitioner, Manchester Royal Eye Hospital

David M Spence BSc(Hons), DipOptom, Optometrist, Devon

Sue Stevens RGN, RM, OND, FETC, Ophthalmic Resource Co-ordinator and Nurse Advisor, International Centre for Eye Health, London School of Hygiene and Tropical Medicine, UK

Gill Taylor BA(Hons), RNT, CertEd, RGN, OND, ENB 176, Cert in Counselling, Lecturer in Adult Nursing, St Bartholomew School of Nursing and Midwifery, City University, London

Bronwyn Ward RGON, BHSc, Charge Nurse, Ophthalmology Department, Auckland Hospital, Auckland

Linda Whitaker RGN, OND(Hons), RCNT, RNT, BA, MA, Research Sister, Cancer Research UK, St James' Leeds

Anatomical Illustrations

Stuart E Lee DipAd, ATD

Acknowledgements

There are a large number of people to thank for getting this book from the idea to the reality – Jim McCarthy for asking me to take the project on (and believing I'd get there eventually), to the chapter authors for putting so much work into passing on their passion for ophthalmic care and for their suggestions and encouragement. To Stuart for the anatomical illustrations and last, but certainly not least, to Dave for putting up with me!

In addition, a number of companies were kind enough to contribute to the project so I'd like to thank.

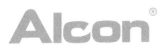

Allergan

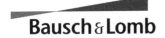

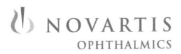

Pfizer

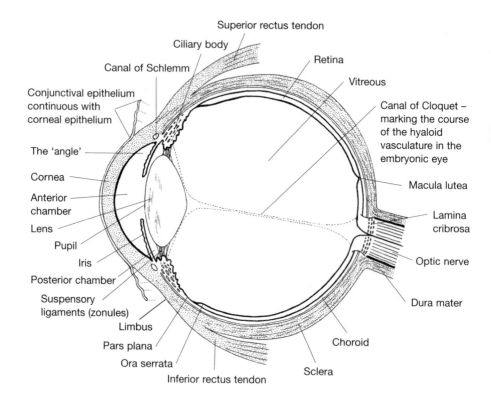

Figure 1 Section through the globe.

CHAPTER ONE

Physiology of vision

RAMESH SEEWOODHARY

The aim of this chapter is to explore the physiology of vision. It is divided into six parts to enable the reader to have an understanding of the concept of sight:

1. Embryological development of the eye
2. Development of visual perception
3. Mechanism of vision in dim light and bright light
4. Light detection and dark adaptation
5. Colour vision
6. Control of eye movements and binocular vision.

Embryological development of the eye

Early eye development starts around day 22 of the embryo's life, and the eye measures 2–3 mm in length. The neural folds fuse to form the neural tube, but, before they complete their closure, the optic sulci appear as shallow grooves or pits in the inner part of the neural folds (Figure 1.1a).

The folds fuse shortly afterwards to form the forebrain, and the optic sulci evaginate to form the optic vesicles (Figure 1.1b). Invagination of the lower surface of the optic stalk and the optic vesicle occurs simultaneously, creating a groove known as the choroidal fissure. At the same time, the lens plate also invaginates to form the lens vesicle. By about 4 weeks, the lens vesicle separates completely from the surface ectoderm to lie free in the rim of the optic cup.

The choroidal fissure allows entrance into the optic stalk of the vascular mesoderm, which eventually forms the hyaloid system. As invagination is completed, the choroidal fissure narrows until it is closed by 6 weeks, leaving one small permanent opening at the anterior end of the optic stalk through which pass the hyaloid artery by the fourth month and the central retinal artery and vein thereafter (Figure 1.1c).

(a)

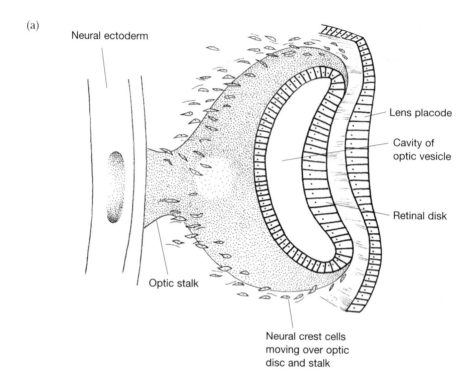

(b)

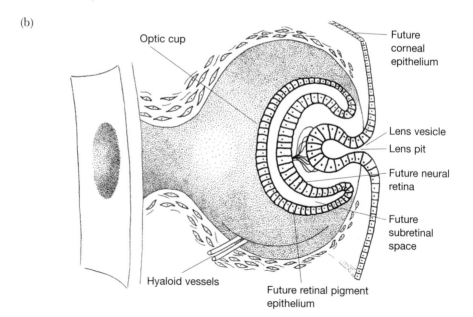

Figure 1.1 The eye at different gestational ages: (a) at 4 weeks; (b) at 5 weeks.

(c)

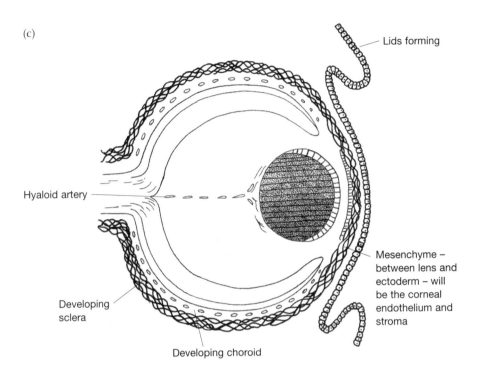

(d)

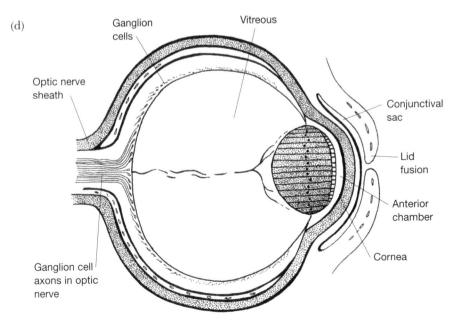

Figure 1.1 The eye at different gestational ages: (c) at 7 weeks; and (d) at 8 weeks.

After the fourth month, the general structure of the eye has been determined. Development after this consists of differentiation into individual structures, which occurs more rapidly in the posterior than in the anterior segment early in gestation and more rapidly in the anterior segment later in gestation (Vaughan et al. 1998).

Generally, the eye is derived from three embryonic layers, namely, surface ectoderm, neural ectoderm and mesoderm:

- The surface ectoderm gives rise to the lens, the lacrimal gland, corneal epithelium, conjunctiva, adnexal glands and epidermis of the lid.
- The neural ectoderm gives rise to the optic vesicle and optic cup, and is responsible for the formation of the retina, ciliary body, pupillary muscle sphincter and dilator, optic nerve and glia.
- The mesoderm contributes to the extraocular muscles, sclera, and orbital and ocular vascular endothelium.

The time line of ocular embryogenesis is summarized in Table 1.1.

Table 1.1 Time line of ocular embryogenesis

Period after conception	Event	Period after conception	Event
Day 22	Optic groove appears	Week 5	Lens pit forms and depends into lens vesicle
Day 25	Optic vesicle forms from optic pit		Hyaloid vessels develop
			Primary vitreous develops
Day 26	Primordia of superior rectus, inferior rectus, medial rectus, and inferior oblique appear		Osseous structures of the orbit begin to develop
		Week 6	Closure of embryonic fissure
Day 27	Formation of lens plate from surface ectoderm Primordium of lateral rectus appears		Corneal epithelial cells develop interconnections Differentiation of retinal pigment epithelium Proliferation of neural retinal cells
Day 28	Embryonic fissure forms Cells destined to become retinal pigment Epithelium acquires pigmentation		Formation of secondary vitreous Formation of primary lens fibres Development of periocular vasculature Appearance of eyelids folds and nasolacrimal duct
Day 29	Primordium of superior oblique appears		Ciliary ganglion appears

Table 1.1 continued

Period after conception	Event	Period after conception	Event
Week 7	Migration of ganglion cells toward optic disc Formation of embryonic lens nucleus Development of choroidal vessels from periocular mesenchyme Three waves of neural crest migration: first wave: formation of corneal and trabecular endothelium second wave: formation of corneal stroma third wave: formation of iris stroma Formation of tunica vasculosa lentis Sclera begins to form	Month 4 *continued*	Development of longitudinal ciliary muscle and processes of ciliary body Formation of tertiary vitreous Bowman's membrane forms Canal of Schlemm appears Eyelids, glands and cilia form
		Month 5	Photoreceptors differentiate Eyelid separation begins
Month 3	Differentiation of precursors of rods and cones Ciliary body develops Appearance of limbus Anterior chamber appears as a potential space Sclera condenses Eyelid folds lengthen and fuse	Month 6	Cones differentiate Ganglion cells thicken in macula Differentiation of dilator pupillae muscle Nasolacrimal system becomes patent
		Month 7	Rods differentiate Ora serrata forms Migration of ganglion cells to form nerve fibre layer of Henle Choroid becomes pigmented Circular ciliary muscle fibres develop Myelination of optic nerve Posterior movement of anterior chamber angle Orbicularis muscle differentiation
Month 4	Formation of retinal vasculature begins Beginning of regression of hyaloid vessels Formation of physiological cup of optic disc Formation of lamina cribrosa Major arterial circle of iris forms Development of iris sphincter muscle	Month 8	Completion of anterior chamber angle formation Hyaloid vessels disappear
		Month 9	Retinal vessels reach the temporal periphery Pupillary membrane disappears
		After birth	Development of macula

Adapted from Yanoff and Duker (1999).

Development of visual perception

Perception of the environment is the end product of the reinterpretation or processing by the visual cortex of the responses made by the retina to visual stimuli. There is no strict separation of cortical and retinal function because some processing takes place in the retina and it is felt that the cortex may not be solely responsible for other processes.

There must be discrimination by means of brightness gradients in the cortex, as well as in the retina. The cortex must be precisely aware of the form and shape of objects and, finally, of the identity of these objects. In the adult, all these processes occur rapidly; we perceive only the objects' identities and react to them automatically and appropriately, often without being fully conscious of them. In the infant, these processes occur slowly and the final stages of form perception and object identification may not occur at all. Although form perception develops automatically with maturation, identification depends on the capacity to acquire and store information and also on the accumulation of experiences on which identification is based.

Retinal response to light and to moving objects by reflex responses of blinking, pupillary contraction and eye movements occurs even in the short gestation infant and is well established in the normal neonate. According to Gesell et al. (1949), during the first few weeks, the infant begins to gaze around him- or herself, and sometimes to fixate objects. Sporadic body activity then ceases and respiration rate alters; there seems to be some awareness of and attention to the environment. This visual exploration of the environment increases with age, especially when infants are handled or situated in complex and unrestricted environments (White and Castle 1964). In young infants the information is fragmentary. Infants aged 2 months cannot store and retain information for more than a very brief period of about 1 second. Each successive appearance of a stimulus is perceived as a new event, so that the environment is experienced in a disconnected manner. At 6 months, the span of attention is so narrow that a single stimulus may capture it entirely. The infant will concentrate on a stimulus in an indiscriminate manner, in order to obtain all possible information from it, and cannot attend selectively.

Awareness of an object involves discrimination between it and its surroundings; brightness and colour discrimination contribute to this also. Infants are known to gaze longer at blue and green stimuli and least at yellow. Experiments by Fantz (1958) suggest that, from a very early age, there is some discrimination between patterns. He claimed that infants within the first week or so of life gazed longer at a picture of a face than at a half-black, half-pink shape. It has been found that infants under 1 month tend to look longer at very simple patterns, such as a half-white, half-black field or one with four quadrants, than at more complex patterns. This is a result of the retinal images being too blurred for finer perception.

Accommodation develops during the second month and it is comparable to that of a normal adult by 4 months. Infants look relatively longer at chequered patterns with four squares by week 3. This increases to 64 squares at week 8 and 576 squares at week 14. Attention to pictures and photographs of faces emerges at 3–4 months. Kagan et al. (1966) found that this is followed by the infant smiling more and more, suggesting that some degree of familiarity is involved.

Development in the accuracy of shape perception takes place in close conjunction with tactile exploration. Before the age of 3 months, the infant is unaware of any association between the visual and the tactile sensory patterns and does not attempt to handle objects that he or she perceives visually, or to examine visually the objects that he or she handles. At 3 months, White and Castle (1964) found that infants stretch out a hand towards an object that they see and glance repeatedly to and fro between the hand and the object. At about 4 months they grasp the object and cease to look at the hand. They explore the object with their fingers, comparing the shape that they feel with the shape that they see (Piaget 1952). Infants thus discover the nature of three-dimensional solid form and also that, as an object is turned round in space, the visual pattern changes regularly, although the object as felt remains the same. It is not until 8–9 months that the infant realizes this fully.

By means of visual and tactile exploration of objects, infants learn not only to discriminate between similar objects but to remember and identify them. In the latter part of their first year, they begin to realize that objects have a permanent identity and that when they are hidden from sight they do not cease to exist but may reappear. Complex shapes are not perceived with complete accuracy until 5–6 years.

Understanding of the relationships of objects to their surroundings also develops gradually. Discrimination of distance, by means of parallactic movement, between fairly near solid objects develops before 2 months (Bower 1965). Infants then learn that they can stretch for and obtain objects within their reach, whereas they can get more distant ones only by crying for someone to give them to them. During the first year of life, infants hardly notice the existence of far-distant objects or else they may suppose that these can also be obtained by crying for them. However, once they begin to move about, infants realize better the relative distances of further objects. The exact nature of environmental spatial relationships is not understood until the age of 6–7 years or even more.

Thus, it is evident that perception of the environment and the objects that it contains, which occurs in older children and adults, is acquired only gradually. The processes of attention, discrimination, form perception, identification and spatial location, requiring both maturation and learning through experience, develop to some extent independently of each other and are not accurately coordinated and integrated, especially with complex precepts, until much later.

Mechanism of vision in dim light and bright light

The mechanism of vision in both dim light and bright light involves the retinal photoreceptors known as rods (for dim light) and cones (for bright light and colour vision). The rod and cone photoreceptors are illustrated in Figure 1.2.

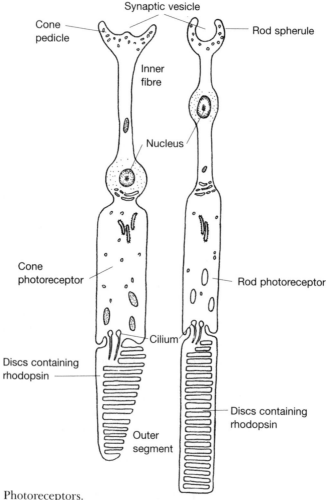

Figure 1.2 Photoreceptors.

Mechanism of vision in dim light

White light is the result of the fusion of coloured lights that can be separated by shining a beam of white light through a glass prism. This is called the visible spectrum (Figure 1.3).

Visual photoreceptors contain pigments that break down chemically in the presence of low illumination. This forms a chemical stimulus, which triggers off nerve impulses that travel from the retina to the cerebral cortex.

Scotopic vision is vision in dim light. It depends on rod photoreceptors. Rods are of one type of photoreceptor and give monochromatic vision. They contain rhodopsin, also known as visual purple. When light of low intensity enters the eye, rhodopsin is immediately changed into lumirhodopsin. However, lumirhodopsin is a very unstable compound that can last in the retina only about a tenth of a second. It decays almost immediately into another substance known as metarhodopsin and this compound, which is also unstable, decays very rapidly into retinene and scotopsin. In the process of splitting rhodopsin, the rods become excited by ionic charges that last only a split second. This results in nerve signals being generated in the rod and transmitted to the brain via the optic nerve.

Red	Orange	Yellow	Green	Blue	Indigo	Violet

Figure 1.3 Visible spectrum of white light.

Figure 1.4 illustrates that, after rhodopsin has been decomposed by light energy, its decomposition products, retinene and scotopsin, are recombined again during the next few minutes by the metabolic processes of the cell to form new rhodopsin. The new rhodopsin can be used again to provide more rod excitation, resulting in a continuous cycle. Rhodopsin is being formed continuously and is broken down by light energy to excite the rods.

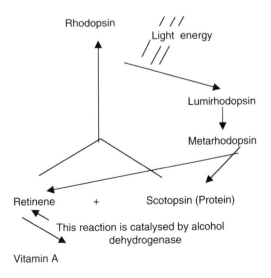

Figure 1.4 The retinene–rhodopsin chemical cycle responsible for light sensitivity of the rods (adapted from Guyton 1979).

When a person passes from a brightly lit scene to darkness he or she is temporarily blinded as a result of the low light levels. In the dark, the eye becomes progressively more sensitive to stimulation by light until a maximum threshold is reached after 30 minutes. The eye then sees much smaller light stimuli than it would in light conditions. This adjustment or increase in sensitivity is called dark adaptation. As light brightness or intensity increases rods lose their sensitivity and cease to respond.

Mechanism of vision in bright light

Photopic vision occurs in bright light and is dependent on cone photoreceptors. Cones are thought to be of three types, thus giving trichromatic vision. Each type has a different photosensitive visual pigment with its own wavelength to which it is sensitive, which it absorbs and by which it is broken down to form the chemical stimulus.

The visual pigments in the cone photoreceptors respond to red, green and blue light (the long, medium and short wavelengths of the visible spectrum). All three types of photopsins are stimulated in roughly equal proportions when white light falls on the retina. The various types of colour blindness could be explained in terms of the absence or deficiency of one or more of these special receptors.

Almost exactly the same chemical processes occur in the cones as in the rods, except that the protein scotopsin of the rods is replaced by one of three similar proteins called photopsins. The chemical differences among the photopsins make the three different types of cones selectively sensitive to different colours. A colour sensation has three qualities:

1. Hue: depends largely on the wavelength.
2. Saturation:
   – a saturated colour has no white light mixed with it
   – an unsaturated colour has some white light mixed with it.
3. Intensity: brightness depends largely on the strength of the light.

As the intensity of light is reduced the cones cease to respond and the rods take over, which explains why, in dark conditions, colour is perceived only very dimly, often just as variations of a shade of grey rather than as a colour.

Exposure of the dark adapted eye to bright light results in a marked decrease in sensitivity to light which takes place over a period of about 1 minute, during which the rhodopsin is bleached and the pupil constricts to let less light into the eye. This adjustment on exposure to bright light is called light adaptation.

Light detection and dark adaptation

The effect of a visual stimulus is not uniform because it depends on the state of adaptation of the retina at the time of stimulus. In a state of light adaptation, vision is mediated largely by the cones, which deal with the appreciation of form and colour. This is known as photopic vision.

In a state of dark adaptation, the vision is mediated by the rod photoreceptors, which are concerned essentially with the appreciation of light and movement. This is known as scotopic vision.

It is a common experience to be almost totally blinded when first entering a very bright area from a darkened room and when entering a darkened room from a brightly lit area. The reason for this is that the sensitivity of the retina is temporarily not attuned to the intensity of the light. To discern the shape, texture and other qualities of an object, it is necessary to see both the bright and dark areas of the object at the same time. Fortunately, the retina automatically adjusts its sensitivity in proportion to the degree of light energy available. This phenomenon is called light and dark adaptation.

When large quantities of light energy strike the rods, large amounts of rhodopsin are broken into retinene and scotopsin and, because rhodopsin formation is a slow process, requiring several minutes, the concentration of rhodopsin in the rods falls to a very low value as the person remains in the bright light. Essentially, the same effects occur in the cones. Therefore, the sensitivity of the retina soon becomes greatly depressed in bright light.

The mechanism of dark adaptation is opposite to that of light adaptation. When the person enters a darkened room from a lighted area, the quantity of rhodopsin in the rods (and colour-sensitive chemicals in the cones) is at first very slight. As a result, the person cannot see anything. Yet, the amount of light energy in the darkened room is also very slight, which means that very little of the rhodopsin being formed in the rods is broken down. Therefore, the concentration of rhodopsin builds up during the ensuing minutes until it finally becomes high enough for even a very minute amount of light to stimulate the rods.

During dark adaptation, the sensitivity of the retina can increase as much as 1000-fold in only a few minutes and as much as 100 000 times in an hour or more. This effect is illustrated in Figure 1.5 which shows the retinal sensitivity increasing from an arbitrary light-adapted value of 1 up to a dark-adapted value of 100 000 in 1 hour after the person has left a very bright area and moved into a completely darkened room. Then, on re-entering the bright area, light adaptation occurs and retinal sensitivity decreases from 100 000 back down to 1 in another 10 minutes which is a more rapid process than dark adaptation.

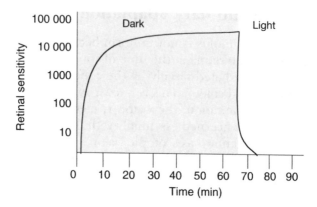

Figure 1.5 Dark and light adaptation. (Adapted from Guyton 1979.)

Colour vision

Colour is detected by cone photoreceptors and it is advisable for colour vision testing to be done in early life, between the age of 8 and 12. Colour vision is important in many occupations, e.g. electronic engineering, air pilot traffic control, ophthalmologist, etc. (see Chapter 7).

Colour vision is not complete until 6 months after birth when, at the same time, the macula is fully developed. Colour appreciation in the retina is ill understood and the only acceptable theory that supports colour appreciation is the Young–Helmholtz theory.

This theory assumes the cone photoreceptors are the perceiving colour elements and are concerned with three essential colours (Figure 1.6a):

1. Red (700 nm light wavelength)
2. Green (600 nm light wavelength)
3. Blue (420 nm light wavelength).

In 1802, Thomas Young proposed that the human eye could detect different colours, because it contained three types of receptor, each sensitive to a particular hue. His theory was referred to as the trichromatic theory:

- Blue pigment absorbing maximally at 420 nm
- Green absorbing at 530 nm (mid-wavelength pigment)
- Red absorbing at 565 nm (long-wavelength pigment)
- (Dotted line in Figure 1.6b represents red pigment = 499 nm.)

There are three types of cone photoreceptors and all colours are produced by varying degrees of stimulation of all three types. The eye can recognize about 150 variations of colour.

(a)

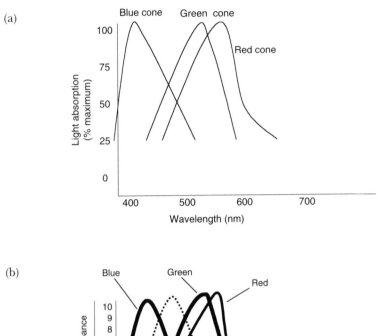

(b)

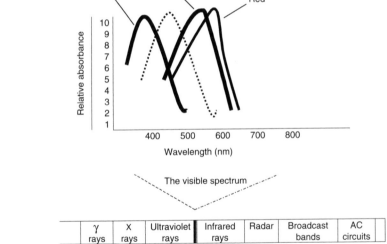

Figure 1.6 (a) Visible light: different cones respond to different wavelengths, e.g. blue cones respond to light of wavelength 400 nm. (b) Retinal colour vision: spectral absorbance curves in the human. (From Tovee 1996.)

A white light is produced when all three are equally stimulated. Therefore, if light of a short wavelength is predominant, blue cone photoreceptors will be stimulated and the person sees a blue colour.

Specific colour is seen if light wavelength is of a specific length, e.g. 700 nm → red colour perception. A person with normal colour appreciation has all three factors present, i.e.

- blue
- green
- red

and is said to have 'trichromatism'.

Colours depend on:

- Hue: this is related to various shades/reflection.
- Saturation: this is an index of purity of a hue, e.g. scarlet is more saturated than pink.
- Brightness: this is related to light intensity.

Colour blindness

- Total colour blindness – is very rare.
- Most colour-blind people have colour deficiency, e.g. the blue factor is weak.
- Most of them have normal visual acuity.

Occasionally, one of the three primary types of cones is lacking because of failure to inherit the appropriate gene for formation of the cone. The colour genes are sex linked and found in the female sex chromosome. As females have two of these chromosomes, they almost never have a deficiency of a colour gene, but, because males have only one female chromosome, one or more of the colour genes is absent in about 4 per cent of all males. For this reason, almost all colour-blind people are males.

If a person has complete lack of red cones, he is able to see green, yellow, orange and orange-red colours by use of his green cones. However, he is not able to distinguish satisfactorily between these colours because he has no red cones to contrast with the green ones. Likewise, if a person has a deficit of green cones, he is able to see all the colours, but is not able to distinguish among green, yellow, orange and red colours because the green cones are not available to contrast with the red. Thus, loss of either the red or the green cones makes it difficult or impossible to distinguish between the colours of the longer wavelengths. This is called red–green colour blindness.

In very rare instances a person lacks blue cones, in which case he has difficulty distinguishing violet, blue and green. This type of colour blindness is frequently called blue weakness.

Abnormal colour appreciation

There are three classifications of abnormal colour vision:

1. Anomalous trichromatism shows an anomaly of one factor.
2. Dichromatism shows an absence of one factor.
3. Monochromatism shows an absence of colour appreciation and the person is therefore totally colour blind.

Figure 1.7 shows the classification. From this, it can be seen that the person with anomalous trichromatism has colour deficiency, which is known as dyschromatopsia. The frequency of this condition is 8% in males and 0.4% in females. The cause is familial with an X-linked recessive trait (the pattern of inheritance of genes located on the X chromosome).

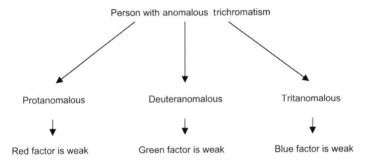

Figure 1.7 Classification of abnormal colour appreciation: anomalous trichromatism – an anomaly in one factor.

Applied genetic criteria for X-linked inheritance

- Phenotypically: physically normal characteristic.
- Genetically: carries the abnormal gene in the sex chromosome.

Male and female sex chromosomes

1 in 23 chromosomes $\rightarrow$ X chromosome

23	+ 23	= 46 chromosomes
Father	Mother	
X/Y	X	
In sperm	In egg cell	= Female (X + X)
		= Male (X + Y)

Human males have 22 pairs of autosomes and 1 X chromosome or 1 Y chromosome in a sperm cell. Human females have 22 pairs of autosomes and 1 X chromosome in every egg cell.

A male receives his Y chromosome from his father and a single X chromosome from his mother, and therefore all of his genes for X-linked traits. The trait controlled by genes located in the X chromosome, e.g. colour blindness, is called a sex-linked trait.

A colour-blind female must have a colour-blind father and a colour-blind mother in order for the disease to be expressed. Such a combination is very unusual. A colour-blind male need have only a mother who has an abnormal gene (heterozygous) for colour blindness. His father can be normal.

- X-linked recessive traits are more common in males (Figure 1.8).
- Disturbance of green factor is more common than red.
- Blue disturbance is very rare.

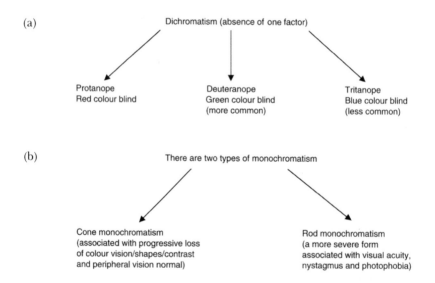

Figure 1.8 (a) Three types of dichromatism and (b) monochromatism – the absence of colour appreciation (totally colour blind).

Control of eye movements and binocular vision

Continuous fine eye movements occur as part of normal viewing. This is an important concept in ensuring that constant stimulation of the photoreceptors maintains image perception – a perception that remains popular. It has been shown that images received by peripheral receptors fade rapidly if fixation is deliberately maintained in one position. Eyes in the alert state are never at rest (Forrester et al. 1999). Eye movements are paired when they move in different directions (see Chapter 22).

Each eye is moved by four rectus muscles (superior, inferior, medial and lateral) and two oblique muscles (superior and inferior). The insertions on the eye of these muscles are such that they have a main and a secondary action. Only the medial and lateral recti move the eye in a simple horizontal direction. The superior rectus muscle elevates the eye and has a secondary action of adducting and intorting the eye.

Torsion of the eye occurs about an anteroposterior axis. While the superior rectus is contracting, the opposite inferior oblique (contralateral synergist) will move the other eye in the same direction. Conjugate movements require reciprocal innervation of the muscles, which can therefore be described as conjugate pairs of muscles for each direction of gaze.

The eye muscles in the primary position of gaze are in a state of tonic activity. Each muscle is, however, activated when the eye moves in its field of action and is inhibited in the opposite direction. The final pathway for neuronal control of eye movement occurs via the cranial nerves, namely the third (oculomotor), fourth (trochlear) and sixth (abducens) cranial nerves.

The extraocular muscles are under both reflex control and higher centre control, with the frontal cortex regulating voluntary activity and the occipital cortex and superior colliculus acting as coordinating centres. The superior colliculus is situated in the midbrain and is the coordinating centre for reflex eye movement. Both eyes normally move together so that images continue to fall on corresponding points of both retinas.

The ability to fixate a bright light is a basic reflex within a few days of birth, but the binocular reflex involving conjugate eye movements and a sustained response takes several months to be fully developed. Foveal fixation is the end point of the searching movement of the muscles and may be considered the point of peak activity in the nerve and muscle response. The nerve response is tuned to foveal fixation. The very small fine eye movements for sustained foveal fixation are the result of reflex attempts by the oculomotor centre to achieve the best perceived image.

Voluntary eye movements are initiated in the frontal cortex. Eye position and fixation are maintained via neural integrators situated in the midbrain. The vertical gaze centre is situated in the reticular medial longitudinal fasciculus, which is above the nucleus of the third cranial nerve. Therefore, loss of supranuclear control by lesions affecting the midbrain and brain stem can give rise to a variety of clinical features, e.g. multiple sclerosis can involve the medial longitudinal fasciculus, resulting in abnormal horizontal gaze.

Binocular vision is achieved by using both eyes together so that the separate images arising in each eye are appreciated as a single image by a process of fusion. Binocular single vision is an acquired ability, not simply an inborn one, and is built up gradually during the early weeks and months of life, provided that there is clear coordination of various abilities:

- The ability of each retina to function properly from a visual point of view, especially the fovea centralis. This requires an intact healthy retina and a clear transparent medium, i.e. cornea, lens and vitreous humour.
- The ability of the visual areas of the brain to promote fusion of the two separate images transmitted to them from each eye, so that a single mental impression of the object is achieved. This is made possible by the forward direction of the eyes in humans, so that the visual field of one eye almost completely overlaps the visual field of the other eye (the binocular field of vision).
- The ability of each eye to lie correctly in its bony orbit, so that the visual axis of each eye is directed to the same object at rest and during movement.
- The ability of the mechanism that turns the eyes inwards to a near object (convergence) or outwards from a convergent position to a distant object (divergence), and the focusing mechanisms of the eye (accommodation) to achieve an adequate degree of harmony.

The advantages of binocular single vision include an enlarged visual field and three-dimensional vision with, in addition, improved visual acuity and compensation for the blind spot of each eye by the other.

Normal binocular vision is acquired by the age of 3 years but alterations in vision can occur up to the age of 7 or 8 years. For this reason, it is essential to manage and correct squints early to prevent amblyopia.

References

Bower TGR (1965) Stimulus variables determining space perception in infants. Science 149: 88.

Fantz RL (1958) Pattern vision in young patients. Psychol Record 8: 43.

Forrester J, Dick A, McMenamin P, Lee W (1999) The Eye: Basic sciences in practice. Edinburgh: WB Saunders.

Gessell A, Ilg FL, Bullis GE (1949) Vision: Its development in infant and child. New York: Hoeber.

Guyton AC (1979) Physiology of the Human Body. Philadelphia, PA: Saunders College Publishing.

Kagan J, Henker BA, Hen-Tov A, Levine J, Lewis M (1966) Infants' differential reactions to familiar and distorted faces. Child Develop 37: 519.

Piaget J (1952) The Origins of Intelligence in Children. New York: International Universities Press.

Tovee MJ (1996) An Introduction to the Visual System. Cambridge: Cambridge University Press.

Vaughan DG, Asbury T, Riordan-Eva P (1998) General Ophthalmology. Norwalk, CT: Appleton & Lange.

White BL, Castle PW (1964) Visual exploratory behaviour following postnatal handling of human infants. Percept Motor Skills 18: 497.

Yanoff M, Duker JS (1999) Ophthalmology. London: Mosby.

CHAPTER TWO
Optics

JANET MARSDEN AND DAVID M SPENCE

Light is a type of energy to which the eye is sensitive. It is an electromagnetic radiation, travelling at 300 000 km/s and is part of a spectrum based on wavelength.

The path of light is always straight unless an obstacle is encountered. It is usually represented by a straight line or ray with an arrow to demonstrate the direction of travel.

Although the nature of light is not, as yet, fully understood by scientists, it is recognized that, rather than behaving only as a ray, light also behaves as though it is made up of particles (photons) and, finally, as a wave. The focus of this chapter is the transmission of light through media – air, eye tissue, etc.; the ray and wave characteristics are most important and the particle characteristics of light are not considered. In general, wave motion is the disturbance of the medium caused by the energy passing through it (Figure 2.1).

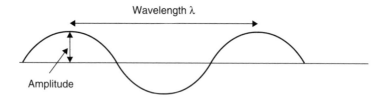

Figure 2.1 Wavelength.

The wavelength is the distance between two symmetrical points on the wave and is often represented by the Greek letter lambda (λ). It is usually expressed in nanometres (nm), a distance that is one-millionth part of a millimetre (10^{-6} mm) or one thousand-millionth part of a metre (10^{-9} m). The electromagnetic spectrum consists of a range of wavelengths of radiation (Figure 2.2).

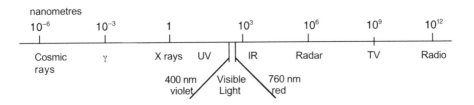

Figure 2.2 The electromagnetic spectrum consists of a range of wavelengths of radiation.

The eye is normally able to discriminate between the wavelengths in the visible spectrum in order to discriminate different colours. The longest wavelength is red and the shortest violet, with the rainbow spectrum in between. White light is an amalgam of all the different colours. The lens absorbs ultraviolet (UV) light and therefore the eye does not normally see UV light. The patient with aphakia often perceives some very violet or blue colours because the UV end of the spectrum is able to impact on the retina.

Waves of light travel randomly. They travel 'out of phase' and in all planes. A single beam of light coming out of the page at the reader would contain waves travelling in all planes. If the beam were cut across it would appear as in Figure 2.3.

Figure 2.3 A section through an unpolarized 'beam' of light.

If light travels through a medium that lets through only those waves travelling in a single plane, the light is said to be polarized – the cross-section of the beam coming towards the reader would therefore be represented as shown in Figure 2.4. Polarizing lenses therefore work by cutting out all light except that going in a single direction; consequently, when used in spectacles, they cut out a degree of the light passing through the lens and remove any scattered light and therefore glare from, for example, water.

Figure 2.4 A section through a polarized 'beam' of light.

Lasers

The word laser is derived from a definition of how they work: light amplification by stimulated emission of radiation. A laser consists of a light source that is usually gaseous. Energy, usually electrical, is 'pumped' into the source. The gas is in a tube with a mirror at each end and the tube has a length equal to a multiple of the wavelength of the light emitted by the gas. The electrons in the gas become 'excited' and are stimulated to emit light, which is in phase. The light emitted is reflected and re-reflected in the tube by the mirrors and, because of the precise length of the tube, the light remains in phase with itself on reflection and therefore reinforces itself. It becomes stronger and stronger while remaining in phase (coherent). If one of the mirrors allows light to leave the tube, the light will be in phase (coherent), monochromatic (of one wavelength) and with all rays parallel (collimated).

Other main types of laser include the following:

- Crystal lasers: light is flashed around a crystal (e.g. ruby or garnet) which produces collimated, coherent light.
- Solid state or semiconductor lasers which are similar to a light-emiting diode or LED. These lasers are found in compact disk players and laser pointers.

The eye focuses parallel light on to the retina. If the laser light is of sufficient intensity, it will cause retinal burns, which is obviously the intention of some ophthalmic lasers. The immensely high-intensity light can also be focused on other structures where it burns or vaporizes tissue in the case of other ophthalmic applications.

The protective goggles used by workers when operating lasers are designed to absorb the wavelength emitted by the laser while transmitting other wavelengths so that the worker can see.

Reflection of light

When light waves hit an object, their behaviour depends on the nature of the medium in which they are travelling and the medium that they 'hit'. Light may be transmitted on through the medium, absorbed by it or reflected back into the first medium. Reflection allows us to see objects around us. There are a number of physical laws associated with reflection:

- The incident ray, reflected ray and normal (a line at 90° perpendicular to the surface at the point of reflection) all lie in the same plane
- The angle of incidence (i) is equal to the angle of reflection (r) (Figure 2.5).

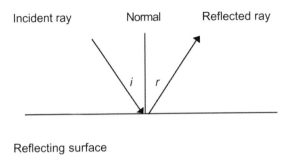

Incident ray   Normal   Reflected ray

Reflecting surface

Figure 2.5 Reflections at a surface – the angle of incidence (*i*) is equal to the angle of reflection (*r*).

Irregular surfaces scatter light in many directions – diffuse reflection. It is by this means that we see objects around us.

Reflection at a flat surface (such as a mirror)

It is easy to demonstrate this reflection if we look at text in a mirror. The text in the mirror is upright, as in the object we are holding up, it is inverted laterally and it appears as far behind the mirror as the book we are holding is in front of it (Figure 2.6b).

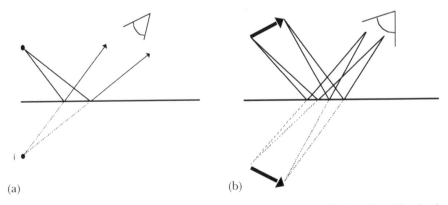

(a)   (b)

Figure 2.6 (a) The rays are reflected according to the laws of reflection. The brain assumes that the point is situated in the direction from which light enters the eye. The eye therefore 'sees' the point behind the surface. There is no real image at point i and it is therefore known as a virtual image. (b) In this case, the reflected object is a solid shape rather than a point. The image is upright, virtual and inverted laterally, and it appears as far behind the surface as the object is in front of it.

Refraction of light

Refraction is the change in direction of light when it passes from one transparent medium to another (it is easier to show this by representing light as a wave). The speed of light depends on the density of the medium in which it travels – the denser the medium, the slower the speed (Figure 2.7).

As the edge of the wavefront is slowed down, as it hits the denser medium, and the opposite side of the beam carries on at the original speed, the beam is deviated towards a line perpendicular to the surface (normal).

The optical density or refractive index of a particular medium is measured by comparing the speed of light through it with the speed of light in a vacuum (air is used under normal circumstances because its optical density is negligible):

$$\text{Refractive index of material} \; = \; \frac{\text{Speed (velocity) of light in air}}{\text{Speed (velocity) of light in medium}}$$

It can be seen therefore that light changes direction at every surface within the eye in order that the light may be focused on the retina.

Some common refractive indexes

Air	1
Aqueous and water	1.33
Cornea	1.37
Physiological lens	1.38–1.42
Glass	1.52

(From Elkington and Frank 1984)

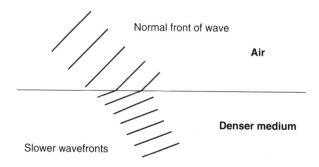

Figure 2.7 Refraction of light: the wavefront changes direction.

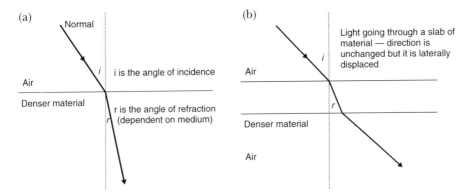

Figure 2.8 (a) Refraction of light showing the change of direction; in (b) the light is going through a slab of material – direction is unchanged but it is laterally displaced. In the figure i is the angle of incidence and r the angle of refraction (dependent on the medium).

Refraction at a curved surface

A convex surface causes parallel light to converge to a focus if the refractive index of the first medium (N_1) is less than that of the second (N_2), or to diverge as if from a focus (Figure 2.9).

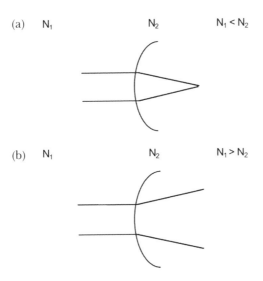

Figure 2.9 A convex surface causes parallel light to converge to a focus if the refractive index of the medium (N_1) is less than that of the second medium (N_2), or to diverge as if from a focus. (a) Air:cornea and (b) glass:air.

Surface power is measured in dioptres (D) – positive for converging surfaces and negative for diverging surfaces. The anterior surface of the cornea is a positive refracting surface and its power accounts for most of the refracting power of the eye. The power of a convex or concave surface or lens is determined by its focal length, which is a measure of the distance from the lens to the point where it focuses parallel rays of light (F) (Figure 2.10).

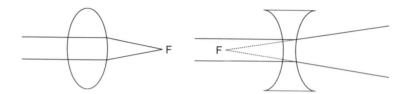

Figure 2.10 The action of a convex and concave lens.

A lens with a focal length of 1 metre is termed a 1-dioptre lens (1 D) and one with a focal length of 0.5 metres, a 2-dioptre lens (2 D):

Dioptric power = 1/Focal length in metres.

So a lens with a focal length of 2 metres will have a power of 0.5 D.

Convex and concave lenses are distinguished from each other by a + for convex lenses and a – for concave lenses.

Optics and the eye

The following are important components in the effective focusing of light on to the retinal receptors:

1. The power of the refractive structures within the eye, the cornea and the lens
2. The axial length of the eye.

The dioptric power of the eye is around 58 D. The cornea contributes about 43 D and the lens 15 D (although its actual power is around 20 D, it is separated from the cornea and therefore the power is not a simple sum) (Snell and Lemp 1998). The lens can change its dioptric power, allowing both distant and near objects to focus on the retina. The lens is normally held in place by the suspensory ligament, which attaches it to the ciliary muscle. Contraction of the ciliary muscle reduces tension on the ligaments and the lens, allowing it to assume a more rounded shape. The curvature of the lens and its thickness increase and therefore its dioptric power increases (accommodation). The range of dioptric power of the lens changes with age – about 8 D at age 40 and only 1 or 2 D by age 60. When accommodation becomes weaker, the eye becomes presbyopic and reading spectacles are needed.

Emmetropia

The eye is considered to be emmetropic if parallel light rays (from infinity or, in effect, greater than 6 m away) are focused on the retina when the eye is in a relaxed state. The eye will have a clear image of a distant object without any adjustment to its optics. Most emmetropic eyes are around 23–24 mm in length (axial length) but smaller or larger eyes may be emmetropic if their optical components are correspondingly stronger or weaker.

Ammetropia

If the rays of light do not fall on the retina, the eye is ammetropic and a refractive error is present.

Refractive errors of the eye

Myopia

When the focused image is in front of the retina, the eye is 'too long' and considered myopic. This is also known as short- or near-sightedness because there is a point less than 6 m away from the eye from which light will focus on the retina when the eye is at rest.

Patient experience

Individuals with myopia will complain of blurred distance vision. Near vision is often much better. They may attempt to see better by narrowing the palpebral fissure or 'screwing their eyes up'. (Myopia is a Greek word meaning to screw up or close the eyes.) This attempts to replicate a pin-hole effect where only a very narrow beam of light enters the eye and does not need focusing, thus negating refractive error.

Causes of myopia

Myopia may be caused by a larger axial length than normal, by a greater curvature of the cornea or lens, or a higher refractive index of the lens. If the eye is longer than normal, the anterior segment will be deeper than normal and therefore there is a lesser possibility of angle-closure glaucoma in myopic individuals. The posterior segment is also affected, choroidal atrophy may occur, usually around the temporal border of the disc, but sometimes around the nasal border or even around the whole disc (peri-papillary atrophy). Degenerative changes may occur in the submacular area after choroidal degeneration in this area and individuals with high myopia are more likely to develop retinal detachments.

Simple myopia

Simple myopia usually develops in childhood or adolescence and needs correcting to ensure that a normal accommodation–convergence reflex develops and to ensure satisfactory progress at school. This type of myopia progresses, necessitating regular testing and changes of specta-cles, but usually stabilizes after adolescence.

Other causes of myopia

- Myopia may be associated with an abnormality in which the axial length of the eye is excessive and continues to enlarge. It is rare and associated with vitreous floaters and chorioretinal changes (pathologi-cal, progressive or degenerative myopia). Myopia carries on increasing and may reach 40–50 D.
- Congenital high myopia is usually a refractive error of around 10 D and can be detected in infants. It is not usually progressive (Pavan-Langston 1996).
- Changes in the curvature of the cornea in keratoconus will lead to myopia.
- Lens curvature changes caused by hyperglycaemia causing lens tumes-cence will give the patient with diabetes myopia. This usually stabilizes as blood glucose levels are controlled.
- Nuclear sclerosis causing an increased refractive index of the lens will also cause a myopic shift.

Hypermetropia

In the hypermetropic eye, the focus point for the parallel light rays is behind the retina so there is no clear image formed on the retina. This may be caused by a shorter axial length than normal, by an insufficient degree of corneal or lens curvature or by a low refractive index of the lens.

Patient experience

The accommodative power of the eye is used to add to the dioptric power of the eye to focus light on the retina and correct the hypermetropia.

Distance vision may therefore be as good as near vision. The eye has to work even harder to accommodate for near vision, so it is often near vision that is blurred if the degree of hypermetropia is more than minimal. The eye is never at rest and the individual may experience headaches associated with reading and other near-vision tasks. Light sensitivity is common in individuals with hypermetropia and is relieved by correcting the hypermetropia. Individuals with hypermetropia may get a spasm of accommodation leading to sudden blurred vision (pseudomyopia). This is also relieved by correction of the refractive error.

Causes of hypermetropia

As hypermetropia may be caused by a shorter axial length than normal or by a lesser curvature of the refracting structures of the eye, the hypermetropic eye is usually smaller than normal. This affects the anterior segment, and the anterior chamber tends to be shallower than normal with a crowded drainage angle that may contribute to the development of angle-closure glaucoma. The posterior segment is also affected and the optic disc may look small or blurred (pseudopapilloedema).

Classification of hypermetropia

• Absolute or total hypermetropia is the amount of hypermetropia with all accommodation suspended as in cycloplegia.
• Manifest hypermetropia is the maximum degree of hypermetropia that can be corrected with a lens when accommodation is active.
• Latent hypermetropia is the difference between absolute and manifest hypermetropia – that part of the refractive error corrected by accommodation (Newell 1996).
• As the person ages, the degree of accommodation possible reduces and thus the degree of manifest hypermetropia will increase.
• Most hypermetropia is 'simple'. Pathological hypermetropia may be caused by microphthalmos, aphakia and forward movement of the retina as a result of a tumour or oedema.

Astigmatism

Astigmatism occurs when the curvature of a refracting surface of the eye varies in different meridians (a toric surface). Light rays passing through a shallow meridian are deflected less than those passing through a steeper meridian, resulting in the formation of a complex image. The directions of greatest and least curvature are usually at right angles to each other. Astigmatism may be associated with emmetropia, myopia or hypermetropia.

Patient experience

The patient often experiences blurred vision and may tilt or turn the head in order to achieve the best image. 'Screwing up the eyes' may occur in order to get a pinhole image and reading material may be held close to the face in order to see the largest, if blurred, image possible. The patient may suffer from 'tired eyes', headaches or transient blurred vision associated with visual concentration. (Astigmat means 'not to a point' – so an individual with astigmatism looking at, for example, a star will observe an elongated streak of light.)

Causes and classification of astigmatism

Differences in the curvature of the cornea in different meridians account for most of the astigmatism of the eye.

Regular astigmatism

On a regular curved surface, the meridians of greatest and least curvature lie 90° apart. If the meridians of ocular astigmatism are constant across the cornea and the amount of astigmatism is the same at each point on the meridian, the refractive condition is known as **regular astigmatism** (American Academy of Ophthalmology 1996). If the vertical meridian is steeper, it is referred to as 'with the rule' and if the horizontal meridian is steeper it is known as 'against the rule'. In the cornea, these meridians are often horizontal and vertical or close to those planes. If the meridians are more than 20° away from the horizontal and vertical meridians, the refractive condition is known as **oblique astigmatism.**

Irregular astigmatism

This occurs when the principal meridians are not at 90° all the way across the cornea or the amount of astigmatism changes from one point to another, i.e. the corneal surface is irregular. The American Academy of Ophthalmology (1996) suggests that all eyes have at least a small amount of irregular astigmatism, but the term is usually reserved for those eyes that have gross irregularities. This may be caused by keratoconus or corneal scarring.

Presbyopia

Presbyopia is a gradual loss of the accommodative response as a result of loss of elasticity of the lens capsule and hardening of the lens. When the eye tries to accommodate, there is less change in the shape of the lens for the same amount of effort. Accommodation decreases with age, and symptoms of presbyopia, when these affect the ability of the patient to carry out normal tasks, begin at around age 40.

Correction of refractive error

Figure 2.11 shows the apparent position of the image, the focus point, in the emmetropic eye (on the retina), the myopic eye (in front of the retina because the eye is too long or its refractive power too weak) and the hypermetropic eye (behind the retina because the eye is too short or its refractive power is too weak). The images in both the myopic eye and the hypermetropic eye are blurred.

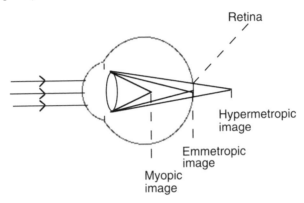

Figure 2.11 Refractive errors.

If the correct lens is placed in front of the ammetropic eye it will change the direction of the light rays entering the eye, enabling the cornea and the lens to focus them at the retina and thus for the person to see a clear image.

In the hypermetropic eye, a convex or plus lens will add to the power of the cornea and lens and enable it to bring the image forward, on to the retina (Figure 2.12).

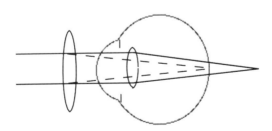

Figure 2.12 Correction of hypermetropia by a convex (+) lens.

In the myopic eye, a concave or minus lens will diverge the light rays before they hit the cornea and the focus point will therefore move backwards to the retina allowing a clear image to be seen (Figure 2.13).

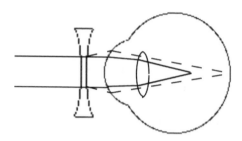

Figure 2.13 Correction of myopia by a concave (–) lens.

Assessment of refractive error

Retinoscopy

Retinoscopy is the objective test that measures the amount of ammetropia of the eye. The retinoscope is an instrument that uses a mirror to reflect light along a line connecting the examiner's and the patient's pupils, and has an aperture in the mirror to allow the examiner to observe the patient's illuminated pupil. The examiner observes the reflex created by light reflected from the retina and refracted by the media of the eye. The area of illumination on the retina moves in the same direction as the retinoscope is moved. The observer, however, sees only a tiny beam of light, which appears to come from the eye's far point: infinity in an emmetropic eye, behind the eye in a hypermetropic eye and in front of the eye in a myopic eye. The observer sees the small reflection from the retina move in the same direction as the retinoscope in the emmetropic or hypermetropic eye and in the opposite direction in the myopic eye. Lenses are placed in front of the eye and the retinoscope beam is moved until the pupil is filled with light that does not move. The lenses have corrected the degree of ammetropia at that point. Positive or convex lenses will neutralize hypermetropia whereas a combination of negative or concave lenses will neutralize myopia.

In practice, the observer is at a distance of 0.5–0.67 m from the eye (arm's length), which induces an error of +2 D to +1.5 D; this will be deducted from the final reading to ascertain the amount of ammetropia. This is called the 'working distance lens'. Thus, an emmetropic eye is one in which the working distance lens causes the neutralization of the movement of the illuminated retinal area.

A similar procedure will be performed at 90° away from the initial meridian to evaluate any correction for astigmatism. A clear medium, good fixation and reasonably sized pupils are prerequisites for accurate retinoscopy so, although the technique can be very accurate, a subjective refraction is usually carried out to ensure that the patient can tolerate the prescription that is eventually prescribed.

Cycloplegic refraction

Cycloplegic refraction is often performed in order to negate the effects of accommodation, so that an accurate refraction, without the eye doing any work, can be obtained. This is used particularly in children who have high levels of accommodation, so that the correct amount of hypermetropic error may be measured but it may also be carried out in adults with hypermetropia to measure the absolute amount of refractive error.

Subjective refraction

Subjective refraction relies on the patient's response to obtain the refractive correction that obtains the best visual results (visual acuity). Retinoscopy findings may be the starting point for subjective refraction or a small dioptre lens, either plus or minus, may be placed in front of the patient's eye while he or she is asked if the distance visual acuity chart becomes more, or less, clear. If there is no astigmatism, the refraction consists of adding more plus or minus lenses until the patient has the best possible correction that is comfortable for him. The eye may be 'fogged' first by using too strong a convex (+) or too weak a concave (−) lens to blur the vision to relax accommodation if the eye is hypermetropic.

Astigmatic correction

Astigmatism requires that a cylindrical lens be added to the basic correction at an appropriate meridian in order to achieve the best correction. One method of ascertaining both the correct meridian of astigmatism and the power of lens needed is to use the 'fogging technique'.

Placing a large plus lens in front of the eye makes the eye artificially myopic and inhibits accommodation. An astigmatic fan (Figure 2.14) is placed in front of the eye and the patient is asked to identify which line on it is darkest and most distinct. This is marked with the angle of the astigmatic meridian.

A minus power cylindrical lens is placed with its axis along this meridian and increases in power until all of the lines on the fan become equal. The patient is kept artificially myopic by continually adding positive spherical lenses. The patient is then asked to look at a distance vision chart and spherical lenses removed until maximum clarity of vision is achieved. If the patient has never worn spectacles before, a reduced form of the

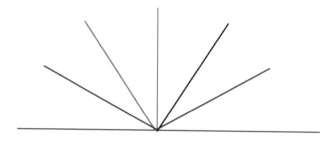

Figure 2.14 The astigmatic meridian (darker line).

prescription may be prescribed initially to avoid intolerance and discomfort, e.g.

+ 2.00 fogs vision to 6/18

120° is the axis on the fan which is clearest

−1.00 at 120° evens out darkness of the fan lines

reducing plus lenses to +0.25 gives sharpest vision on distance reading chart

Reading 'add'

The patient with presbyopia will need a correction to replace that part of the accommodative reflex that is no longer available. This is done with plus lenses that supplement the remaining accommodative power of the eye. The person with emmetropia will need a correction for reading only. If a person has myopia or hypermetropia, he or she will need a near vision prescription to add to the prescription for distance. This is known as the reading 'add'.

Autorefraction

Sophisticated instruments are available that are able to refract patients and felt to be reasonably accurate. Alignment of the eye with the machine is critical as is fixation, which makes these instruments less useful for some patients. Some refractors measure only through very small portions of the optics of the eye, achieving a result that may not be representative of the eye as a whole. The tendency to accommodate when looking into instruments has also proved problematic, but fogging techniques may be used to overcome this. The autorefraction readings must be checked by retinoscopy and refined by subjective testing before prescribing. Failure of this to be carried out by an appropriate professional (registered optometrist, ophthalmic medical practitioner or an ophthalmologist qualified to refract) is a breach of the law.

Prescriptions

As in the astigmatism example (+0.25 −1.00 × 120) it can be seen that the final written prescription is interpreted as follows: the first figure is a spherical lens to correct myopia or hypermetropia depending on whether the symbol in front of it is minus (myopia) or plus (hypermetropia). The second figure is the correction, in the form of a spherical lens, for astigmatism (again, either positive or negative), which is added to the initial correction. The third figure is the axis at which the lens is placed in order to correct the astigmatism. The reading add is documented separately.

Correction of refractive error in practice

Spectacles

Most ammetropia may be corrected with spectacle lenses. As stated previously, convex (plus) lenses are used to correct hypermetropia and presbyopia and concave (minus) lenses are used to correct myopia. Although lenses ore often drawn as biconvex or biconcave, other forms of the lenses exist – planoconvex and planoconcave – and those that are most often used for spectacle lenses to reduce distortion and, for best cosmetic effect, meniscus lenses (Figure 2.15).

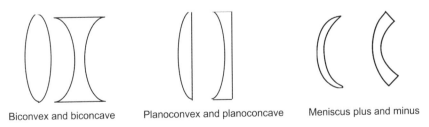

Biconvex and biconcave   Planoconvex and planoconcave   Meniscus plus and minus

Figure 2.15 Types of lenses.

Lenses prescribed for one distance (reading or distance vision) are termed 'single vision lenses'. Bifocal lenses have a reading add in addition to the distance vision part of the lens and this is placed inferiorly in the lens so that the person may look down to read. Progressive addition lenses or PALs have a distance correction in the superior portion of the lens and then a zone of gradual reduction in distance power, leading to a reading zone inferiorly.

Spectacle lenses may be made in glass or various forms of plastic material. Glass does not usually scratch as easily as plastic but is less impact resistant unless toughened and therefore less safe in case of accident. Plastics are much lighter and therefore less tiring to wear.

Lenses need to be centred both horizontally and vertically in their frame and on the patient's face to ensure that the patient is looking through the correct portion of the lens. The intrapupillary distance must also be taken into account.

Contact lenses

The major use of contact lenses is for the correction of refractive errors. They may be used therapeutically, as in the case of bandage lenses that protect the cornea from external factors and allow healing of corneal disorders, or cosmetically to cover an unsightly damaged eye or to enhance eye colour.

The prime motivating factor for contact lens correction of refractive errors in most patients is cosmetic, in that they are less obvious and cumbersome than spectacles. Contact lenses will improve the quality of vision for individuals with high myopia in particular and the field of view is enhanced for all users. A contact lens aids in the 'smoothing out' of an irregular corneal surface and thus in the enhancement of the retinal image formed, and rigid or hard contact lenses may also help to eliminate astigmatism. Contact lenses are also very useful in the initial correction of keratoconus. All contact lenses can cause a reversible change in the curvature of the cornea, which may resolve within minutes of removing the lenses or may take a number of days. Patients may find that their vision is slightly blurred for a while when they swap from contact lenses to their normal spectacle prescription.

Types of contact lens

Contact lenses are categorized by size and material. The smallest of the lens types are corneal lenses, which are confined to covering the cornea. These are generally hard lenses, made of polymethylmethacrylate (PMMA), or gas-permeable lenses, which are also hard and made out of materials such as cellulose acetate butyrate (CAB), silicone and other similar materials. Slightly larger than these are semiscleral lenses, which bridge the limbus and lie partially on the conjunctiva that overlies the sclera at the limbus.

These are soft lenses that are made from a variety of polymers and are all hydrophilic to various degrees (hydrophilic means having an affinity with or taking in water). The water content of these lenses may be anything from 30% to around 85%. The final classification of lens based on size is the scleral lens, which covers the cornea and most of the conjunctiva overlying sclera. These are usually made of PMMA but newer developments include gas-permeable scleral lenses. Extended wear lenses are often used when the patient's ability to use daily wear soft lenses is impaired.

Each type of lens works in a slightly different way. Hard lenses float on a film of tears, which also forms a type of lens. In this way, corneal irregularities are evened out and astigmatism may be corrected up to a certain level. After about 2 D of astigmatism, a cylindrical or toric lens must be incorporated into the back surface of the lens. Soft lenses adapt to the shape of the cornea without a tear film layer and so will not correct any degree of astigmatism unless a toric lens is incorporated into them.

Lenses and corneal oxygenation

PMMA lenses, the traditional hard lens, floats on a film of tears, which provides the cornea with an oxygen supply. They are in themselves impermeable to oxygen. The lenses need to fit correctly with an adequate space between the edge and the cornea to allow for an exchange of tears between the lens and the cornea, and to allow a comfortable fit. Corneal epithelium has a very high metabolic rate and therefore needs high levels of oxygen. Oxygen solubility in the tear film is limited and, therefore, unless a very good flow of tears is maintained, oxygenation of the corneal tissue is limited by PMMA lenses. Lactic acid and carbon dioxide can accumulate under the lens. Moderate oxygen deprivation of the cornea can lead to degrees of corneal oedema, associated with blurring of vision and haloes around lights. Damage to epithelial cells may lead to punctate corneal erosions on the cornea and, consequently, a degree of pain.

Gas-permeable lenses have varying degrees of permeability to oxygen and therefore interfere less with corneal epithelial metabolism. Little or no corneal oedema results, although a decrease in corneal sensitivity occurs which is common to all types of contact lens.

Soft lenses retain a large amount of water and therefore cause minimal problems associated with lack of oxygen. They are much easier to adapt to than hard lenses where tolerance has to be built up over a number of days. They are also much more comfortable to wear than hard lenses and there is less chance of their becoming accidentally dislodged. They are, however, much more easily damaged by handling. Overwear is more likely to cause physical or pathological changes than with other lens types.

Care of contact lenses

All lenses accumulate deposits of lipid, proteins, minerals and other matter. These deposits may result in reduction in vision, poor contact lens fit, infection caused by the presence of organisms adhering to the lens and decreased oxygen transmission, and therefore any potential problems associated with this. A variety of solutions and systems for use in the care of contact lenses are available and are broadly split into four categories.

Cleaning agents

These remove deposits from the lens. Surfactants dissolve and clean off adhered protein, lipid and minerals from the surface of the lens, and enable more effective disinfection. Enzyme cleaners digest the deposits.

Disinfecting agents

Various systems are available but are divided into three common methods:

1. Thermal disinfection involves boiling the lenses but has the disadvantage that, if inadequately cleaned before boiling, any deposits of protein on the lens will become permanent. Thermal disinfection is not recommended for high water content soft lenses because it changes their molecular structure.
2. The effectiveness of hydrogen peroxide disinfection depends on the soaking time of the lens in the solution. More than 20 minutes is necessary for adequate disinfection (American Academy of Ophthalmology 1996). The hydrogen peroxide must then be neutralized.
3. Chemical disinfection systems take much longer to remove all contamination from the lens and require good cleaning of the lens beforehand.

Rinsing agents

A rinsing solution is necessary after cleaning or disinfecting the lens. Unpreserved sterile saline is commonly the solution of choice and is widely available in a variety of presentations such as single-dose containers and aerosols.

Wetting agents

Wetting agents are use to lubricate PMMA and gas-permeable lenses before insertion into the eye.

Contact lens cases are a common source of corneal infection. There is little point in cleaning a lens adequately if it is immediately put back into a contaminated container. Lens cases must be disinfected along with the lens and changed regularly.

Potential problems associated with contact lens wear

Epithelial problems

Contact lenses may cause thinning of the corneal epithelium (and areas of variable density that are seen as microcysts), along with reduction in the density of structures anchoring it to its basement membrane (hemidesmosomes and anchoring fibrils), and therefore cause reduced adhesion to the basement membrane (Forrester et al. 1996). Corneal abrasions may be caused by mechanical damage and punctate epithelial erosions by overwear or chemical damage caused by poor neutralization of cleaning or disinfecting solutions.

Corneal infection

Infected corneal ulcers are a very serious complication that may be associated with contact lens wear. They occur with all types of lenses but are much more frequently associated with soft lens wear. Many factors are linked to the development of corneal infection and include poor hand washing technique, inadequate lens disinfection, overwear leading to corneal epithelial problems, and contaminated solutions and contact lens cases. Although many corneal ulcers are bacterial in origin, a growing cause of corneal ulcers associated with contact lens wear is *Acanthamoeba* sp. The main source of contamination is the fluid in the contact lens case. Acanthamoeba keratitis causes pain out of all proportion to the clinical findings and responds very slowly to therapy (Forrester et al. 1996).

Corneal neovascularization

This is caused by chronic hypoxia associated with contact lens wear, especially if the lenses are thick, or badly fitting, or lens cleaning is inadequate over a period of time. New vessels may extend onto the visual axis if ignored, causing an impairment in vision. Discontinuation of lens wear often leads to regression of the new vessels although ghost vessels may still be seen on the cornea.

Other methods of ammetropia correction

A number of other methods of ammetropia correction are possible.

Orthokeratology

This is a technique where a contact lens is fitted that is flatter than the corneal curvature, in order to induce corneal flattening and so reduce myopia. The patient may have to wear lenses for only part of the time in order to induce the changes in the cornea all the time. The effect is only transient and will disappear if the lens is not worn for the necessary time.

Corneal surgery

For corneal surgery, see Chapter 16.

Correction of aphakia

Correction of aphakia may be achieved by replacing the crystalline lens with a strong convex (+) lens in front of the eye in the form of a spectacle lens. Moving the refracting surface to the front of the eye results in a change in the size of the image of 25–30% (Pavan-Langston 1991). Coming to terms with this new image needs considerable adaptation on the part of the patient and, if only one eye is aphakic, this adaptation is impossible because the brain is incapable of coping with the two different sized images. Strong plus lenses also cause a lot of visual distortion.

Contact lenses are a better solution to aphakia correction. Magnification is reduced to 5–10%, which causes the brain fewer problems. Elderly people who have undergone cataract extraction may be unable to handle contact lenses easily, leading to the necessity for extended wear lenses with their inherent problems.

Intraocular lenses are the most common means of correcting aphakia.

Intraocular lenses

The cataractous lens is replaced by one made usually of PMMA or compounds containing this material. The lens power needed to correct aphakia is calculated using measurements of the curvature of the cornea (ascertained by keratometry), the axial length of the eye (by A-scan biometry), the expected position of the intraocular lens (using a constant for a particular type of lens) and the refraction required after surgery.

Intraocular lenses may be situated in the anterior chamber with the optical part of the lens (optic) in front of the pupil and the supporting structures (haptic) in the anterior chamber angle. The more common position is in the posterior chamber, which is more anatomically correct. The lens is supported by its haptic, which is placed in the capsular bag or ciliary sulcus. Iris clip lenses are used less often. Multifocal intraocular lenses are available, often designed with concentric zones of different powers. Foldable lenses are becoming more common for use in small incision surgery that results in less astigmatism.

References

American Academy of Ophthalmology (1996) Optics, Refraction and Contact Lenses. San Francisco, CA: American Academy of Ophthalmology.

Elkington AR, Frank HJ (1984) Clinical Optics. London: Blackwell Scientific.

Forrester J, Dick A, McMenamin P, Lee W (1996) The Eye: Basic sciences in practice. London: WB Saunders.

Newell FW (1996) Ophthalmology: Principles and concepts. St Louis, MO: Mosby.

Pavan-Langston D (1996) Manual of Ocular Diagnosis and Therapy, 4th edn. Boston, MA: Little, Brown.

Snell RS, Lemp MA (1998) Clinical Anatomy of the Eye, 2nd edn. Oxford: Blackwell Science.

CHAPTER THREE

Pharmacology

SHARON ANDREW

Pharmacology is the study of how drugs act in the body. This chapter is concerned with the action and interaction of drugs on the eye. The main categories of ophthalmic drugs and their uses, the delivery methods of ophthalmic drugs, along with the major adverse side effects are covered. The chapter concludes with a discussion about the nurse's role in relation to the effective use of eye treatment and an overview of the current UK legislation on prescribing.

In general terms pharmacology can be divided into two parts: pharmacodynamics and pharmacokinetics.

Pharmacodynamics

This deals with the effects of the drug and where and how these effects are produced. Attention must also be given to the relationship between adverse drug actions and interactions.

To achieve their effects drugs act on receptors; these can be inside the cell or on the cell membranes. The receptors can be stimulated or inhibited by the drug and the effect is determined by: the concentration of the drug, its affinity for the receptors (strength of attraction) and the presence of other drugs that may be in competition for the receptors.

Unwanted side effects elsewhere in the body may also occur such as dyspnoea with timolol and paraesthesia with acetazolamide, resulting from the high affinity of these drugs for their receptors.

Pharmacokinetics

This deals with the role of various factors in controlling rates of absorption of drugs from the sites of administration, distribution within the body or eye, metabolism and elimination.

The response to a drug and any adverse effects will vary from person to person and factors such as age, general health, genetic background and the presence of other drugs must be taken into account.

Delivery methods

Systemically administered drugs such as antibiotics, anti-inflammatories, analgesics

Absorption

The route of administration will play a major role in the absorption of a drug. Most drugs are given orally and are absorbed mainly in the stomach and small intestine. Factors such as the solubility of the drug, the dissolution rate of the tablet or capsule, the gastrointestinal enzymes and pH, and the presence of food will determine the degree and rate of absorption.

Some drugs are given by injection (intravenously, intramuscularly, subcutaneously). If given intravenously the total amount of drug reaches the bloodstream, and to a slightly lesser extent if given by the other two routes. However, higher, consistent and more predictable plasma levels can be maintained by these routes than by the oral route.

Distribution

Many drugs bind to plasma proteins such as albumin and establish a balance between the bound and unbound fractions of the drugs. Only the free (unbound) fraction of the drug is able to move out of the bloodstream. The amount of the drug in the free form can be influenced by the amount of drug given and other drugs present in the plasma competing for the binding sites on the plasma proteins.

Most drugs can penetrate from the bloodstream into extracellular tissues, except for the brain, aqueous humour and retina where they must have some fat solubility (blood–brain and blood–eye barrier).

Metabolism

Most drugs given systemically are broken down in the liver, either by conjugation or by various chemical reactions such as oxidation and reduction. Some drugs, however, such as acetazolamide, are not metabolized at all and are excreted unchanged in the urine.

Excretion

The kidneys excrete most water-soluble drugs and the biliary system the large-molecular-weight compounds. Some drugs such as aspirin appear in the tears (which is important for contact lens wearers to be aware of). Other drugs are excreted in saliva and breast milk and even though the quantity may be small it may affect the breast-fed baby, a factor that must be taken into account when a drug is prescribed to a nursing mother.

After absorption, the time for one-half of the plasma concentration of the drug to be eliminated is called the biological half-life $(t_{1/2})$. This has important implications when considering frequency of doses in order to achieve steady-state plasma concentrations, rather than peak (high) and trough (low) plasma levels.

Locally administered drugs

Topical application

Topical drugs for extraocular conditions such as conjunctivitis are effective if their concentration is maintained. The concentration will be affected by dilution with tears, drainage through the nasolacrimal duct, and loss through the blood vessels of the conjunctiva and eyelids into the systemic circulation.

For the treatment of intraocular conditions, the topically applied drugs are required to penetrate into the eye and must therefore be capable of crossing the cornea. The areas that they have to cross include the pre-corneal film, corneal epithelium, stroma and endothelium. To do this the drug has to be available in both the un-ionized (lipid-soluble) and the ionized (water-soluble) forms. Initially, to pass through the corneal epithelium it needs to be in the un-ionized form and then in the ionized form to pass through the stroma, before changing again to the un-ionized form to pass through the endothelium into the aqueous.

The penetration of any topically administered drug will alter if there is damage or inflammation of the cornea, e.g. fluorescein exists only in the water-soluble form and will not normally penetrate the cornea, so it is used to assess whether there is any corneal damage.

Topically administered drugs may have an improved penetration if applied as an ointment as a result of the extended ocular contact time. To maximize benefits and minimize adverse effects from topical administration, it is recommended that systemic absorption through the nasal mucosa be minimized by occlusion of the punctum or simply closing the eye for a count of 60. Leaving a sufficient interval between drops to minimize dilution and overflow, and adherence to recommendations about order of application (a synergistic action effect occurs in some cases, e.g. by using pilocarpine after latanoprost), will help to maximize benefits.

The uptake of a drug by ocular tissues is also regulated by the amount of time that it sits in contact with the epithelium. Aqueous solutions will stay within the lower fornix and tear film for less time than suspensions (particles suspended in fluid rather than dissolved in it). Drugs in more viscous carriers such as polyvinyl alcohol, hyaluronic acid or gels have a prolonged contact time and the highest contact time may be achieved by the use of an ointment. Although ointments may not release lipophilic drugs well, gels allow five times more drug to enter the cornea and act as a reservoir, gradually releasing the drug and prolonging its effect (Fechner and Teichmann 1998).

Subconjunctival injection

Drug penetration is by local diffusion through the tissues. There are advantages and disadvantages of this route of administration:

* Advantages include high local concentrations, high tissue concentrations and possibly avoiding the necessity of topical or systemic medication.
* Disadvantages include very low tissue concentrations between injections, local side effects and perhaps most importantly patient apprehension.

Metabolism

Local agents applied to the eye are metabolized by enzymes within the globe, although the exact mechanisms are unknown.

Properties of topical preparations

Preservatives

Preservatives, e.g. benzalkonium chloride and thiomersal, are germicidal at very weak concentrations and so preserve the sterility of eyedrops. In a single drop dispenser unit, such as Minims, a preservative is unnecessary because the unit is disposable. Eye preparations containing preservatives should not be used by contact lens wearers because some preservatives can accumulate in hydrogel lenses and may induce toxic reactions.

Isotonicity

Isotonicity with tear fluid is desirable because it facilitates the acceptance of the eyedrop by the patient.

Oxidation

Some substances, e.g. phenylephrine, are oxidized and so a reducing agent, such as sodium metabisulphite, is added.

Hydrogen ion concentration (pH)

The H^+ concentration is expressed as the pH with the neutral value being 7.4. The eye can withstand a pH range of 4.5–10, but extremes are to be avoided, so solutions known as buffers, e.g. sodium citrate, are used to remove excess H^+. It is not only for ocular comfort that a desirable pH is needed; some drugs are physiologically active only at a particular pH, so a balance has to be struck between comfort and activity.

Viscosity

As a result of tear drainage, overflow and blinking, a topical agent remains in the lower fornix for only a short time. To prolong the presence of a drug and enhance corneal uptake, substances with a higher viscosity than tear fluid, e.g. polyvinyl alcohol and methylcellulose, are added to drops.

Light

Light may cause oxidation or hydrolysis. Some products therefore need to be packaged in dark, light-resistant containers.

Sterility

Drops/Ointments

Those products intended to be sterile should be terminally sterilized in their final container. Where it is not possible to carry out terminal sterilization by heating as a result of formulation instability, a decision needs to be taken to use an alternative method of terminal sterilization such as filtration and/or aseptic processing. It has been accepted that other factors such as the type of container, route of administration and patient benefit have contributed to the choice of a particular container type that will not withstand terminal heat sterilization. Certain ophthalmic products are therefore manufactured by validated aseptic processing. The European Agency for Evaluation of Medicinal Products (EMEA) has set out decision trees for selection of sterilization methods, involving sterilization by moist heat at 121°C for 15 min, by dry heat at 160°C for 120 min or by filtration through a microbial retentive filter.

Drugs for injection

These come in ampoules, either in powder form for reconstitution with appropriate diluent, such as water, for injection, or in liquid form. All of these have to be prepared aseptically, filtered and sterilized.

Recommended expiry dates

It is generally recommended that eyedrops and ointments for domiciliary use by patients are used for no longer than 1 month after opening (28 days).

For hospital ward use by patients, they are used for no longer than 1 week (7 days) after opening, with individual containers for each patient.

For hospital outpatient clinic and theatre use, they are used once and then the remainder discarded.

Classification of ophthalmic drugs

Drugs acting on the eye may be classified under a variety of headings and in this chapter have been classified as:

• Antimicrobial agents, including antibiotics, antiviral and antifungal agents
• Anti-inflammatory agents, including steroids and antihistamines
• Drugs affecting the autonomic nervous system
• Drugs used in the treatment of glaucoma
• Ocular lubricants
• Local anaesthetic agents
• Diagnostic agents.

Antimicrobial agents

Antibiotics

These can be classified as either bactericidal or bacteriostatic:

• Bactericidal is when the drug destroys the bacteria during active multiplication.
• Bacteriostatic is when the drug diminishes the rate of multiplication.

Antibiotics may act by one or more bacteriostatic means:

• Interference with the synthesis of the cell wall of the bacterium, e.g. penicillin.

- Prevention of protein synthesis inside the micro-organism, e.g. erythromycin.
- Disturbance of cell wall permeability so that the bacteria lyse, e.g. polymyxin B.
- Inhibiting the enzyme responsible for supercoiling of the DNA helix (DNA gyrase), e.g. ofloxacin.

Most acute superficial eye infections can be treated topically, although systemic treatment may occasionally be required.

Antibiotics can have a narrow or broad spectrum of activity; those with a narrow spectrum are effective against a specific type of bacterium (such as Gram positive); those that have a broad spectrum are effective against a wider range of bacteria. It should be noted that resistance to antibiotics can develop quite quickly and therefore antibiotics should be used only when an accurate diagnosis has been made and ideally after antibiotic sensitivity has been determined. In practice a broad-spectrum antibiotic such as chloramphenicol is usually prescribed in the first instance for a presumed bacterial infection and is generally well tolerated by the patient. There have, however, been recommendations that topical chloramphenicol should be avoided because of an increased risk of aplastic anaemia but this does not appear to be well founded at present (Field et al. 1999). It may, however, be worth avoiding if the patient has a family history of blood dyscrasias.

When prescribing systemic antibiotics various factors should be taken into consideration including the age of the patient, any liver or kidney problems that the patient may have and pregnancy/breast-feeding.

As with all classes of drugs adverse effects can occur with antibiotics and these should also be taken into account when prescribing treatment, e.g. gentamicin is ototoxic and penicillin may cause serious allergic reactions in susceptible patients. Local toxic reactions may also occur in response to the presence of preservative in the eyedrops, especially after prolonged use. Many antibacterial preparations also incorporate a corticosteroid (e.g. Betnesol-N), but these should **not** be used unless a patient is under close specialist supervision because they may mask a more serious condition. In particular they should not be used for an undiagnosed 'red eye', which is sometimes caused by the herpes simplex virus and may be difficult to diagnose.

Eyedrops can be used up to every 2 hours with the frequency reducing as the infection is controlled although it should be continued for 48 hours after resolution. Eye ointments should be administered either at night when used in conjunction with eyedrops or three to four times daily if used alone.

Antivirals

Viruses proliferate inside cells, so antiviral agents must be able to penetrate the cells to prevent viral multiplication. There are several viruses that may affect the eye but effective treatment is available for only the herpes viruses.

The drugs work by inhibiting the viral deoxyribonucleic acid (DNA) synthesis, including aciclovir and trifluorothymidine (F_3T). Aciclovir acts by blocking viral replication within the infected cells only because it needs an enzyme produced by the virus to convert the drug into its active form and is the treatment of choice in ointment form for herpes simplex keratitis. Trifluorothymidine acts by bringing about the substitution of a base in the chain for DNA synthesis; however, it acts on uninfected cells too and is therefore more toxic, but is a useful alternative in those patients who are intolerant of (for whatever reason) or unresponsive to aciclovir.

Ganciclovir and fomivirsen are two drugs used in the treatment of cytomegalovirus (CMV) retinitis. Fomivirsen is administered by intravitreal injection whereas ganciclovir is available as a slow-release ocular implant. It must be remembered that local treatments do not protect against systemic infection or infection in the other eye.

Antifungals

These are rarely required in ocular disease. However, fungal infections can occur after agricultural injuries, especially in hot and humid climates. Many different fungi are capable of producing ocular infection and they should be identified by appropriate laboratory procedures. Antifungal preparations for the eye are not generally commercially available, so treatment will need to be carried out at specialist centres, although requests for information about supplies of preparations should be addressed to the local health authority or the nearest hospital ophthalmology unit. Antifungal drugs that have been used in ocular infections include amphotericin and miconazole.

Anti-inflammatory drugs

Corticosteroids

Steroids are substances that are normally produced in the cortex of the adrenal gland. Cortisol or hydrocortisone is the important steroid in this context and is released in response to a pituitary hormone, adrenocorticotrophic hormone (ACTH), with negative feedback between the level of hydrocortisone and ACTH in the circulation, which is monitored by the hypothalamus. Hydrocortisone has many physiological effects but the one with which we are concerned here is its anti-inflammatory effect. This effect is used in the treatment of many different inflammatory disorders, but generally large doses need to be used; however, newer agents are now available that have greater potency but with accompanying adverse effects.

Local and systemic steroids are used in the treatment of eye disease. Corticosteroids administered locally (as eyedrops, eye ointments or subconjunctival injection) have an important place in the treatment of anterior segment inflammation, including that which results from surgery.

Local steroids

Drops

There are many different preparations available such as prednisolone, prednisolone acetate, betamethasone, dexamethasone, fluorometholone and rimexolone. Rimexolone appears least likely to cause a rise in intraocular pressure.

Steroids can also be combined with an antibiotic (e.g. betamethasone and neomycin).

Ointments

Ointments stay longer on the corneal surface hence increasing the retention time and effect of the drug, though some temporary visual disturbance will be experienced. Again many different preparations are available with or without antibiotic components.

Subconjunctival injection

There are two commonly used preparations: betamethasone (useful for short-term effect – 24 hours) and methylprednisolone (for longer effect – about 10 days or more).

Systemic steroids

Oral

Prednisolone is the usual oral anti-inflammatory of choice in the treatment of ocular inflammation. The starting dose in certain conditions is high – up to 80 mg daily. Enteric coated tablets are available and are preferable to minimize the risk of intestinal ulceration. Reduction in dosage has to be gradual, but the degree of dose reduction and for how long each reduced dose is taken will vary according to the individual patient's condition and response. All patients on oral steroids should be issued with a steroid card detailing their current dose and regimen duration.

Adverse effects of steroids

Topical corticosteroids should normally only be used under expert supervision. There are three main dangers associated with their use:

1. A 'red eye' where the diagnosis is unconfirmed may result from herpes simplex virus and a corticosteroid may aggravate the condition, leading to corneal ulceration, possible damage to vision and even loss of an eye. Bacterial and fungal infections pose a similar hazard, because not only may the corticosteroid mask symptoms but it may also predispose a patient to these infections if used long term.
2. 'Steroid glaucoma' may follow the prolonged use of a corticosteroid and therefore it is important that the intraocular pressure (IOP) of patients on long-term steroids be monitored.
3. 'Steroid cataract' may follow prolonged use.

About 30% of the general population will respond to steroids with a rise in IOP of 6–15 mm. Four to five per cent will have a marked IOP rise > 15 mmHg. This steroid response may occur immediately, or after 2–3 weeks of topical application. There may be a delay of 4–6 months. Discontinuing steroids generally results in a reduction of pressure elevation (Fechner and Teichmann 1998). Other side effects include thinning of the cornea and sclera.

Withdrawal of topical steroids in certain conditions should be gradual if a relapse or rebound effects are not to be seen (e.g. in anterior uveitis). Some patients may even have to remain on a very weak-strength preparation indefinitely.

Prolonged systemic treatment will be accompanied by exaggerated physiological effects of steroids (cushingoid appearance, raised blood sugar); this may also be accompanied by dramatic mood changes. The high level of steroids in the circulation also leads to disruption of the negative feedback mechanism between the adrenal cortex and the anterior pituitary, which if the treatment is prolonged may lead to atrophy of the adrenal cortex; this, in turn, could necessitate the patient taking lifelong replacement therapy. Other adverse effects that can be expected are osteoporosis, peptic ulcers and retarded growth in children. In the eye, systemic corticosteroids have a high risk (75%) of producing a 'steroid cataract' if the equivalent of more than 15 mg prednisolone is given daily for several years.

Non-steroidal anti-inflammatory drugs

These are drugs that block the effects of prostaglandins, which are found in almost all tissues including the eye. Prostaglandins are released in inflammatory reactions and are said to be mediators in the process.

Several drugs have been shown to block the synthesis of prostaglandins such as indometacin and flurbiprofen. These are generally given systemically, although indometacin, diclofenac, flurbiprofen and ketorolac are available as topical eyedrops. It is becoming common practice for these to replace the use of topical steroids in the treatment of episcleritis, and they have also been shown to be very useful in the treatment of corneal pain after trauma.

Drugs for the treatment of allergy

Allergy is a common cause of conjunctivitis and the cause of signs and symptoms is principally the release of histamine. Treatment can be offered in two ways:

* Using drops that block histamine receptors, e.g. emedastine (antihistamine)
* Using drops that prevent the release of histamine, e.g. lodoxamide, sodium cromoglicate (mast cell stabilizer).

Once an allergic reaction has taken place, an antihistamine will block histamine receptors, thus preventing or relieving the symptoms of the allergic reaction. This action is relatively rapid. It will take some time for the mast cell membrane to stabilize and therefore a mast cell stabilizer will have no immediate effect and it is likely to be 7–10 days before its effect is noticed. For patients who have seasonal allergic disorders such as hay fever, therefore, a mast cell stabilizer should be used from the beginning of the season to its end, in order that the cell membrane does not break down, releasing histamine and causing the symptoms of allergy. Once this has happened, an antihistamine is useful to prevent symptoms. Newer preparations are said to have both properties, e.g. olopatadine.

Drugs affecting the autonomic nervous system

Anatomy

The autonomic nervous system is divided into the sympathetic and parasympathetic pathways. The sympathetic pathway originates in the hypothalamus, passes down the spinal cord and emerges in the thorax. The fibres then pass upwards, towards the superior cervical ganglion lying at the carotid bifurcation where they synapse. The neurotransmitter here is acetylcholine. The postganglionic fibres run towards the eye, wrapped round the internal carotid artery, and finally reach the eye via the ophthalmic artery. They supply the dilator pupillae, the trabecular meshwork and the blood vessels in the eye. The chemical transmitter is noradrenaline (norepinephrine), which acts on both α and β receptors.

The parasympathetic pathway originates in the midbrain; fibres run in the third nerve towards the eye and synapse in the ciliary ganglion, which lies within the muscle cone between the lateral rectus muscle and the optic nerve. The transmitter is acetylcholine. The postganglionic fibres then innervate the constrictor pupillae and ciliary muscle as well as sending branches to the lacrimal gland and trabecular meshwork:

- A drug that mimics the action of the chemical transmitter of the sympathetic nervous system is called a sympathomimetic, e.g. brimonidine.
- One that mimics the action of the chemical transmitter of the parasympathetic nervous system is called a parasympathomimetic, e.g. pilocarpine.
- One that blocks the action of the sympathetic nervous system is called a sympatholytic, e.g. guanethidine.
- One that blocks the action of the parasympathetic nervous system is called a parasympatholytic, e.g. atropine.

Drugs affecting the sympathetic nervous system

Sympathomimetic agents mimic the actions of the transmitter and so will produce some or all of the following effects:

- Dilatation of the pupil
- Reduction in the rate of production of aqueous humour
- Increase in outflow through the trabecular meshwork by lowering outflow resistance
- Constriction of the conjunctival vessels.

Phenylephrine reduces IOP but is more often used as a mydriatic. It should be used with care in patients with hypertension because it may interact with systemic monoamine oxidase (MAO) inhibitors. It is usually recommended that the 2.5% strength be used, with care in hypertension.

The only sympatholytic agent of note is guanethidine which is present in Ganda eyedrops alongside adrenaline (epinephrine) and is used to enhance and prolong the effect of adrenaline (a sympathomimetic).

Drugs affecting the parasympathetic nervous system

The parasympathomimetics (miotics) may work either:

- directly, e.g. pilocarpine, which causes miosis – increased outflow of aqueous by opening up the inefficient drainage channels in the trabecular meshwork resulting from contraction or spasm of the ciliary muscle
- indirectly, e.g. by acting on enzymes that normally metabolize acetylcholine and therefore potentiate its action.

The parasympatholytic (antimuscarinic) agents work by blocking acetylcholine. Hence, they cause pupil dilatation and varying degrees of cycloplegia. They vary in potency and duration of action. Atropine is the most powerful, long-acting agent; tropicamide is a short-acting drug that dilates the pupil but has limited effect on accommodation and is therefore an ideal agent for examining the fundus.

It should be remembered that a darkly pigmented iris is more resistant to pupillary dilatation and caution should be exercised to avoid overdosage. Patients should also be warned not to drive for 1–2 hours after mydriasis.

Treatment of glaucoma

Glaucoma is usually (but not always) associated with an abnormally high IOP. The rise in pressure is almost always the result of reduced outflow of aqueous humour, the inflow remaining constant. Treatment is aimed at reducing IOP.

Sympathomimetics and miotics, as detailed previously, are used in the treatment of glaucoma for their effect on increasing outflow of aqueous humour through the trabecular meshwork. Other drugs used in the treatment of glaucoma include the following.

β Blockers

Topical application of a β blocker reduces IOP effectively probably by reducing the rate of production of aqueous humour. Topical β blockers include betaxolol, timolol, carteolol.

Systemic absorption and subsequent side effects may follow topical application and therefore eyedrops containing β blockers are contraindicated in patients with bradycardia, heart block or uncontrolled heart failure. The Committee for Safety in Medicine has also advised that β blockers, even those with apparent cardioselectivity, such as betaxolol, should not be used in patients with asthma or history of obstructive airway disease unless no alternative treatment is available.

β Blockers have a number of important properties in addition to β-adrenoceptor blockade. These include intrinsic sympathomimetic activity (ISA), cardioselectivity and membrane-stabilizing activity, which are all of importance when considering the side effects seen with these agents.

The property of membrane stabilization is relevant to the incidence of ocular side effects. The absence of anaesthetic properties reduces the number and severity of foreign body and dryness sensations, anaesthesia of the cornea and dry eye syndrome. It has been suggested that those β blockers that show ISA are less likely to produce bronchospasm and peripheral side effects. The selectivity of cardioselective β blockers diminishes with increasing dosage, even within the therapeutic range. A degree of brady-cardia and hypotension is commonly seen with all β blockers but is more marked with non-selective agents.

The precipitation of bronchospasm in susceptible patients can occur with the administration of as little as one drop of timolol. Those β blockers that show cardioselectivity or ISA are less likely to cause bronchoconstriction.

Ocular β blockers are generally not contraindicated in diabetes, although a cardioselective agent may be preferable. However, they are best avoided in patients who have frequent hypoglycaemic attacks because they do produce a slight impairment of glucose tolerance.

The long-term benefits of β blockers on visual field preservation have been shown to be less than would be expected. This may be a result of adverse effects on the ocular microcirculation whereby the β blockers interfere with endogenous vasodilatation and cause optic nerve head arteriolar vasoconstriction. The various β blockers demonstrate marked differences in their vasoconstrictive effect, with betaxolol possibly showing the least vasoconstriction.

Adrenergic agonists

The adrenergic system consists of both α_1 and α_2 receptor cells as well as β_1 and β_2 receptor cells. Adrenergic agonists work by decreasing aqueous production mediated by the β-adrenergic system and an increase in outflow is mediated by the α-adrenergic system. The two most common adrenergic agonist drugs are apraclonidine and brimonidine. Both of these drugs are selective α_2 agonists. Apraclonidine carries a high allergy rate and has been restricted to short-term therapy such as postoperative laser trabeculoplasty and YAG (yttrium–aluminium–garnet) laser iridotomy. Brimonidine, on the other hand, possesses a good safety profile as well as a good efficacy level. It may also provide an intrinsic neuroprotective property. Some of the side effects include headache, insomnia, nervousness, depression and anxiety attacks. Ocular side effects include follicullar conjunctivitis, ocular dryness and conjunctival oedema.

Carbonic anhydrase inhibitors

These act by reducing aqueous humour production through blockage of the carbonic anhydrase enzyme involved in aqueous humour production in the ciliary body. Two carbonic anhydrase inhibitors are available for topical use: brinzolamide and dorzolamide; of the two, brinzolamide appears to cause less burning and stinging on instillation. Acetazolamide is available for systemic use in the form of injection, tablets or slow-release capsules. Although this agent is among the most potent ocular hypotensive agents available, it has limited use in the long-term management of glaucoma as a result of poor patient adherence after the occurrence of side effects such as paraesthesia and gastrointestinal complaints.

It must be remembered that drugs of this class are sulphonamides and that blood disorders (such as thrombocytopenia), rashes and other sulphonamide-related side effects occur occasionally, which, if severe, may require discontinuation of the drug.

Prostaglandin analogues

Prostaglandins are hormones found in most tissues and prostaglandin analogues are biologically active products of arachidonic acid. These drugs act by increasing the uveoscleral outflow and three drugs are commercially available: travoprost, latanoprost and bimatoprost. They are all administered once daily at night and are generally well tolerated. They are relatively free of systemic side effects but have some interesting local side effects such as pigmentation of the iris, which occurs in patients with mixed colour irides and is a result of increased deposition of melanin in the melanocytes. An increase in the length and thickness of the eyelashes and pigmentation of the palpebral skin are also noted side effects.

Hyperosmotic agents

These substances are used effectively to reduce IOP in the short term in emergency situations because of their speed of action; they include intravenous mannitol and oral glycerol (50% solution, 1 g/kg), which is usually given with orange juice or ice to disguise its unpalatable taste. Isosorbide is also used, because it has no caloric value, in patients with diabetes. Hyperosmotic agents increase the osmotic pressure of plasma in relation to aqueous and vitreous, the effect of which is to draw fluid out of the eye and so decrease IOP. The maximal effect of glycerol is seen within 1 hour and lasts for about 3 hours, whereas mannitol acts within 30 minutes with effects lasting for 4–6 hours.

Ocular lubricants

The precorneal tear film is made up of lipid, aqueous and mucin components. The lipid layer is on the outside (helps to decrease evaporative loss), the aqueous layer is in the middle and the mucin layer is on the epithelium to provide a hydrophilic surface, allowing the aqueous layer to maintain contact with the cornea. Disturbance in any one of these layers affects the function of the others, leading to a dry eye condition.

There is an abundance of preparations designed to treat dry eye states and the severity of the condition should guide the choice of preparation:

- Hypromellose: traditional choice, may need to be instilled frequently, useful when aqueous deficient
- Polyvinyl alcohol: hydrophilic, mucomimetic
- Carbomers: cling to corneal surface, improve tear film stability and prolong tear break-up time
- Paraffin eye ointments: decrease evaporative loss, useful in corneal erosion
- Systane: HP guar with demulcents, a gelling and lubricating polymer system.

The ideal solution would be one that normalizes tear film to prevent evaporative loss, increases hormonal support for the lacrimal glands, meibomian glands and other ocular structures, restores the health of the ocular surface, decreases or eliminates ocular surface and lacrimal gland inflammation, and increases tear production.

Local anaesthetic agents

The topical agents are all useful for examination and treatment of simple procedures such as removal of foreign bodies from the cornea, but they should never be used for the management of ocular symptoms.

Oxybuprocaine (benoxinate) and tetracaine (amethocaine) are probably the most widely used topical local anaesthetics. Oxybuprocaine or a combined preparation of lidocaine (lignocaine) and fluorescein is useful in tonometry. Tetracaine produces a more profound anaesthesia and is suitable for use before minor surgical procedures; however, it does have a temporary disruptive effect on the corneal epithelium. Proxymetacaine causes less initial stinging and is useful for children. Side effects of topical anaesthetics include dose-related toxicity to corneal epithelium causing superficial punctate epithelial defects to occur, although oxybuprocaine appears to be less toxic to epithelium than tetracaine or lidocaine. Topical anaesthetics also inhibit epithelial healing as a result of their interference with cell mitosis. Use of topical anaesthetic for anything other than examination purposes is contraindicated.

Lidocaine, with or without adrenaline, is injected into the eyelids for minor surgery, whereas retrobulbar or peribulbar injections are used for surgery of the globe itself.

Diagnostic agents (dyes)

Fluorescein sodium

This is the most commonly used diagnostic agent and is available in a number of different forms:

- A 1% or 2% solution for topical use
- Dry paper impregnated with 1 mg fluorescein
- In combination with lidocaine for tonometry
- An intravenous form that can be obtained in various strengths.

The principle on which it is used comes from the fact that it absorbs light of a certain wavelength and emits light of longer wavelength, i.e. it fluoresces. The principal clinical uses are:

- demonstrating surface defects on cornea and conjunctiva
- Seidel's test (for penetrating injury)
- applanation tonometry (with topical anaesthetic)
- demonstrating patency of nasolacrimal ducts
- fluorescein angiography.

Rose Bengal

This is more efficient for the diagnosis of conjunctival epithelial damage than fluorescein sodium, but it stings excessively (more so in those patients with dry eyes) unless a local anaesthetic is instilled beforehand.

Adverse effects of systemic drugs

As a result of its rich blood supply and relatively small mass the eye exhibits an unusually high sensitivity to adverse drug reactions (ADRs). ADRs can occur to systemic medications as they may enter the bloodstream, from where they can reach ocular structures across the limbal, uveal and retinal vasculature. An important mechanism for ocular ADRs is the selective deposition of drug molecules in the specialized ocular tissues including the cornea, lens and retina, which may therefore show individual susceptibilities to toxicity.

There are various determining factors when looking at the possibility of ADRs occurring; these include the physicochemical properties of the drug itself: protein binding, lipid solubility, molecular size, active transport. Also, the integrity of the blood–ocular barriers is important because, when the eye is inflamed, the blood–aqueous barrier becomes more permeable, allowing increased amounts of the drug to enter the eye from the bloodstream.

Numerous drugs used in general medicine may cause ocular ADRs and here are some examples according to the part of the eye that is affected.

Cornea

- Amiodarone: whorl-like corneal epithelial opacities
- Ciprofloxacin: epithelial deposition

- Chlorpromazine: pigmentation of corneal endothelium
- Indometacin: corneal stromal opacities.

Lens

- Corticosteroids: cataract and lenticular deposits
- Phenothiazines: anterior cortical opacities.

Conjunctiva

- Isotretinoin: blepharoconjunctivitis
- Chlorpromazine: deposition.

Lacrimal apparatus

- Antihistamines: tear production
- Rifampicin: coloration of tears.

Retina

- Tamoxifen: maculopathy
- Vigabatrin: field defects
- Digoxin: colour vision defects.

There are certain drugs that are known to cause significant ocular ADRs and these are as follows.

Vigabatrin (antiepileptic)

ADRs reported with vigabatrin include:

- Colour vision deficiencies: selective short wavelength impairment consistent with GABAergic (GABA is γ-aminobutyric acid) inhibition at retinal level.
- Contrast sensitivity impairment.
- Visual field abnormalities: up to a third of patients receiving vigabatrin at a normal therapeutic level will have these. This visual field loss appears to be dose dependent and permanent. It usually presents as concentric, binasal, peripheral constriction with temporal and central sparing.
- Retinal disorders: narrowing of retinal arterioles, atrophy of the peripheral retina, surface wrinkling retinopathy of the macula, abnormalities of retinal pigment epithelium, irregularities of macula reflex and optic disc pallor.

The Committee on Safety of Medicines has advised that onset of symptoms varies from one month to several years after starting treatment. In most cases, visual field defects have persisted despite discontinuation. Visual field testing is therefore recommended before treatment commences and at 6-monthly intervals. Patients should be warned to report any new visual symptoms that develop and those with symptoms should be referred for urgent ophthalmological opinion.

Levodopa (anti-parkinsonian)

Adverse drug reactions reported with levodopa include:

* mydriasis, visual hallucinations, ptosis and/or blepharospasm
* hallucination sufferers had abnormal rapid eye movement (rem) sleep patterns
* may lead to melanomas in any part of the epithelial or ocular pigmented tissues
* secondary Meigs' syndrome with long-term usage (ocular dystonia).

Hydroxychloroquine/chloroquine (antimalarials)

ADRs reported with hydroxychloroquine/chloroquine include:

* Irreversible retinal damage
* Corneal opacity.

Patients on these drugs should have their eyes checked annually and the Royal College of Ophthalmologists has advised that a screening protocol for chloroquine should be negotiated with local ophthalmologists. Recommendations also exist for those patients on hydroxychloroquine, with examination suggested both before treatment is started and once it has started.

Oculogyric crisis

A number of drugs may precipitate oculogyric crisis, a condition characterized by maximal upward deviation of the eyes, associated with backward, lateral flexion of the neck, an open mouth with tongue protrusion and ocular pain. Other features may include an increased blood pressure and heart rate with flushing, and psychiatric symptoms such as depression, paranoia and anxiety.

Precipitating drugs include neuroleptics, benzodiazepines, carbamazepine, chloroquine, metoclopramide, nifedipine, tricyclic antidepressants and cetirizine. Treatment in the acute phase involves reassurance, diphenhydramine and/or diazepam or lorazepam. Recovery is rapid after treatment.

Adverse effects of ophthalmic drugs

It must also be remembered that drugs applied topically to the eye may also cause systemic ADRs. The occurrence of systemic ADRs may be decreased but not eradicated by occlusion of the punctum or by closing the eye for a count of 60 following administration, to minimize systemic absorption.

Topical β blockers

Systemic ADRs reported following use of topical β blockers include:

- bronchoconstriction
- hypotension
- bradycardia
- nausea/diarrhoea
- anxiety/depression
- hallucinations
- fatigue.

Topical sympathomimetic agents

Systemic ADRs reported after use of topical sympathomimetic agents include:

- dry mouth/nose
- headache
- asthenia
- bradycardia
- depression.

Topical carbonic anhydrase inhibitors

Systemic ADRs reported after use of topical carbonic anhydrase inhibitors include:

- fatigue
- headache
- dry mouth
- nausea
- dyspnoea
- taste perversion.

Drugs and the nurse

The Nursing and Midwifery Council's (NMC) *Guidelines for the Administration of Medicines* (NMC 2002, p. 6) are clear that:

> As a registered nurse or midwife, you are accountable for your actions and omissions. In administering any medication, or assisting or overseeing any self-administration of medication, you must exercise your professional judgment and apply your knowledge and skill in the given situation.

They go on to state that (NMC 2002, p. 6):

> In exercising your professional accountability in the best interests of your patients, you must know the therapeutic uses of the medicine to be administered, its normal dosage, side effects, precautions and contra-indications.

Although this applies only to nurses registered in the UK, it forms a general statement of good practice for the use of good professional judgement in relation to the administration of prescribed drugs.

Prescription, supply and administration of drugs by nurses in the UK

Recent and proposed changes in policy and legislation allow some nurses in the UK to prescribe drugs. Previously, this facility was limited to medical practitioners and dentists, but it is planned that prescribing will be extended to other professionals allied to medicine.

Two types of prescribing are possible. After a prescribed educational programme and assessment, nurses may prescribe, independently, all pharmacy (P) medicines and a range of prescription-only medicines (POMs) from a limited formulary. Independent prescribing means that the prescriber takes responsibility for the clinical assessment of the patient, establishing a diagnosis and the clinical management required, as well as responsibility for prescribing where necessary and the appropriateness of any prescription. The independent prescribing formulary is very limited and is designed to be used mainly in minor illness and minor injury. Supplementary prescribing builds on this and may be more use to nurses in specialist areas.

Supplementary prescribing

Supplementary prescribing is defined as:

> . . . a voluntary partnership between an independent prescriber (a doctor or dentist) and a supplementary prescriber, to implement an agreed patient-specific Clinical Management Plan with the patient's agreement.
>
> Department of Health (2004, p. 1)

There are no legal restrictions on the clinical conditions that may be treated under supplementary prescribing, although it is intended by the Department of Health that supplementary prescribing will be used mainly for the management of chronic medical conditions and health needs.

Provided that medicines are prescribable by a doctor, and that they are referred to in the patient's clinical management plan, supplementary prescribers are able to prescribe any general sales list (GSL) and P medicines and all POMs including those used 'off label' and those unlicensed drugs used as part of a clinical trial.

Training for supplementary prescribing for nurses is the same as for independent nurse prescribing, with the addition of a short module covering the context and concept of supplementary prescribing.

There are some situations where patients may have a POM supplied and/or medicine administered directly to them by a range of health-care professionals without the legal necessity of a signed prescription. This can be achieved in one of two ways.

Patient group direction

Patient group directions (PGDs) were introduced in August 2000 to replace standing orders and constitute a legal framework that allows certain health-care professionals to supply and administer medicines to groups of patients who fit the criteria laid out in the PGD. A health-care professional can supply (e.g. provide tablets) and/or administer a medicine (e.g. give an injection or eyedrops) directly to a patient without the need for a prescription or an instruction from a prescriber. Where medicines are supplied in this way, patients must be counselled and provided with a patient information leaflet. The PGD applies to groups of patients who may not be individually identified before presenting for treatment.

PGDs fit best within services where medicine use follows a predictable pattern and are generally most appropriate to manage a specific treatment episode where supply or administration of a medicine is necessary. In ophthalmic practice, PGDs might be used for administration of eyedrops for ocular examination and for defined situations such as provision of topical antibiotics after corneal abrasion or removal of a corneal foreign body.

The list of practitioners who may use PGDs is defined at present as: nurse, midwife, pharmacist, optometrist, orthoptist, podiatrist, radiographer, physiotherapist, ambulance paramedic, dietitian, prosthetist, occupational therapist, and speech and language therapist.

This list may be extended in the future and it must be noted that unregistered practitioners such as health-care assistants and assistant practitioners are not included. Individual practitioners using the PGD must be named on a list kept by the employing authority (National Prescribing Centre 2004).

Patient-specific direction

A patient-specific direction (PSD) is used once a patient has been assessed by a prescriber and that prescriber instructs another health-care professional, in writing, to supply or administer a medicine directly to that named patient or to several named patients. This might be an instruction in the patient's notes or an instruction on a clinic list containing names of patients attending that clinic. PSDs do not require an assessment of the patient by the health-care worker instructed to supply and/or administer the medication. Where a PSD exists, there is no need for a PGD. This might be used for a clinic list of patients whose pupils need to be dilated before examination.

The role of the clinician

The ophthalmic clinician has a major role in ensuring that patients receive optimum drug therapy for their condition. The roles include the obvious instillation or provision of prescribed medication, but also as a patient educator to ensure that the patient is not only able to use the medication, but also understands the consequences of using it or of choosing not to. Patients cannot be expected to agree with our conclusions about their therapy if they do not understand them.

Compliance is a term often used by clinicians, but compliance has connotations of power – we, the ophthalmic clinicians, tell the patient what they should do and they do what we say. Compliance and non-compliance are both patient-related phenomena and non-compliant behaviour may represent a conscious decision or choice by the patient (Kyngas et al. 2000). Concordance is an approach to the prescribing and taking of medicines that suggests an agreement reached after negotiation between a patient and a health-care professional who respects the beliefs and wishes of the patient in determining whether and how medicines are to be taken (Wilson and O'Mahoney 1999). Often, the biggest factor in concordance is nurses – we too must ensure our understanding, the understanding of the patient and the patient's ability to undertake the tasks that we ask of them. The message should be consistent regardless of whether the patient is being cared for by specialist ophthalmic clinicians, or those in other settings. The message about all therapy, ophthalmic and general, needs to be consistent so that trust in the information is maintained and the patient is enabled to make the best personal choices (Marsden and Shaw 2003).

General rules for optimal topical drug therapy

- The patient must be enabled to have adequate knowledge of each drug, the intended therapeutic effect, possible side effects and how to deal with them, as well as the optimal timing between doses and any particular order in which drugs should be used.
- One drop into the lower fornix is enough – excess will overflow from the fornix, down the cheek and will also exit the fornix via the puncta and canaliculi into the nasolacrimal duct. Excessive systemic absorption may take place through the nasal mucosa.
- Ideally 5 but at least 3 minutes should be left between drops to the same eye – otherwise, the previous drop will be washed away and not absorbed in any therapeutic amount.
- All drops should be instilled before any ointment – ointment 'waterproofs' the eye and any drops instilled will not be absorbed but will overflow and the drug will be lost to the eye.
- Adverse systemic effects can be minimized by asking the patient to close the eye gently and count slowly to 60 after drop instillation or by occluding the punctum.
- In elderly people or a disabled population, physical disability may be responsible for lack of concordance – instillation aids are available and the clinician should be aware of different types, what might work best for the patient and where to obtain them.

References

Department of Health (2004) Mechanisms for Nurse and Pharmacist Prescribing and Supply of Medicines. London: DoH.

Fechner PU, Teichmann KD (1998) Ocular Therapeutics. Thorofare, NJ: Slack.

Field D, Martin D, Witchell L (1999) Ophthalmic chloramphenicol: friend or foe? Ophthal Nursing 2(4): 4–7.

Kyngas H, Duffy ME, Kroll T (2000) Conceptual analysis of compliance. J Clin Nursing 9: 5–12.

Marsden J, Shaw M (2003) Correct administration of topical eye treatment. Nursing Stand 17(30): 42–4.

National Prescribing Centre (2004) Patient Group Directions: A practical guide and framework of competencies for all professionals using patient group directions (www.npc.co.uk/publications/pgd/pgd.htm).

Nursing and Midwifery Council (2002) Guidelines for the Administration of Medicines. London: NMC.

Wilson CG, O'Mahony B (1999) Non-compliance in glaucoma management. Eye News 5: 6.

CHAPTER FOUR

Examination of the eye

MARY E SHAW

Although examination of the eye is at the forefront of the mind of the health professional, it is important in making a diagnosis to consider the patient as a whole. The general impression of the patient gained by the examiner can provide clues or cues to subsequent action.

Checking patient demographic details is not only essential to ensure that you have the correct patient but also helps to break the ice and establish the first line of communication. When doing this take care not to breach confidentiality or embarrass the patient. Identification of patient should include:

- Name
- Date of birth
- Age
- Address
- Source of referral
- Reasons for referral.

When you greet a patient, make a general assessment of the patient taking into consideration the following:

- The general appearance of the patient.
- Mobility: whether in a wheelchair or using walking aids. This not only could give clues to systemic conditions that affect the eye, but will also alert the examiner to whether the patient requires assistance to the position at the slit-lamp or examination chair. Are moving and handling equipment or techniques needed to maintain safety for patient and examiner?
- Race/ethnicity: some races are more susceptible to some ocular diseases than others, e.g. people of African–Caribbean origin are more susceptible to developing primary open angle glaucoma (POAG).
- Gender is significant with some hereditary conditions and susceptibility to some diseases.

- Any visible physical impairment that might interfere with compliance, especially with topical medications.
- Large/small stature relative to age.
- Overweight/underweight: this could affect mobility but could give cues to ocular pathology in some cases.
- General state of the patient: is he or she calm/nervous/agitated. Agitation or nervousness may affect the patient's ability to communicate effectively. Put the patient at ease. You will get more out of your encounter with him or her.
- Whether the patient is accompanied by a care-giver or relative: does the patient want the care-giver/relative with him or her in the consultation? They do not have an automatic right to be there. The patient should be asked if they want to be accompanied.
- Mental capability of the patient: a difficult judgement to make – learning disability may be obvious in the case of the patient who has Down's syndrome, but it does not mean that the patient is not capable of complete engagement in the consultation.
- Sensory deficit: look out for evidence of poor hearing; a hearing aid is an obvious cue but do not assume that it is working properly! If you suspect poor hearing, speak clearly and directly to the patient. If it is known ahead of the appointment that the patient is profoundly deaf, arrange for an interpreter or facilitator to sign for the patient. Respect patient confidentiality; do not use relatives, especially children. They may not be giving accurate information.
- Speech impairment or impediment may not be an obvious thing to consider, but it could affect how well you communicate with the patient. If the patient stutters, avoid closing their sentences or filling in words.
- Communication issues including language barriers. If you are aware of any such barriers ahead of time, an official interpreter can be arranged.

The examination room

The room should afford privacy for the patient. Attempting to examine the patient in an open environment is not recommended unless it is an emergency/first-aid measure, because the patient needs to feel secure, not embarrassed, e.g. the patient whose first language is not English or is illiterate will not enjoy others knowing of these difficulties during vision testing.

Ideally the examination room should have good lighting and a comfortable chair for the patient to sit in that affords head and neck support.

Equipment needed

For a simple examination, a good quality pen-torch will suffice. An ophthalmoscope provides added magnification, light filters and cobalt blue. A slit-lamp biomicroscope is a most adaptable piece of equipment.

Charts to test visual acuity of the Snellen (Figure 4.1) or logMAR (logarithm of the minimum angle of resolution) (Figure 4.2) type should be available, along with near vision and colour testing equipment. An occluder, or occluder combined with pinholes (more usual), should also be available. Pinholes rule out refractive error when testing visual acuity.

The test chart should be 6 metres distant from where the patient will sit or stand; alternatively a mirror at a distance of 3 m reflecting the chart should be used. Thomson (2003) states that testing charts are also available on computers.

Diagnostic fluorescein strips, sterile saline, dilating drops as well as cotton buds, used to facilitate eversion of the eyelids when examining the subtarsal conjunctiva, are required.

It should be possible to dim the lighting in the room.

Preparing the patient

The patient should be comfortable and ideally pain free to facilitate a good examination. If the patient is in pain following trauma, instillation of topical local anaesthetic may improve compliance. This will of course have to be prescribed if the examiner is not qualified to prescribe. With some conditions such as iritis, it is not appropriate to instil local anaesthetic drops because they will not affect the pain but, as the examiner is not making a diagnosis at this stage, it may not be obvious that the patient has iritis and a drop of topical anaesthetic will do no harm to a painful eye.

The patient needs to be informed about what to expect in the examination to ensure informed consent and cooperation.

Taking a history

The process of history taking and clinical examination performs several vital functions:

- Helps to establish a rapport between the examiner and the patient
- Establishes physical contact between the examiner and patient

- Enables the establishment of an accurate diagnosis (about 70–90% of all diagnoses are established by the end of the history and examination and before tests are performed)
- Identifies the severity of signs and symptoms
- Determines diagnosis
- Commences treatment if appropriate
- Monitors treatment.

Patient evaluation always begins with a careful history. The order of history taking is usually as follows:

- Presenting symptoms: find out from the patient if he or she is experiencing any problems with vision. Check what the visual acuity or refraction is for both distance and near. Is the patient myopic or hypermetropic?
- History of presenting illness (if any, as glaucoma patients may be asymptomatic): find out if the patient's visit to the optician is a routine appointment or if he or she has gone to the optician for a specific reason. If patients are experiencing visual problems, establish the onset/duration/severity and location of symptoms.
- Past medical/surgical history paying particular attention to any history of hypertension/hypotension, diabetes, history of vascular disease such as hypertension or myocardial infarction, cerebrovascular accident and cholesterol problems. Attention must be paid to any respiratory disorders such as asthma or chronic obstructive airway disease. History of any renal problems or blood transfusion should also be noted, because they could influence diagnosis and decisions about relevant treatment.
- Ask whether the patient suffers from migraine, cold hands or feet (sign of vasospasm attack).
- Past ophthalmic history: any history of trauma, ocular disease such as iritis, previous ophthalmic surgery? Is he or she registered blind or partially sighted?
- Family history of eye problems including glaucoma.
- Current medication: systemic, intramuscular, intravenous, subcutaneous or topical.
- Allergies.
- Social history: smoking habit (cigarettes, pipe, cigars), illegal substances, consumption of alcohol, occupation, interests, whether or not lives alone, vehicle or machine operator.

Testing visual acuity

A record of visual acuity (VA) should be taken for each patient presenting with an ocular condition. This is to provide a baseline for later comparisons

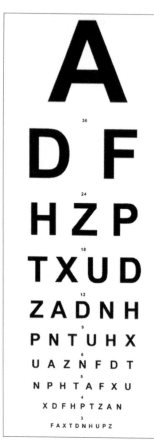

↑ **Figure 4.1** Snellen visual acuity chart.

↓ **Figure 4.2** LogMAR (logarithm of the minimum angle of resolution) visual acuity chart.

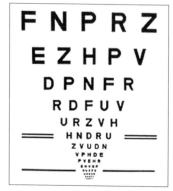

to be made and may also assist diagnosis. VA is normally done after taking an ocular history.

Privacy is essential to prevent embarrassment and also to prevent patients from learning the chart.

If the patient normally wears distance glasses, he or she should continue to wear them, a note being made when recording VA that glasses were worn. Where glasses are worn, record the VA with and without them.

Be systematic with your testing, testing the right eye (oculodexter or OD) first, then the left (oculosinister or OS). If the patient presents with a problem, it is usual to test the 'bad' eye first and the 'good' eye after to prevent the patient remembering some of the letters seen with the 'good' eye.

The examiner should observe the patient during the test and not the chart; the examiner will therefore need to know the test chart by heart. This is to ensure that the patient does not try to 'cheat' and thus provide an erroneous result.

If the patient cannot read letters they may be able to read a number chart. If they can do neither because of language or literacy problems, the 'E' test can be used, where each letter on every line is an E but in a different position. The patient is asked to point to a sheet of Es and indicate the corresponding position of the E. Alternatively, they could be given an E to hold and position appropriately. VA is recorded as usual. It is not appropriate to use an interpreter because he or she could bias the test. Matching may also be undertaken using a template for the normal Snellen (Figure 4.1) or logMAR letter (Figure 4.2) chart or for a number chart, and this may be considerably easier than trying to decide whether the patient is matching an E incorrectly or whether the operator has lost his or her place on the chart! Charts are available with images/pictures of familiar objects but an adult may see the use of this as demeaning.

The patient should be 6 m distant from the chart. They should be instructed to cover the left eye with the occluder, not to squint and to read every letter on each line out loud. (It has been known for patients to mind read!) Encourage the patient to try to read as far down the chart as possible, noting the smallest line that the patient can read. Also note if the patient misses or gets a letter(s) wrong. Do the same steps, occluding the right eye, to note and record VA in the left eye. VA should be recorded, e.g. VA; R(OD) 6/6 L(OS) 6/6. The numerator is the line on the test chart and the denominator the distance from the chart, 6 m in this case.

If the patient cannot read the largest letter on the chart from 6 m, move the patient nearer to the chart, usually in 1-m increments. The distance from the chart is duly noted, e.g. VA; R 3/36 L 3/60, indicating that the chart was read at a distance of 3 m.

If the patient cannot see the top letter even when moved nearer the chart (e.g. 1 m), ask the patient to count the number of fingers (CF) that you are holding up. The test distance is usually 1 foot or 30 cm. If the patient can count fingers, record as CF in the notes (this should be undertaken more than once because guessing can sometimes be very accurate).

Should the patient not be able to count fingers, he or she should be asked if he or she sees any hand movement (HM). Again this is done at 1 foot (30 cm). Record as HM for that eye. If HM cannot be noticed by the patient, ask him or her to locate a light source such as a pen-torch. Hold the light at about 2 feet (60 cm) from the patient, asking him or her to look at the light, which is moved into different areas of the patient's field of vision. If the patient can see the light, record as PL (perception of light). In the event that light cannot be seen, record as NPL (no perception of light).

Where VA is less than 6/9 in either eye, pinhole (PH) VA should be recorded. Pinhole acuity will give an indication about whether vision can be corrected with spectacles or contact lenses, which is indicated by the VA improving with pinholes.

Use of pinholes

If worn, the patient should wear distance spectacles. He or she should be asked to hold the pinhole to the right eye and the occluder over the left, and to adjust the position of the pinhole until he or she can view the chart through it and read the smallest line of letters that is visible. It may be necessary to encourage the patient to try a smaller line of letters even if he or she makes some errors.

Record VA as before but adding PH to the measurement. Note that some clinical areas have space affording less than the 6 m or do not have 3 m with a mirror, necessary for the test. A 3-metre Snellen chart is available for use in confined places. It gives the result as if at 6 m.

The Snellen chart has some limitations in that the number of letters per line varies from one letter on the 6/60 line to many on lines for higher acuities, and the change in letter size across the chart is not even. There is no systematic or logical spacing between letters. This ensures that the visual task is not the same at each level of acuity. The logMAR chart was designed to take this into account and is used much more frequently both in eye clinics and in eye research now.

LogMAR charts and testing

Charts are designed so that the letters are of almost equal legibility and there are five letters on each row. The spacing between each letter is equal and the spacing between rows is equal to the height of the letters on the smaller row. The letter size follows a geometric progression with a ratio equal to 0.1 log units (1.26). The chart is designed for a standard testing distance of 4 m which is much more manageable in most settings than 6 m. The chart is marked on the left with the equivalent Snellen notation; on the right, the notation is the logMAR of the letters concerned. The value of 0.0 logMAR is equivalent to 4/4 or 6/6.

The patient should be asked to read from left to right from the 0.5 logMAR, or the 4/2 line if the VA is sufficient. The patient should be encouraged to continue to read down the chart until he or she fails to identify any letters on one line.

Scoring allows the inclusion of each individual letter missed or read incorrectly. Each line is 0.1 logMAR and so each letter is 0.02 logMAR. In practice, the total number of letters read incorrectly is noted and 0.02 logMAR unit assigned to each. This sum is added to the logMAR value for the last line on which any letters were read correctly and recorded as the final logMAR score.

To use the chart at 3 m, 0.1 logMAR unit should be added to the final score; at 2 m, 0.3 should be added and at 1 m, 0.6. The equivalent of 0.0 logMAR is 6/6 Snellen; 0.3 is equivalent to 6/12, 0.6 to 6/24 and 1 to 6/60.

Colour vision testing

Colour vision is tested to determine whether there is any acquired and/or hereditary defect of colour vision. Testing colour vision will enable the examiner to determine whether there are problems with the macular or optic nerve.

Some jobs depend on the person having normal colour vision, e.g. British train drivers. According to Birch (2003) there is a duty to ensure that colour vision testing equipment meets quality standards and must therefore be 'fit for purpose'.

The patient should wear his or her near-vision spectacles for the test. The most common colour vision test is the Ishihara plates. More detailed examination tools are available to determine hue discrimination, but the operator must have specialist skill.

Eye examination

Examination of the eye is essential to the diagnosis and management of ocular disease and trauma. While within a specialist ophthalmic unit, the health professional will have access to a slit-lamp (Figure 4.3); this is likely not to be the case in other settings such as the doctor's surgery or the treatment room. Anyone caring for an ophthalmic patient should be able to perform a basic systematic examination of the eye, adnexae and anterior chamber.

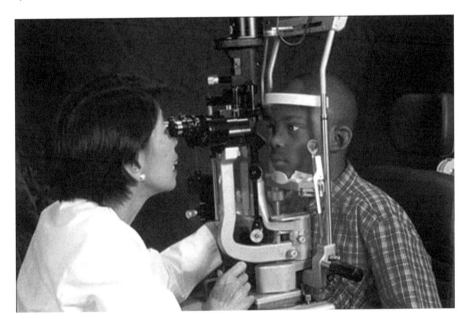

Figure 4.3 Slit-lamp examination.

Pen-torch examination of the eye

Pen-torch examination of the eye can reveal findings that are significant to making a diagnosis. It may demonstrate that the eye is in fact healthy or diseased, or detect the presence of trauma or a foreign body (FB).

Equipment needed

A good pen-torch is essential, with batteries that are well charged. Dull light will not highlight anomalies and will prevent adequate examination of the pupil response.

A source of magnification will enable the examiner to view and, if appropriate, remove FBs. It will also enable the examiner to view structures better.

The examination

Much of the patient's confidence in the practitioner comes from the practitioner having a good examination technique but, in addition, the ability to explain clinically what is seen during the examination process needs to be developed, so that the giving of a step-by-step account of what is seen will help to explain the symptoms experienced by the patient as well as the subsequent rationale behind treatment choices. It is helpful to use simple diagrams/leaflets to aid explanations, or to develop drawing skills in order to be able quickly to produce simple sketches of what is seen to share with patients and help understanding. The diagrams can then be given to patients to take away with them.

Examination of the eye should be systematic. It is usual to look first at the eye that is thought to be diseased or injured; if it is a general check follow the systematic process and examine the right eye first. Beforehand, the patient's face should be considered. Does it look normal? Is there facial symmetry? Are there any signs of disease or trauma, e.g. port wine stain, the presence of which could indicate a risk of glaucoma? Are the eyes proptosed? Is the patient using the brow to open the eyelids? Does the patient adopt a particular inclination of the head that could be an indicator of visual problems such as macular degeneration?

Before you shine the torch directly into the patient eye, warn him or her to prevent screwing up of the eyes.

Eyelids

Observe the lids for anomalies, if present, such as: ptosis, inflammation, redness, oedema, trauma (old and new) such as lacerations, cysts, lesions, and swelling, particularly over the lacrimal sac. Examine lid margins for: redness, scales, dandruff, orientation of the eyelashes – are they turning in (entropion) or out (ectropion) – are they scant? Are the margins swollen? Are live lice or nits present or absent.

Ask the patient to close the eyes gently, and observe whether the margins are in apposition or if closure is incomplete. Is the blink rate normal (every 3–6 seconds) or is there some blepharospasm? Check that the lids and puncta are in good apposition to the globe.

Conjunctiva

Each of the following areas of the conjunctiva should be examined carefully: bulbar area, palpebral area and area of the fornices (Figure 4.4).

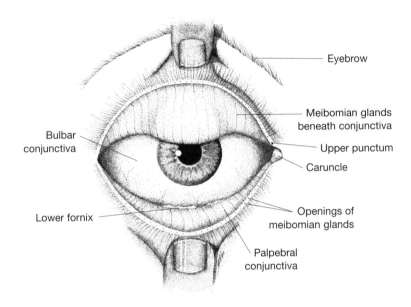

Figure 4.4 Eversion of the upper and lower lids.

Everting the upper lid

Ask the patient to look down and grasp the lashes of the upper lid with the thumb underneath the lashes. Hold the lid, down and slightly away from the globe, taking care not to pull it tight. Using the tip of a cotton-tipped applicator, held in the other hand like a pen, press down on the centre of the lid. The lid will evert along the edge of the tarsal place. The cotton bud may be removed as the thumb presses the everted part of the lid backwards and anchors it against the upper orbital rim.

To examine the bulbar conjunctiva, gently pull down the lower lids to expose the lower bulbar conjunctiva. After viewing this area, gently push up the upper lid, asking the patient to look down to expose the superior bulbar areas. By asking the patient to look in all directions of gaze, you can view all the area. The conjunctiva is normally transparent. Some patients have visible conjunctival blood vessels. The sclera should be visible below and is normally white in appearance.

To view the palpebral conjunctiva it is necessary to evert the lids. The lower lid can be gently pulled down to expose the conjunctiva although it is necessary to evert the upper lid manually. Look for papillae, follicles and cysts.

In a healthy conjunctiva you should be able to view the vasculature clear of signs of injection. Note the presence, degree, depth and location of hyperaemia. Note that the superficial vessels are motile whereas the deeper vessels are not. Such differentiation will assist the diagnosis of the type of conjunctivitis or whether you are observing episcleritis. Differential diagnosis may necessitate slit-lamp examination. Look for cysts, lacerations, papillae, pinguecula, pterygium and FBs.

Episcleral vessels are visible below the conjunctiva and should normally show no signs of injection.

Sclera
The sclera should be white. It is hyperaemic in cases of episcleritis, scleritis or uveitis. In the case of scleritis, the sclera appears to have a bluish/purple tinge.

Cornea
A healthy cornea should appear clear, with no opacities or vasculature and no encroachment of conjunctival tissue. Note the curvature: is it abnormally conical as in keratoconus?

Anterior chamber
Anterior chamber (AC) examination is possible using a pen-torch. Each eye is assessed individually. Shine the torch on the cornea centrally and observe the AC from the temporal aspect; this gives a rough estimate of AC depth but not how shallow the angle may be. The angle is better estimated using the slit-lamp, although a rough estimate can be made by shining the pen-torch on to the nasal side of the cornea and noting the angle depth.

Viewing through the cornea to the AC, you should normally have an uninterrupted view of the iris and pupil. After blunt or penetrating trauma, including surgery and laser, hyphaema may be present. You should note how much of the AC is filled. In extreme cases, the whole of the AC may be filled.

In infected conditions, including corneal ulcer and endophthalmitis, hypopyon may be detected. Sterile hypopyon may also be present.

The iris
Note the colour – usually both irises are a very similar colour. Look for presence of iris atrophy or evidence of trauma such as iris prolapse. Iridodonesis may be noted if the patient has had an intracapsular cataract extraction. Note sphincter tears.

Assess the pupils by:

- shape and size – compare with the other eye
- reaction to light (direct and consensual)
- pupil response
- relative afferent pupillary defect
- subjective assessment of brightness.

Pupillary assessment It is important to evaluate the pupillary reaction between the two eyes because a relative afferent pupillary defect may indicate that there is an inequality in the severity of glaucomatous optic nerve damage between the two eyes of a patient. Careful evaluation and documentation serve as a baseline for future evaluations.

Lens
Some lens opacities can be viewed with the naked eye through the pupil. Note whether the patient is aphakic or pseudophakic (you may be able to see a reflection from a posterior chamber intraocular lens).

Tear film
It is difficult to estimate tear film break-up time with a pen-torch unless you have a blue filter cover. Instil fluorescein into the lower fornix. Ask the patient to blink. Shine the pen-torch on to the cornea, observing how long it takes before the tear film starts to break up and disperse. The break-up time is normally 15–20 seconds, after which streaks are noted in the fluorescein. Applanation tonometry is explained in Chapter 20.

A more in-depth examination of the ocular structures requires a source of magnification, ideally with a stereoscopic view using a slit-lamp or an indirect ophthalmoscope for the posterior segment.

Slit-lamp examination follows a similar pattern of examination. Do not expect to achieve competence with the use of a slit-lamp after a single practice. It may take weeks or months of practice under supervision before confidence is gained to begin to use it independently as a diagnostic tool.

It is not possible to provide a short, succinct description of how to set up and use a slit-lamp. Any reader wishing to learn more about setting up the slit-lamp should review the manufacturer's handbook.

Slit-lamp examination
It is important to practise and become familiar with the slit-lamp; it is not a test that can be performed just once to make you competent. It needs to be used regularly and feedback from an expert on performance can be helpful. It is rather like driving a car and getting used to the controls, highway code, road conditions and other road users. Confidence will be gained gradually. If you are a novice, it may be helpful to find a willing

volunteer to sit on the other side of the slit-lamp and go through the practical aspects of setting the slit-lamp to your requirements and getting the individual sitting correctly at the slit-lamp.

The principle of the slit-lamp is the narrow 'slit' beam of very bright light produced by the lamp. This beam is focused on to the eye, which is then viewed under magnification with a microscope. The following are key points in slit-lamp examination:

- The patient's comfort and your comfort at the slit-lamp are of utmost importance.
- Provide a good explanation of the procedure to ensure the patient's cooperation.
- Use a systematic and methodical process in your slit-lamp examination to reduce the likelihood of missing something.
- Ensure that the eyepieces are correctly adjusted to your prescription before commencing the examination, e.g. your refractive errors (if any) are accounted for and that you have adjusted your pupillary apertures accordingly.
- Document findings accurately and legibly.

The slit-lamp has many uses including examination and monitoring of:

- ocular adnexae including lids, lid margins, punctum, lashes.
- ocular structures: cornea, anterior chamber, iris, lens, lens capsule and anterior vitreous face.
- signs, symptoms and progress of anterior segment disease or injury.
- posterior segment of the eye by the use of auxiliary lenses.

Further 'special' investigations
- Goldmann tonometry
- Van Herick's estimation of anterior chamber depth
- Gonioscopic examination of the angle.

Components of the slit-lamp
- The microscope, which houses the viewing system, composed of the oculars and the magnification changers.
- The illumination arm, which houses the illumination system.
- The remainder of the instrument, e.g. chin rest, fixation light.

The microscope and adjustment of ocular eyepieces The slit-lamp is a binocular microscope, which means that it gives the examiner a three-dimensional view of the eye and surrounding structures. The prime advantage of a three-dimensional view is that ocular abnormalities can be detected with greater precision. All slit-lamps are slightly different – the explanations here should be modified to suit individual slit-lamps.

The viewing system of the microscope can be adjusted to account for any refractive error; alternatively you may choose to wear glasses during the examination. If you are unsure what your refractive correction is, a focusing rod, which is supplied with the slit-lamp, can be used to measure your refractive error. Slide off the footplate and insert the focusing rod with the flat side facing you. Turn on the slit-lamp and using a slit beam of light (about 1–2 mm in width) focus the light on to the rod. Close one eye and with the other eye look through the slit-lamp and start turning the wheel of the ocular eyepiece from the plus side of the scale, stopping immediately once the image of the light through the eyepiece is clear and in focus. Where possible (if you know your own refraction readings), check whether the scale readings in dioptres actually correspond to your own spectacle correction.

You will have to adjust the interpupillary distance of the eyepieces to your own eyes. Some people's eyes are more widely spaced apart or closer set than others. To adjust the eyepieces to suit your interpupillary distance, first take a look down the binocular eyepieces of the slit-lamp. You should not be aware of seeing any black shading in your field of vision; this indicates poor adjustment. If black shading is noted, you will need to adjust the interpupillary aperture by either squeezing the eyepieces together or pulling them further apart. When the pupillary apertures are correctly set, you will have an unobstructed view when looking through the eyepieces.

Magnification adjustment of the binoculars of the microscope depends on the model or manufacturer; some have a flip switch whereas others have a dial. If your magnification changer is a lever switch, you will have two different settings on $10 \times$ and $16 \times$. If your magnification changer is a knob, you will normally have five different magnification settings: $6 \times$, $10 \times$, $16 \times$, $25 \times$ and $40 \times$. Magnifications of $10 \times$ and $16 \times$ are adequate for most examination purposes.

The illumination arm houses the light source. The illumination arm is capable of being moved from $0°$ to $90°$ on either side of the microscope. The illumination arm houses the following components:

1. Two slit controls which have the capability to vary the height and width of the slit beam. In addition, the orientation of the beam can be altered from a vertical to a horizontal plane. The slit control is also used for interposing the blue filter.
2. Filters are available that control the heat and light intensity of the beam. In addition, colour filters (cobalt blue and cyan) are available and these are used are in conjunction with different eyedrops.

The position of the illumination system to the observation system can be measured by a graded index, which is located at the bottom of the illumination column. Knowledge of the angle of the illumination to the illumination column is important for examining/grading certain structures of the eye.

The movement of the slit-lamp is controlled by the joystick, which is situated on the base of the slit-lamp; by moving the joystick left to right and back to front, movement of the slit lamp is achieved. The slit-lamp is raised or lowered by turning the joystick clockwise (to elevate) or counterclockwise (to lower).

Further adjustment to the slit-lamp can be achieved by a lever located at the base of the slit-lamp table. By releasing the lever, the height of the whole table (including the slit-lamp) can be adjusted to accommodate the height of the individual patient. Take care to control this movement because you could cause the patient some injury.

Patient comfort at the slit-lamp can be further achieved by moving the chin rest up and down by means of the adjustment knob located on the side frame of the slit-lamp. When the patient is in the correct position, the patient's outer canthus will be aligned with a black mark or notch on the headrest bar. The patient's forehead should be snug against the forehead rest.

An explanation of the examination to the patient is vital in order to ensure cooperation and to obtain informed consent from the patient. It can also be explained that, although the machine may look formidable, it is only a glorified microscope or pair of binoculars used to magnify the different structures of the eye.

Advise patients that to facilitate accurate examination they need to ensure that their forehead rests against the bar and that their chin should be in the chin rest; they should keep their mouth closed and both eyes open. Note also that they should be warned that the light from the slit-lamp can be bright; this is especially important if the patient is already photophobic.

The position of the slit-lamp is equally important to ensure cooperation. Be patient with elderly and very young people. If the patient is in a wheel-chair, where possible transfer him or her to an examination chair. If this is not possible, manoeuvre the slit-lamp as close as you can to the patient by removing the arms and footrests of the wheelchair. For shorter patients or children, it may be possible to examine them standing right in front of the slit-lamp. Patients with head tremors should have their head supported from behind by an assistant. Above all, be patient. Align the slit-lamp to the patient and make yourself comfortable. Set your slit-lamp on the lower magnification and turn it on at the control box to the lowest voltage setting. Use one hand to operate the joystick and the other to operate the illumination arm. If examining the patient's left eye have the illumination unit on the left-hand side, and vice versa for the right eye.

To focus the light onto the slit-lamp, you can look at the patient's eyes by looking from the side of the slit-lamp machine and grossly aligning the eye. Then look through the oculars and fine-tune the focus by using the joystick and movement of the illumination arm. The second method of alignment is to look through the oculars from the start and, by using the joystick, move the slit-lamp and illumination arm until the eye is in focus. For beginners, this may require some practice before confidence is developed. Do not despair if you do not get the hang of this skill at the first few attempts. Use of the slit-lamp gets easier with practice. An important early lesson to learn is to be methodical in your examination. In this way, you are less likely to miss something. You can then start your examination.

Some tips for using the slit-lamp Fixation: ask patients to look at your right ear when you examine their right eye and at your left ear when you examine their left eye. Some machines have a fixation light, which is useful when removing FBs. There is a latch that tilts the slit-lamp, which is useful for posterior examination work or to see the depth of FB penetration.

Ophthalmoscope
Fundal examination can be by direct ophthalmoscopy using an ophthalmoscope (providing a binocular view) or by indirect methods that often provide a stereoscopic view as with a slit-lamp. An ophthalmoscope is a useful piece of equipment because it provides sources of magnification, illumination and light filters (usually cobalt blue and cyan – blue–green). It is also portable.

* Ensure that the ophthalmoscope is working properly: check the light source is working (battery charge and light bulb) and ensure that the light source is the largest circle at the beginning of your examination. Adjust the lens setting to 0.
* Hold the ophthalmoscope in your right hand when examining the right eye and the left hand when examining the left eye. In either hand, adjustments to the lens rotator of the ophthalmoscope are made using the index finger.
* Fundal examination is made easier if the pupil is dilated with short-acting drops such as tropicamide 0.5% or 1%, although some would suggest that this is not essential.
* The patient should be sitting comfortably in a chair that affords you ease of access to both eyes; they should be asked to remove their spectacles or contact lenses.
* The examination room should be dimly lit, and the patient be asked to focus on a set distant target. Patients need to be encouraged to maintain their gaze throughout the examination.

- When examining the patient's left eye use your left eye, and your right eye to examine the right eye. Hold the ophthalmoscope comfortably against the arch of your eyebrow.
- You should look towards the patient's eye through the aperture of the ophthalmoscope, directing the light onto it. Aim to move closer towards the patient's eye in a mid-vertical plane, and at about 30°laterally.
- At between 50 and 30 cm distance from the patient, and as you move closer, you should be able to observe the 'red light reflex'. If there are any lens or corneal opacities, these will appear black against the red reflex. As you draw closer to the patient, you may find placing your hand on the patient's head makes it easier to hold up the upper eyelid.
- As you keep moving closer with the ophthalmoscope, you will find that the retina will come into focus. If you cannot then find the clearest image, use the lenses to assist you. Try to locate the optic nerve head.
- Observe the margins of the disc and note whether they are well defined or notched.
- Look at the colour of the rim, noting its colour.
- Estimate the size of the optic disc and the cup:disc ratio, noting whether or not the cup takes up a large part of the disc.
- Note the presence of optic disc haemorrhages, peripapillary atrophy and bared circumlinear blood vessels.
- Move on to examine the macula. This is the area of the retina with the highest visual resolution, corresponding to central vision. It is found lateral to the optic disc itself. Any abnormalities such as haemorrhages, exudates or cotton wool spots should be noted.
- Identify the retinal arteries and veins.

Record your findings, separately for each eye, accurately in the patient's case notes, usually with a diagram.

Indirect ophthalmoscopy
This piece of equipment is a binocular, stereoscopic, head-set device that allows the examiner to gain a wide-field view of both the vitreous and the retina. Some indirect ophthalmoscopes have a teaching mirror attachment. This allows learners to 'see' the same view as the examiner who can describe what they are viewing.

It is usual to dilate the patient's pupils before the examination. As a result of this it is important to ensure that the anatomical angle of each eye is not narrow or closed. It has been suggested that, if narrow angles are present, the examination is best performed in the morning because emergency back-up is more readily available.

It is usual to have the patient lying recumbent on an examination couch with the examiner at the head of the couch. If the patient cannot lie flat, the head of the couch can be raised slightly.

A light source from the indirect ophthalmoscope, positioned on the examiner's head, is directed into the patient's eye by an adjustable mirror; the reflected light is then gathered by a condensing lens to provide an image of the retina. Note that this image will be inverted. The oculars should be close to the examiner's eyes.

As a general principle the low-powered condensing lenses must be held further from the eye while stronger condensing lenses need to be held closer, because of the focal length of the condensing lens. Aim to focus the light from the condensing lens perfectly within the centre of the patient's pupil. As a consequence the condensing lens will form an image of the retina, in front of the condensing lens, which fills the whole lens.

There are several factors that could affect the field of view including: the size of the patient's pupil; the power of the condensing lens used; the size of the condensing lens; any refractive error; and the distance the condensing lens is held from the patient's eye.

To help ensure that the condensing lens is properly directed it should be noted that most lenses are coded with either a white or a silver ring, indicating that that side should be on the side of the patient's eye. Another tip is that, if the light reflection images from the front and back surfaces are of equal size, the lens is being held correctly.

Both eyes should be examined at the same time to enable comparison of both peripheral fundi, including pigmentation and appearance. It may be necessary to elevate the head of the patient in order to examine the superior fundus, thus allowing for a maximum superior view by the examiner. The nasal region, temporal region and retina directly above and below the posterior poles are examined, followed by the inferior fundus. The posterior pole of the optic nerve and macula are usually examined last.

Beginners should practise on non-dilated eyes. Initially, practise with ophthalmoscopes that have converging systems. As a steady hand is essential, try resting part of the hand on the patient's forehead. This is particularly so with non-dilated pupils.

A better peripheral view will be obtained using a +28-D or +30-D lens and scleral indentation. Note that a higher-power lens will reduce magnification. Conversely, a better view of the optic disc will be gained using lenses of a power in the +15 D range.

Scleral indentation

Indentation is a technique that moves areas of retina into the field illuminated by the indirect ophthalmoscope through pressing (indenting) the sclera. It is not nearly as difficult or as uncomfortable for the patient as might be imagined. It should be noted that indentation will not worsen or cause retinal detachment.

Clinical examination can be as simple or as complex as time or equipment allows. However, even the simplest of tools, in the right hands, can be used to aid diagnosis and to facilitate treatment interventions.

References

Birch J (2003) Colour vision examination. In: Doshi S, Harvey W (eds), Investigative Techniques and Ocular Examination. Edinburgh: Butterworth-Heinemann, pp. 13–26.

Thomson D (2003) Use and development of computer-based charts in the assessment of vision. In: Doshi S, Harvey W (eds), Investigative Techniques and Ocular Examination. Edinburgh: Butterworth-Heinemann, pp. 7–12.

CHAPTER FIVE

Visual impairment

LINDA WHITAKER

Visual impairment can have a profound effect on individuals, both in their own lives and in having to come to terms with the stigma attached to 'disabled' people by society. Visual impairment has been shown to reduce a person's functional status and well-being, with a magnitude comparable to that of a major medical condition, and to have a major impact on quality of life (Chia et al. 2004).

Many visually impaired people may have been so since childhood and have learned to adapt to living in a world where we take sight for granted and cannot envisage being without visual stimulus, on which we place such a high priority.

Those people losing their sight later in life can often find it difficult to cope with, and visual impairment is associated with lower subjective well-being, reduced competence in everyday activities and greater depression in older people. For those visually impaired from childhood, they have grown up in a non-sighted environment and are usually able to cope with their daily lives independently with little or no assistance from sighted individuals. Wahl et al. (1998) found that they were generally better adapted than older adults who had impairment in later years. It may be, however, that, as a person ages, other factors or illnesses may lead to increasing problems with maintaining that independence, similar to those of the ageing population as a whole. Whenever visual impairment occurs, being aware of issues and suitable coping strategies can often aid a person in coming to terms with his or her impairment, and assist in his or her rehabilitation.

Myths and folklore

It is a myth that most people registered as blind cannot see. Most will have some residual vision, and will use that in learning to cope with the environment and its hazards. It is also a myth that visually impaired people have better hearing than sighted individuals, and they are no more musically gifted than the sighted population. Visually impaired people therefore have similar characteristics to the sighted population, and as such they are pleasant, grumpy, musical, non-musical, academic, non-academic, sports enthusiasts, non-sports enthusiasts, home owners and non-home owners whom one would expect to find in the population as a whole. It is also a myth that blindness results from 'being evil' and that blindness can be 'passed on' through touch. These are some of the issues that are raised in relation to folklore in blindness by Wagner-Lampl and Oliver (1994, pp. 275–6), who point out that: 'the general dichotomy of positive and negative beliefs about blindness is exemplified by such ideas as that, on the one hand, blind people have superior hearing, touch, and smell and, on the other hand, are often talked to loudly as though they were hearing impaired'. It is important therefore that we determine factors on an individual basis. We need to ascertain how much residual sight, if any, a blind person has, and whether he or she does have any hearing problems, which may in fact be the result of ageing rather than of association with the visual impairment. People need to be treated as individuals, and not to be expected to behave as we might believe or expect them to.

Stigma and blindness

In society as a whole, people who are blind are often treated as being different from 'normal' members of society. A stigma is usually attached to a person with some sort of a distinguishing mark, especially disgrace, and leads to disapproval and exclusion from society. This is usually a view reflected in society of disabled people generally, which leads to the non-integration of those people into society as a whole, and which can have an effect on their personal self-esteem. As Allen and Birse (1991, p. 147) suggest, 'even positive attributes of the individual may be minimized and overruled by the negative assessments others make as they assess the disabling conditions'. Stigma therefore is a labelling by society, whereby generalizations are made about individuals in a particular group, usually based on minimal experience of either the group or the individuals who make it up. It is linked to the stereotyping and labelling mentioned earlier, which can have a negative effect on the individual coming to terms with a visual loss. Common strategies used by visually impaired people to minimize the impact of visual impairment include folding the cane out of sight in the presence of others, wearing dark glasses to disguise an abnormal appearance of the eyes and maintaining eye contact during conversations with others (Allen 1989). Health-care workers are also members of society and must therefore face up to the values and attitudes that they have in relation to people with a visual impairment. Society holds a responsibility to recognize the process by which it stigmatizes individuals. The focus must change from an emphasis on the blindness to an emphasis on the person who happens to be blind.

Altered body image

Linked to the notion of stigma and visual impairment is the concept of body image. When a person is visually impaired, there can often be an obvious defect of the eyes, which is noticeable to the sighted person. This can pose problems to the visually impaired individual, because they are often aware of their altered body image and can become uncomfortable with it. Sometimes this discomfort stems from other people's reactions and not just those of the person with the altered body image, which is why it is linked to the notion of stigma.

It is well documented that society views attractiveness in a positive light and ugliness tends to be treated with derision. Whitehead (1995) suggested that attractive people are more likely to receive greater consideration. Less attractive people are more likely to experience lower self-esteem and this must surely be associated with the way that they are treated by others. As members of society, it is up to us to attempt to educate people who may 'make fun' of those with altered body image and use of the media, such as newspapers, magazines, television and radio, and ourselves as role models to get the message across, could do this. Many visually impaired people will choose to attempt to conceal their appearance by wearing dark glasses and, if they are comfortable with this option, they should be encouraged. We should, however, be under no illusion that this option is for the benefit of sighted individuals, because the wearing of dark glasses has no therapeutic effect on the visually impaired person other than to prevent others discussing their appearance.

One of the most obvious instances that can lead to problems with altered body image is when a person has an eye surgically removed. This can present great challenges to the individual, because it is not as easy to hide defects involving the face as it can be with other parts of the body. People needing to have an eye removed for whatever reason will need a great deal of psychological support from nurses involved in their care. With today's advances in technology, it is usual to anticipate a good cosmetic effect from artificial eyes and this can be conveyed to the patient. It can be of benefit to have an ocular prosthetist visit the patient preoperatively if there is one available to discuss any concerns that the patient may have. Similarly, patients who have had similar surgery and who have a good cosmetic appearance are often willing to visit patients who are faced with these operations, and this could be encouraged.

Registration

In considering registration for blind and visually impaired people, it is necessary to be aware of the legislation involved in this area. The legal definition of blindness is 'to be so blind as to be unable to perform any work for which eyesight is essential'. There is no statutory definition of partial sight, but it is generally accepted that registration as partially sighted can occur if the person is 'substantially and permanently handicapped by defective vision'.

Registration in the UK has changed recently. The old form, the BD8, grew out of the National Assistance Act of 1948 and was seen as a starting point for access to services and a register of visual impairment and to gather epidemiological data. It is widely recognized that there is massive under-registration of blind and partially sighted people. This is partly because of the unwieldiness of the system, which required a visit to a consultant ophthalmologist before any stage of registration, but also because many people preferred not to register. This could be for a number of reasons, including the fact that registration was seen as an end point – the end of the road for hopes of better sight. People also felt that, because they would be registered 'blind', this was an indication that any or all of their remaining vision would be expected to disappear. Issues of labelling and stigma could also be a problem.

In order that people with visual impairment are able to access the assessments and services to which they are entitled as quickly as possible, a revised system of registration is now in place in the UK. It consists of three documents, any of which can be an 'end point' in registration for the patient:

1. Letter LV1 'Optometrist Identification of a Person with Significant Sight Problems': this is a letter concerning visual impairment needs and is given by optometrists to relevant patients so that they can self-refer for social care. It enables patients to be aware of what types of help there may be so that they or their carers are able to ask for help from Social Services or voluntary agencies. There is no diagnostic information included and these patients will continue to be referred for medical investigation in the usual way.
2. Referral form RV1 'Hospital Eye Service Referral of Vision Impaired Patient for Social Needs Assessment': this is a form issued by staff in the hospital eye services to refer patients (with their consent) for assessment of their social needs. Eye clinic staff should use the form and it can be used where registration is not currently appropriate (e.g. where medical intervention in future may alter the situation but there are problems in the meantime), or where the patient has declined registration but still wants or needs advice about difficulties.

3. Certificate of Vision Impairment CV1: this directly replaces the BD8 and is the document that establishes formal eligibility for registration and any benefits that are directly linked to registration. There is revised terminology on the form. The two categories are now 'sight impaired or partially sighted' and 'severely sight impaired or blind', which recognizes that many people have some residual vision. There is a diagnostic section with tick boxes for the most common causes of sight loss, an expanded section about the patient's needs (emotional, physical and social) and circumstances, which can be filled in by eye clinic staff, and a section where clinical staff can express an opinion about the urgency for social needs assessment.

This new regimen means that patients can choose not to be registered (although the new terminology takes much of the stigma of 'blindness' away, so perhaps more people will feel able to take this step) and still access services.

Clinical staff at all levels within ophthalmic services must be aware of new registration processes and what they mean for patients, and be able to direct patients to local, appropriate services. According to Donnelly (1987), in a survey considering the impact of blind registration on an individual, 56% of the sample were upset by the registration process. She suggested that there is a need for information, advice and emotional support at the time of registration. It is helpful to the individual to have as short a period as possible between registration and support from Social Services. Although provision of services via Social Services can vary from one district to another throughout the UK, there are now standards in place that local authorities must endeavour to achieve in relation to the care of those with visual and other sensory impairment.

Rehabilitation

To survive in the real world, it is important to consider issues such as rehabilitation, work and leisure for the visually impaired person. To be rehabilitated, as a visually impaired person, it is necessary for the individual to come to terms with the impairment. It is not uncommon for people losing their sight to experience anxiety about what the future might hold for them, their family and friends. The personal experience of visual impairment varies but adjustment is progressive, with stages identified as pre-impact, realization of loss and the decision to live with the impairment, concluding with adjustment and readjustment (Allen 1989).

The stages described are not unlike those found in the grieving process generally. Ultimately, the visually impaired person will learn to adjust skills previously learned, or adapt coping strategies in order to carry out daily living activities. This will, however, be an ongoing process, because individuals will continue to be faced with new situations to which they have not previously been exposed. In this way there will always be an ongoing situation for visually impaired people of continually learning to adjust.

It is also necessary to consider the family in relation to individuals with visual impairment, because it is a situation that can affect all family members. The family will need to be involved at all stages in the care and rehabilitation of visually impaired members. Any questions and needs that the family have will need to be identified and discussed, and solutions sought and offered so that the family (and other significant people in the patient's life) do not feel isolated and subsequently become stressed by the situation, hampering the rehabilitation and adjustment of the visually impaired family member to their loss. This must all be done with sensitivity to the needs of the visually impaired person first and, at all times, with their explicit consent.

As the population is generally living to a greater age, the number of visually impaired people can be expected to rise along with the age of the general population. It is therefore of concern that elderly visually impaired people may experience problems associated with the ageing process as well as with their visual problems. This can have a double effect on them. A study by Barron et al. (1994) considered the marital status, social support and loneliness in visually impaired elderly people, and proposed that, at a time of increased need, elderly people may experience a loss of social support, and that low vision may affect mobility and access to communication, with a resulting social isolation. Although it may be true to say that elderly people generally can experience this loss of support at a time when they most need it, visual impairment problems place an additional burden on the individual, who may feel quite isolated if his or her partner who has been sighted and therefore is his or her 'eyes on the world' dies. Loneliness has been estimated as being as high as 40% in elderly people (Creecy et al. 1985), and it has been reported as a significant health problem in visually impaired elderly people (Evans et al. 1982). It is suggested, therefore, that assessment should be made of the support network for visually impaired people and that interventions directed at enhancing the size of this network may be helpful in preventing and alleviating loneliness. It may be feasible to consider the use of support groups in helping people who are visually impaired to adjust to their impairment, and this is an issue identified by Van Zandt et al. (1994).

Mobility

Another issue concerns the elements of mobility for visually impaired people. In considering mobility, it is necessary to remember, as mentioned earlier, that most individuals will have some residual vision, and this should be used in order to promote orientation and mobility. The most significant factor in orientation and mobility performance has been identified as the visual field, with the central 37° radius zone and the right, left and inferior midperipheral zones being the most important (Haymes et al. 1996). Orientation and mobility are, however, complicated areas and can be influenced by the amount of light that is available. The indoor environment can be more easily manipulated to create the best possible conditions for the visually impaired person for orientation and mobility, but it is not possible to manipulate the external environment to any great degree and, therefore, it may be that individuals have good indoor orientation and mobility, but poor outdoor orientation and mobility. In addition, the personality and intelligence of the person can have a bearing on how he or she copes with orientation and mobility, and so physical factors such as amount of visual acuity, visual field and lighting issues may only be part of the puzzle.

Yet, practical issues that should concern us are to do with making the environment less hazardous for those with a visual impairment who are travelling. Obstacles that we take for granted and avoid because we can see them can be dangerous for the visually impaired traveller. Car parking, half on the road and half on the pavement, is a danger to the visually impaired person attempting to negotiate the environment. In addition, pedestrian areas in a lot of city centres are made visually more acceptable by placing rubbish bins in the middle of the pavement, which again can prove hazardous for visually impaired individuals. Road works and drain maintenance with barriers around them also provide an additional hazard, as do overhanging tree branches at the side of roads or in parks.

Indoors, wet floors obviously present a hazard as do the signs that are usually left behind to indicate that the floor is wet. By taking care in considering safe environments and involving visually impaired people in community issues, such as access provision to buildings, designing of pedestrian precincts, informing about road and pavement works with essential service maintenance, a lot of the problems could be addressed. Some start has been made with 'talking lifts' in buildings, providing railings and bevelled surfaces at pedestrian crossings, as well as audible warnings, but there is still a long way to go.

Individuals still, however, need instruction in independent travel before they can endeavour to negotiate the external environment independently. For this reason, mobility officers are usually employed by local authorities to assist with mobility training, especially the use of the long cane, so that individuals can learn to negotiate the environment. The visually impaired person with a white stick is a familiar sight but there is an important distinction between white sticks and a long white cane. A stick may be painted white to show that the person is visually impaired but its function is still support. A white cane is used only as a mobility aid. It is necessary for the visually impaired person mobilizing with the long cane to use it to detect any obstacles in his or her path. To do this the cane is swept in an arc in front of the person's body, with the cane touching the ground in front of the 'trailing foot, rather than the forward foot'. This is identified as the single most important point in the best use of the cane. By doing this, the individual is able to determine any obstacles in the path of where his or her next foot will fall.

An additional problem experienced by visually impaired people in relation to orientation and mobility is that of veering or moving away from their intended path. This can obviously have repercussions for safety if the individual veers into the road and towards the traffic. According to Guth and LaDuke (1994, p. 391) 'orientation and mobility instructors teach a variety of strategies by which to recover from a veer after it has been discovered, but few strategies by which to prevent a veer'. It is reported that the use of spatial relationship strategies can be employed to prevent veering. These can include using physical contact such as with walls and acoustic information such as sounds bouncing off buildings, traffic sounds and pedestrian crossing signals as beacons. In addition, it has also been found that walking at normal speed results in less veering than walking at a slow speed. However, Guth and LaDuke (1994) do point out that individuals who walked faster tended to veer less than those who walked more slowly, not that an individual can reduce his or her veer by walking faster. It is evident that further research is needed in this area, because the amount and direction of veering can be individual to the particular person, so it is not possible to accept a global strategy to prevent it.

Guide dogs can be a useful aid to mobility, but they are not suitable for everybody, because the visually impaired person will need to have good balance. Also, the individual and family must be prepared to accept the dog into the family, and there must be an area for the dog to play and exercise just like any dog, because they cannot be expected to be working at all times. Guide dogs cannot see and interpret the world as a human can; they are trained to respond to instruction, and the visually impaired person is normally expected to attend a training programme, often residential, before he or she can acquire a guide dog.

Sighted guiding

There are times when visually impaired people may need help from sighted people to enable them to move around. This is known as 'sighted guiding'. Visually impaired people should always be asked if they actually want help. Some may neither need nor want it. It is not appropriate to assume, or to 'grab' the person and take charge.

To guide someone, it is necessary to allow the visually impaired person to take the arm of the sighted guide. This will place him or her slightly behind the sighted guide and so he or she will be more confident that he or she will not be guided into any obstacle. It also allows the person to feel the body movement of the guide, and so he or she will be able to turn to the left or right with minimal verbal instruction.

When guiding someone on a level surface, it is usually necessary to verbalize any change in floor surface or obstacles in the path so that no collisions or falls occur. It is important to remember, as a sighted guide, that the minute the visually impaired person is allowed to bump into an object, he or she will loose all faith in you as a guide, and any trust he or she had in you will be difficult to retrieve.

When guiding someone to a chair, it is necessary to verbalize to him or her about the type of chair it is, whether or not it has arms, and how it is positioned. If the chair is against a wall, it will be necessary to guide the person to it from a front facing position, and then allow him or her to feel the chair and, unless there are any mobility or balance problems, allow him or her to sit down independently. If the chair is not against a wall, it may be better to approach the chair from the rear, and again allow the individual to feel the chair before sitting down.

When guiding through a doorway, it is usual to allow the visually impaired individual to be on the hinge side of the door, so that he or she can have control of it and shut it behind him or her, without your having to stop, turn around and shut the door yourself. Before passing through the door, you need to verbalize whether the door opens to or away from you and whether or not it is a spring-loaded door, in order to avoid accidents.

When negotiating stairs, it is necessary to verbalize whether the stairs are ascending or descending. If a rail is present, allow the visually impaired person to hold the rail so that he or she feels more secure. At the beginning of the stairs, it is prudent to pause, and for the sighted guide to explain that they will go onto the stairway first. After stepping onto the first step, again pause, so the visually impaired person can feel for the edge of the step with a foot, before proceeding. Keep one full step ahead of the visually impaired person, and verbally indicate when the end of the stairs is imminent. If there are only a small number of stairs, it may be possible to count them and verbalize this to the individual. If there are a lot, it is of more use if you explain that you will say when you are nearing the end rather than waste time and effort counting.

The main point to remember is that, when acting as a sighted guide, anything you see should be related verbally to the visually impaired person. It is often the case that we will see any obstacles and hazards and avoid them without too much thought, but to a visually impaired person, the hazards and obstacles are not always apparent, and so must be verbalized.

Communication

The presence of a visual impairment does not in its own right prevent that individual from communicating. Although deafness can be apparent in a visually impaired person, not all blind people are deaf, nor have they suddenly lost their mental faculties because of their visual loss. It is therefore wrong to assume that a person with visual impairment is mentally affected or that you need to shout to make yourself heard.

It is true, however, that people with a visual impairment may not be as aware of the aspects of non-verbal communication that we take for granted. They may not be able to see clearly the face of the person to whom they are talking and consequently may not be able to rely on the visual cues presented during normal conversation, e.g. it is normal when talking to increase the amount of eye contact as a clue for that individual that it is his or her turn to speak, and this may not be apparent. Also, we normally tend to watch the face and mouth of the person who is speaking, especially in noisy situations. These facial cues are sometimes not applicable for those with a visual impairment, and this can exacerbate the myth of deafness and mental insufficiency if the individual does not understand what we are saying initially. It is important therefore to be aware of the environment, because undue noise can affect the transmission and reception of information.

We have all probably been in the position of answering a question, or responding to a statement when it was not directed at us, and the subsequent embarrassment that can ensue. By using the individual's name when addressing someone, this potential for embarrassment can be avoided. Similarly, when talking to a visually impaired person, it is important to indicate if you have to leave the vicinity, because again it can be embarrassing if that person finds that he or she is talking to him- or herself.

Visual impairment in children

When a visual impairment is present or occurs in childhood, it is essential to consider the parents' requirements as well as those of the child. Babies can be born with visual problems, which can have a devastating effect on the family. Most parents just wish for their children to be healthy and, if a child is born with a visual impairment, they suffer the same grieving process that accompanies adult sight loss. They will grieve for their normal child and will go through processes including denial, anger and blame. The blame will be directed at themselves for producing an unhealthy baby, at chance and possibly at the medical profession. Support is therefore essential in helping them come to terms with the problem, and with providing information and support in raising their visually impaired child.

Most parents would prefer to receive information about their child's problems as soon as possible (Speedwell et al. 2003). They need to know about the degree of visual disability and the possibilities and probabilities for the future. Clinicians should be extremely sensitive to the needs of the family and the information needs of the parents in order to be able to equip them with the knowledge that can help in planning for the future. This may be by referral to specialist social workers, education teams, or local and national support groups. Although this information may not be appropriate immediately on diagnosis, parents will need to know very soon afterwards where to go for help.

It is generally accepted that children who are blind will lag behind their sighted counterparts in attaining motor skills. They will take longer to reach developmental milestones such as reaching for objects, sitting up independently, crawling and walking. Further milestones attainable throughout the child's development will subsequently be delayed.

Children with a visual impairment cannot always mimic the behaviour of others, which is a normal process of learning while growing up. Most sighted children will mimic adult behaviour in their play by, for example, dressing up, making cups of tea and meals, pretending to serve in a shop, using biscuit tins as drums, dancing. A study by Troster and Brambring (1994) suggested that sighted children engaged in more complex levels of play at an earlier age than did blind children. They found that blind children interacted less frequently with other children than the sighted children did and that blind children preferred games and toys involving touch and sound rather than those involving imagination. It is therefore a necessity to structure a blind child's play and provide playthings that are meaningful in order to develop the child's cognitive, social and emotional skills. Examples of suitable materials would include auditory toys such as musical chimes, building blocks, electronic musical keyboards and non-toxic play materials that can be manipulated. They should also be encouraged to mix and play with other children, to develop their social skills. This may prove to be a trying period for them, as a result of the different play styles of sighted and blind children (Rettig 1994).

Visually impaired or blind children usually have to be shown things by touch, before they can be learnt, which will involve a lot of handling of objects. They will also need to handle materials to give them a perception of the world. They will need to handle, for example, sand, sugar, flour and water to learn what is meant by the different words given to the different objects.

Nielsen (1996) suggests a note of caution in guiding the hands of a visually impaired child on to specific objects or different parts of the environment. She suggests that this can disturb children's opportunities to build up strategies for themselves. She suggests that it is better to allow children to reach and feel the objects so that they can take the time needed to make sense of the object themselves. She concludes that, if visually impaired children have the opportunity to explore objects without interference, a strategy for mapping will be developed, which can later be corrected and developed according to enhanced motor capability, enhanced capacity for memorizing and enhanced cognitive development.

Visual impairment in childhood affects development and education in the way that the child is cared for, and shapes the adult that the child becomes. It is imperative that each child receive the best possible care, information and education, and be enabled and encouraged to achieve his or her aspirations, rather than having those aspirations limited by the disability.

The visually impaired person in hospital

All of the topics dealt with in this chapter are relevant to nurses when caring for visually impaired patients in any health-care setting. It is not only specialist ophthalmic units that deal with patients with a visual problem. As has been explained, the population is generally living to a greater age, and therefore other health-related problems might necessitate hospital admission for those with sight problems. The orientation to the hospital ward is of paramount importance and the use of normal sighted guide techniques should be used. It is often the case that the normal mobility techniques of the individual may not be of use to them during an inpatient stay, because the use of long canes may prove to be hazardous for other patients, and guide dogs may not be welcome in surgical units because of infection control risks. This can result in a loss of independence for the individual and therefore needs to be considered by the nursing staff.

If people have difficulty seeing the food on their plate, this can cause embarrassment to the individuals at mealtimes. A strategy that may alleviate the problem is to use the clock face to describe the location of food on the plate: potatoes at 12 o'clock, meat at 3 o'clock and vegetables at 8 o'clock. By using this strategy, independence in eating can be maintained.

Communication strategies outlined earlier should also be used while the patient is in hospital. The problem of undue noise interfering with the communication process is one that is readily apparent in the hospital setting, because noise levels tend to be rather high at times. Strategies should therefore be implemented to assist the process of communication between health-care staff and visually impaired patients.

Further discussion of the visually impaired person in hospital is available in Chapter 8.

References

Allen MN (1989) The meaning of visual impairment to visually impaired adults. J Adv Nursing 14: 640–6.

Allen M, Birse E (1991) Stigma and blindness. J Ophthal Nursing Technol 10: 147–51.

Barron CR, Foxall MJ, von Dollen K, Jones PA, Shull, KA (1994) Marital status, social support, and loneliness in visually impaired elderly people. J Adv Nursing 19: 272–80.

Chia EM, Wong JJ, Rochtchina E, Smith W, Cumming R, Mitchel P (2004) Impact of bilateral visual impairment on health related quality of life: the Blue Mountains Eye Study. Invest Ophthalmol Vis Sci 41: 171–6.

Creecy RF, Berg WE, Wright R (1985) Loneliness among the elderly: a causal approach. J Gerontol 40: 487–93.

Donnelly D (1987) Focus on disability: registered hopeless? Nursing Times 83(24): 49–51.

Evans RL, Werkhoven W, Fox HR (1982) Treatment of social isolation and loneliness in a sample of visually impaired elderly persons. Psychol Reports 51: 103–8.

Guth D, LaDuke R (1994) The veering tendency of blind pedestrians: an analysis of the problem and literature review. J Vis Impair Blindness 88: 391–400.

Haymes SA, Guest DJ, Heyes AD, Johnston AW (1996) The relationship of vision and psychological variables to the orientation and mobility of visually impaired persons. J Vis Impair Blindness 90: 314–24.

Nielsen L (1996) How the approach of guiding hands of the visually impaired child can disturb his opportunity to build up strategies for tactile orientation. Br J Vis Impair 14: 29–31.

Rettig M (1994) The play of young children with visual impairments: characteristics and interventions. J Vis Impair Blindness 88: 410–20.

Speedwell L, Stanton F, Nischal KK (2003) Informing parents of visually impaired children: who should do it a and when? Child Care Health Dev 29: 219–24.

Troster H, Brambring M (1994) The play behaviour and play materials of blind and sighted infants and preschoolers. J Vis Impair Blindness 88: 421–32.

Van Zandt PL, Van Zandt SL, Wang A (1994) The role of support groups in adjusting to visual impairment in old age. J Vis Impair Blindness 88: 244–52.

Wagner-Lampl A, Oliver GW (1994) Folklore of blindness. J Vis Impair Blindness 88: 267–76.

Wahl HW, Heyl V, Oswald F, Winkler U (1998) Visual impairment in old age. Ophthalmologe 95: 389–99.

Whitehead E (1995) Prejudice in practice. Nursing Times 91(21): 40–1.

CHAPTER SIX

Patient education

HELEN DAVIES

Introduction: the need for patient education

In the new millennium ophthalmic nursing has seen a dramatic shift in the nursing approach to the needs of ophthalmic patients. Surgical techniques and technical developments such as foldable intraocular lenses have allowed ophthalmic nursing to embrace day surgery as the preferred option of care and still attain improved visual outcome and safe practice (NHS Executive 2000).

Day surgery can result in a high throughput of patients if approached in an organized fashion. An increase in patient volume, however, also has the potential to increase possible risk factors to patient outcomes. To compensate for any increased surgical risks clear performance specifications are required. The development of performance specification structures in both professional and organizational advancement can in turn clarify work roles and education programmes, and ultimately meet patient needs. The term more commonly used to describe such performance specifications is an 'integrated patient care pathway'. The essence of such a pathway is to standardize care and record a patient's progress in a manner that can be used to audit the effectiveness of the care. Evans (2002) identifies that the fundamental principle of integrated care pathways is to make explicit the most appropriate care for an identified patient group based on available evidence and consensus of best practice. Agreed standardized care will, through consistent management, result in a reduction in unnecessary variations in treatment and outcome. Within the development of patient pathways should also be incorporated all aspects of care aimed towards patient education.

Throughout the history of ophthalmic nursing the importance of the role of patient education has been recognized. This role has now somewhat overtaken many aspects of traditional ophthalmic nursing care and taken precedence. Today's emphasis by nurses on patient education is largely born out of the consequence of reduced patient–nurse contact time. Two decades ago most ophthalmic units would admit patients for cataract surgery for a 3 to 5 day admission period. The average length of patient stay in most units today may be 3–5 hours! Such a reduction in contact time highlights the need for good quality patient information to ensure that a positive outcome is achieved from a surgical intervention. The document *Action on Cataracts* (NHS Executive 2000) provides a clear guide that is the way forward in service delivery in England and a model for streamlined care with the aim of reducing the number of visits a patient makes to the hospital setting. The streamlining of ophthalmic service contact emphasizes the importance of nurses' effective use of time spent with the patient and other family members when visiting the ophthalmic department. Opportunity for patient education can therefore be limited and needs to be sensitively included into all areas of practice to support and enhance information gathered at each stage of the patient's care pathway.

It is at this stage that the terminology used to distinguish 'patient education' should be discussed in more depth. To achieve any degree of patient education the general aims and purpose of the action should be addressed. In most cases any nursing intervention aimed at patient education relates to maintenance or improvement of their health status. Defining health is not a simple exercise because it involves personally held values, beliefs and experiences. The concept of health is multidimensional and may contradict or alter over time. Health has both an objective and a subjective dimension. The objective dimension of health provides a solid fundamental approach to health care and health education. Although it is important that the objective dimension of health be acknowledged, the nurse must also consider the patient's interpretation of health within its subjective dimension. Health holds a fundamental position in the discipline of nursing, although lay beliefs about health vary and may differ from those of health professionals. It is important then to reflect on the complexity of health in order to develop the nursing interventions that encompass health (Larson 1999); thus, the definition of health can direct the education of nurses and other clinicians and the application of patient education within clinical practice.

Once the difficulties in identifying a standardized definition of health are acknowledged, the complexities of a conjectural approach to patient health education and health promotion are not made any easier for the ophthalmic nurse. Patient education is seen as integral to the ophthalmic nursing role; however, Norton (1998) suggests that it is sometimes difficult to distinguish clearly enthusiastic education, persuasion and manipulation when health professionals attempt to promote the health of their patients. Fathers (1998) has for a long time been an advocate for nurses taking responsibility for promoting health and health education to ophthalmic patients. Nursing practice and development of the nurse's role ensure that nurses are best placed to recognize patients' potential health deficits or needs and are able to provide positive opportunities to inform patients sufficiently for them to make their own personal choices in their health management.

Strategies for patient education

Patient education is a dynamic process that is conducted in a variety of settings both formally and informally, with numerous interactions between patient and nurse appearing to occur in an ad hoc manner – as is sometimes the case! Although this informal approach can complement the nursing and medical approach to patient education, it remains important for ophthalmic nurses to follow a strategic framework to achieve optimum patient interaction and health decision-making. The foundation of nursing practice is made up of a combination of beliefs, values, knowledge, practice and skills. Nursing models utilized by ophthalmic nurses provide an influential basis on which patient health education and health promotion approaches can be structured. As in nursing there is no single model or approach to patient education that can act as a 'one size fits all' solution. In comparison to other established fields, such as psychology, medicine or nursing, the specialism of health promotion and patient education has only recently established itself.

Health promotion has its roots in a variety of specialist fields and eclectically uses elements from medicine, psychology, nursing, sociology, epidemiology and political awareness. Approaches to positive patient education can involve information giving, teaching or preventive measures or be driven legislatively. The health promotion model developed by Tannahill demonstrates this wider application for health promotion by incorporating three overlapping spheres of health education, prevention and health protection (Figure 6.1). Stuckey (1999) promotes the application of Tannahill's model on health promotion in its attempt to enhance health and prevent ill-health through the overlapped parameters of education, prevention and protection (Downie et al. 1992), although Stuckey goes on to point out that even this model has its difficulties despite its application to the wider audience by its involvement in public health, community and political issues.

There are numerous models of health promotion in existence for nurses to apply when planning a strategic approach to patient education; some are descriptive, others prescriptive in style with the trend in patient education now adjusting from a top-down approach to that of the democratic involvement of the individual.

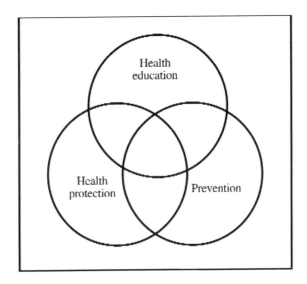

Figure 6.1 A model of health promotion. (From Downie et al. 1992.)

One of the earliest models used in patient education was the traditional-ist medical model of prevention. The approach of the model largely focuses on activity aimed at reducing morbidity and premature mortality rates. The model encourages dependency on medical knowledge, requiring a coercive approach for compliance from the patient as advised/prescribed by the pro-fessional medic – this in turn reinforces the medical hierarchical system, creating a model in which victim blaming can occur. Although many aspects of ophthalmic treatment and care rely on medical intervention and diag-nostic techniques, it is the role of the nurse to ensure that patients receive a holistic approach to their care and provide wider educational opportunities to ensure that patient empowerment and choice can occur despite the dependency of medical colleagues on this medical model approach.

Human behaviour is complex and an individual's health behaviour is determined in many ways. In the field of health promotion and patient education interest has been concentrated on an individual's motivational and attitudinal determinants to health and health behaviours. The health belief model (Rosenstock 1966, Miaman and Becker 1974) was formulated to explain preventive health behaviour and examine the interaction of val-ues, beliefs and the perception of cost versus benefit. The model highlights the role of beliefs stimulating preventive health actions with the provision of a cue to change an individual behaviour. The health belief model hypothesizes that health-related action would depend on the simultaneous occurrence of sufficient motivation, levels of vulnerability and belief of per-ceived benefit. It is very clinically oriented because disease or fear of potential illness is again the motivating factor, relying on perceived threat and susceptibility, and was the approach used in the early 1980s to inform the public about HIV and AIDS.

Over the past decade the concept of voluntarism has since developed within the field of patient education and this approach encompasses the philosophy to facilitate patient choice and encourage individualism more widely. Tones's empowerment model (Tones and Tilford 1996) combines educational and radical aspects in its approach for the nurse to provide information to increase patients' knowledge and raise consciousness of any potential problem areas. Tones's approach to patient education enables a bottom-up strategy to assist patients with skills in decision-making. For effective patient education self-empowerment skills are essential and more ethically justifiable.

Sadly, in Ward's study (1997) of nurses' perceptions of health promotion and professional nursing practice, few identified their development beyond relating their practice using only the preventive medical model. It may be viewed that as nursing works so closely alongside medicine its environment and infrastructure create little opportunity for adapting views from the traditional, medically oriented, preventive approach to those of the alternative holistic models, which encompass radical and empowerment issues. Realistically true freedom of patient choice remains a rare commodity – even in ophthalmic nursing practice. With the application of a sound theoretical basis relating to patient education approaches, nurses can more fully understand and focus on the needs and desires of the individual patient, adopting a flexible approach that is best suited to and selected for each situation.

Written information

Patient education is a valuable part of professional nurses' practice. In their study on nurses' perceptions of patient education, Marcum et al. (2002) reported that over 90% of nurses identified patient education as a priority of the care giving. Written information is a cost-effective intervention that complements verbal advice offered by nurses and other health professionals. With increased access to the internet, the public are provided with an opportunity to seek information about their condition. Some sites are highly professional and informative, whereas others can be misleading. The need for patients and the public to have accurate and clear written information relevant to their condition is therefore obvious and should reflect local services available (Nicklin 2002). Appropriate information that is understood by the patient can encourage participation in the decision-making process. Semple and McGowan (2002) found that many patient information leaflets are produced using a language that is difficult for the public to understand. As part of the nurses' assessment it is important also to recognize the level of individual patient participation and desire for knowledge expressed by the patient about his or her condition. All patients' coping mechanisms vary and information overload can become destructive.

In practice, the patient–nurse contact time is limited and is dependent on the provision of written information as an accurate reference and back-up to any verbal information that has occurred during the ophthalmic consultation. National organizations in the UK, such as the Royal National Institute for the Blind (RNIB) and the International Glaucoma Association (IGA), provide written information on ophthalmic conditions. This material can provide a wealth of generic information written within the confines of best practice (Table 6.1). Such information is, however, produced with a national audience in mind and patients and their relatives also require specific information relevant to their condition to avoid conflicting information. Printed information is of little use if the patient is unable to read it; consideration must therefore be given to the size of font used in booklets, with photocopies avoided because distortion can occur. Any visual impairment can reduce the effectiveness of written information if it is produced in the incorrect format.

Table 6.1 Recommendations for written information

Type size	A minimum of font typeset 14 (4 mm in height), although consider using 16–22 size font for some readers
Contrast	Black text on white background
Typeface	Select Arial/Univers or New Century schoolbook
Type style	Avoid CONTINUOUS CAPITAL LETTERS
	Avoid *italics*
	Choose **bold** or **semi-bold** type to emphasize point
Print material	Use non-glossy paper to print information

Skills technique/training

The provision of information is merely a foundation for good patient education. For some patients additional skills have to be learnt in order to maintain a healthy continuum, such as hand washing, the safe insertion of contact lenses, prosthetics or the ability to instil eyedrop medication. Once a patient has accepted that he or she needs to replicate such a skill independently, it is the role of the nurse to ensure that retention and motivation to learn and assimilate are achieved (Bandura 1977).

Safe eyedrop instillation is a fundamental aspect of many ophthalmic patients' treatment regimens. For this to be successfully adopted by patients, a combination of clear information about why medication is prescribed and the technique for administering it needs to be imparted. Demonstration of a skill is useful; however, the ophthalmic nurse needs to develop lateral thinking in the educational approach. The patient's home environment should be considered, as should physical abilities, lifestyle and time. These should be taken into account with the aim of introducing as few changes as possible into a person's daily routine. When nurses assist their patients in developing a practical skill such as drop instillation, not only does communication become relevant but the empathetic qualities of the nurse are also drawn upon. It is important for the nurse to be able to consider how the patient feels about learning new skills. If a patient or relative is anxious about the process the nurse will need to alter her or his approach in teaching the skill. Confidence building therefore becomes an integral part of health education. To develop a patient's skills requires the nurse to demonstrate the task, to rehearse and then to practise. As this involves patient interaction, it is important that the environment is conducive to allow the patient to see the demonstration, hear the instructions and understand the process. Ideally, the environment chosen can replicate a similar area that the patient may select at home or in the work area. It is important therefore for the nurse to build up a picture with her or his patients as to where they would be when instilling their eyedrops: at home, on the train, in the office, in a mechanic's garage or on a building site – each will require adaptation from the process carried out in a clinical environment. Other considerations include:

- hand-washing facilities
- lighting
- availability of shelving or a mirror
- seating/standing
- whether head and neck support is required
- storage of drops in-between administration
- finger and thumb movement
- grip
- special awareness when instilling drops
- technique
- memory and suitable triggers to remind when medication is due.

In a clinical setting the nurse follows clear guidelines to maintain safe practice and reduce risk. For the patient, it is important that the nurse provide advice and guidance while accepting that patient compliance may occur only if the patient chooses to take this advice. As mentioned earlier, the approach selected towards educating patients may not result in their selecting the nurse's favoured option; this is a difficult adjustment for some nurses to make. In the world of potential litigation relating to practice, clear legible documentation of verbal advice given and/or written documentation (include version or edition number) should be made with a dated signature to identify your practice. By taking an empathetic approach the nurse can target advice more realistically, e.g. timing of drop administration may be adjusted for the construction site worker if the potential for cross-infection may occur as a result of the environment and hand-washing facilities. By making adjustments to recommended treatment regimens the likelihood of the patient completing the course of treatment can be increased (McKie 1994).

In the event of long-term drop instillation in the form of medical treatment, the nurse is limited in the options available to offer patients, e.g. in the control of glaucoma. For this group of patients, compliance plays a significant part in their lifestyle adjustment. Some medically driven studies have concluded that patients who are treated with latanoprost monotherapy drops were more likely to comply with their treatment regimen than patients prescribed combinations of other glaucoma medication. The number of adjustments made to a patient's medication creates a confusing message to patients. It is therefore useful for the nurse to discuss these multi-options and treatment approaches with the patient at the outset. Taking time to get to know the patient's day-to-day lifestyle can help the nurse advise on drop instillation times to coincide with a radio or television programme or a regular activity such as shaving.

Although this section has concentrated on skills training relating to instillation of eye medication, it is important to acknowledge that eyedrops and ointments are governed by the same controls as other medications. It is therefore important that the nurse be able to inform the patient of the proposed effect of the medication. Information on the duration of treatment, frequency and possible side effects should all be imparted to the patient so that he or she can share the responsibility of care (Nursing and Midwifery Council (NMC) 2002).

Opportunities for patient education

The Royal College of Nursing (RCN) recognizes that the ophthalmic nurse has the knowledge and skills to provide educational guidance and opportunities to the ophthalmic patient and the wider population in the aim to maintain ocular health (RCN 2000). Nurses therefore have a professional duty to ensure that patients have sufficient understanding about their treatment to be able to make the decision whether to comply with recommended therapy.

An area in which ophthalmic nursing has led the way for a long time is preoperative nursing assessment. For most ophthalmic departments or even larger specialist units, the fundamentals of ophthalmic nursing relate to surgical intervention. Recent focus on health care in the UK has been directed at patient-centred care and education. Casey and Ormrod (2003) recognize the development and value of nurse-led surgical preassessment clinics for a variety of surgical procedures, although this role for ophthalmic nurses has long been established. For ophthalmic nurses, involvement in the preoperative assessment process through a planned systematic approach is a major part of their role (Fathers 1998).

For much of the population the prospect of undergoing surgery is daunting; raised anxiety levels can cause stress which in turn may result in an increased length of stay in hospital (Beddows 1997). The much publicized effects of inpatient surgery include: communal sleeping arrangements, deprived sleep, poor hospital food, risk of hospital-borne infection – all these makes day-care surgery appear far more attractive (Solly 2004). However, with the decrease in length of stay comes a decrease in actual nurse–patient contact. The challenge then is for good preoperative nursing assessment to occur to ensure that patients and their families are suitably prepared physically, psychologically and socially to cope with their postoperative needs. Patient education and counselling are the focus of preoperative nursing assessment. Preoperative assessment opportunities vary widely in design; the most effective will be structured and built into the routine working day to become an integral part of the nursing process and patient surgical care pathway (Garretson 2004). Structured within the process should be nurse–patient interviews, discussion about choices, provision of written information to support verbal interaction, diagnostic testing and documentation, skills training or viewing of postoperative equipment if required and a departmental tour that may include the relatives' waiting room, patient seating/bedded areas, locker/storage facilities and treatment area.

The benefits of a well-structured preoperative assessment can include a streamlined service for the patient on the day of surgery, an increase in surgical throughput, and hence a reduction in the surgical waiting list and increased patient satisfaction.

In some instances patients do not have the luxury of planned surgery and in the case of some retinal conditions patients are admitted to hospital for emergency treatment. In the case of retinal detachments it is the aim of the surgeon to identify the cause of the detachment and respond by closing or sealing the tears/holes or relieving any vitreoretinal traction. Although the procedures carried out to rectify the condition are relatively routine in some ophthalmic units, the experience is usually unique for the patient. The anticipation of surgery and fear of permanent loss of vision create added stress to the patient's situation. The nurse has to ensure that all relevant information is presented to the patient in an orderly and succinct manner. In an urgent surgical situation patients need to be aware of potential outcomes, risks and benefits in order to make informed decisions with as balanced a view as possible. Psychological support and time made to discuss issues are important factors of the patient education process.

Patient education and involvement increase patient awareness and understanding of postoperative expectations such as positioning and medication regimens (Shelswell 2002), thus increasing the opportunity of compliance. For subspecialties such as vitreoretinal nursing the level of nursing knowledge on the topic can vary and result in conflicting communication. In McLauchlan et al.'s study (2002) patients cited that lack of preoperative information exacerbated some of the problems related to postoperative posturing. The study identified that standardization of information is imperative and, in this instance, acknowledged the appointment of a nurse specialist as a positive move towards addressing patient and staff education deficits.

When surgical intervention is not an option or at least a later consideration, many ophthalmic patients find themselves attending the eye outpatient department. This area in ophthalmic services is synonymous with lengthy clinic waits spent sitting in corridors or cramped waiting areas – few ophthalmic units have managed to overcome this problem for patients. For the glaucoma patient the visit will include a number of interventions such as recording distance vision and a peripheral field test. At some point during the visit such patients may also need pupillary dilatation for an examination of the optic disc; all this adds to the patients' time in the clinic. For Oermann et al. (2001) this provided an opportunity to explore the potential benefits of structured patient education about glaucoma. The exposed group were played video-taped information during the clinic visit and provided with audiotapes and information booklets. Using the time spent waiting to see the practitioner or medical officer in a structured manner, to enhance patient understanding about the eye condition, appeared to be effective and increased the patients' knowledge about glaucoma. There are a number of ways in which patient education can be structured to give patients information during their wait in clinics. Videotape instruction offers one option because it is cost-effective, reaches a wide audience and provides consistent advice. Teaching videos are available that depict practical advice on the administration of eyedrops and ointment, rehabilitation and mobility, such as those from the London School of Hygiene and Tropical Medicine. When selecting patient videos it is important to ensure that they are aimed at the public audience and not health professionals because this can lead to confusion and misunderstanding for some listeners. Video instruction does have limitations, including limited interactive opportunities and difficulty in hearing any advice given. As with all patient education approaches, it is important to provide a diverse approach to enhance care rather than restrict patient choice.

It is not unusual for the ophthalmic patient to be under the care of numerous health-care professionals involved with maintaining a balance of health; this may include gerontology, respiratory, cardiac, rheumatology or endocrinology. Consideration should therefore be given during all patient education interactions to the provision of congruent and non-contradictory information. In this way, each individual patient will be enabled to make the best decision about care and treatment, based on the best available information in a supportive environment provided by all clinicians involved in the care.

References

Bandura B (1977) Social Learning Theory. Englewood Cliffs, NJ: Prentice-Hall.
Beddows J (1997) Alleviating pre-operative anxiety in patients: a study. Nursing Stand 11(37): 35–8.
Casey D, Ormrod G (2003) The effectiveness of nurse-led surgical pre-assessment clinics. Professional Nurse 18: 685–7.
Downie RS, Fyfe C, Tannahill A (1992) Health Promotion Models and Values. Oxford: Oxford University Press.
Evans T (2002) An Introduction to Surgical Care Pathways. Conference lecture notes. London: Royal College of Surgeons.
Fathers CP (1998) Health promoting by nurses in the ophthalmic care setting. Ophthal Nursing 1(4): 13–17.
Garretson S (2004) Benefits of pre-operative information programmes. Nursing Standard 18(47): 33–7.
Larson JS (1999) The conceptualisation of health. Med Care Res Rev 56: 123–36.
McKie L (1994) Risky Behaviours – Healthy Lifestyles. Lancaster: Quay Publishing Ltd.
McLauchlan R et al. (2002) Using research to improve ophthalmic nursing care. Nursing Times 98(2): 39–40.
Maiman LA, Becker MH (1974) The health belief model: origins and correlates in psychological theory. Health Education Monographs 2: 336–53.
Marcum J, Ridenour M, Shaff G, Hammons M, Taylor M (2002) A study of professional nurses' perceptions of patient education. J Continuing Educ Nursing 33: 112–18.
NHS Executive (2000) Action on Cataracts: Good practice guidance. London: Department of Health, p. 7.
Nicklin J (2002) Improving the quality of written information for patients. Nursing Stand 16(49): 39–44.

Norton L (1998) Health promotion and health education: what role should the nurse adopt in practice? J Adv Nursing 28: 1269–75.

Nursing and Midwifery Council (2002) Guidelines for the Administration of Medicines. London: NMC.

Oermann MH et al. (2001) Filling the waiting time in the clinic with education about glaucoma. Insight 26(3): 77–80.

Rosenstock IM (1966) Why people use health services. Millbank Memorial Fund Q 44: 94–127.

Royal College of Nursing (2000) The Nature, Scope and Value of Ophthalmic Nursing. London: RCN.

Semple CJ, McGowan B (2002) Need for appropriate written information for patients, with particular reference to head and neck cancer. J Clin Nursing 11: 585–93.

Shelswell NL (2002) Perioperative patient education for retinal surgery. AORN J 75: 801–7.

Solly J (2004) A nursing leader in surgery. Nursing Stand 100(32): 26–9.

Stuckey B (1999) Health promotion for cataract day-case patients. Professional Nurse 14: 638–41.

Tones K, Tilford S (1996) Health Education: Effectiveness, efficiency and equity, 2nd edn. London: Chapman & Hall.

Ward M (1997) Student nurses' perceptions of health promotion: a study. Nursing Stand 11(4): 37.

CHAPTER SEVEN

Work and the eye

JANET MARSDEN

Work is what many people do for a significant proportion of their day, for many days of the year and for many years. Work is therefore a very important part of people's lives and the need to see to be able to work effectively is implicit in many roles. This chapter describes some aspects of the eye and vision related to the working environment. The first section describes the functions of the visual system related to work, the second considers aspects of health and safety related to the protection of the eye and vision in the working environment. Driving is also covered here as an integral part of working life. As regulations tend to be specific to the countries in which they apply, aspects of this chapter are likely to be UK or Eurocentric. The reader should apply local conditions, laws and regulations to the principles considered here.

Visual performance

The person must be able to see adequately in relation to the demands of a particular task. Each task will require different standards. Functions of the visual system can be divided into four main groups:

(1) detection
(2) recognition
(3) colour discrimination
(4) depth perception.

Detection

Detection includes many factors such as the visual field. The normal stationary eye can detect visual stimulus within an defined area – a total horizontal field of around 190°. This consists of a 145° monocular field and a 120° binocular overlap. The eye can see an area of about 60° superiorly, 70° inferiorly, 95° laterally and 60° medially (quoted figures vary). The retina is most sensitive at the macula and least at the periphery, and the blind spot is situated in the temporal visual fields, 15° temporal to fixation and just below the horizontal meridian. Some occupations require a full field of vision whereas others, perhaps involving close work, make little use of the peripheral field. Age influences the visual field; senile enophthalmia results in contraction of the lateral field. The visual field may also be reduced mechanically, by spectacles or lens types, or by types of protective eye wear. Monocular vision results in a loss of visual field and many people need a considerable adaptation period before resuming previous tasks. Detection ability is enhanced by head and eye movements. Different types of eye movement include saccadic (fast eye movements that locate an object on the macula) and smooth pursuit movements (that maintain fixation on the object). The vestibular system enables stabilization of the eyes with respect to the environment when the head moves and the vergence system allows accurate fixation at any distance in the visual field, acting as a range-finding system (North 1993). There are different amounts of accommodation and convergence needed for viewing objects at different distances and tasks that require a frequent change of direction of gaze can be fatiguing and cause discomfort. Conversely, tasks such as visual display unit (VDU) operation, which require a fixed direction of gaze and fixed accommodation for long periods, can also cause some problems.

Other aspects of detection include the light levels at which the person perceives light (light perception) and the adaptability to different levels of light (visual adaptation including dark adaptation – see Chapter 1). Contrast sensitivity allows the person to detect border contrast – the object against its background and flicker frequency to resolve a rapidly flickering object into a fused one.

Recognition

The main component of recognition is the static visual acuity, which is discussed more fully later in the book. Static visual acuity is influenced by luminance – visual acuity is increased in brighter situations until a threshold is reached, at which point glare may actually reduce acuity. Contrast also has an effect on the ability of the eye to discriminate between two objects, and has its maximum effects at low levels of illumination and its least at high levels. Visual acuity is also influenced by the time available to recognize the object to be seen. The longer an object is visible for, the more likely the person is to be able to recognize it. Rapidly moving or changing objects may, therefore, be seen less easily than static ones and this dynamic visual acuity is not directly related to static visual acuity

(North 1993). Pathology may reduce visual acuity and therefore the recognition component of visual performance.

Colour discrimination

The physiology of colour vision is discussed more fully in Chapter 1. The identification of colour is subjective but can be analysed in terms of hue, saturation and luminous intensity (North 1993). The human visual system can detect and discriminate between millions of colours and this discrimination depends on the following:

- The state of adaptation of the retina: in photopic or light conditions the retina is best able to detect colour.
- The region of retina stimulated: colour vision extends only 20–30° from the fovea where the cones are situated. Other areas of retina are not able to distinguish colour.
- Contrast: the ability to detect a colour depends to a great extent on the colour of the background. The greater the contrast between the colour and its background, the greater the ability to distinguish it. The colour perceived may change depending on the background (simultaneous contrast) – the colour of the object tends to appear as a colour nearer to the complementary colour of the background (a grey spot viewed against a red background may appear slightly green) (North 1993). After-images may also appear after exposure to colour, the after-image taking the appearance of a complementary colour to the initial image (successive contrast).

Depth perception

Both monocular and binocular cues are used by the visual system in order to judge depth. Binocular clues are the most sensitive and therefore it may take some time for a person to adapt to perceiving depth correctly after the loss of vision of one eye. Monocular depth perception relies on perspective, parallax (the movement of an object in relation to another object), and the appearance of light, shade and size. As the two eyes see slightly different images that are resolved by the brain, binocular clues are based on this stereopsis and also on convergence. Depth perception can be affected by a large variety of factors including uncorrected refractive errors and squint. In low light levels, depth perception is also reduced.

As well as the capability to see an object, its visibility has an effect on the ability of the person to see it. Many factors influence visibility, including size, colour, contrast, the illumination of the object or the area, the distance of the object from the eye, the movement and speed of the object and the conditions in which it is seen. This applies to any object, but also to any task that must be undertaken. The visual ability of a person to perform a task (visual performance) therefore relies on both the visual capability of the person and the visibility of the task.

The visibility of a task is often fixed, dependent on the task, so the factor that impacts most on a person's ability to undertake a task or occupation is their visual capability. Some tasks and, therefore, occupations need a very high level of visual performance and some less.

Occupational visual standards

This list of visual standards for different occupations is not comprehensive but represents British requirements for some occupations at the present time. They are adapted from those published by the Association of Optometrists (2004).

The Royal Navy (Table 7.1)

Table 7.1 Visual standards for the Royal Navy

| | **Requirements** | | |
	Right eye uncorrected– corrected	*Left eye uncorrected– corrected*	*Refraction limit*
Royal Navy standard I	6/12–6/6 N5	6/12–6/6 N5	+3 sphere +1.25 cylinder –0.75 sphere or cylinder
Standard II (entry standard)	6/24–6/6 N5	6/36–6/9 N5	+3 sphere –2.5 sphere or cylinder
Standard II (serving personnel)	6/60–6/6 N5	< 6/60–6/9 N5	± 6 sphere or cylinder
Standard III	6/60–6/6 N5 6/60–6/9 N5 6/60–6/12 N5	< 6/60–6/24 N10 < 6/60–6/18 N10 < 6/60–6/12 N10	± 6 sphere or cylinder

Different levels of visual requirement apply for different areas of speciality, e.g. bridge watchkeepers are required to have standard II and many other officers need standard III whereas flying officers need standard I. Snipers need standard I without corrective lenses and divers standard III.

The Navy also has different levels of colour perception requirements graded 1 (the correct recognition of coloured lights on a Holme–Wright lantern at low brightness) to 4 (correct recognition of colours used in relevant trade situation). Some pathologies are a bar to acceptance for entry to the Navy, including penetrating injury, retinal detachment, post-keratotomy and photorefractive keratectomy.

The Army

Officer candidates for some regiments must have 6/9 corrected in their worst eye whereas others require 6/6 in one eye and not less than 6/36 in the other. Normally the right eye must be correctable to 6/6, except in some areas such as signals or the army medical service where the right eye may be the worse. Soldiers are accepted with minimum corrected acuity of between 6/6 R and 6/36 L depending on the regiment or corps. Some trades must be correctable to 6/6 in each eye. High levels of myopia or hypermetropia preclude acceptance. Lack of colour perception is not necessarily a bar in some areas. Testing is undertaken with spectacles rather than contact lenses and candidates who have had photorefractive keratectomy (PRK), laser in situ keratomileusis (LASIK) and intrastromal corneal rings are accepted in some areas. Ocular pathology normally precludes acceptance to the Army.

The RAF

A history of refractive surgery is a bar to entry for all aircrew and specialist branches but is allowed in some areas. Standards for entry are very variable, depending on the trade of the individual, but both ground crew and officers must be correctable to 6/9 in both eyes on entry. Some areas require correction to 6/6 in both eyes and fire-fighters must have 6/6 uncorrected vision bilaterally. Colour standards are similar to the other branches of the Services.

Flying

Flying in the UK is controlled by the Civil Aviation Authority and their standards generally apply. Class 1 medical assessments apply to commercial pilots and transport pilots and class 2 to private pilots. The class 1 test is 'that there shall be no abnormality of the function of the eyes or their adnexae, or any active pathological condition, congenital or acquired, acute or chronic, or any sequelae of eye surgery or trauma which is likely to interfere with the safe exercise of the privileges of the applicable licence' (Association of Optometrists 2004). Distance visual acuity must be 6/9 or better monocularly and 6/6 or better binocularly and vision tests take place regularly, every 2 years after age 40. The refractive error at initial examination must not be more than ± 3 but may be slightly more if it is proved to be stable. Diplopia or significant binocular vision defect is a bar to this type of licence and normal colour perception is required. For a class 2 licence, vision must be 6/12 or better monocularly and 6/6 or better binocularly. The refractive error must not be more than ± 5 D with no more than ± 3 D of astigmatism and no more than 3 D of anisometropia. Amblyopia is allowed but the amblyopic eye must be 6/18 or better and normal colour perception applies. Both these regulations may be varied slightly if the pilot is examined for re-certification. Other flight officers may have slightly lower levels of corrected acuity (6/9) and normal binocular vision; radial keratotomy (RK) or photorefractive keratoplasty (PRK) will lead to the person being grounded for a year before he or she can fly again. All applicants who wear contact lenses must carry a spare pair of spectacles. Glider pilots flying solo must meet driving standards and class 2 flying standards if carrying passengers.

Seafarers and coastguards

Most seafarers have visual acuity and colour vision testing as part of their medical examinations. Standards vary but 6/6 and 6/12 apply for some duties, 6/18 and 6/18 for others with a reading acuity of N8. The final standard is 'sufficient to undertake duties efficiently' (Association of Optometrists 2004). Binocular vision is normally necessary and full colour vision is required. The test is valid for 2 years. The standard for coastguards is, again, sufficient for them to do their duties. Lifeboat crew members must have 6/12-6/12 uncorrected and 6/6-6/9 corrected (under 22) and 6/12-6/24 correcting to 6/6-6/9. Spectacles are provided by the Royal National Lifeboat Institution but may not be worn on the lifeboat. Contact lenses are not permitted in lifeboats at sea.

The offshore oil and gas industry specifies corrected vision of 6/12 in the better eye and monocular vision as acceptable as long as job performance is satisfactory. Colour perception must be adequate for the type of employment undertaken.

Police force

Different standards may apply in different branches of the service, e.g. for the mounted branch or driving, or in different areas of the UK. Generally, however, the standard is as shown in Table 7.2.

Table 7.2 Visual standards for the police force

System	Reject	Consider carefully	Comments
Vision	Squint History of detached retina History of glaucoma Radial keratotomy Photorefractive keratoplasty	Latent squint Lens implant Corneal graft with good acuity	
Visual acuity unaided	< 6/24 either eye	6/18–6/24	Some force standards are more strict in special circumstances, e.g. firearms
VA aided	Worse than 6/12 in either eye with binocular worse than 6/6		
Colour vision	Failure on City University test	Failure in Ishihara test	

Prison officers

Prison officers have a requirement for 6/24 or better in each eye correcting to 6/12, or 6/6 in one eye and 6/36 in the other, correcting to 6/12.

Fire officers

Fire officers need uncorrected acuity of 6/6 in both eyes with N12. Refractive surgery is not necessarily a bar to employment.

Railways

Drivers must have a minimum of 6/9 corrected in one eye and 6/12 in the other. Unaided vision must be more than 3/60 and near vision N8. Bifocal lenses, but not Varifocal, are allowed as are contact lenses although spectacles must be carried. Guards, and other railway workers, have the same requirements except for the near vision requirement. The London Underground has slightly different regulations: corrected vision is similar to that for other drivers but uncorrected vision must not be less than 6/60 and they should read N6. Fields are specified here and must be full and colour vision normal. Contact lenses are not permitted.

Electrical engineering

Electrical engineering as a speciality contains a lot of colour coding of components and wires. Lack of colour vision could therefore have serious consequences; no other vision tests for the industry are specified, although trainee engineers undertaking apprenticeships must have colour vision testing.

Teaching

There are no standards for vision in teaching. Although it is clear that teachers with visual impairment are not barred from teaching, qualified teacher status (QTS) requires individuals with sensory impairment to teach mainstream classes. An individual assessment of teachers with impairment would be necessary, bearing in mind that reasonable adjustments to the environment, including the provision of support staff, can be made to facilitate the teacher's practice.

Protecting the eye(s) at work

The Health and Safety at Work Act was implemented in 1974 and replaced a number of acts including the Factories Act (1961), which had become rather dated, confused and confusing. The Protection of Eyes Regulations were drawn up in 1974 to complement the new Act. They were replaced in 1992 by the Personal Protective Equipment at Work Regulations, which drew together all aspects of protective equipment in the workplace. These have been amended by the Personal Protective Equipment Regulations (2002) but remain substantially as they were written in 1992. The Management of Health and Safety at Work Regulations (1992) (MHSWR) require all employers to identity and assess the risks to health and safety in the workplace, so that the most appropriate means may be taken to reduce those risks to acceptable levels. This suggests that there is a hierarchy of control measures and personal protective equipment (PPE) should always be regarded as a last resort when all other systems, engineering controls and safe systems of work have failed to protect against a risk. This is because PPE protects only the person wearing it where other methods of risk control may protect everyone in the workplace. PPE is effective only if suitable, correctly fitted, maintained and, above all, worn. Maximum protection levels are seldom achieved. PPE may also restrict the wearer by limiting visibility and therefore introduce new risks. In many cases, however, PPE is still required and employers must provide employees with adequate equipment and train them in its use wherever there is a risk to health and safety that cannot be controlled by other means. Employees must have access to the equipment and, although most must be provided on a personal basis, some might be shared if it is used for only limited periods. No charge can be made to the worker for the provision of PPE that is used only at work. PPE should offer the best protection in the circumstances and it must not be worn if the danger of using it is greater than the risk against which it is worn to protect. PPE should comply with UK and European legislation.

In the context of eye protection, the employer should first identify the types of hazard present, such as dust, projectiles or chemical splashes, and then assess the degree of risk (in terms of size and velocity of projectile). They can select the suitable PPE from a range of approved equipment which should be comfortable for the person for whom it is chosen. PPE should always be in good order and well maintained, and should be replaced as soon as it becomes unfit for its purpose.

Eye protection serves to guard against the hazards of impact, splashes (from chemicals or molten substances, liquid droplets, mists and sprays), dust, gas, welding arc, radiation (non-ionizing) and laser light.

Safety spectacles are similar in appearance to prescription spectacles but may have lateral shields incorporated to prevent impact from the side. To prevent against impact, lenses are made from tough, optical quality plastics such as polymethylmethacrylate (PMMA) and polycarbonate, which has the highest impact resistance of all lens materials and is very light. Plastics tend to be quite soft so they are easily scratched. They age well and do not warp or discolour. They are easily made with an integral prescription.

Eye shields are like safety spectacles but heavier, in one piece and frameless. Vision correction is not usually possible although many types of eye shield can be used over prescription lenses.

Safety goggles are heavier and less convenient to use than either safety spectacles or eye shields. They give the eyes total protection from all angles because the whole periphery of the goggle is in contact with the face. They may have toughened glass or plastic one-piece lenses. As a result of the seal around the face, goggles are more prone to misting than spectacles and some may have built-in vents, which must be specially designed if they are to protect against liquids, dust, gas or vapour. Double-glazed goggles with anti-mist coatings are also used.

Face shields are heavier and bulkier than other types of protector but can be comfortable if fitted with an adjustable head harness. They protect the face but do not fully protect the eyes and will not therefore protect against dust and gases. Thy can be worn over prescription spectacles and do not generally mist.

Helmets may be worn when welding and protect the head and face from radiation and spatter. The light filter for welding may be adjustable so that the wearer can move it in order to see for grinding or chipping purposes.

Accident and incident reporting

The Reporting of Injuries, Diseases and Dangerous Occurrences Regulations 1995 (RIDDOR) dictate that certain classes of accident at work must be reported to the Health and Safety Executive. RIDDOR (1997) applies in Northern Ireland. All employers have a legal duty to report the following work-related health and safety incidents:

* Deaths
* Major injuries
* Three-day injuries, where an employee or self-employed person has an accident resulting in him or her being off work – or unable to do the work – for more than 3 days
* Injuries to members of the public that result in the need to go to hospital
* Work-related diseases
* Dangerous occurrences which could potentially have resulted in a reportable injury.

All other accidents should be recorded by an employer and the employee should make sure that they are recorded in case there are any long-term sequelae. If the employee is injured as a result of dangerous or faulty equipment or premises, unsafe working practices or lack of supervision, training or instruction on lifting, or as a result of inadequate safety equipment or protective clothing, they may be able to claim compensation. In actions for damages for personal injury, the limitation period is 3 years, starting either from the date on which the injury occurred or from the date the person first had knowledge of the injury; the courts have a wide power to extend the normal time limits.

Ophthalmic clinicians see the results of many accidents at work, most of them relatively minor. It is important, however, that correct information be given to the ophthalmic patients about their rights to adequate protection against work-related injury, and clinicians should take every opportunity to reinforce information about safety eyewear and the possible consequences to the eye, vision and person of accidents at work.

Life out of work also presents many hazards for the eye. Do-it-yourself (DIY) and sport in particular present emergency departments with large numbers of eye injuries each year, with potential long-term visual problems for some of these patients. Ophthalmic clinicians are often unable to give advice about eye protection before the injury takes place, but must take every opportunity to aid the person to make decisions about eye protection to prevent injury in the future. One of the most important ways in which clinicians can help is perhaps by setting an example by wearing appropriate eye protection in situations where it is necessary.

Display screen regulations

The Health and Safety (Display Screen Equipment) Regulations (1992) are for the protection of people, both employees and the self-employed, who habitually use display screen equipment as a significant part of their normal work. The regulations apply to protect them, whether they are at an employer's workstation or a workstation at home. A display screen user is one who uses equipment where the job depends on the use of the equipment, they use it for continuous spells of an hour or more and there is no alternative to its use. Workstation analysis must take place and the employee must be provided with enough equipment to enable him or her to use the equipment for long periods without risk of harm (footrests, appropriate chairs, wrist supports, etc.). The aspects of the regulations relating to vision include the employer ensuring that the employee is provided with an eye test at his or her request and then that he or she would have further tests of an appropriate nature at regular intervals. Display screen users are not obliged to have eye tests but, when they wish to, the examination should be by an optometrist or a doctor with suitable qualifications. If the employee is found to need correction for display screen use, it must be provided by the employer.

People who use display screens often complain of fatigue that is generally unrelated to the need for correction. A fixed focus for long periods can lead to fatigue and it should be suggested that users take advantage of breaks and changes of work, and regularly change the focus of the eyes, looking beyond the screen in front of them, to avoid fatigue. Concentration on a single object tends to reduce blinking. This can lead to dry eyes and, again, feelings of eye fatigue. This can be alleviated by ocular lubricants in severe cases or in patients with existing dry eye. Often just the knowledge that reduced blinking can lead to these symptoms can help the user remember to change focus and blink.

Vision and driving

The single most important sense for driving is vision. It is estimated that the driver receives up to 90% of the information needed to carry out this task safely through the visual system. It is clear, then, that people without vision should not drive. There is a continuum, however, between poor or no vision and perfect vision, and there need to be standards so that, at some point along this continuum, a person is deemed fit to drive with respect to vision. In the UK, the single test of visual ability to drive is undertaken at the time of the driving test. The law states that the driver must be able to read (with correction if required) a registration plate, attached to a vehicle, with letters 79 mm high and 57 mm wide at a distance of 20.5 m (if the vehicle was registered before September 2001) or letters 50 mm wide at 20 m (if registered during or after September 2001) – equating to around 6/10 acuity. This is the only eye test that drivers in the UK are likely to take to assess vision for driving, unless they come to the attention of the Driver Vehicle Licensing Authority (DVLA) for some reason. Although the standard for the UK appears clear, Currie et al. (2000) found that 26% of patients with 6/9 vision failed the number plate test, and 34% with 6/12 vision passed it. They also found that optometric, ophthalmological and GP advice on whether or not the person could drive was inconsistent.

Other countries use more rigorous tests including visual field, stereopsis, glare recovery and dark adaptation, and measure vision periodically throughout the person's driving 'career'. One of the problems with visual acuity and driving is that there are no agreed international standards and the research on what constitutes adequate vision for driving is incomplete. In an extensive literature review, Charman (1997) found that, although visual performance by most tests declines at middle age and beyond, older drivers have fewer accidents than their younger counterparts, whose visual performance is better.

The review concluded that, although correlations between poor vision as assessed by some tests and accident rates can be shown in large samples of drivers, there are many factors other than simple acuity involved in driving performance; no single test or combination has been able effectively to screen out those more at risk of accidents without disqualifying a substantial number of potentially safe drivers. In a later study, Owsley and McGuin (1999) found that visual acuity was only weakly related to a driver being involved in crashes and felt that peripheral vision plays a more critical role. They also felt that colour vision problems are not in themselves a threat to safe driving and this stance is taken by the DVLA in the UK.

Although older people perform less well in visual performance testing, West et al. (2003) found that many elderly drivers appear to recognize their limitations and restrict their driving, even though they may not attribute this to visual impairment.

Although the acuity test for driving in the UK is simple, drivers are obliged to report any change in their circumstances, such as eye disease or injury, to the DVLA so that a decision can be made about fitness to drive. The regulations are divided into two groups, corresponding to licence type.

A group 1 licence includes cars, motor cycles and light goods vehicles, whereas a group 2 licence includes large (previously heavy) goods vehicles, passenger-carrying vehicles, medium goods vehicles and minibuses (Table 7.3).

Table 7.3 Visual standards for driving

	Group 1 entitlement	Group 2 entitlement
Visual acuity	Able to meet the number plate test	New applicants are barred if the acuity using corrective lenses is worse than 6/9 in the better eye or 6/12 in the other eye. Uncorrected acuity must be at least 3/60
Monocular vision	Complete loss of vision in one eye. The person must inform the DVLA but will be able to drive when advised that he or she has adapted to the disability and acuity in the remaining eye fulfils the requirement, and there is a normal monocular field in the remaining eye	Complete loss of an eye or vision of less than 3/60 uncorrected in one eye. Applicants are barred from holding a group 2 licence
Visual field defects, glaucoma, retinopathy, retinitis pigmentosa, hemianopia, etc.	Driving must cease unless the person is confirmed to have a field of at least 120° on the horizon, measured using a target equivalent to the white Goldman 1114e setting. There should be no significant defect in the binocular field which encroaches within 20° of fixation above or below the horizontal meridian	A normal binocular field of vision is required
Diplopia	Cease driving on diagnosis – resumption on confirmation to the DVLA that diplopia is controlled by spectacles or a patch that the driver undertakes to wear while driving. In exceptional cases, a stable diplopia may be compatible with driving, with consultant support	Permanent refusal or revocation of licence. Patching is not acceptable
Night blindness	Cases considered on an individual basis	Cases considered on an individual basis
Colour blindness	Need not notify the DVLA	Need not notify the DVLA
Blepharospasm	Consultant opinion is required. Control with botulinum toxin may be acceptable	Consultant opinion is required. Control with botulinum toxin may be acceptable

It is clear from the field requirements that many patients should be screened for field defects, particularly those with neurological problems such as stroke who may not normally be screened, because homonymous or bitemporal field defects that come close to fixation are a bar to driving. Certain static defects that have been present for a long time may be considered as exceptional cases. For some holders of group 2 licences, grandfather rights apply. If they have had a type 2 licence before the more stringent regulations came into force (particularly those about complete loss of vision in one eye), licences were not revoked.

People who should not be driving

In practice, it is likely that clinicians will encounter people who should not be driving. Certain groups are more easy to deal with than others, including those with temporary visual impairment.

Padding

If a patient has an eye padded for any reason, he or she should not drive. Such individuals have effectively been rendered monocular and the regulations state that they should not drive if monocular until they have adapted to the disability. Driving while padded is likely to render them open to prosecution because their licence to drive is compromised by this change in circumstances and, if they are involved in an accident, it may invalidate any insurance because the company are likely to state that the person's visual status has changed and they were not informed.

Dilatation

The only standard for driving in the UK is the number plate test (and field of vision). A dilated pupil does not affect the patient's distance visual acuity and therefore he or she is likely to be able to fulfil the requirements for driving. A recent study (Potamitis et al. 2000) suggested that pupillary dilatation may lead to a decrease in vision and daylight driving performance in young people, but it considered only a sample of 12 people. At present, therefore, there is no regulation that stops people with dilated pupils from driving, although they should be warned about glare and lack of accommodation and that, if they do not feel able to drive, they should not do so.

Reduced acuity resulting from lack of correction

Patients should be informed that, without correction, they do not have visual acuity of a legal standard for driving. Unfortunately, unless they have an accident and someone actually checks their acuity at the scene, this is not likely to be picked up by any authority. However, the legal aspects of driving should be highlighted along with the consequences for insurance and the safety of other road users.

Visual acuity and field loss

It is the responsibility of patients to inform the DVLA of any changes in their visual function. If they do not, clinicians have a problem about what to do. Patient confidentiality undoubtedly applies in this case and the clinician should not, without a great deal of consideration, inform the DVLA unilaterally.

It is debatable whether the breach in confidentiality is justified on the grounds of the possibility of harm to others. It is difficult to know what to do in these cases, but multidisciplinary discussion should take place, and be recorded, including any decisions made. Patients should be told of any decision made to enable them to decide to inform the DVLA themselves.

References

Association of Optometrists (2004) Visual Standards: www.assoc-optometrists.org/services/visual (last accessed 29/3/05).

Charman WN (1997) Vision and driving – a literature review and commentary. Opthal Physiol Opt 17: 371–91.

Currie Z, Bhan A, Pepper I (2000) Reliability of Snellen charts for testing visual acuity for driving: prospective study and postal questionnaire. BMJ 321: 990–2.

North RV (1993) Work and the Eye. Oxford: Oxford University Press.

Owsley C, McGuin G (1999) Vision impairment and driving survey. Ophthalmology 43: 535–50.

Potamitis T, Slade SV, Fitt AW et al. (2000) The effect of pupil dilation with tropicamide on vision and driving simulator performance. Eye 14: 302–6.

West CG, Gildengorin G, Haegerstrom-Portnoy G, Lott LA, Schneck ME, Brabyn JA (2003) Vision and driving self-restriction in older adults. J Am Geriatr Soc 51: 1348–55.

CHAPTER EIGHT

Care of the adult ophthalmic patient in an inpatient setting

MARY E SHAW

The aims of the chapter are to help the reader to understand the general needs of ophthalmic patients admitted for medical and surgical interventions and to address their specific needs relative to their condition and treatment. The health education needs of the patient, the family/significant others and the carers are also considered.

General introduction

Despite the growing trend to treat most patients in outpatient or day-case settings, many people will still need to be admitted for their treatment. This may be because of the complexity of the treatment or surgical intervention, e.g. a patient admitted for intensive treatment of a corneal ulcer or someone with type 1 diabetes attending for vitreoretinal surgery. On the other hand, patients may have been selected purely, and perhaps unnecessarily, on the grounds that they have a 'social' problem – perhaps living alone or with mobility problems. Throughout this chapter, the reasonableness or otherwise of such decisions is explored.

It is recognized that activities and approaches to patient management will be strongly influenced by the nature and location of the ophthalmic unit. Smaller units may have no inpatient facilities at all, referring those who require a hospital stay to other centres. Other hospitals may have beds for ophthalmic patients attached to other specialities, meaning that the nurse caring for the ophthalmic patient may not have any ophthalmic training but only experience gained 'on the job'. In addition, some smaller units are likely to refer complex cases to specialist tertiary referral hospitals. Government policy, including matters relating to patient choice, affects how treatment centres are organized (NHSE 2000, Royal College of Ophthalmologists 2002).

Regardless of where they are nursed, ophthalmic patients should be cared for by nursing staff with appropriate competence and experience, which ideally should include an ophthalmic qualification. Many inpatients are those people requiring surgical interventions. These can range from cataract extraction to more complex oculoplastic surgery as well as surgery for ocular trauma. Other people are admitted for medical management of ocular disease such as acute glaucoma, corneal ulcer and orbital cellulitis.

Any nurse working in an inpatient ophthalmic unit is required to have a broad range of highly specialist knowledge and skills relating not just to ophthalmology but also to medicine, social work, care of elderly people and those with learning disabilities, and counselling. On a daily basis, they will be challenged with what is likely to be an unpredictable workload. Although most patients may be admitted for routine surgery and procedures, they frequently bring with them complex medical and social histories which will impact on their nursing and medical management. Frequently, out of normal hours, the ophthalmic ward-based nurse will be triaging ophthalmic emergencies or fielding calls from patients or relatives worried about postoperative problems or difficulties. The age range of people admitted to the ward for treatment can be from age 16 to over 100 years. This range of clients clearly calls on all of the ophthalmic nurse's skills and judgement. Inpatient children and infants must be cared for in paediatric centres and by specialist paediatric nurses.

Selection for inpatient stay

In many ophthalmic units, the decision to admit to a hospital bed is determined by agreed protocols. These relate to decisions to admit as a medical emergency or for routine surgery. It is not unusual for a decision to admit to be taken as a last resort, all other options having been considered. The following are examples of criteria for ward admission:

- Patient is not happy to have day surgery
- Adverse health problems, e.g. heart disease, unstable diabetes mellitus
- Surgical intervention requires careful monitoring postoperatively
- Poor fitness and poor health
- No adult support at home if general anaesthetic
- No access to a telephone for use in an emergency
- Patient has no transport.

The ward environment

Many wards are designed to accommodate both men and women. It is imperative that all patients are afforded the opportunity to maintain their privacy and dignity at all times. Separate toilet and bathroom facilities must be available for each of the sexes and signed appropriately so that people with visual problems can access them. Ideally, rooms should have en-suite facilities; this can help prevent the spread of infection and makes the isolation of infected cases easier to manage.

It should be emphasized that the need to care for the patient in a single room should not result in any patient feeling isolated or neglected, albeit unintentionally, by nursing, medical or other staff.

Inevitably many patients attending the ward for medical and surgical interventions will have some degree of problem with their visual acuity and/or field of vision. Ophthalmic outpatient facilities have been criticized for failing to meet the needs of those with visual impairment in terms of both the service they offer and the environment in which care takes place (McBride 2000, 2001). Ward settings are equally open to criticism if the facilities and staff fail to meet the needs of the ophthalmic patient. Staff should be encouraged to review the care setting and ensure that it meets the special needs of people with visual problems. It should be borne in mind that the patient may be admitted to the ward with good vision but that treatment and interventions may temporarily affect vision, e.g. the patient who had lid surgery may return to the ward with a pad and pressure bandage. Such patients will have had no time to adapt to their new situation. Another example is the patient undergoing vitrectomy and repair of detachment who has silicone oil inserted intraoperatively. How well will he or she be able to navigate around the ward with the resulting distorted vision unless support is provided?

Consider practice routines for which a reasonable amount of vision may be needed, such as patient education or obtaining written informed consent from the patient. If patients are having dilating drops instilled for examination of the posterior segment just before they are expected to read some important information about their condition or treatment, they may not be able to read any documents shown to them easily.

Letters inviting the patient to attend should be clear, and of size 14 point. The detail within the letter should be sufficient for the patient to be able to respond to any specific instructions such as date and time of admission, and fasting requirements. Also, the patient will need clear directions to the ward and there should be adequate signage at the hospital to direct the patient. McBride (2000) recommends that the patient should also be able to access the information in Braille or on tape.

Cross-checking the findings of the case note review (see highlighted box) against admission lists and theatre lists will enable judgements to be made and help identify priorities for staff to address in the morning.

Case note review

Before admission (perhaps the night before admission), a review of the patient's case notes could highlight important matters that will enable staff to ensure that admission and transfer to surgery goes smoothly on the day. Issues for consideration include: diagnosis; type of surgery; whether the patient is arriving by hospital transport (and so may be late in arriving); mobility problems; special needs, including link worker and/or carer requirements; co-morbidity issues; relevant investigations performed or not; fasting instructions; consent to procedure.

The reception staff should greet the patient and anyone with him or her in an efficient and welcoming manner. If the bed is not immediately available, the patient should be shown to the waiting room/admission lounge and advised as to how long a wait he or she will have. Any specific instructions must be given before leaving the patient, such as not to eat or drink until advised otherwise. All patients must be shown how to call for assistance if needed and where the nearest toilet facilities are.

The waiting area should be uncluttered, well lit and with sufficient materials to prevent boredom while waiting. Diversion activities can include television or radio but this should not cause nuisance.

Care should be taken to keep those waiting up to date on the length of any ongoing delays. This is because their level of anxiety is likely to increase if they are kept in the dark. The general care on admission is shown in the box, below.

General care on admission

- Greet the patient and relatives or friends, making them feel welcome and at ease
- Introduce yourself
- Identify named nurse
- Ensure that the patient or escort is aware of your presence and also when you are leaving
- Confirm patient identity
- Escort patient to the bed
- Orient to the ward environment, including meal times and drink arrangements
- Ensure patient confidentiality
- Maintain patient dignity at all times

- Ensure that patient is shown where the toilets and bathroom/shower nearest to the room are located
- Show call bell system and how to work this to contact staff when needed, including in an emergency
- Give advice on visiting times and telephone contact details
- Infection control matters, including staff and visitor hand washing and visitor numbers, minimum age for visitors (if appropriate)
- Allow time to place clothing and other items in locker
- Advise about local policy relating to storage of valuable items
- Advice to patient on and instigation of self-medication policy, if appropriate, or remove medication for safe storage and dispensing
- Apply identity bracelet, having confirmed patient identity
- Apply wrist bracelet to alert to known allergies
- Undertake moving and handling risk assessment
- Measurement and recording vital signs: temperature, pulse, respirations, blood pressure
- Record visual acuity

Discharge planning

If not already started at the pre-assessment clinic appointment, discharge arrangements must be reviewed at the earliest opportunity after admission with the following being assessed:

- Transport arrangements: how will the patient get home? Relatives or friends can be of help; remind the patient to make such arrangements. In some cases, with criteria determined locally, patients may be provided with hospital transport.
- Availability of responsible adult in the event of an emergency after a general anaesthetic.
- Availability of telephone at home to ring for advice.
- Drop instillation and/or ointment application: can the patient manage or is help available or district nurse required?
- Eye care/first dressing.
- Eyelid hygiene (if necessary).
- Wound care (in the case of lid surgery or other oculoplastic surgery).
- Ability to recognize and respond appropriately to complications.
- Ability to manage everyday activities of living.

Patients undergoing surgical intervention – general points on admission

- Verbal fasting instructions are given to the patient or, if admitted already fasting, note when last ate or drank
- Nil-by-mouth signage, as appropriate
- If on medication, establish whether omitted or taken as normal that day. Some medications need to be taken as usual, e.g. anti-hypertensives, whereas others need to be omitted
- Take and record the weight of patient (if necessary)
- Change into theatre gown, if local policy to do so
- Needs of persons with disability met
- Needs of ethnic minority groups met, e.g. official interpreter
- Written consent to procedure confirmed

Organizing patient care priorities on admission

The nursing goal will be to admit patients quickly and efficiently, while making them feel welcome and assured that those involved in their care understand their specific needs. The speed with which admission activities are carried out will be dictated by patient need and when the patient is having surgery. So, the patient who is admitted at 08:00 for surgery at 08:30 will be dealt with before the patient arriving at the same time but whose surgery is not until later that same morning. In either case, letting the patients know what is happening and why is important to ensure cooperation and to reduce anxiety.

The nurse, doctor or anaesthetist may need to spend extra time with a patient to examine and prepare him or her for the operation. This could affect the theatre list schedule and so it is imperative that staff in the theatre are kept informed about patient progress.

The patient's preoperative assessment should be reviewed and any changes or additional matters duly recorded in the care pathway document. Pre-assessment ensures that vital information and investigations are carried out ahead of time so that appropriate action, based on findings, can be taken in a timely manner. Where there is no pre-assessment, the necessary information gathering and investigations must take place as quickly and efficiently as possible.

Assessment on the day of surgery, although sometimes happening, is not recommended because there is a risk that important and relevant matters may be missed or that findings could result in delays in transfer to theatre. Vital signs are usually taken and recorded on the day of admission as a baseline for comparison in the immediate postoperative period. Any abnormal findings are re-checked before appropriate action is taken.

Patients with diabetes should have their blood glucose monitored hourly while fasting preoperatively. Postoperatively, patients should be monitored at least hourly until eating and drinking normally. If patients have type 1 diabetes, the usual insulin is resumed when they are eating and drinking normally. Locally, regimens will be available for the management of unstable diabetes pre- and postoperatively and these should be followed.

Where hearing aids are worn, the patients should be reassured that they can wear them to theatre so that they can hear and join in conversations and follow instructions in the anaesthetic room. Patients may wish to keep spectacles on until they are in the anaesthetic room, to retain independence and to facilitate good communication with others. If they are having a general anaesthetic, the nurse/care worker should ensure that the hearing aid and/or spectacles are safely returned to a patient's locker and are available for the recovery period.

Link workers are vital where English is not the first language of the patient. The use of relatives or friends to translate is not to be recommended for reasons of confidentiality and accuracy of information. Local clinical governance guidelines must be followed.

Contact lenses, if worn, should be removed and placed in the appropriate receptacle in cleaning/storage fluid.

The nurse must ensure that the necessary tests and investigations have been performed and that the results are available in the case notes.

Care and management of the patient undergoing cataract extraction

Cataract, opacity of the crystalline lens, is a common cause of treatable blindness. Cataract extraction is one the most commonly performed ophthalmic operations; most people with this condition are treated as day cases. The most common operation is phacoemulsification of the lens with implant of an artificial intraocular lens (IOL). This surgery may be done under general, local or topical anaesthetic. (Further details of this can be found in Chapter 18.)

To be admitted for this type of surgery, there is generally some relevant history such as a health and/or social problem(s). Despite these problems, admission to the ward may be on the actual day of surgery, with discharge later that evening or the next morning. In such circumstances it could be argued that the ward is in effect acting as an extension of the day-surgery unit. Occasionally, admission will be organized for the day before surgery for reasons such as the need to stabilize brittle diabetes mellitus. One could question the reasonableness of treating the person with diabetes as an inpatient on the grounds that admission itself could contribute to the destabilization of their diabetic state. Other reasons for pre-admission relate to ensuring that transport difficulties do not interfere with surgery, or the patient requires some other test or intervention preoperatively.

Preoperative assessment is likely to have been completed at the out-patient stage in a pre-assessment unit. Nursing, medical and ocular history will have already been obtained and specific investigations already undertaken.

Local protocols or guidelines will dictate which other tests and investigations are carried out, e.g. electrocardiogram (ECG), blood tests such as urea, electrolytes, full blood count, chest radiograph and screening for methicillin-resistant *Staphylococcus aureus* (MRSA), and whether the results are available or need to be obtained. The nurse must ensure that the necessary tests and investigations have been performed and that the results are available in the case notes.

To view and access the cataract during surgery, achieving pupillary dilatation (mydriasis) in the eye to be operated on is essential. This is the case even if the patient is undergoing a combined procedure, e.g. phacoemulsification and IOL with trabeculectomy (drainage surgery).

The type of drops to achieve pupil dilatation will vary depending on local patient group direction (PGD) or consultant requirement in the form of a prescription (see example below). On no account should verbal instructions be taken (Nursing and Midwifery Council (NMC) 2004). Obtaining standard dilatation instructions is by far the safest system because multiple systems will add to the risk of error. PGDs have their limits in that they can be used only in the circumstances for which they have been prepared, and only by staff groups able to use them. Any variation in requirement will necessitate an individual prescription. So, for example, if a PGD was for dilatation before phacoemulsification and an IOL, it could not be used for a combined procedure.

A typical preoperative prescription for dilating

Cyclopentolate 1% × 3 to right eye and

Phenylephrine 2.5% to right eye × 3

or

Tropicamide 0.5% or 1% to right eye × 3

An estimate of the depth of the anterior chamber will indicate whether it is safe to go ahead and dilate the pupil. A simple test is the shadow test, for which you will need to use a good pen-torch. The van Herick test, using the slit-lamp and a narrow beam, or the Shaffer grading system using a gonioscope, will give an indication about the likelihood or otherwise of a rise in intraocular pressure (IOP) if the pupil is dilated.

Whatever drops are prescribed, the nurse or other member of staff instilling them must follow relevant checking procedures to ensure that the right patient gets the correct drops at the correct time, and that they are instilled into the correct eye. The consent-to-operation form should be examined for patient and doctor/nurse signature and details of the eye to be operated on. A verbal check, asking the patient which eye is being operated on, may also be undertaken to confirm that the patient is aware which eye it is. The drops should be in date and the patient should not be allergic to them or have a medical condition contrary to their use. It is usual to use Minims rather than bottled drops, because they are free of preservative and single use.

It is becoming increasingly common to give the patient dilating drops at the pre-assessment clinic and to ask him or her to begin instillation before coming into the hospital on the day of surgery. The patient should be allowed to void urine before being taken to theatre.

If the patient has a urinary catheter, this should be emptied or, where incontinence briefs are worn, the patient should be given the opportunity or assistance to change. If the patient has a stoma bag, he or she should also be given the chance to ensure that it is empty and secure. Assistance should be provided as appropriate, taking care to maintain privacy and dignity.

Where used, the preoperative theatre communication sheet/checklist should be completed. This can assist handover of important information to the anaesthetic/theatre team. This, in turn, can be a source of reassurance to the patient.

The patient undergoing general anaesthetic may require a pre-medication and this should be given at the time prescribed. For those having a local anaesthetic, a pre-medication is rarely prescribed because the patient's cooperation is needed and, in addition, it is potentially catastrophic should the patient fall asleep and suddenly awaken during surgery. However, if the patient is particularly anxious, local anaesthetic with sedation may be arranged.

During transfer to theatre, the patient may walk there if able or be transferred in a chair or on a theatre trolley. The staff escorting the patient should maintain direct communication with the patient. This helps to calm the patient.

Postoperatively the patient will require the standard routine care relative to the type of anaesthetic used. The operated eye will be protected with only a cartella shield, secured with non-allergenic tape. This allows for some useful vision, which can be of particular importance if the fellow eye has poor vision or no useful vision at all as in a previous enucleation. Excess blood-stained tearing on to the cheek is often seen; this is normal and should be dabbed away (ensure that the patient does not rub the skin because this leads to excoriation) using tissues. As this is body fluid, standard precautions (gloves and correct disposal) should be used to prevent cross-infection. Hand washing is essential before and after patient contact.

The cartella shield is removed the next morning before the eye is cleaned for the first time. The shield should be washed in warm soapy water and stored dry. It is reapplied each night for 1 or 2 weeks, secured with tape. The purpose is to prevent rubbing of the eye, reducing the risk of dislocating the IOL.

Pain is normally minimal after cataract extraction and yet it must be addressed. A pain score should be taken, asking the patient about the location, nature and type of the pain. This can also assist the diagnosis of postoperative complications, especially raised IOP. Appropriate analgesia should be given. For minor discomfort, paracetamol 1 g can be given as per local PGD or formulary for nurse prescribing.

Vision in the operated eye is likely to show improvement soon after the operation. After some types of local anaesthetic, this improvement may be delayed, but only by a matter of hours. In the interim period the patient should be assisted with activities of daily living as necessary, based on assessment of need. This includes mobility, personal hygiene, elimination, and eating and drinking.

The patient should have access to a call bell at all times. Postoperative complications, although rare, none the less do occur and include:

- iris prolapse
- striate keratopathy
- endophthalmitis
- hyphaema
- hypopyon
- allergy to topical medication
- subluxation of the IOL.

In the immediate postoperative period, those caring for the patient should be alert to any of these complications. The patient and/or carer should be made aware of how to recognize complications and action to be taken should they arise. Signs and symptoms to look for include:

- eye ache/pain not relieved with paracetamol
- reduction in vision
- other visual disturbance including flashing lights
- conjunctival injection (redness)
- conjunctival oedema
- corneal oedema
- sticky eye.

The patient or carer should be advised to contact the ward should any symptoms appear after discharge. The ward staff should maintain a telephone triage record (Figure 8.1) of the presenting complaint and current treatment and patient details. It is imperative that details of any advice given are recorded and retained.

```
Date.........................Name of patient.................................

Name of caller......................... Time of call................................

Patient problem.................................................................

Information/advice given............................................................

Signed..........................................................................
```

Figure 8.1 Telephone triage record.

On the first day postoperatively, the eye should be cleaned. As the wound is on the globe, not on the lids, the nurse is essentially performing lid hygiene. Cotton-wool balls can safely be used for cleaning the eyelids. It is usual to use an aseptic technique in hospital to prevent cross-infection. Patients should be encouraged to clean their own eyelids under supervision and to instil their own drops. This will enable the nurse to determine whether patients need additional help or support to instil their drops. Hospitalization is not a rationale for automatic referral to the district nursing service. Such referrals should be a last resort and must be carefully considered. Drop aids may make it easier for the patient to maintain independence. As there is no single style of drop bottle, there is as yet no single universal drop aid, so a patient on multi-drop therapy may need more than one type of drop aid.

If, having been assessed, the patient is found to have difficulty with memory, memory aids can be tried.

Once cleaned, the eye can be examined using a good pen-torch or a slit-lamp. Examination of the eye is necessary before any postoperative drops are instilled because some findings may contraindicate drops, e.g. if a prolapsed iris is seen, cyclopentolate should not be instilled. Eyedrops are instilled as per prescription. It is usual to use anti-inflammatory drops combined with a broad-spectrum antibiotic.

Discharge to the usual place of residence is normally the day after surgery. Patient education beforehand is essential. Information should be given verbally and also in writing, on managing the drops, cleaning the eye, specific instructions relating to identifying complications and what

action to take should they occur, getting back into normal routine and follow-up appointment.

Generally speaking, the patient should be able to resume normal activities within 24–48 hours. Swimming and contact sports should be avoided
for 3 weeks. Some centres no longer routinely see patients postoperatively but rather advise them to visit their optometrist for refraction and,
where appropriate, corrective lenses. Others see the patient at 3 or 4
weeks. Telephone pre-assessment for listing for the second eye is becoming quite routine practice.

Care and management of the patient

Trabeculectomy

This aim of this type of operation is to create an artificial drainage outlet
for aqueous humour to reduce IOP. A scleral flap is made and a sclerecto-
my performed to improve aqueous outflow into the suprachoroidal space.
In addition, a peripheral iridectomy is performed to ensure that the internal opening is not obstructed by peripheral iris. The scleral flap is sutured
but, as it is hoped that it does not heal, the result is a filtration bleb that
can be seen under the conjunctiva. Filtration surgery is usually performed
when conservative treatment or laser trabeculoplasty has failed to stabilize the IOP or where the patient's health, age or circumstances dictate.
This may or may not be used in conjunction with antimetabolites such as
5-fluorouracil (5-FU) to prevent healing of the scleral tissue (Kanski
2003). (See Chapter 20 for more details.)

Specific preoperative care

Trabeculectomy may be performed under local or general anaesthetic.
The patient will require little specific preparation for this type of surgery.
Topical or oral medication to reduce the production of aqueous humour
should not be taken on the day of the operation. This helps to increase the
amount of aqueous filtering through the bleb. The patient requires a full
explanation of the procedure and postoperative care. A care pathway or
theatre communication sheet should be completed by the nurse. The surgeon will determine whether any drops are required preoperatively, such
as pilocarpine, but these are by no means given routinely.

Specific postoperative management

On return to the ward the patient will have a cartella shield in place over
the operated eye. This will be removed the next morning and is normally

discarded because it is no longer required. Assistance with activities of daily living is as required. Pain, which is normally minimal, should be addressed, making an accurate assessment as to the nature and type of pain; where present, treat with appropriate analgesic agents and/or refer to the medical staff in the case of suspected elevated IOP.

Complications after surgery include:

- leaking bleb
- flat anterior chamber
- elevated IOP
- infected bleb.

The patient should be monitored for any signs of complications, especially elevated IOP. Accurate pain assessment will help to determine the cause of pain and result in timely and appropriate treatment. Elevated IOP is usually characterized by brow ache or headache, nausea and vomiting. If IOP is thought to be elevated, urgent medical intervention should be sought.

Repair of perforating injury

The patient with a perforating injury will normally be admitted as an emergency. He or she may be in shock as well as being overwhelmed by the speed of events as they have occurred. The patient will be anxious about what is happening with the eye as well as, perhaps, home or work matters. The trauma could have occurred at home, work or in an accident while travelling. Whatever the cause of the trauma, the patient will require expert nursing attention.

The patient needs to be admitted to the ward and made comfortable, including provision of pain relief where appropriate. The nurse needs to introduce her- or himself and if not done already ask the patient if he or she wants anyone notifying about admission. If the patient has been scheduled for surgery, he or she needs to be physically and psychologically prepared for this and nursing assessment completed before transfer to theatre. Additional tests and investigations ordered should be completed; these may include photographs, scans and blood tests. If transfer to surgery is imminent, sufficient nursing assessment to ensure patient safety should be undertaken and completed in a timely fashion upon return from theatre.

Postoperatively, the patient must be safely transferred into bed, vital signs being monitored and a pain assessment undertaken. Analgesia, which may be intramuscular, is given in a timely fashion. If intravenous antibiotics are in progress, these should be given as prescribed and the infusion site monitored for signs of extravasation or inflammation. If the antibiotic is being given via a volumetric pump, this should be set at the correct rate and it too should be monitored for accuracy. Postoperative care will depend on the nature and type of injury.

Vitrectomy

Vitrectomy (see Chapter 21) is the surgical removal of vitreous. It is performed for a variety of reasons including repair of retinal detachment and macular hole. This type of surgery is performed on a planned, routine basis unless there is an ocular emergency. This gives the opportunity to pre-assess and plan the admission and postoperative management. As with other ocular surgery, the trend is towards day case, so inpatient admission is usually associated with other medical, social or logistical issues.

The operation can be performed under local or general anaesthetic. The patient needs to be carefully assessed about whether they can manage to lie flat and remain still for a prolonged period (sometimes for as much as 3 hours).

Routine preoperative care should be instigated by the nurse. As the surgeon needs to have a good view of the retina, preoperative dilating drops will be prescribed. It is not unusual for dilating drops to be prescribed for the fellow eye to give the surgeon the opportunity to examine for the presence or otherwise of ocular pathology, but this will need to have been part of the patient consent process.

If there is a need to posture the patient postoperatively to maintain tamponade on a particular area of the retina, the patient can be given the opportunity to practise and experience the effect on his or her body and activities of living. Occasionally, the nature of the condition may actually indicate the need to posture preoperatively. In either case the patient needs to be prepared psychologically and physically to posture, because the regimen could be for up to 6 weeks. If available, specific equipment for support should be utilized or, where not available, safe adaptation to existing equipment (e.g. pillows on a lowered bed table) and use of aids such as pillows could be deployed to support face-down posturing.

Patients should be consulted and involved in planning to prevent the complications of immobility, as well as how they will manage their activities of living in the postoperative period. Boredom, difficulty eating and drinking, rest and sleep are all areas of life that will be affected.

Postoperative management will be routine nursing management plus supporting the patient with any posturing requirement. Positioning the patient who is posturing in the immediate postoperative period can prove challenging for the nursing team. The posture to be adopted should be ordered by the surgeon, e.g. strictly face down or upright cheek to pillow. If patients have had general anaesthetic and/or postoperative analgesia, they may forget they have to posture and need to be reminded to adopt their posturing position. Should it be necessary to assist the patient to adopt a posturing position, safe moving and handling principles must be followed, including the use of mechanical lifting aids as appropriate.

Pain management is essential to ensure patient comfort and to detect early complications, including elevated IOP. Appropriate action should be taken and care documented.

Routine postoperative care should be carried out, including monitoring and recording vital signs. Fluids and diet should be introduced as appropriate. Note whether there is any nausea and vomiting and assess whether this is likely to be a response to anaesthetic or elevated IOP. Take appropriate action in either case to make the patient comfortable. It is challenging for the nurse to support the patient experiencing such complications while assisting them to maintain posture to assure positive outcome of surgery. If patients do vomit, they will need to have vomit bowl and tissues close at hand, plus a call bell to get prompt assistance. A mouthwash should be offered afterwards.

For the first 24 hours or overnight, a double pad is worn on the operated eye. (Occasionally a cartella shield is used instead.) This is removed the following day, and the first dressing and pen-torch or slit-lamp examination of the eye performed and drops instilled. This is an opportunity for the nurse to educate the patient about aftercare, especially drop instillation.

The patient will, in all probability, be discharged on the first day postoperatively; having been examined by the doctor and declared fit for discharge, plans made preoperatively need to be implemented. The patient or carer needs to be instructed on eye care and also given verbal and written information on the drop and posturing regimens. Patients need to be aware of the complications of surgery and posturing, how to prevent and detect the same, plus they need a 24-hour contact number so that they can discuss progress. An appointment should be given for them to return for routine postoperative review.

Oculoplastic surgery

Although oculoplastic surgery may be performed on a day-case basis, there are times when, for clinical reasons, the patient will need to be admitted for pre- and postoperative management. Some surgery requires careful postoperative monitoring of the patient to prevent and detect complications of surgery.

Entropion

This is involution of the lids resulting in the patient experiencing tearing and pain (because of corneal irritation). The cornea may also become ulcerated and ultimately opacity may result. Causes include age-related, spasticity and cicatricial ones. The lower lid is affected but, in the case of cicatricial entropion, the upper lid may also be involved.

Ectropion

This is drooping of the lower lid, resulting in tearing that can lead to excoriation of the skin on the cheek, corneal exposure and corneal ulceration.

The following are specific needs with both types of surgery:

- A careful preoperative assessment to prepare the patient and/or the carer for the surgery and postoperative period of care.
- If both eyes require surgery, patients may have pads on both eyes postoperatively to prevent haemorrhage. This will render patients temporarily blind. In such circumstances they need to be certain that they can get assistance when required. A call bell must be at hand and the patient needs to know how to use this. Preoperatively, the patient needs to be oriented to the ward, the nursing and support staff and the routine of the ward.
- Standard preoperative preparation is needed.

Postoperative management will be the routine needs, including monitoring vital signs and observing for signs of haemorrhage. However, it will be affected by the dressing or lid oedema and how this impacts on the patient's visual acuity and/or depth perception.

If patients are not used to having little or no vision, they will be very nervous and anxious about such catastrophic lack of independence, albeit temporary. They need assurance that they will be assisted to manage their routines in the immediate postoperative phase. Expert care is essential. Patients need to know why the dressings are needed and that assistance with eating and drinking, toileting, etc. will be provided.

Mohs' reconstruction

This type of surgery is undertaken in order to treat basal cell carcinomas (rodent ulcers) affecting the eyelids. The surgery is in two parts: first, removal of the carcinoma and, second, reconstructive surgery.

The patient usually attends the ophthalmic ward after the excision of the ulcer and will have a pad in place on the operated eye to prevent haemorrhage. Patients need routine preoperative care and management supplemented with support and explanation about what must be a frightening experience for them. Despite reassurance that this type of cancer does not usually metastasize, patients are frequently worried about the long-term implications as well as what they will look like after the surgery.

Nursing staff need to provide honest explanations to patients about their condition and care, reinforcing detail given by medical staff. As part of pre-operative care, patients need to have visual acuity taken and recorded – note especially that of the opposite side to the surgery because, if vision is poor in this eye and it cannot be corrected, this will influence nursing management.

If not already undertaken, the patient's face and surgical wound will need to be photographed, which means that the dressing has to be removed by a nurse (following standard precautions) who also knows how to manage should a haemorrhage occur. Unless they have been especially trained, it is not appropriate to expect ophthalmic imaging staff to manage the dressing.

Many specialist centres have nurses who specialize in oculoplastic nursing. The expertise of these individuals should be routinely called upon to support the patient's care. They can advise patients and carers about the surgery and aftercare.

The reconstruction may require tissue to be taken from a graft site. This means that, in the postoperative period, the nurse will have at least two operation sites to monitor. It is also not unusual for the graft site to cause the patient more pain and discomfort than the site of the reconstruction.

Both sites need to be monitored for signs of haemorrhage and, if noted, pressure pad and bandage to be applied over the existing dressing and the medical staff contacted as a matter of urgency. The patient's general health and vital signs should be recorded and documented during this period. Often, the pressure bandage is sufficient to halt the bleeding, but occasionally it is necessary to return to theatre to stop the bleeding.

Pain management is essential postoperatively. Patients need to be aware that the dressings will normally be left in place (undisturbed) for a week. They will be given routine analgesia to take home as well as oral antibiotics. They need to be pain free for their journey home. Verbal and written instructions should be given about aftercare and complications. A contact number to use for emergencies and other enquiries should be given.

As they temporarily have monocular vision, patients need to be advised that they may not be able to judge depth that well.

Dacryocystorhinostomy

Blockage within the nasolacrimal apparatus causes tearing that is constant and results in patient discomfort and irritation of the cheek. Surgery is carried out either via the external route or as an endoscopic procedure.

Other than routine preparation for surgery plus physical and psychological preparation, no specific preparation is needed. The patient should be visited by the oculoplastic nurse specialist to discuss postoperative management.

In the postoperative period, the external approach to surgery will require pad and bandage with or without a nasal pack; the patient having endoscopic surgery will normally have a nasal pack *in situ*. As haemorrhage is a possible complication, a tray should be set up for dealing with epistaxis in an emergency, with a nasal pack (may be kept in refrigerator), nasal forceps and nasal speculum.

In the postoperative period, but for routine management, the patient needs to be monitored for signs of haemorrhage. This could be from the external wound or from the operative site as epistaxis. Epistaxis can be severe, and in any case it must be treated as a medical emergency with appropriate first-aid action taken. Epistaxis may not be overt through the nose; it could be trickling down the back of the throat. The patient must be kept calm, sitting upright (not flat), leaning slightly forward and pinching the bridge of the nose. Tissues and a receptacle should be used to collect any blood (not to be discarded until seen by the medical team) to estimate total blood loss. The emergency epistaxis tray should be brought to the bedside. The medical staff will pack the wound in an attempt to halt the bleeding. If this is not successful, the patient may have to return to theatre. Routinely, the dressing and nasal pack are removed before discharge home.

Written and verbal instructions should be given to the patient on how to manage care at home. Antibiotics and analgesia are given as prescribed to take home. With an external dacryocystorhinostomy, chloramphenicol ointment may be given with which to massage the wound. Appointment for follow-up will also be given.

Enucleation

This involves complete removal of the globe but with conservation of the remaining orbital content, including the extraocular muscles.

Evisceration

This involves removal of the contents of the globe, retaining the sclera. This type of surgery provides for better long-term success of any implant and prosthesis because the body is less likely to reject the implant.

Exenteration

This involves surgical removal of the globe and the orbital content. In some cases it may include the loss of bone. If the lids can be conserved, they may be used to line the cavity.

Throughout the admission the nursing staff should implement the care prescribed by the specialist nurse. Waterman et al. (1999) found that patients undergoing these types of surgery experienced marked postoperative nausea and vomiting and were often in pain. For this reason, these patients will normally remain in hospital for up to 48 hours postoperatively. During this time they can be supported to begin to overcome some of the physical and psychological trauma associated with the loss of an eye. Postoperative pain and nausea should be assessed and treated appropriately.

The patient should be monitored for haemorrhage. This will manifest overtly through the pressure pad and dressing, which should not be disturbed. If bleeding is noted, an additional pad and bandage should be applied and the patient should rest, semi-recumbent, in bed. Urgent medical assistance is required.

Analgesia, anti-inflammatories and antibiotics should be given as prescribed. Pain assessment should be made and recorded. The patient should be subsequently approached to ensure that the analgesics are working.

It has been identified that there is a paucity of research in relation to the type of postoperative dressing to use with such wound cavities because often there are fissures and cavities connecting to other structures. Although the dressings are normally left in place for 1 week, the nurse needs to understand the dressings used, both to inform practice and so that correct information and advice can be given to the patient.

On the day of discharge, the patient needs written and verbal postoperative advice, including what to do if the dressing comes loose (contact the ward and return for it to be re-applied). The patient or a family member should be able to help re-apply the bandage only. They need to know that the dressing will ooze and may have a slight odour; however, if there is any cause for concern, such as fever or uncontrollable pain or bleeding, the patient should be instructed to contact the ward as a matter of urgency.

Admission for medical treatment

Such admissions tend to be unplanned and such patients come via accident and emergency or outpatient departments. Pre-assessment is unlikely to have been undertaken so the nurse needs to complete one in order to determine the care needs of the patient.

MRSA status may be significant in determining where to nurse the patient. It may be necessary to isolate the patient until his or her status is known; this will be determined by local and/or national policies.

Hyphaema

Hyphaema, blood in the anterior chamber, may be the result of accidental injury such as blow to the eye with squash ball, or surgical trauma. It is also seen occasionally following YAG (yttrium–aluminium–garnet) laser iridotomy.

Admission is not usual unless there are exceptional circumstances such as elevated IOP or total hyphaema, and depending on the cause, e.g. associated with penetrating injury. The patient could be cared for at home, provided that he or she is prepared to rest in an upright position and is able to return for a follow-up appointment. Total hyphaema will affect the patient's vision.

If admitted, the patient will be anxious and will require explanation as to why he or she has to rest in bed, nursed upright. Keeping a young fit person at rest is not the easiest task but, if complications such as raised IOP are to be avoided or detected early, the patient needs to be supported to rest. Remember, this could be the person's first experience of hospital admission.

Unless on strict bedrest, the patient should be allowed to mobilize to the toilet to void urine or open their bowels and to the bathroom to wash. While on bedrest, patients are at risk of the complications of immobility so a suitable assessment should be made together with the patient and a care plan developed to prevent their occurrence. Diet and fluids must be considered in such assessment to prevent dehydration and constipation. The latter could be compounded by codeine-based analgesia given for pain relief.

Corneal ulcers (see also Chapter 16)

This is a regular reason for admission to the ophthalmic ward. Patients may be elderly, confused and disoriented. In addition, they may also have other health problems that need to be addressed during the admission. Younger patients with severe corneal ulcers may also be admitted but are usually supported or self-caring at home. Patients with corneal ulcers need not necessarily be isolated as part of their care. This is necessary only if the ulcer is infected with a virulent organism. In such a situation patients need to be isolated in a single room with en-suite facilities. Staff and visitors need to know how to follow standard precautions to prevent cross-infection. It is vital that medical isolation does not lead to social isolation. The patient should have access to TV, radio and books/newspapers, but most importantly to people during their stay in hospital.

Pain needs to be managed. The cornea is very sensitive and acute or chronic pain must be managed with oral medication given in response to pain assessment. Pain may arise from other causes, which must be identified and dealt with appropriately. Discomfort may be an issue rather than overt pain; patients occasionally need education about not having routine ocular discomfort, but trying mild analgesics or anti-inflammatories to relieve it.

Frequent/intensive drop therapy will normally be prescribed, the antibiotic being determined by culture of a swab or corneal scrape. The nurse may be instilling drops as frequently as every 15 minutes, day and night, for the first 24 hours. This can lead to sleep disturbance, poor appetite, and resentment of the care regimen and the people delivering it. The patient needs to understand the rationale for this care. Intravenous or oral antibiotics should be given as prescribed.

Sleep disturbance may have been a feature of the patient's problem before admission, compounded by the intensive drop regimen. The nurse must not omit drops if the patient is sleeping; such action could unwittingly prolong the need for such treatment.

The patient needs to have an adequate intake of fluids and a nutritious diet. It may be necessary in some cases to refer the patient to the dietitian. The patient is likely to feel generally unwell on admission and will need nursing interventions as appropriate while avoiding unnecessary dependence on others.

Patient education is essential. Take the opportunity to assess the patient's drop technique during his or her stay once he or she is well enough. In chronic ulcer management, acute episodes could be the result of the patient missing drops or not being able to instil drops for physical/mechanical reasons or memory loss. Drop and memory aids could be tried. If these do not work, alternatives need to be considered, including district nurse or care manager (social worker) review.

Loneliness and social isolation could be at the root of the acute episode of corneal ulceration. The care manager and voluntary agencies or support groups may assist in developing a care package if the patient will permit it.

Discharge planning will have started on admission and the plan should be implemented in a timely fashion to support transfer home or into temporary or permanent residential or nursing home care. A follow-up appointment must be given, along with consideration about transport to the appointment.

Acute glaucoma

As suggested, the onset is acute, the IOP elevated, the glaucoma is usually unilateral, and there is a fixed semi-dilated pupil and reduced vision because of corneal oedema, which is also responsible for the patient seeing haloes around lights. As well as feeling generally unwell, the patient is likely to be frightened or anxious about the admission.

Patients will probably still be in some pain or discomfort despite emergency treatment. They should be assessed for pain and if necessary analgesia given as prescribed, which could be intramuscular pethidine, often accompanied by an antiemetic.

Nausea and vomiting are a feature of acute glaucoma and so a vomit bowl and tissues should be available in easy reach if the patient needs them. Should the patient vomit, it may relieve some of the discomfort. They should be offered a mouthwash or the opportunity to brush their teeth. Patients should be nursed in a side room with dim lighting because of the photophobia experienced.

Reduction of IOP with drop therapy should be continued as prescribed. Fluids and diet should be encouraged, and definitely fluids to prevent dehydration.

Preparation for laser iridotomy the following day is done by explaining the procedure to patients and answering any queries that they may have. If assessed as needed, oral analgesia should be given before the procedure to ensure cooperation. The pupils should already be constricted by the pilocarpine drops. The patient should be reassured that the procedure is relatively pain free but that topical analgesia will be administered in the laser department.

Discharge advice and information should be given verbally and in writing. (See Chapter 20 for more details of glaucoma.)

Orbital cellulitis

This is a rare but distressing condition that may be bilateral. If severe enough, admission to hospital is warranted. The patient will be generally debilitated and also pyrexial. Assessment on admission and planning of care is essential to improving well-being.

Patients need to be nursed in a quiet, dimly lit room; however, if hourly visual acuity and test for relative afferent pupillary defect (RAPD) have been requested, illumination will be necessary. Warn patients about the change in light intensity so that they can prepare for it.

Pain management is essential as is the introduction of topical and intravenous antibiotics as prescribed. Cold compresses are normally found to be soothing and can relieve some ocular discomfort. Moistened eye pads can be utilized, using clean pads each time, and safely discarding the used pads.

If the lids are crusty or purulent, they need to be cleansed using an aseptic technique. Swabs should ideally be taken before any antibiotics are started. As the patient will be in pain, ensure that adequate analgesia has been given before performing eye care. The decision of whether or not to isolate the patient will be determined by the cause of the cellulitis, but this is not usual.

Physical care should include care related to rest and sleep, adequate oral fluid and nutrition intake, personal and oral hygiene, temperature regulation and elimination needs. Bed rest is indicated in the first 24 hours until the patient is well enough to sit out for increasing periods of time, and then until well enough to return home.

As the cause of orbital cellulitis is not always known, the patient should be assured that recurrence is rare. Prompt and timely intervention can prevent permanent damage to visual function. Discharge home is normally being planned from admission so that systems are in place to support the patient as required. Unless advised by the doctors, patients should refrain from work until they have been discharged by the hospital.

Although care of the ophthalmic patient as an inpatient is less and less common as a result of a reduction of inpatient beds and the recognition of the benefits of day surgery, there are a number of occasions, as demonstrated here, when inpatient care is essential. Good care for the ophthalmic patient in hospital requires a battery of skills and knowledge that are less and less available to the ophthalmic unit, and this area should be recognized as a highly specialized domain of ophthalmic nursing.

References

NHSE (2000) Action on Cataracts: Good practice guidance. London: DoH.

Kanski JJ (2003) Clinical Ophthalmology, 5th edn. London: Butterworth-Heinneman.

McBride S (2000) Patients Talking: Hospital outpatient eye services – the sight impaired user's view. London: RNIB.

McBride S (2001) Patients Talking 2: The eye clinic journey experienced by blind and partially sighted adults. London: RNIB.

Nursing and Midwifery Council (2004) Guidelines for the Administration of Medicines. London: NMC.

Royal College of Ophthalmologists (2002) Clinical Governance and Ophthalmology. London: RCOphth.

Waterman H, Leatherbarrow B, Slater R, Waterman C (1999) Post-operative pain, nausea and vomiting: qualitative perspectives from telephone interviews. J Adv Nursing 29: 690–6.

CHAPTER NINE

The care of the child undergoing ophthalmic treatment

JILLY BRADSHAW

Florence Nightingale's remark that the first requirement of a hospital was that 'it should do the sick no harm' (1863) is familiar to generations of nursing and medical staff. It is never truer than when caring for sick children. Nursing children is a great challenge in many ways, and children's nurses must act as the child's advocate, particularly when caring for infants and pre-verbal children. Recent government legislation in the UK has clearly identified the rights and needs of children in hospital and laid down guidelines for good practice.

Principles of care of children in hospital

The aim of care should be effective, complete care of the whole child and his or her family (the child is, for convenience, referred to as he throughout this chapter).

Environment

Each department should be a safe and cheerful environment with a friendly and relaxed atmosphere in which to look after children and their families. Inpatient children and day-case children should be nursed in a dedicated children's area, away from adult patients, and if possible with day cases being cared for away from acutely ill children. In the accident and emergency department (A&E) or a clinic, a specially designated, safe area for children to play and relax is necessary. It has long been recognized that play is of crucial importance to children; it is their normal activity, and helps them work through fears and cope with stressful situations (see Doverty 1992). In each department there should, therefore, be the provision of a wide variety of toys and games suitable for all age ranges.

Nursing

In line with legislation over several decades, most recently the National Service Framework (NSF or DoH 2003a), children should be nursed by specially trained children's nurses. Wherever possible, particularly on the ward, there should be some continuity of nurses caring for the child, otherwise children can easily meet many different staff during one hospital visit or admission, which is very unsettling for them.

Paediatric nurses who look after children are educated to be aware of the many significant differences between children and adults – children are certainly not 'mini adults' in any way.

Paediatric nurses are not always available and nurses looking after children should be aware of the significant differences between them and adults (DoH 1991, Thornes 1991). It has long been recognized that children have complex emotional needs, particularly when they are in stressful situations, such as being hospitalized (Shuttleworth 2003).

The overwhelming benefits of effective preoperative preparation are well researched, so a preoperative admission programme should be in place for all children who have to undergo any type of elective surgery, as well as for their families (Dearmun 1994, Shuttleworth 2003).

All staff in every department that treats children should be aware of child protection issues and the procedures laid down in their trust policy. There should also be a system of referrals for children to the GP, health visitor, school nurse or Social Services. All referrals must be carefully documented as emphasized in the guidelines in the Lambing Report (DoH 2003b), following the Victoria Climbié Inquiry.

The child

All children should be involved in the process of their care while in hospital, as appropriate for the individual child. Rushforth (1999) shows that this concept is underpinned by the growing recognition of children's rights in more recent legislation. Similarly, many children are able to arrive at the point of giving informed consent, provided that they are given information and made aware of the particular issues, in an appropriate way for their age, stage, knowledge, life experience and culture (DoH 2003a).

Effective communication among child, family and staff should be established from the first hospital visit onwards. Young children often have a limited vocabulary, may have their own personal words for things, and use non-verbal communication to express themselves. The significance of and the need to employ therapeutic play cannot be over-emphasized (Chandler 1994). Clear information giving, in a way appropriate to the individual child, to aid understanding and minimize anxiety, promotes patient confidence and trust in the staff, and lessens children's feelings of powerlessness and loss of control. Thus, Rushforth (1999) states that the multidisciplinary team are obliged to inform the child fully before admission and before each procedure that causes stress.

It is important to recognize that adolescents (about 11–18 years) have distinct and varying needs to adults and younger children, requiring careful communication and a different approach to planning and negotiating care (Deering and Jennings 2002). Great tact and sensitivity are required by all clinical staff who care for young people. Recognizing this, some children's hospitals now have dedicated adolescent units.

Children and babies can and do feel pain, although knowledge and awareness are needed to evaluate this, particularly in pre-verbal children. It is imperative for nurses caring for children in all departments to have pain assessment tools in use to medicate children effectively – paediatric analgesia/antiemetic 'ladders' – and to promote the use of many non-chemical methods to reassure and help children (RCN 1999).

Family

Nurses should have a good understanding of and adhere to delivery of child- and family-focused care, with an emphasis on their involvement in that care (RCN 2003). Clinical staff should appreciate the natural anxiety and fear of all parents coming into hospital with their child, however minor the reason may seem, and, importantly, the crucial importance of parental presence to the child. This alliance between nursing staff and parents can be problematic if there are misunderstandings between parents' expectations and nurses' expectations of the care to be given to their child (Kristensson-Hallstrom 2000), so good verbal and written communication is essential.

Parents must be supported and helped through each stage of their child's time in hospital, however short. Nurses should discuss with parents about how much nursing of the child they feel comfortable doing, but never assuming that the worried parent can give all the care during their hospitalization. The more secure and informed the parents feel, the more likely they are to nurse their child in a way that supports the child effectively during hospitalization (Kristensson-Hallstrom 1999).

Parents must be offered regular breaks and meals and 'time off' as appropriate, with staff recognizing their needs and also the demands of the rest of the family, particularly the child's siblings. Parents appreciate time taken by the nurse to empathize with them and show that they care (Shandor Miles 2003).

Special considerations

There are key differences for the families and children who are to undergo eye surgery. First, when asked, most children say that they 'live' in their eyes and that vision is their most important sense; importantly the eyes offer the face beauty and they give character and expression to the face. Children can be very distressed if there is disruption to their vision after the instillation of eyedrops or postoperatively. Children of all ages are frequently teased about their appearance, e.g. if they have a squint or cyst, which can make them unhappy and sometimes withdrawn. Parents are usually extremely concerned and emotional about surgery on such a small yet vital organ and frequently assume, with horror, that the eye will have to be removed during surgery. Parents and children, too, worry about the cosmetic result of surgery, the healing process and the visual outcome. Finally, what may seem just routine eye surgery to staff is always a major event to the child and his family.

The care of the child undergoing day surgery

Reasons for admission

Many children are admitted to the ophthalmic unit as day cases for elective surgery, usually under a general anaesthetic. Day surgery is beneficial to children in several ways. First, it minimizes the overall emotional stress and disruption to the child and his family. Second, it facilitates the continual presence of the parent, so vital to every child's well-being. Third, the cost to the hospital is considerably reduced. However, if the psychological advantages are to be maximized, it is very important that day-case children are properly prepared preoperatively and looked after efficiently throughout their day in hospital (Kelly and Adkins 2003).

The most common conditions that require day surgery are squints, suspected blocked lacrimal ducts and meibomian cysts in the eyelids:

- A squint is a malalignment of one of the three pairs of extraocular muscles that hold the eye within the bony eye orbit. A squint in childhood, which affects about one in four to five children, is commonly associated with a refractive error. Correction of this error with orthoptic exercises, occlusion therapy if one eye is amblyopic and spectacles may play a part in the management of squint, but surgery may be indicated to try to achieve binocular vision and improve the cosmetic appearance. However, surgery cannot improve binocular vision once it has been lost (Stollery 1997) (see also Chapter 22).
- A blockage of the lacrimal duct, which carries tears to the nasolacrimal duct in the nose, causes the eye to become persistently watery and pus

is expelled through the punctum, leading to infection. Commonly the symptoms have been present since birth. The blockage may be the result of the failure of canalization of the lacrimal duct, a narrowing of the duct through a membrane left over from fetal life, the presence of pus or, in rare cases, the absence of the duct. Surgery aims to assess the duct, clear the blockage and restore effective tear drainage (see Chapter 14).

- A meibomian cyst, or chalazion, is a sebaceous swelling of one of the meibomian glands in the eyelid. This may cause discomfort, itchiness and pain, and can interfere with vision. Cysts can be present on either lid and several may occur at once. If conservative treatment fails to improve the condition, surgery is carried out to incise and evacuate the cyst (see Chapter 14).

Pre-admission assessment

The first crucial step in planning the care of a child to be admitted as a day case is a pre-admission visit to the ward, and an assessment of each child and his parents by a paediatric nurse (Kelly and Adkins 2003). Research over many years has confirmed that good preoperative preparation reduces perioperative problems, e.g. pain and anxiety, and hastens discharge. The nurse is therefore uniquely placed to agree an individualized plan of management with the parents as partners in the care (Kenyon and Barnett 2001). Ideally, the visit should take place 1–2 weeks before admission and will offer the child a safe time to play, meet his nurses and have fun! This can effectively help the child feel secure and realize that time in hospital can be enjoyable. The nurse should be relaxed, friendly and unhurried. The nurse should record information about the child's individual routine and personality, past medical history, his weight, allergies, immunization status and medication. The parents must be given clear, accurate verbal and written instructions about the preparations at home before admission – most importantly how to manage the preoperative starvation period successfully, parents of babies being most concerned on this particular aspect. They need to know the course of events on the operation day, especially the anaesthetic procedure. A thorough plan for discharge and care at home to ensure seamless care must be established at this stage. This will include sorting out domestic arrangements, parental jobs, time off playschool/school for the child, care of siblings and all aspects of caring for the child at home afterwards (Caring for Children in the Health Services or CCHS 1991).

An explanation must be given to the child about his role when he comes back into hospital for surgery, appropriate to his age, stage and life experience. This is best explained to children by allowing them to play with teddies and dolls displaying equipment that they are likely to see, e.g. theatre gown, anaesthetic mask and tubing, syringe and stethoscope. This type of therapeutic play significantly helps the child to understand what is to happen to him, assimilate information and cope better with hospitalization (Dix 2004). Adolescents need more detail and choices about what is to happen to them, in order to feel more confident and in control. All children should be treated with respect and their opinions and wishes taken into consideration when planning care with them. There is a comprehensive website for children called 'Children First', which offers a wide range of health information to all age groups (Shuttleworth 2003).

Much reassurance must be given to families, because a prospective hospital admission can be distressing for them and may also bring back memories of a bad experience for one of the family. However, young children often see things differently from adults, and they may be very excited indeed about the visit and a whole day on the ward! Indeed, some children enjoy themselves so much during this visit that they do not wish to leave!

The family must be shown around the ward and the available facilities explained. If appropriate, they may be shown into the anaesthetic room, which is usually less threatening than people imagine and can effectively allay fears before the 'big day'.

The day of surgery

The child should be admitted early on the morning of surgery. It is preferable for children to be placed first on the morning, not afternoon, operating list whenever possible. This avoids long, anxious waiting times and reduces preoperative fasting. The child should be greeted by name, shown his bed and introduced to other families. The children's ward should be safe, homely and cheerful, and offer a wide range of toys and games for all age groups. Parents should be encouraged to be with their child for all procedures.

Any changes in the child's circumstances since the pre-admission visit are noted and the child's fitness for surgery ascertained. Parents should support their child for all procedures, however seemingly minor, and implement care with help from the nurse. Identity bands are checked and put round the child's ankles, leaving the hands free. The child may need to put on a theatre gown and a baseline set of vital signs is recorded. A local anaesthetic cream, e.g. Ametop, is applied over veins on the back of the hands at the correct time before surgery; parents are asked to help ensure that the young child does not tamper with this 'magic' cream so that it stays in situ. The child should be sensitively reminded about what the operation will involve, and how he is likely to feel afterwards, in a way appropriate to his age and stage. This will help the child feel less alarmed later on. Appropriate explanations should be given to the child and his parents as necessary throughout the day, whilst always maintaining confidentiality.

The child will be examined by the doctor/nurse practitioner, his relevant medical history reviewed and informed consent from parents and child/young person for surgery recorded. A pen mark on the forehead will denote the correct eye for surgery; it is essential to check this carefully against the consent form, medical notes and operating list, identifying the correct child too, because they do run about the ward and sit on each other's beds!

Any prescribed preoperative premedication, e.g. midazolam 0.5 mg/kg, and any preoperative eyedrops must be administered at the correct time. Children and parents must understand the reason for and effects of all medication given. The nurse may need to use play and distraction techniques in order to succeed with this! Verbal informed consent from the child and parents will be needed if 'holding still' techniques need to be employed. Often, however, if the child is given adequate explanation and encouragement, he will cooperate. Throughout these preparations, the paediatric nurse should treat the child with tact and sensitivity. His natural need for privacy and dignity must also be taken into consideration in all circumstances. In this way the nurse will increase the child's trust and confidence in what is happening to him, help him feel happy and in control, and therefore more likely to be cooperative.

One or both parents and the child's teddy or snugly blanket may accompany the child and nurse to go directly into the anaesthetic room. There should be no waiting around at any point during this journey, because this heightens the inevitable stress felt by child and parent. The nurse should help during the anaesthetic process as required and must support the parent after the child is anaesthetized, usually a very upsetting stage for parents, however smoothly the anaesthetic procedure has gone. It is good practice to accompany parents discreetly back to the ward and, after being told approximately how long the operation will take, they should be advised to take a break for a drink or fresh air.

Postoperative care

Before the child's return to the ward parents should be forewarned about what to expect in the child's appearance and behaviour. Many anaesthetists welcome parents into the recovery room to comfort the child and accompany him back to the ward with the nurse. If possible, the bed area or room should be kept quiet to promote sleep, and darkened to minimise sensitivity to light. Parental presence and their caring for the child are vital components of relieving the child's discomfort and distress postoperatively

(RCN 1999). Parents are usually anxious to see their child after surgery, but are also nervous about how he will be. Support of parents involves advising them how to care for their child by reassuring him, lying on the bed and cuddling him, stroking his forehead and wiping his face with a cool flannel, and gently distracting him with a story or a nursery rhyme. These interventions work well and the child will usually sleep with the parent close by.

Postoperative observations are essential to monitor the child's recovery and promptly identify problems in the early stages (Tume and Bullock 2004). Assessment is made of the following: child's consciousness level and skin colour; pulse, respiratory rate/effort and temperature. These are recorded until the child is conscious. Further observations of O_2 saturations, peripheral pulses and capillary refill time should be taken and medical staff alerted if the child's condition deteriorates in any way (McAllister 2001). The condition of the eye should be monitored – the presence of any swelling or haematoma, blood in the tears noted or remarks indicating that the child has diplopia (double vision). Eye movements should be discreetly observed and concern about any aspect of the eye discussed with the surgeon. The child is to be gently discouraged from rubbing the eye.

Rectal analgesia, e.g. diclofenac (Voltarol) 1–3 mg/kg or paracetamol 10–15 mg/kg, can be given intraoperatively, with good effect, to minimize postoperative pain. An intravenous antiemetic, e.g. ondansetron 100 μg/kg for over-2-year-olds, may be given at the same stage. Any further discomfort later on can be treated with a simple analgesic, e.g. paracetamol elixir. Parents must be informed about the medication given and its effects.

As the child recovers, tepid drinks and light snacks are offered. When the child wakes and is feeling better, gentle play is allowed and activity re-established while maintaining safety. The intravenous cannula is removed only once the child's overall condition is good, mobility is regained and fluids/diet tolerated. Before going home the eye and eye movements are checked.

Planned discharge

The parent and child, as appropriate, must understand the process of how the eye will recover after surgery and be shown how to clean the eye and administer eye drops, e.g. chloramphenicol 0.5% w/v, 1 drop four times daily. Little children loathe eyedrops and the gentle restraint often needed, and strategies must be given to parents for this to be successful, getting a relative or friend to help if possible. Instructing the child to look at a toy held above him and counting to 20 after the eyedrops to focus his attention and giving a small reward (chocolate or stickers) for compliance all help.

Parents also need advice about administering appropriate regular analgesia for 2–4 days postoperatively, an important aspect of care to minimize discomfort and stop the child rubbing the eye, making it sore. Being free of pain also helps the child re-establish his normal level of play and activity, and helps him look back more favourably on his recent experience in hospital.

Advice must be given about recreation, activities and schooling. Swimming and contact sports should be curtailed until the eye has settled, usually 2–6 weeks depending on the surgery performed. All aspects of care of the eyes, and general child care, are discussed with the parent and child before discharge. Teenagers should be advised not to wear eye make-up for 2–3 weeks after surgery.

Research shows that children can be disrupted by even a short stay in hospital, especially the under-5s, and parents should be made aware of this (While and Wilcox 1994). This may be manifest by clingy and tearful behaviour, which will pass if plenty of extra love, praise and encouragement are offered to the child. Attention should be given to siblings too and small tasks devised for them to 'help', so that they do not feel left out. Therefore, parents should be advised to plan a quiet few days based at home after surgery, allowing each member of the family to settle down, and limiting visitors and long trips.

A useful strategy is to ensure that the family receive a postoperative telephone call from the ward the day after surgery, to ensure that all is well and provide further advice where necessary; this is always greatly appreciated by the family (Feasey 2000). They should have a hospital contact telephone number and be assured that they may ring at any time for advice about the eye.

The child will usually have a follow-up appointment after surgery, and further help and support for families may be sought from the community paediatric nurses, the health visitor and family doctor, and must be organized before discharge.

The care of the child as an inpatient

Reasons for admission

After day surgery

On some occasions a child who has undergone eye surgery as a day case does not meet the discharge criteria and needs to stay overnight. This delay may be the result of postoperative problems, e.g. failure to tolerate fluids, the need for further observation or a domestic situation that warrants a longer stay in hospital. Other indications for inpatient care include the following.

Severe infections

Orbital cellulitis is a potentially life-threatening and vision-threatening condition, arising from bacterial infection in the nasal sinuses, after a penetrating injury or eye surgery (Khaw et al. 2004). It is more common in children than adults and causes an acute, purulent infection of the tissue of the eye orbit, resulting in a tender, swollen and painful eye. Proptosis of the affected eye may occur, as a result of inflamed tissue behind the eyeball, which can lead to abscess formation. Early diagnosis and treatment is crucial and is made on the history and clinical examination. Computed tomography (CT) is performed for a localized abscess that requires surgical drainage and to look for sinus disease.

The child will be febrile and unwell, with a painful eye and altered vision (Evans 1995). Treatment will involve regular and effective analgesia (a child will often refuse medication if he does not think it works) and antipyretic medication, systemic antibiotics intravenously or orally, and antibiotic eyedrops. Nursing care of this child includes allowing adequate rest, gentle play, careful cleansing of the eye and face, instillation of eyedrops and organizing work brought in from school if his stay in hospital is prolonged. As always parents fall into the remit of care.

Ophthalmia neonatorum is any eye infection that occurs within 21 days of birth and is notifiable. It may be caused by bacteria such as gonococci or pneumococci, but most commonly by *Chlamydia* sp. (see also Chapter 15). Gonococci cause a severe bacterial eye infection and requires urgent admission to hospital. The infection is transmitted to the baby during vaginal delivery. Sexually transmitted disease in the parents must be excluded.

Gonococcal infection causes the eyelids to swell with a profuse, purulent discharge from the baby's eyes, and there is a real risk that the cornea may become ulcerated or even perforate. The baby's eyes require hourly bathing, intensive treatment with antibiotic eyedrops and often a systemic antibiotic as well. Scrupulous attention to the hygienic care of the infant, including care of the umbilicus, is essential, to prevent cross-infection. Attention must also be paid to all the other needs of a newborn baby, including nutrition, adequate warmth and the comforting of a baby who may feel unwell. Chlamydia infection is less dramatic, causing a sticky eye that may be treated on an outpatient basis.

If a young baby is admitted, the mother of the baby also needs careful nursing. She may well be feeling the physical and emotional effects of the birth, and may require a midwife's attention. If the mother has chosen to breast-feed she will need guidance and support, because establishing breast-feeding is demanding and tiring. The mother needs regular updates about her baby's condition and support to allow her to contribute in her baby's general care, to promote bonding and affection between mother and baby.

This family will need very sensitive emotional support through this upsetting and difficult time and appropriate support and follow-up planned before discharge.

Retinoblastoma

Retinoblastoma is a highly malignant retinal tumour of childhood affecting children under 5 years of age. It occurs in 1/20 000 live births, is often hereditary and may be present at birth. Usually one eye is affected, but in about 30% of cases the primary tumour affects both eyes. The child may present with a squint, an abnormal papillary reflex or a painful red eye (Moore 2000), or the child's eye may display a white pupil, instead of the normal red reflex. A squint may herald the presence of retinoblastoma (Khaw et al. 2004). Investigations will include an examination of the fundus of the eye, a CT scan, ultrasound scan of the eye and an examination under anaesthetic, performed to confirm the diagnosis. Children can find a CT scan very alarming and must be well informed and prepared beforehand; very young children will usually be sedated or given a general anaesthetic for the procedure.

If the tumour is advanced, the eye will be enucleated. If the tumour is small, chemotherapy, laser treatment, cryotherapy or radiotherapy may be used to preserve the eye and hopefully some vision (Moore 2000). Close follow-up will involve further examinations under anaesthetic to monitor progress. Children who are cared for at a specialist centre have a cure rate for the primary tumour of over 95% (Moore 2000), but a proportion of patients will go on to develop another malignancy in early adult life (Evans 1995).

Children born to survivors of retinoblastoma, or those who have a close family relative who has had the disease, will be monitored throughout their first 5 years of life and, along with the survivors of the disease, will be offered genetic counselling.

Eyedrop therapy

A child may be admitted as an inpatient for the instillation of essential eyedrops if he is refusing to cooperate with treatment at home, the parent is unable to cope, or the social situation is such that the treatment is difficult or impossible. Sometimes a child who has just undergone a cataract extraction will require frequent eyedrop administration (e.g. Pred Forte 1–2 hourly for 24 hours) and this can be demanding and difficult for some parents to achieve at home. The nurse will require great patience and ingenuity to teach parents and the child the best way to cope with the eyedrop routine at home and thus ensure a good outcome from this admission. Further support at home may be offered by health visitors, school nurses and community paediatric nurses.

Occlusion therapy (see also Chapter 22)

Amblyopia, or 'lazy eye', is reduced visual acuity in an affected eye that lacks visual experience and use in early life, when the visual pathways are developing. There may be a squint or refractive error also present but otherwise the eye is structurally normal. This condition is the most common visual ailment in children, occurring in 1.2–4.4% (Royal College of Ophthalm-ologists or RCOphth 2001).

Vital occlusion treatment has been successfully used for over 200 years and involves use of an occlusive patch to cover the unaffected eye, thus encouraging the amblyopic eye's use and function. This is possible up to the age of 8 years, but it is generally accepted that, after that age, the visual system has matured and visual acuity cannot be improved upon. Compliance with treatment is pivotal to treatment success (RCOphth 2001) and failure to develop binocular vision has psychosocial effects and limits certain career options in adult life.

Most children will tolerate 'patching' at home, but some resist strongly, exhibiting very 'challenging' behaviour if parents even attempt to apply the patch! Some hospitals admit non-compliant children for a few days with the aims of teaching them to wear an eye patch and establish a routine for them to wear it for the designated time each day (Dorey et al. 2001). Parents must fully understand the aim of occlusion therapy and how this will be achieved. Success depends very much on the good information given to parents and teaching them effective practical strategies to use at home with their child.

Parents often feel a strong sense of failure and exasperation at not succeeding in carrying out such seemingly simple treatment at home, and need much support and encouragement themselves during admission and afterwards at home.

It is also crucial for a parent to stay with their child in hospital, first to support him but crucially to learn how to manage the occlusion at home after discharge. The child's normal routine and discipline – mealtimes, bathing, bedtimes, etc. – should be maintained as far as possible while he is in hospital, to help him feel secure.

It is essential to work directly with the child throughout the period of treatment. A simple, clear explanation must be given to him and he must understand why he has to wear an eye patch and that he may not be able to see very well at first. But with lots of fun, different toys, puzzles and games, the exposed eye will work hard and vision can, on occasions, improve enough on the first day, making the wearing of the 'patch' more tolerable. The first few hours are usually the most demanding for the nurse and parent or carer, persuading and enticing the child to leave the patch alone – constant distraction is essential!

The use of a simple reward scheme, perhaps using a colourful chart and an attractive book to stick used patches in and record the patching time achieved, will often appeal to the natural competitiveness of the young child. While the child is on the ward, he should be kept fully occupied with good play facilities. Close work encourages the eye to work hard but frequent breaks for walks or more active play should be given to prevent boredom. It is often boredom or frustration that can make a child remove his patch, in order to gain the adult's attention. There may well be certain times that the child may find particularly difficult to cope with wearing the 'patch', such as at playschool, and strategies should be sought to improve matters. Siblings are encouraged to visit, to prevent them worrying about the parent and child in hospital. Parents should be offered frequent breaks, because this is a demanding and emotional time for them.

Following on the admission, children are closely monitored in the orthoptic clinic, to assess improvement, avoid amblyopia in the occluded eye, and offer parents and indeed the child further support.

The health visitor should be made aware of the admission, because she is well placed to continue advising parents about problems at home. If the child is of school age, the school nurse and teacher can be instrumental in helping the child succeed with 'patching' at school.

Trauma (see also Chapter 12)

Trauma is one of the most common reasons for a child's admission to the eye ward. Trauma can cause a wide range of injuries to the eye itself and to the surrounding area. These injuries usually fall into two types:

1. Blunt injury, e.g. from a blow from a games racquet or ball.
2. Penetrating injury, e.g. from a stick or pencil entering the eye.

Both types of injury can cause severe disorganization of the structures of the eyeball, including haemorrhage and oedema, tears of the iris or lens, retinal detachment and damage to the optic nerve. If damage has occurred to the aqueous drainage system, the pressure in the eye may rise, causing glaucoma. If the lens is involved, a cataract may develop. Most ocular tissue has very little or no regenerative ability. A minor injury may be extremely painful, because the surface of the cornea is very sensitive to pain. But a deeper wound may cause no pain, be easily overlooked and noticed only when complications arise. Therefore, an injury that would cause only a minor laceration on the body may affect the eye far more seriously and cause blindness.

Children are at special risk from eye injuries because they are less aware of potential dangers and are often fearless in their outlook. They love to experiment and can easily stray into dangerous situations. The injuries sustained by children are usually unilateral and often severe. About one-third of these injuries lead to the loss of an eye, so that more children lose an eye in the first 10 years of life than would happen in any other period in their lives (Roper-Hall 1987). The human eye is protected from trauma by the eyelids and the blink reflex, the lids closing spontaneously if a hazard threatens, and by movement of the head to avoid injury. The eye is also protected by the orbital bones and a surrounding layer of fat, but the orbit of a child's eyes is also smaller than an adult's, offering relatively less protection.

Emergency admission

On admission the ophthalmologist will see the child immediately. It is essential that an accurate history of the incident be obtained so that no injury is missed. This may prove difficult because young children in particular may not be able to articulate or to recall the circumstances of the injury, and older children may give a vague account of events, wanting to protect themselves or friends from blame.

The ophthalmologist will aim to assess all structures of the eye carefully (Stollery 1997) and then decide how to manage the injury. This may involve an examination under anaesthetic (EUA), immediate surgery to repair the injury or a period of observation. The nursing staff can help facilitate this examination by taking a few minutes to talk to the child in a straightforward way and familiarize him with the consulting room: the slit-lamp and lights; how and why he will have to sit, perhaps on Mummy's knee; why he must sit still. Again, turning this into a game, examining 'teddy' first and using distraction toys, can effectively promote a quick and successful examination, whereas 'muddying the water' by missing out this valuable stage can cause real problems. It is important to give the child and parents a clear explanation of the chain of events at an early stage; they will all require much support and reassurance to lessen stress at this worrying time.

When a child is admitted to the eye ward with a serious eye injury, he will be frightened, quiet and pale, and may vomit. He should be nursed in a quiet, darkened room and encouraged not to rub the affected eye. As his sight has been adversely affected, maintaining a safe environment is crucial, particularly because the child will be relying more on his non-visual senses than usual.

The nurse must observe the eye carefully and immediately report any change to its appearance, swelling, the level of vision, diplopia, an increase in pain or discomfort and any other symptoms. In particular, she must observe and report any change in the child's level of consciousness and pupil reaction, or general condition that may indicate the presence of another injury, particularly a head injury.

The child may need to have a period of bedrest, particularly if a hyphaema (a bleed into the anterior chamber of the eye) has been sustained. Rest will promote absorption of blood and reduce the chance of a re-bleed. The importance of rest may be difficult for a young child to comprehend and it will require a resourceful nurse and family to keep him happy and occupied.

A child in discomfort or pain will be distressed and uncooperative; this must be avoided. Effective analgesia is therefore important and needs close monitoring using the hospital pain assessment tools and analgesia/antiemetic ladders. If the child is comfortable, he will be more relaxed and tolerate treatment better. He may also feel frightened and confused, especially if vision is much reduced or absent, and he will need regular, straightforward, appropriate explanations about what is happening, helped by diagrams and models. He will also need much support and emotional care. It is important that the child be encouraged to be as independent in washing, dressing and eating as his condition allows. Play, which is so vital to children's well-being, can be gently introduced when the child is well enough. This will help normalize a strange and stressful situation for the child and distract him from the more unpleasant aspects of his care.

The child will usually require eyedrops, e.g. antibiotics, steroids and possibly a mydriatic; these may need to be given every hour or two at first. Young children do not like having eyedrops. They may sting and blur vision, and often taste nasty. It often takes much ingenuity on the nurse's part to administer them accurately and without undue distress to the child. Supervising a willing parent may be the best way; distraction techniques and play may help, together with much praise and encouragement. The eye will also require regular gentle cleansing using an aseptic technique; this may be more easily done with a young child if his own teddy has his eye cleaned first.

If the ophthalmologist decides surgery is indicated, preoperative preparation (including psychological preparation) of the child is needed. It is essential to obtain informed consent to surgery from the child, who is often very frightened, and the adult with parental responsibility. It must be accurately established at what time the child last ate and drank, and the required period of starvation observed. The child is then prepared for theatre in the usual way, including applying a local anaesthetic cream, such as Ametop, over veins on the hands before cannulation. Even if time is limited, play therapy using equipment that the child will see (syringe, anaesthetic tubing and mask, plaster, etc.) will help familiarize him with anaesthetic procedure. Time spent in this way is really valuable in helping the child to cope with a stressful situation.

Postoperative nursing care should be followed, as suggested previously, with special attention to the emotional well-being of the child and parent, and regular updates about progress to both child and parent. As the child recovers further, his general hygiene, elimination, nutrition, activity, play and possibly school work also need the attention of the nurse. Boredom should be avoided but sufficient rest taken too.

It is hard for parents to see their child in pain, and they often feel guilty or angry about how the injury occurred, so they too need much sensitive help and support. Such support will include clear and accurate information, reassurance and strategies on how to give the best emotional and physical help to their injured child. They may also need guidance about their domestic situation and the care of any other children at home, who will be worried about their sibling.

As discussed, the care of the child must be talked over with him and his parents so that they can participate in that care at a level with which they are comfortable, bearing in mind the type and nature of the injury, and that they are all upset and worried.

Parents should be encouraged to stay with their child, as far as is practicable, particularly when the child undergoes *any* nursing procedure or treatment, however small. Parents need to be shown ward facilities, offered accommodation and meals, and enough time to rest and look after others of their family.

Before the discharge, the parents must be fully advised about the care of the child at home. Written information can be taken home and referred to, which is helpful for busy parents. Parents should be proficient at cleansing the eye and administering eyedrops and analgesia. They need advice about what kinds of activity, recreation and schooling are appropriate for the child. Parents should also be made aware that, after being in hospital, their child's normal behaviour may well be disrupted, especially after such a traumatic event, but with plenty of love and attention, any 'clinginess' and tearfulness should pass (While and Wilcox 1994). The child himself may feel dispirited and sad, especially if visual loss is permanent, and he will need much sensitive support.

The child who experiences a significant loss of vision, his parents and siblings will need much ongoing practical help and psychological support from the various health agencies. Ongoing support from the hospital and the availability of a telephone number with which to access this will also be welcomed and support groups may be helpful. The child will also be closely followed up as an outpatient. Various charities such as the RNIB have many excellent publications and offer a wide range of help, including websites for children to access support (see Appendix).

Minor trauma

Many children with eye complaints visit the eye A&E or indeed the main A&E department of a hospital without a dedicated eye unit. As discussed above, children are inexperienced individuals, prone to experimentation with all sorts of household and garden objects that they perceive as intriguing and fun to play with. Accordingly, with this spirit of adventure, little children in particular can be injured quickly and easily and a wide range of accidents does happen, including: the child spraying an aerosol into his eye – deodorant, polish, cleaning fluid etc.; scratching the eye with his own – or his friend's or sibling's – finger, a stick or a toy; rough play; a toy or game with mobile pieces that cause injury; pens and pencils scratching the eye; climbing on to furniture or trees and falling; or playing with inappropriate things in the garden.

Foreign bodies can also enter the eye or get trapped under the eyelids (Stollery 1997), e.g. dust or pieces of stick used during play. Trauma sustained to the eyelids is relatively common, because the lids protect the globe of the eye. Commonly, the claws of dogs and cats 'jumping up' to greet the child can lacerate the eye or surrounding area, which may damage the lacrimal system.

It is important to examine the eyes of the child carefully, to establish the nature and extent of the injury. However, this is often easier said than done, because superficial injuries to the eye can be exquisitely painful and often cause the eye to 'water' profusely. So the young child arriving in the department is often fractious, tired and uncomfortable, and unwilling to let anyone near him!

Under these circumstances, it is wisest to attend to the child's basic needs before attempting to examine his eye – if his condition allows. This involves ensuring that he is not overheated in a thick jumper, that he has a drink and a snack if he is hungry (and surgery is not imminent), that he uses the lavatory if needed, and that he is distracted with toys and books while his weary parents are offered a drink, reassured and given an explanation of the management of the child and how they can help. But, perhaps most *importantly*, especially if the child is in pain or discomfort – usually obvious by his body language and challenging behaviour, i.e. crying, grumpy, head down, eyes screwed up and arm shielding face – is to give a simple analgesic, e.g. paracetamol syrup, *first*. The child can then be left to play and get used to his surroundings and the staff and the parents to relax a little. This is time well spent, because it is far more likely that the child will cooperate with the staff once he is comfortable.

Lastly, *before* examination and treatment, it is necessary to sit with the child and explain what is going to happen to him and, thereby, if possible gain informed consent. He must understand exactly what is to happen, particularly if eyedrops are involved (either analgesic drops and/or fluorescein drops to distinguish an abrasion), and what he will feel; encourage him to look at and touch equipment, and see teddy go through it all first! The child should be talked through each step of the examination, to maintain cooperation, by a member of staff who has got to know the child a little and hopefully established some rapport with him. The second person can then more easily carry out the examination.

This whole respectful planned approach, enlisting the help of the child and parent, with the assurance of stickers or a bravery award afterwards, can very often win the child's favour, with the examination being carried out successfully on the *first* attempt and with minimal fuss.

The care of the child in the outpatient department

It is important to remember that a child's referral to the outpatient department may well be his first personal experience of entering a hospital. How he interprets this experience may affect him considerably, so it is vital to make the time as positive and enjoyable as possible. Depending on his age and life experience, he may feel frightened and anxious or, conversely, quite excited about the visit. He and his family will need a sensitive and confident approach from the clinical staff to gain his cooperation and help him feel at ease.

The waiting area should be safe from the many hazards found in a busy department – unlocked cupboards containing urine-testing equipment, chemicals or eyedrops, and wet floors. It should be borne in mind that other people attending the department are often elderly and poorly sighted.

After arriving in the department the child should be addressed by name and the nurse should aim quickly to establish a rapport with him and show interest in him, yet not seek to remove him from his parent(s).

There should be a special, cordoned-off play area and a good supply of toys, puzzles and books suitable for all children's age groups. (There should also be evidence of a regular cleaning and checking programme for the toys.) There should be easy, well-signed access to lavatories and nappy-changing facilities, and a private area for breast-feeding mothers. A nearby snack bar/WRVS canteen will provide a welcome drink and snack for weary families – but care should be taken with people wandering around with hot drinks in their hands and warning signs to this effect should be clearly visible.

The waiting time, for young children in particular, should be kept to a minimum to prevent their becoming bored and miserable. A board with waiting times should be visible and parents kept informed as to any changes. Parents will often have other children with them, and children to collect from school, or be travelling on public transport, so a lengthy wait may make them feel more anxious.

The nurse may be required to assist in recording the visual acuity of the child and help the doctor or orthoptist examine him, with the parent present for support. Before the test or examination begins the child, whatever his age, must be given an explanation about what is about to happen to him. This should be delivered in a language-appropriate way, in short sentences, with clear and straightforward instructions. The child needs a little time to think about what has been put to him and should not be rushed. Involvement of the child may be enough to expedite the examination. If eyedrops need to be given, verbal informed consent must be obtained and 'holding still' techniques discussed with parent and child, should he not be in a cooperative mood The resourceful nurse can often distract the child sufficiently to facilitate the examination by turning it into a game, perhaps with the child's teddy and the use of 'distraction toys' – toys that can immediately capture a child's attention; such toys may be kept in each consulting room. The nurse can also appeal to the child's competitive side by offering him 'fun' stickers and a bravery certificate after the examination! Positive praise and encouragement will also help.

When the doctor speaks to the parents afterwards, especially if it is about a deterioration in the child's condition, or the possibility of surgery, the nurse should be available to take the child aside gently with some toys, so that the parents can listen carefully to what the doctor is saying. Teenagers really value their own opinions and wishes being taken into account and may have many questions to ask. Again, a large model of the eye or large diagrams can help in explaining the condition to families.

The nurse should ensure that the family fully understands what has been said before they leave. They can be given information leaflets on the various eye conditions that are helpful to refer to at home. If their child is to be listed for surgery, the family should be told that they will receive a date for a pre-admission visit, where all the procedures and details will be explained to them, which reassures them.

Contact with, and referrals to, other health professionals may be needed, and this link should be well established in the outpatient department as in any other dealing with children. Information should be passed both to and from the hospital service by all professionals concerned with the care of the child, so that a seamless service can be ensured.

References

Caring for Children in the Health Services (1991) Just for the Day: Children admitted to hospital for day treatment. London: CCHS.

Chandler K (1994) Play preparation for surgery. Surg Nurse 7(4): 14–16.

Dearmun A (1994) Defining differences: children's day surgery. Surg Nurse 7: 7–11.

Deering C, Jennings D (2002) Communicating with children and adolescents. Am J Nursing 102(3): 34–41.

Department of Health (1991) Welfare of Children and Young People in Hospital. London: HMSO.

Department of Health (2003a) Getting the Right Start: National Service Framework for Children in Hospital. Standard for Hospital Services. London: The Stationery Office.

Department of Health (2003b) The Victoria Climbie Inquiry: report of an inquiry by Lord Lambing. Presented to Parliament by Secretary of State for Health Department and for Home Affairs. London: The Stationery Office.

Dix A (2004) Let us play. Health Service J 22: 26–7.

Dorey S, Adams G, Lee J, Sloper J (2001) Intensive occlusion therapy for amblyopia. Br J Ophthalmol 85: 310–13.

Doverty N (1992) Therapeutic use of play in hospital. Br J Nursing 1(2): 77–81.

Evans N (1995) Ophthalmology. Oxford: Oxford University Press.

Feasey S (2000) Quality counts: auditing day-surgery services. J Child Health Care 4: 73–7.

Kelly M, Adkins L (2003) Ingredients for a successful paediatric pre-operative care process. AORN J 77: 1006–11.

Kenyon E, Barnett N (2001) Partnership in nursing care: the Blackburn model. J Child Health Care 5: 35–8.

Khaw P, Shah P, Elkington A (2004) ABC of Eyes, 4th edn. London: BMJ Books.

Kristensson-Hallstrom I (1999) Strategies for feeling secure influence parents' participation in care. J Clin Nursing 8: 586–92.

Kristensson-Hallstrom I (2000) Parental participation in paediatric surgical care. AORN J 71: 1021–9.

McAllister S (2001) Paediatric risk assessment in an adult setting. Nursing Times 97(50): 40–1.

Moore A (2000) Paediatric Ophthalmology. London: BMJ Books.

Nightingale F (1863) Notes on Hospitals, 3rd edn. London: Longmans Green & Co.

Roper-Hall M (1987) Eye Emergencies. Edinburgh: Churchill Livingstone.

Royal College of Nursing (1999) ASC. Report of a Qualitative Study of Children's Pain Experience. Clinical Practice Guidelines. London: RCN.

Royal College of Nursing (2003) Clinical Governance: An RCN Resource Guide. London: RCN.

Royal College of Ophthalmologists (2001) Annual Report. Guidelines for the management of Strabismus and Amblyopia in Childhood. London: RCOphth.

Rushforth H (1999) Communicating with hospitalised children: review and application of research pertaining to children's understanding of health and illness. J Child Psychol Psychiatry 40: 683–91.

Shandor Miles M (2003) Support for parents during a child's hospitalisation. Am J Nursing 103: 62–4.

Shuttleworth A (2003) A health website for children. Nursing Times 99(44): 18–19.

Stollery R (1997) Ophthalmic Nursing, 2nd edn. London: Blackwell Science.

Thornes R (1991) Just for the Say. Caring for Children in the Health Services. London: National Association for the Welfare of Children in Hospital.

Tume L, Bullock I (2004) Early warning tools to identify children at risk of deterioration: a discussion. Paediatr Nursing 16(8): 20–3.

While A, Wilcox V (1994) Paediatric day surgery: day-case unit admission compared with general ward admission. J Adv Nursing 19: 52–7.

CHAPTER TEN

Developments in care in day surgery for ophthalmic patients

MARGARET GURNEY

The trend towards day surgery for ophthalmic patients in the UK has grown rapidly following the development of:

- new technology
- evidence-based practice
- new approaches to local anaesthesia
- changes in the way the NHS delivers care
- the influence of politics
- patient expectations.

Day case is now the norm for many ophthalmic procedures; the following indicates the range of procedures now deemed suitable for day surgery:

- cataract extraction
- strabismus correction
- corneal grafts
- trabeculectomy for glaucoma
- some lid and oculoplastic surgery.
- some vitreoretinal procedures.

The history and context of day surgery in ophthalmic practice

Day-case surgery has a much longer history in the UK than many realize. An early proponent of day-case surgery was Nicholl, a paediatric surgeon who reported regularly to the British Medical Association between 1899 and 1908 on his success with operations on 9000 children as day cases at his Glasgow hospital. Despite this pioneering work day-case surgery was extremely slow to develop in the UK.

An enquiry into the 'Management of the NHS' (the Griffiths Report – Department of Health and Social Security 1983) identified an urgent need to reform the NHS in order for it to become a more effective service able to meet the challenges of the twenty-first century. One area identified as needing urgent review was the length of time people stayed in hospital before and after surgery for routine procedures.

This was followed by a number of studies in the early days from the Audit Commission (1990, 1991) and the NHS Management Executive (1991). An investigation into the provision of day-case surgery (Audit Commission 1990) identified that at least 40% of ophthalmic operations could be undertaken as day cases. When the Audit Commission reviewed costs, it estimated in 1990 that a shift in emphasis towards day surgery would save between £10 million and £19 million annually. Day surgery was regarded by health service economists as an opportunity for reducing expenditure and as a method of reducing waiting lists. These studies determined that increased use of day surgery would lead to improved organization in the delivery of care and would be tailored to suit the needs of the individual.

The benefits of day surgery have been well documented as a:

- shorter wait for treatment
- reduced costs
- shorter procedure time
- better postoperative recovery
- minimum waits and cancellations
- higher technical expertise by surgeons and anaesthetists
- less psychological trauma to elderly people and children
- minimum disruption to normal lifestyle
- more holistic nursing care.

A political change in 1997 introduced sweeping changes to the NHS in a 10-year plan of modernization – *A First Class Service* (Department of Health or DoH 1998). This was followed by *Making a Difference* (DoH 1999) which set out to strengthen the contribution of nursing, midwifery and health visiting in a restructured NHS. These documents gave nurses the opportunity to take forward new approaches to care that previously would have been frustrated by our professional partners in care. Ophthalmology services have been greatly influenced by these documents and even more so by the publication of *Action on Cataracts* (NHS Executive 2000) and *The NHS Plan* (DoH 2000), which identified wide areas in ophthalmology that can be better provided by nurses.

Qualitative studies conducted since the move to day surgery have demonstrated very high levels of satisfaction with it. In a survey by the Audit Commission (1991) over 80% of respondents reported that they preferred day surgery and would recommend it. More recent studies by Law (1997) and Otte (1996) continue on that theme but found that there was still a lot of work to be done in the area of giving information in the right manner and in alleviating patient anxiety.

Throughout the country day-surgery units were being set up to cope with the increasing demand. Although there were many positive reports at first, it soon became evident that this change in culture had raised a number of issues in relation to the quality of care and nurse–patient contact time.

Markandy and Platzer (1994) expressed concern that reports such as those by the Audit Commission (1990, 1991) ignored the role of nurses in patient selection and pre-assessment. These reports focused on cost-effectiveness and efficiency, whereas Markandy and Platzer (1994) identified areas of concern such as patient anxiety, information giving and education. The reduced contact time between nurse and patient meant that clearly defined roles for nurses were needed in order to maintain quality in nursing care.

Day-case ophthalmic surgery

Cataracts and strabismus operations were the first operations to be identified as suitable for day-case admission. Reports discussing the merits of day-case ophthalmic surgery by Gregory and Lowe (1991) and Smith (1993) indicate that patients displayed high satisfaction levels. In addition, research by Strong et al. (1991) on the clinical effectiveness of an ophthalmic day surgery unit (ODSU) demonstrated that a carefully planned service could deliver an increased throughput of patients with improved quality of care and outcomes cost-effectively. This model formed an example of good practice that was drawn on by other ophthalmic departments wishing to change.

Cataracts form the bulk of day-surgery ophthalmic procedures, so the issues arising from this are discussed in some depth.

Action on cataracts

The implications for ophthalmology in the UK changed dramatically in February 2000 with the publication of *Action on Cataracts* (NHS Executive 2000). This guidance to good practice set out to reduce the very long waits that were occurring for patients needing cataract surgery; worst case scenarios were patients waiting as long as 2 years.

A new model of care was proposed that aimed to:

• reduce the wait for outpatient appointments
• make surgery more accessible

- reduce the number of visits to hospital
- introduce an integrated pathway of care
- provide a booked admissions project
- streamline the role of the nurse in pre-assessment and pre- and post-operative care.

Large sums of money were made available to enable ophthalmic departments to introduce the necessary changes. This theme of streamlined care is echoed in ophthalmic settings everywhere, with the realization of the possibilities of day surgery. Whatever model is chosen, however, it must ensure that although the patient's journey is streamlined, patient care is not compromised, remembering that most day-care ophthalmic patients are elderly, and many are frail with concurrent medical conditions. They may need to take things rather more slowly than models of streamlined care allow.

For many patients with ophthalmic conditions, however, day surgery is preferable to inpatient surgery for all the reasons identified and gives satisfaction to all the staff involved in its delivery. There appear to be huge benefits to service providers and patients alike and these are well demonstrated by the NHS Centre for Reviews and Dissemination (1996) and Cooper (1996). Qualitative studies by De Jesus et al. (1996), Law (1997), and Heseltine and Edlington (1998) have all identified that patient satisfaction is high.

Changing the model of care

Early models of ophthalmic day care were seen to be protracted, e.g. the pathway in Figure 10.1 was the traditional pathway model adopted when day-case ophthalmic surgery was introduced. This was a long drawn-out process and was a service-focused model rather than a patient-focused one.

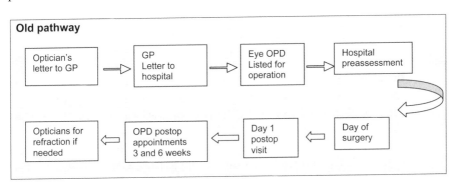

Figure 10.1 Old pathway for model of care for ophthalmic day-care surgery. OPD, outpatient department.

With the introduction of *Action on Cataracts* (NHS Executive 2000) and a streamlined pathway, clinicians are required to spend less time than ever on patient assessment and care. Criteria for day surgery vary wildly and, in order to enhance throughput and fulfil targets for day-surgery rates, they have often changed to allow more vulnerable patients access to day surgery. Although this is not necessarily a bad thing, packages of care must be in place to ensure that day surgery works for the patient rather than just for the ophthalmic unit.

In the more modern day-surgery pathway, it is possible to see how short the contact time has become (shown in Figure 10.2).

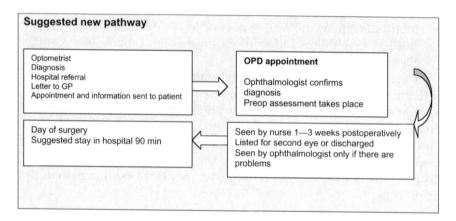

Figure 10.2 Suggested new pathway for model of care for ophthalmic day-care surgery. OPD, outpatient department.

The role of the nurse in pre-assessment

Nursing practice is influenced greatly by the need to concentrate on the clinical suitability of patients, to the extent that emphasis was placed in this area rather than on therapeutic nursing interventions. In a study on approaches to pre-assessment, Cahill (1998), like previous researchers, identified flaws in the quality of information delivery and management of anxiety.

Ideally *Action on Cataracts* (NHS Executive 2000) wants one-stop cataract clinics that combine diagnosis and preoperative assessment. Ophthalmic nurses are now the pivotal point in the pre-assessment of patients for day-case surgery. Many patients have their entire assessment carried out by ophthalmic trained nurses and the appointment usually occurs 2–3 weeks before surgery. Each ophthalmic unit will have developed its own criteria and protocols, which reflect the organization's philosophy and the needs of the population that it serves. In particular there will be different criteria for patients having general or local anaesthesia (Table 10.1).

Table 10.1 Common criteria for ophthalmic day surgery

Inclusion criteria
Patient must want day surgery
Patient must be able to understand the self-care that is expected
Patient must have access to a telephone
Patient must be able to lie still for the required operative period
Patient must have transport arranged if necessary
Patient must have someone at home if surgery is under general anaesthesia

Exclusion criteria
Patients with complex health problems
Patients with body mass index (BMI) > 36 if having general anaesthetic
Patients with uncontrolled diabetes
Patients with only one useful eye

The involvement of anaesthetists on lists adopting local anaesthesia varies across the country. When anaesthetists are involved protocols tend to be less flexible, despite guidance in *Action on Cataracts*. The consequences for patients of not being able to access day-surgery procedures may be a longer wait for surgery. Patients may therefore give false or misleading information to the nurse at pre-assessment to ensure that they fit the criteria. Accurate assessment is therefore the key to safe day surgery.

Assessment of the patient

An ophthalmic nurse with recognized competencies in ophthalmic assessment and examination should carry out the ophthalmic pre-assessment. The timing of pre-assessment varies from hospital to hospital and may be conducted as a purely nurse-led service or may be incorporated into a one-stop clinic involving the ophthalmologist for patients going through a cataract pathway. For other ophthalmic conditions the pre-assessment will generally be 1–3 weeks before surgery.

Traditionally a nursing model of care has formed an intrinsic part of a framework of care, but formalized care pathways and personal constructs are replacing these models. This does not, however, negate the nurse's responsibility to assess and plan the appropriate care for the individual. The use of pathways can make clinicians complacent because they try to fit the patient into the pathway rather than adjusting the pathway to suit the needs of the patient.

It is easy to assume, when pre-assessing, that patients already know why they have come to the clinic, but it is surprising how many people do not understand what their ocular problem is. Patients with complex conditions, such as those with oculoplastic or vitreoretinal problems, have often not had their eye problem explained to them comprehensively or have not understood or remembered the information, so time will need to be set aside for explanation before full assessment begins. Many patients with a cataract may still be unaware of their actual problem. Although assessing planning and implementing care is a core nursing activity, it is useful to have guidelines to follow when assessing suitability for ophthalmic day surgery.

Pre-assessment considerations

General

The patient's general mobility and safety are a consideration at all times. Co-existing medical conditions, such as poorly controlled diabetes and frequent hypoglycaemic attacks, might suggest that the patient would be at less risk if an overnight stay were considered (although admission to hospital may also destabilize previously stable situations). Patients who are frail, with no support at home, whose vision in their unoperated eye is poor, so that they might be unsafe at home after their surgery, should also be considered for an overnight stay or robust packages of care must be in place preoperatively to facilitate day surgery.

Many areas now use care pathways in which nursing assessment is reduced to the minimum and focus on general health, medications, allergies, communication, breathing and mobility, so pre-assessment acts as a data collection point from which interventions will be planned.

Unless nurses are prepared to individualize care pathways where appropriate, this minimalist approach fails to recognize that patients are individuals with a variety of needs and may lead to less than optimum care in the very fast pace of the day-surgery setting.

Suitability for local anaesthesia

To be able to achieve successful surgery under local anaesthetic, the patient must be able to lie flat for 30 minutes. A 'trial lie' at pre-assessment may help to confirm this. Patients with Parkinson's disease or uncontrolled head tremor may not be suitable for local anaesthetic and, because of this, a general anaesthetic may be considered.

Learning disability or confusion/dementia may also preclude the use of local anaesthesia. Similarly, the inability to communicate with patients as a result of language barriers, verbal or non-verbal in the case of patients with deafness, may be alleviated by arranging for an interpreter to be present at surgery.

Anticoagulant therapy

Patients on warfarin need an international normalized ratio (INR) < 3.5, so the last result should be reviewed at pre-assessment and checked on the day of surgery. If the last result is within the level, check on the day of surgery. Patients with levels consistently > 3.5 should be discussed with the ophthalmologist, anaesthetist and haematologist if necessary.

Patients needing surgery for oculoplastic problems also need to stop aspirin before surgery and advice needs to be sought for those on other anticoagulants.

Blood pressure

When diastolic pressure is 100 or above the patient should be referred to his or her primary care physician or nurse for a check before admission. Studies suggest that raised blood pressure is not a valid reason for cancelling ophthalmic surgery. However, local policies should be followed if the diastolic pressure remains > 100.

Pulse

An ECG may be indicated if the patient's pulse is irregular or if he or she is bradycardic or tachycardic. If the ECG is abnormal, an anaesthetic opinion should be sought.

Urinalysis

Although it would be most helpful if this were assessed in the primary care setting, before pre-assessment, urinalysis is a good indicator of diabetes, renal function and infection. Findings at pre-assessment, such as blood, nitrates or glucose in urine, should precipitate a referral back to primary care so that these can be investigated further.

Open wounds

Open wounds should be swabbed and cultured, and abnormal results should be managed accordingly.

Haematological investigations

Although there is little evidence of the need for preoperative blood tests before local anaesthesia unless there is a clinical need, anaesthetists undertaking the management of local anaesthesia often require haematological tests. Local policy should therefore be followed but clinicians should endeavour to modify non-evidence-based practices!

Blood tests are indicated in the following circumstances.

Full blood count (FBC)

- Patients with anaemia
- History of alcoholism, liver disease, or on warfarin or chemotherapy
- Haematuria.

Urea and electrolytes (U&Es)

- Patients with diabetes having general anaesthetic
- Multiple drug therapy
- Significant diuretic therapy.

Technical assessment

Many nurses acquired the technical skills of keratometry and biometry when pre-assessment for ophthalmic patients became a fundamental part of care. With a multidisciplinary approach and the growth of one-stop clinics, this is increasingly being undertaken by hospital opticians, orthoptists and technicians.

Clinical governance has also had an impact on who performs keratometry and biometry, as continuous audit reports have highlighted variances in the refractive outcome of patients after cataract surgery. Accuracy is of paramount importance and ophthalmic surgeons are therefore demanding consistency in this skill and prefer specifically identified staff to carry it out.

Slit-lamp examination at pre-assessment

Slit-lamp examination of the patient is essential, because many patients have not been seen for many months. Systematic examination will highlight problems such as blepharitis, dry eyes and any variations in intraocular pressure from previous examinations. Findings should be documented and any necessary health education or treatment requirements can be instigated. The fundus should be assessed at some point before surgery because this may have implications for visual outcome, and the patient needs to know of any changes in the retina (such as age-related macular degeneration) before surgery if at all possible, so that truly informed consent can be given for the surgery and expectations for the visual outcome after surgery are realistic.

Informed consent

The term 'informed consent' is an ethical one that underpins the legal requirement of health professionals to obtain consent for any procedure undertaken on a patient and is valid only if you have explained properly. Clinicians are required to inform patients about the procedure to which they are being asked to agree and to explain the risks, benefits and alternatives available to them. Failure to do this negates the validity of consents and leaves both the patient and health professional in a vulnerable position.

Although it is best for the person carrying out the procedure to obtain consent, this is often delegated to others trained to seek consent for that procedure, such as pre-assessment nurses. It is useful to confirm the 12 key principles of consent (Table 10.2) (DoH 2002).

Table 10.2 Twelve key principles for informed consent: the law in England and Wales

When do health professionals need consent from patients?
1. Before you examine, treat or care for competent adult patients you must obtain their consent.
2. Adults are always assumed to be competent unless demonstrated otherwise. If you have doubts about their competence, the question to ask is: 'Can this patient understand and weigh up the information needed to make this decision?' Unexpected decisions do not prove the patient is incompetent, but may indicate a need for further information or explanation.
3. Patients may be competent to make some health-care decisions, even if they are not competent to make others.
4. Giving and obtaining consent is usually a process, not a one-off event. Patients can change their minds and withdraw consent at any time. If there is any doubt, you should always check that the patient still consents to your caring for or treating him or her.

Can children give consent for themselves?
5. Before examining, treating or caring for a child, you must also seek consent. Young people aged 16 and 17 are presumed to have the competence to give consent for themselves. Younger children who understand fully what is involved in the proposed procedure can also give consent (although their parents will ideally be involved). In other cases, someone with parental responsibility must give consent on the child's behalf, unless they cannot be reached in an emergency. If a competent child consents to treatment, a parent cannot over-ride that consent. Legally, a parent can consent if a competent child refuses, but it is likely that taking such a serious step will be rare.

Who is the right person to seek consent?
6. It is always best for the person actually treating the patient to seek the patient's consent. However, you may seek consent on behalf of colleagues if you are capable of performing the procedure in question, or if you have been specially trained to seek consent for that procedure.

Table 10.2 continued

What information should be provided?
7. Patients need sufficient information before they can decide whether to give their consent, e.g. information about the benefits and risks of the proposed treatment and alternative treatments. If the patients are not offered as much information as they reasonably need to make their decision, and in a form that they can understand, their consent may not be valid.
8. Consent must be given voluntarily, not under any form of duress or undue influence from health professionals, family or friends.

Does it matter how the patient gives consent?
9. No! Consent can be written, oral or non-verbal. A signature on a consent form does not itself prove that the consent is valid – the point of the form is to record the patient's decision, and also increasingly the discussions that have taken place. Your trust or organization may have a policy setting out when you need to obtain written consent.

Refusal of treatment
10. Competent adult patients are entitled to refuse treatment, even when it would clearly benefit their health. The only exception to this rule is where the treatment is for a mental disorder and the patient is detained under the Mental Health Act 1983. A competent pregnant woman may refuse any treatment, even if this would be detrimental to the fetus.

Adults who are not competent to give consent
11. No-one can give consent on behalf of an incompetent adult. However, you may still treat such a patient if the treatment would be in their best interests. 'Best interests' go wider than best medical interests, to include factors such as the wishes and beliefs of the patient when competent, their current wishes, their general well-being, and their spiritual and religious welfare. People close to the patient may be able to give you information on some of these factors. Where the patient has never been competent, relatives, carers and friends may be best placed to advise on the patient's needs and preferences.
12. If an incompetent patient has clearly indicated in the past, while competent, that he or she would refuse treatment in certain circumstances (an 'advance refusal'), and those circumstances arise, you must abide by that refusal.

It is important to remember that consent is an ongoing process and may be withdrawn at any time. It is advisable to check that consent is still current on the day of admission. It is incumbent on the person obtaining consent to ensure that the individual is competent to consent to treatment.

Educational and psychosocial needs of patients having day surgery

With the decreased time of contact between patient and nurse, it is important that the psychological needs of patients are not overlooked (see also Chapter 6). Research by Mitchell (2002) highlighted the need to manage preoperative information, anxiety and postoperative recovery to a high standard, because care will become less directly supervised in the future. Written and verbal information about the ophthalmic problem and treatment should be given to the patient and any concerns explored fully. Visual presentations such as the use of an eye model or video increase interest and often aid retention of information.

The use of a framework for health education/health promotion such as that of Downie et al. (1992) to enhance patient knowledge and awareness of preventive measures is useful in practice. This model asserts that health education empowers individuals by providing information that helps them develop skills and self-esteem.

One of the most important components of patient education is the teaching of eyedrop instillation. Assessment of the patient's ability to do this is essential because postoperative drops are generally required for several weeks after surgery. If a patient cannot safely perform this or is confused, arrangements need to be made with a relative, carer or district nurse before admission. If practice with drops is required, ocular lubricants could be given under an agreed patient group direction or other appropriate strategy.

Agree the date and time of admission and provide a contact number for patients and relatives should they have any questions. Discharge planning should commence at pre-assessment and any transport or social care needs should be agreed at this time, along with arrangements for district nurse care if required. Follow your local policies in relation to this.

Day of admission

Ideally patients should be given a time of admission that is staggered and convenient to them. Unfortunately this does not happen in many instances. For the convenience of the service and to reduce delay and optimize theatre time, patients for surgery in the morning may all be told to arrive at 07:30 and afternoon patients at 12:30 or 13:00. This causes a number of problems for patients and can increase anxiety levels as some people are waiting 3–4 hours before their surgery.

Provision of a welcoming environment with good facilities will help to reduce the stresses on patients. On admission patients should receive a warm welcome and have their details checked and baseline observations taken and documented, ideally by the nurse who pre-assessed them. Familiarization with the environment is necessary to enhance safety, particularly if there is a significant degree of visual impairment.

Preparation for theatre should follow local policies. Patients having cataract extraction or retinal/vitreoretinal procedures will need dilating drops and the safety of patients following this needs careful attention. For cataract patients it is vital that keratometry and biometry readings are in the notes.

Although cataract pathways are often robust, patients undergoing other types of surgery may not have attended a pre-assessment clinic and this must be taken into account so that they have adequate information and support at this time.

Patients having a general anaesthetic for ophthalmic surgery must have the results of any tests or investigations available with their notes and a check on the last time food or drink was taken. Preoperative fasting remains a contentious issue despite research and best practice evidence, and local policy should be followed.

Intraoperative period

Patients having local anaesthesia often feel vulnerable; to alleviate this many areas adopt the use of therapeutic touch, which can be carried out by the nurse who is caring for the patient or a member of the theatre team. It also provides a communication link for the patient (see Chapter 11).

Postoperative period

The postoperative period after ophthalmic surgery is often very short before discharge; it is therefore important to observe patients carefully. On return to the ward or day-case area after local anaesthesia, patients should be able to recover in a chair and be offered refreshments. Blood pressure and pulse should be taken and documented. Patients who have had general anaesthesia need to recover safely in a bed.

Analgesia and antiemetics should be available if required.

Discharge

Good discharge of ophthalmic patients is imperative and should encompass the following:

- Provision of eyedrops and any oral medications
- Full verbal and written instructions on the actions and any expected side effects of the medications
- Written advice that is relevant and can be easily read and understood

- Advice about return to normal daily activities
- Contact number for any problems or advice
- Outpatient appointment.

Many departments operate a follow-up service by telephone to check on the patient's well-being. This might be felt to be an example of good practice, although the patients should give consent for the call and a convenient time should be arranged.

Outpatient appointment

Previously patients were reviewed the following morning by both the nurses for a 'first dressing' and then by the doctor for clinical review. In most departments this no longer happens and the negative aspect of this is that a valuable teaching point has been lost to nurses. The potential for reassurance on the first postoperative day is also lost at a time when many patients may feel anxious about their ability to look after themselves.

For patients who have had uncomplicated cataract surgery many hospitals have a nurse-led discharge service that sees the patient once and discharges them from hospital care or places them on the waiting list for second eye surgery. Anecdotally this is very successful but as yet no studies evaluating its effectiveness have been published. Patients who have undergone other surgical procedures are generally seen the following day, in either the day-stay unit or the clinic. It is important to ensure that patients/ relatives know this and can attend.

Conclusion

Day-case surgery in ophthalmology has been very successful in reducing the time patients wait for treatment. Innovative ophthalmic nurses who have created new roles in practice to enhance patient care and develop professional practice have driven a large part of that success. It is clear that, to be successful, day-case surgery should be in the best interests of the patient as well as the service and the needs of elderly and frail people must be paramount in this fast-paced setting.

References

Audit Commission (1990) A Short Cut to Better Services: Day surgery in England and Wales. Abingdon: Audit Commission Publications.

Audit Commission (1991) Measuring Quality: The patient's view of day surgery. NHS Occasional paper 3. London: HMSO.

Cahill H (1998) It isn't what you do but the way that you do it: nurse practitioners in day surgery. J One Day Surg 8(3): 11–12.

Cooper JM (1996) Surgical nursing. Development of day case cataract surgery: a literature review. Br J Nursing 5: 1327–8, 1330–3.

De Jesus G, Abbotts S, Collins B, Burvill A (1996) Same day surgery: results of a patient satisfaction survey. J Qual Clin Practice 16: 165–73.

Department of Health (1998) A First Class Service – quality in the new NHS. London: DoH.

Department of Health (1999) Making a Difference – strengthening the nursing, midwifery and health visiting contribution to health and healthcare. London: DoH.

Department of Health (2000) The NHS Plan. London: DoH.

Department of Health (2002) 12 Key Principles of Informed Consent. London: DoH.

Department of Health and Social Security (1983) NHS Management Inquiry. London: DHSS. (Griffiths report.)

Downie RS, Fyfe C, Tannahill A (1992) Health Promotion Models and Values. Oxford: Oxford University Press.

Gregory D, Lowe K (1991) An enhanced role for the ophthalmic nurse. Professional Nurse 1, 43–50.

Heseltine K, Edlington F (1998) A day surgery post-operative telephone call line. Nursing Stand 13(9): 39–43.

Law M (1997) A telephone survey of day-surgery eye patients. J Adv Nursing 25: 355–63.

Markanday L, Platzer H (1994) Brief encounters. Nursing Times 90(7): 38–42.

Mitchell M (2002) Guidance for the psychological care of day case surgery patients. Nursing Stand 16(40): 41–3.

NHS Centre for Reviews and Dissemination (1996) Management of cataract. Effective Health Care 2(3).

NHS Executive (2000) Action on Cataracts: Good practice guidance. London: DoH.

NHS Management Executive (1991) Day Surgery: Making it happen. Value for Money Unit. London: HMSO.

Otte DI (1996) Patients' perspectives and experiences of day case surgery. J Adv Nursing 23: 1228–37.

Smith H (1993) Day release cataracts. Nursing Times 89(39): 29–33.

Strong JP, Wigmore W, Smithson S, Rhodes S, Woodruff G, Rosenthal AR (1991) Day case cataract surgery. Br J Ophthalmol 75: 731–3.

CHAPTER ELEVEN

Ophthalmic theatre nursing

PATRICIA EVANS AND GILL TAYLOR

Patients undergoing ophthalmic surgery enter a stressful and highly technical environment where the outcome of their surgery may have a significant impact on the future quality of their lives. Theatre nurses daily face the challenge of balancing the demand of providing a therapeutic and communicative approach in caring for patients within an increasingly technological environment. The impact of political and economic pressure to meet the demands of 'high-volume, high-quality' surgery (NHS Executive 2000) has increased this challenge. Waterman and Grabham (1995) describe how patients undergoing ophthalmic surgery are in a situation where they are largely dependent on ophthalmic theatre nurses for their safety and well-being. It is during this perioperative phase of treatment that patients experience extreme vulnerability and the need for advocacy is essential (Schroeter 2000). The nurse's role also includes other demands such as risk assessment, managing resources, assisting with the surgical procedures and working within a multiprofessional team.

This chapter identifies the key issues for ophthalmic theatre nursing practice, with an emphasis on risk management and the nurse's role within the multiprofessional team. Professional and technical aspects have been integrated to reflect clinical practice. It has not been possible to address everything in detail, but references for further reading are given where possible to other key texts, articles and websites. The focus is on the day-to-day considerations of practice, which directly affect patients. Further information on the organization and management of the department, legal aspects of operating theatre practice and design considerations can be found in *Brigden's Operating Department Practice* (Clarke and Jones 1998).

The success of the intraoperative phase depends on an accurate and holistic preoperative assessment (see Chapter 10) in identifying potential problems and taking appropriate steps to prevent them. This also maximizes effective use of theatre time and avoids unnecessary cancellations.

The importance of team working, communication and problem-solving is central and threaded throughout the three overall concepts:

1. Principles of patient care in the ophthalmic operating theatre, including the role of the nurse in patient assessment and local anaesthesia.
2. Risk management issues in ophthalmic surgery.
3. Specific nursing considerations of common surgical procedures including the scrub practitioner role.

Principles of patient care in ophthalmic surgical departments

Several points should be highlighted for consideration when caring for ophthalmic surgical patients:

• Patients may be visually impaired as a result of their underlying pathology, the use of miotics or mydriatics, or surgery on the eye with best vision.
• The patient may be anxious as a result of the forthcoming surgical procedure.
• Local anaesthesia is becoming the norm for many adult ophthalmic procedures and the patient is required to keep still for the surgery.
• Day-case surgery is also the norm and therefore timely communication is paramount to support patient safety and continuity of care from assessment through to discharge.

Planning care in the ophthalmic theatre

Preoperative assessment aims to identify and minimize risks, together with patient education to ensure that the patient presents for surgery as fully prepared and fit as possible (Southampton University 2002). The Royal College of Ophthalmologists and Royal College of Anaesthetists (RCOphth/RCA 2001, p. 10) suggest: 'Preoperative assessment is essential to imbue a sense of confidence in the patient and minimize unexpected problems and late cancellation of the procedure.' It is also essential to assess the patient's anxiety level in relation to suitability for local anaesthesia. The assessment process provides the opportunity for information sharing, ensuring that the patient understands not only the surgical procedure and intended outcome, but also what is required from him or her during the local anaesthesia procedure. This should include a realistic explanation of what this experience is like. It is an essential step in gaining informed consent and managing risk. Perioperative visiting by a member of the theatre team may be ideal to support the ongoing nature of assessment and care planning. Crawford (1999) suggests that the aim of visiting is to relieve patients' anxiety and assess patients' underlying medical conditions in order to plan care. It also supports recent trends towards a patient-oriented approach. However, in day-case practice the feasibility of this is controversial (Williams 2002) and the benefit to the patient needs further research. The implementation of rotational working within the patient pathway could encourage better communication and improve the quality of information given to the patient.

Ophthalmic surgical patients are often highly anxious (Katzen 2002), not only because they are undergoing a surgical procedure but also because the success of the surgery may be directly linked to the visual prognosis. 'Sight is the sense over 90% of us say we most fear losing' (Royal National Institute for the Blind (RNIB) 2002, p. 1) and a 'majority of patients embarking on ocular surgery do so to improve their sight in some way' (Dobson 1991, p. 4).

It is an essential element of the ophthalmic theatre nurse's role to make an individual assessment of each patient's level of anxiety on arrival in the department and plan care accordingly within the multiprofessional team. As a result of the short duration of the modern surgical care pathway, this may often be a quick but vital assessment using verbal and non-verbal cues because the patient may have arrived for admission as little as 15 minutes before transfer to theatre.

Anxiety during the perioperative phase can be reduced with the use of therapeutic touch, hand-holding and music (Dobson 1991, Allen et al. 2001, Moon and Cho 2001, Katzen 2002). An individual assessment of each patient's choice should be made, because this may not always be appropriate or appreciated.

As ophthalmic patients are often visually impaired, special care needs to be taken with mobility and communication within the department. An understanding of visual acuity measurements (such as Snellen and perimetry) is a useful preliminary guide to the extent of an individual's visual impairment, but must not be used without consideration of the underlying condition, e.g. patients with macular degeneration may not be able to see facial expression although they may have useful peripheral vision. Theatre nurses should include this in their information gathering during patient handover. Dobson (1991) suggests that care should be taken to introduce self and others, announcing when entering or leaving the room, using touch, explaining noises, not leaving the patient on his or her own and allowing extra time for transfer from the preop area.

Nursing considerations for anaesthesia

Anaesthesia for ophthalmic surgery has become an increasingly complex topic as a result of a wide range of influences: changes in techniques both local and general, the individual patient's needs and expectations, surgical demands and the change in health service provision. Most ophthalmic procedures are carried out under local anaesthesia so general anaesthesia is not covered in this chapter. Advocacy is an essential aspect of the nurse's role and includes accepting responsibility for safeguarding the rights of surgical patients in negotiating a plan for care including the choice of anaesthesia. The *Action on Cataract* document (NHS Executive 2000) identified that 57% of patients having cataract surgery have another medical condition. Of these 30% have hypertension, 18% arthritis and 11% diabetes. Effective communication by the nursing team is essential to identify potential high-risk cases and manage them accordingly.

Table 11.1 shows the specific medical conditions highlighted by the Royal College of Ophthalmologists and the Royal College of Anaesthetists (2001) for consideration with patients undergoing local anaesthetic ophthalmic surgery and the potential problems and actions required to manage these.

Table 11.1 Potential risks associated with local anaesthetic ophthalmic surgery on patients with specific systemic medical conditions and suggestions for managing these risks

Medical condition	Potential risk and management plan
Hypertension	*Risk of expulsive haemorrhage in intraocular surgery*: uncontrolled hypertension should be referred to the GP for management before admission. Check BP before sending for the patient. Ensure patient has taken any antihypertensive medication as normal. Ensure supply of necessary equipment available in the event of an incident and that the scrub nurse is aware of action to take
Myocardial ischaemia	*Risk of angina attack during procedure*: induced by stress and anxiety. Patient should not have surgery within 3 months of a myocardial infarction. Patients should bring any glyceryl trinitrate (GTN) spray to theatre with them. Monitor with ECG and pulse oximetry. Intravenous access available. Ensure that all staff attended regular Basic Life Support (BLS) training. Anaesthetic cover available if required. Nurses should be aware of the controversy surrounding the use of phenylephrine 10% to dilate the pupil in this group of patients and follow local guidelines

Table 11.1 continued

Medical condition	Potential risk and management plan
Diabetes mellitus	*Risk of hypoglycaemic attack during the procedure*: monitor blood sugar level immediately before procedure whether local or general anaesthetic. For patients undergoing local anaesthetic their usual regimen is maintained. Hypostop® gel may be administered if required according to local patient group directives (PGDs)
Anticoagulation therapy	*Risk of bleeding*: ensure recent international normalized ratio (INR) level within therapeutic range before sending for the patient, particularly relevant to orbital/lid surgery
Chronic obstructive pulmonary disease	*Inability to tolerate lying flat and surgical draping covering the face*: check if the patient has practised lying flat before coming to theatre and evaluate findings. Careful positioning of the patient to support breathing and comfort. Ensure adequate O_2 supply under the drape. Monitor with pulse oximeter. Arrange for patient to bring usual inhaler to theatre

Options for local anaesthesia include topical, sub-Tenon's, peribulbar and retrobulbar anaesthetic, with sedation as an adjunct. The percentage of patients undergoing local anaesthesia varies from one unit to another and may be as high as 100% for adult day-case cataract surgery.

For surgery under local anaesthesia the patient's involvement in care is essential and this is facilitated by explanations of what is happening. Ongoing evaluation of how the patient is coping is also important and the care plan may need to be altered in response to changes. Although a thorough explanation should have been given to the patient before arrival in the department, it is beneficial to reiterate the essential points again to ensure comprehension and compliance. This should be brief and carried out with a professional and calming voice to inspire trust and confidence in the patient. Initially, an explanation about attachment of any monitoring equipment and its benefits for safety is recommended and this should be followed by an explanation about the administration of the anaesthetic. The anaesthetic should be administered in a quiet room with the minimum of staff present, i.e. anaesthetist/surgeon and an anaesthetic nurse/operating department practitioner (ODP) (King, cited in Clarke and Jones 1998, p. 95).

Standards for monitoring have been specified by the Royal College of Ophthalmologists and the Royal College of Anaesthetists (2001) and are as follows:

- A dedicated and trained member of staff to take responsibility for remaining in contact with the patient and reporting any adverse events.
- Clinical observation including patient's colour, response to surgical stimuli, respiratory movements and palpation of the pulse.
- Pulse oximetry to detect cardiac and respiratory problems promptly.
- Intravenous access is essential if peribulbar or retrobulbar techniques are used or if sedation is used.

This monitoring should start before the administration of the anaesthesia and continue until the surgical procedure is ended. Depending on the patient's medical condition additional monitoring may be required, such as ECG or blood pressure measurements. This should be indicated in local guidelines.

Table 11.2 Specific nursing considerations with each type of ophthalmic local anaesthesia

Type of local anaesthesia	Nursing implications
Topical: instillation of local anaesthetic drops	Patient's eye will be fully mobile; so vital that patient is given a full explanation of the need to keep both eyes open and still
Sub-Tenon's: anaesthetic placed in potential space between globe and Tenon's fascia surrounding the globe using a blunt cannula	Spring scissors needed to create opening in conjunctiva and Tenon's, local anaesthetic drops are required before start. Provides good anaesthesia and akinesia. This may be a nurse-led procedure (Waterman et al. 2002)
Retrobulbar: a small amount of anaesthetic is introduced behind the globe in the intraconal space	Topical anaesthesia may be used before administration of retrobulbar. The patient may experience discomfort because of pressure during administration. The risk of haemorrhage, perforation of globe and brain-stem anaesthesia is increased because a long sharp needle is used. Close monitoring during and after administration essential (Foss 2001). A Honan's balloon may be used to facilitate diffusion of the anaesthetic agent. This procedure is surgeon or anaesthetist led
Peribulbar: similar to retrobulbar but uses a shorter needle, placing anaesthetic more anteriorly and using more volume	Topical anaesthesia may be used before administration of peribulbar. A Honan's balloon may be used. A small time gap between administration and start of surgery is recommended by Foss (2001). Same risks as retrobulbar so close monitoring is also recommended. This procedure is surgeon or anaesthetist led

Intravenous sedation may be used during local anaesthetic ophthalmic surgery, although this is controversial. Nordlund et al. (2003) recommend the use of light, short-acting sedation, but Katz et al. (2001) showed that the use of intravenous sedation significantly increased the risk of adverse events, with arrhythmia and hypertension being the most common. The guidelines of the Royal College of Ophthalmologists and the Royal College of Anaesthetists (2001, p. 17) say that sedation 'should only be used to allay anxiety and not to cover for inadequate blocks'. This guideline suggests the use of 'conscious sedation', which minimizes the chances of a sleeping patient suddenly waking during surgery and being startled, disoriented and moving (Nordlund et al. 2003).

Once the patient is transferred to the operating theatre an explanation about the skin preparation and draping arrangements should be given. A transparent drape is helpful for claustrophobic patients. It is common practice to elevate the drape away from the patient's mouth and secure it to a pole. An adequate oxygen supply can then be maintained by administrating 35% oxygen via the Venturi system under the drape and the partial oxygen pressure (Po_2) levels can be monitored by the pulse oximeter. Time spent ensuring that the patient is positioned comfortably will also help the patient to keep still. This should not be rushed because it contributes to a successful outcome. Most ophthalmic procedures require the patient to be supine. A pillow placed underneath the knees may be more comfortable and alleviate back strain. Patients should be warned of any sensation that they may experience (Cooper 1999), e.g. fluid trickling down the side of the face after corneal wetting during surgery. Research has shown that most patients will experience some visual stimulation, e.g. bright white light or a kaleidoscope of colours (Murdock and Sze 1994), and the patient may continue to have sensation in the eye (Duguid et al. 1995, Newsom et al. 2001) during the operation. They should be informed how to communicate if assistance is required (Reeves 1993). The procedure may become painful or the patient may need to cough or urinate. It is essential that the 'alarm' mechanism be fully understood by the patient to prevent complications and help the patient feel more in control of the environment (Nordlund et al. 2003).

Risk management and environmental issues in ophthalmic surgery

Risk management is a central part of the ophthalmic theatre nurse's role. Some of the main areas for concern are:

- ventilation
- correct eye/correct patient

* positioning
* infection control
* noise
* using microscopes
* laser safety
* radiation safety
* pharmacological issues
* instrumentation.

Ventilation

Ophthalmic theatres should be designed to the same high specification as other theatres (Clarke and Jones 1998), ensuring that pressure inside the theatre is higher than outside so that air flows in one direction away from the theatre and 20–30 air exchanges occur each hour. At the beginning of each session, the nurse must ensure that this system is working. Adequate checks should be carried out regularly to ensure that the air conditioning system has not been contaminated, e.g. monitoring for contamination, changing filters. There is a lower limit recommendation for ambient temperature in operating theatres, i.e. 18°C, but no upper limit is set currently (Clarke and Jones 1998). Warming blankets may be required even within these limits, particularly for children. Recommendations suggest a 25°C upper limit for staff and patient comfort and infection control reasons. If the system is not functioning the nurse is responsible for taking appropriate action because this is an essential aspect of infection control and safety.

Correct eye/correct patient

The nurse has a professional responsibility to ensure that the correct patient is identified in the reception area according to local guidelines. This should include checking full name, date of birth and hospital number both verbally and against the patient's identity band (National Association of Theatre Nurses or NATN 1998).

The nurse also has a responsibility to ensure that the correct eye is marked and prepared, the type of procedure is identified and the results of any relevant tests are present and that consent has been obtained according to the Department of Health guidelines for consent (DoH 2001).

Positioning

The operating table needs to be very stable, because slight movements are magnified during microsurgery. Care should be taken not to lean against the table, the surgeon's chair or the microscope. The correct position for most ocular surgery is absolutely horizontal, i.e. chin and forehead at the same level or height because fluid will pool if the head is tilted (Foss 2001). The exception to this supine position is during some adnexal procedures when head tilt or reverse Trendelenburg is required to aid haemostasis. Minor adjustments can be made using Gamgee/pillows to ensure patient comfort for the duration of the procedure. Heel support or other equipment may be required to prevent venous stasis in the lower limbs. Access underneath the draping to endotracheal tubes or laryngeal mask airways needs to be considered during positioning for general anaesthetic.

A number of different headrests are available with a variety of different features to aid positioning and surgical access, e.g. Ruebens and Halliday. The operating table may have a head clamp attachment against which the patient can rest his or her head to help keep still.

Infection control

Safety while undergoing ophthalmic surgery is of paramount concern for the perioperative nurse. One major potential problem for every patient who undergoes surgical intervention is that of infection. Intraocular infection (endophthalmitis) is one of the most serious complications after eye surgery and can be devastating for both the patient and the team (Stanford-Kelly 1997). Infection control measures are a team responsibility and good practice aims to minimize potential sources of infection. These will be addressed in relation to the patient, the team and the equipment, including handling technique and universal precautions. Environmental issues have already been mentioned.

The patient's own eyelids and conjunctival flora are a major possible source of wound contamination. The most common causative organism of bacterial endophthalmitis is *Staphylococcus epidermidis*, which is a commensal of the eyelids (Roach 1989). Povidone–iodine antiseptic solution in a 5% dilution (or less) has been proved effective against common commensals of the skin and certain spores (Kent 2000). It is also non-toxic to the eye and is the antiseptic of choice.

Careful draping, taking the time to tuck the patient's eyelashes under the drape, to prevent contamination by the patient's own microflora (Nordlund et al. 2003), will establish a sterile field and prevent contamination from unprepared areas (NATN, 1998, p. 41). It is good practice to use disposable drapes and equipment where possible because of the higher risk of contamination with Creutzfeldt–Jakob disease (CJD) associated with ophthalmic surgery (RCOphth 2002). The ambient air under the drapes can be supplemented with oxygen in a variety of percentages and delivery methods. The potential fire hazard associated with this has been explored (Ho and French 2002) but to date no incident has been reported in the literature.

There is no conclusive evidence relating to best practice for scrubbing and gowning of staff before surgery although the purpose of scrubbing with an antibacterial scrub solution is considered necessary to reduce the micro-organism load on the hands of the surgical team. Each department should have guidelines to provide detail for this procedure (NATN 2000). Foss (2001) suggests that the ideal gloves for ophthalmic surgery should be a non-toxic barrier to cross-infection with touch sensitivity being of particular importance.

Decontamination and sterilization

Special precautions with decontamination and sterilization of equipment are necessary, particularly with regard to CJD, because ocular tissues, in particular retinal and corneal tissue, are thought to be high risk for transmission of this disease (RCOphth 2002). Sterilization is usually defined as the inactivation of all living organisms, but this may need to be reconsidered with the discovery of prions. These proteins are not fully understood, but are thought to be destroyed only by incineration. Where possible ophthalmic surgery now utilizes single-use disposable instrumentation for this reason. Attempts are made to identify high-risk category patients at the time of preoperative assessment. Any non-disposable instruments used during high-risk cases are then taken out of circulation for an undetermined period to prevent any risk of cross-contamination. For latest guidance on practice for non-disposable items readers should access the Department of Health (website at www.dh.gov.uk) and the Spongiform Encephalopathy Advisory Committee (www.seac.gov.uk). Current practice appears to contradict the guiding principle behind universal precautions, which is to assume that everyone is a potential risk and take action accordingly. The potential cost implication of any radical recommendation is enormous and without a sound evidence base current opinion seems to adopt a 'wait-and-see' approach to certain practices.

Before sterilization can start all the instruments used need to be decontaminated. This is defined as the process of cleaning instruments that have a heavy bioburden (American Society of Ophthalmic Registered Nurses or ASORN and Burlew 2002). Decontamination reduces the bacterial load, removes organic material that could interfere with sterilization and, if not removed although killed by the sterilization process, could still cause intraocular inflammation as a result of the presence of endotoxins. Decontamination starts during the surgical procedure after the surgeon hands the instrument back to the scrub nurse. The scrub nurse should manually clean these as soon as possible after use to prevent drying of blood and other organic debris. ASORN recommend that the scrub nurse should rinse instruments between uses in sterile distilled water. It is vital that no water is left on the instrument if the surgeon wishes to place it back inside the eye again. Water damages the corneal endothelium, because it is not an isotonic solution. Rinsing the instrument in irrigation solution such as Balanced Salt Solution (BSS) kept in a syringe for this purpose is usually sufficient. Physiological or 0.9% saline is not recommended for rinsing instruments because it can damage instruments by staining and leaving a saline residue. Decontamination continues in the 'dirty area' after the procedure. Staff involved in manual decontamination need to wear personal protective clothing, goggles and masks as a health and safety measure. This is usually followed by mechanical decontamination using ultrasonic washers.

Several methods for sterilization exist and the most common nowadays is heat, either dry in hot air ovens or wet in autoclaves. Flash sterilization in 'Little Sisters' is no longer recommended, because sterility cannot be proved and their use can encourage bypassing of the decontamination process. Certain ophthalmic instruments cannot withstand autoclaving or are not suitable for other reasons, e.g. small-bore cannulae, and alternative methods are required. Ethylene oxide was traditionally used but has been phased out because of health and safety risks (explosive and toxic to skin and mucous membranes). Incidents of toxic endothelial cell destruction (TECD) and toxic anterior segment syndrome (TASS) have been reported after gas plasma sterilization, which has been used as an alternative to the above methods (Smith et al. 2000, cited by Gimbel and Pereira 2002). TECD is characterized by a profound corneal oedema and opacification within 24 hours of surgery (Duffy et al. 2000). TASS is a non-infectious intraocular inflammation, which occurs after the introduction of a toxic agent intraocularly during anterior segment surgery (Clouser 2004). It should be noted that several incidents of TASS have been attributed to residual detergents left on instruments because of inadequate rinsing after their use in ultrasonic washers or inadequate training of staff in their use (Clouser 2004). Ophthalmic theatre personnel should be aware of these risks and take appropriate action to overcome them.

These issues have led to increased use of single-use items whenever possible. Whichever method of sterilization is used, a recording and tracking mechanism is an essential risk management strategy, to prove sterility of instruments used and identify the cause should any problems arise.

Noise

Noise should be kept to a minimum because sudden patient or surgeon movement could have serious consequences for the surgical outcome (Phillips 1991, Foss 2001). The patient needs to be able to identify the surgeon's voice in order to follow instructions. Whispering should be avoided, because it may be a distraction for both patient and surgeon. A normal tone of voice is preferable and limited to passing on relevant information.

Microscopes

Modern theatres are usually equipped with overhead microscopes, which provide illumination as well as magnification essential for microsurgery. In addition, they are useful for camera attachments for video recording, audit and teaching purposes. Nurses need to be competent in setting up, using and preventing accidental injury when using microscopes. It is good practice to check that the microscope is clean and in full working order and ensure that safety locks are tightened, cabling is not a hazard and the foot controls are waterproof. Most modern microscopes have a built-in filter to protect against ocular damage to the user during laser treatment. Nursing staff need to be aware if the microscope being used has a built-in filter or how to attach a filter if necessary. Sufficient sets of sterile microscope handles should be available.

Care should be taken to reduce the incidence of retinal toxicity from prolonged exposure to the focused light beam (Michels and Sternberg 1990). A skilled and efficient nursing team will facilitate minimum surgery time. Corneal light shielding and reducing the light intensity of the beam will also contribute to preventing toxicity during lengthy procedures. The light beam also increases corneal drying which can be overcome by the application of irrigating solutions or viscoelastic agents to maintain a healthy epithelium and a good surgical view. The use of a Halladay pillow or armrests will facilitate good positioning and prevent tremor when using the microscope. Positioning is also important for the team to prevent back strain.

Lasers

Nursing staff have an important role to play in ensuring good laser practice to prevent hazards to the patient and team. Hill (1998) outlines three potential hazards:

1. The direct beam can damage the eye so appropriate protective eye wear and filters on microscopes are necessary. As a result of the variation in laser wavelength and power, not all safety eye wear is suitable for all lasers. The standards for laser safety eye wear are based on key international standards.
2. Any kind of reflection of the beam can damage the eye so non-reflective surfaces in the surgical field are required for safety.
3. The laser is a fire hazard so regular maintenance and careful storage are important.

The nurse needs to work within local laser safety rules in line with international guidelines and obtain training where required. All staff should be aware of the emergency shutdown procedure. Suitable warning signs at entrance doors and regulation of staff movement are required to avoid accidental exposure. A useful source of advice on laser safety is the National Radiological Protection Board.

Radiation safety

Radiotherapy is used therapeutically in medicine to achieve controlled cell destruction in certain conditions such as malignancies, e.g. malignant melanoma, or to alter wound healing, e.g. pterygium (Foss 2001).

'Brachytherapy' is the term used when the radioactive source is held close to the body to deliver the dose. Ophthalmic brachytherapy is delivered by applying a radioactive plaque to the sclera adjacent to the tumour for a specified period of time. The plaque is applied and removed surgically in the surgical department. Radioactive sources currently in use are ruthenium-106 (plaque) and strontium-90 (less common). Both mainly emit β radiation and therefore do not radiate any great distance. However, they do pose a potential health and safety risk, and certain precautions are recommended for storage, handling and monitoring. The use of radioactive sources in medicine requires a licence, naming the person who has permission to use it. Further information is available from the National Radiological Protection Board (www.nrpb.org.uk). Any centre using radioactive sources should also have 'local rules' in place. Regular training and updating, and safe handling techniques, local radiation protection officers and reporting mechanisms should all be addressed in the local rules. It is the responsibility of each nurse to ensure that she or he is familiar with safe use of radioactive sources.

During insertion and removal of the ruthenium-106 plaque, the scrub team should wear lead aprons and thyroid shields underneath the sterile gowns for protection. The plaque should not be removed from its lead container until ready for insertion. Therefore, the surgeon usually uses a plastic 'dummy' to prepare the area before insertion. Once the plaque is in place, regular monitoring of its presence and position using a Geiger counter is recommended. The scrub team should never handle the plaque directly with fingers, but only with plain plastic forceps. The plaque has an inner concave area, which is the main radiation emission site. The silver outer convex surface absorbs 95% of the beam so the plaque should always be handled with this side facing the user, to further reduce the likelihood of any radiation.

Careful documentation to track plaque usage is required. A lead eye shield should be applied over the eye dressing at the end of the insertion and a Geiger counter should accompany the patient to the ward afterwards. The ruthenium-106 plaque is a reusable silver button. The issue of sterilization is controversial. It is suggested that any micro-organisms will be destroyed by the radioactivity. However, this does not address the need for decontamination to prevent build-up of biomaterial which, although it may not be capable of causing infection, may act as an allergen.

Pharmacological issues

There are several important points to remember about pharmacological agents and fluids used in ophthalmic theatres. Two main points are stressed when using drugs and fluids during ocular surgery. First, preparations with preservatives should not be used inside the eye because of the risk of damage by toxicity. Second, fluids used inside the eye should be isotonic and preferably buffered.

Specifically designed intraocular irrigating fluids and viscoelastic agents have been developed to help maintain stable intraocular pressure and the anterior chamber during intraocular surgery, thus preventing haemorrhage and damage to the corneal endothelium. (The corneal endothelium has no regenerating properties and severe damage leads to loss of the essential 'pump mechanism' that maintains corneal fluid balance and therefore transparency.) These solutions are isotonic in that they mimic the balance of salts within the aqueous. If the fluid used is not isotonic an imbalance can occur between the ocular cells and the fluid. Fluid and electrolytes may cross cells' semipermeable membranes in an attempt to achieve a balance, and the cells may be destroyed as a result. Certain salts are added such as potassium and calcium to help maintain this balance and keep ocular tissue alive. Buffers are usually also added because the effect of a change in pH can be just as damaging. Common buffers used are lactate (in Hartmann's solution) and acetate or citrate (in BSS). A new intraocular irrigating solution should be used for each patient. Additives should not be used with the exception of adrenaline (epinephrine) to BSS for phacoemulsification surgery or Hartmann's solution for vitreoretinal surgery if the surgeon requests it to maintain mydriasis.

Viscoelastics have all the properties of fluids, making them easy to manipulate, and one of the advantages of solids, in that they can provide support. They are very useful during intraocular surgery to help the anterior chamber to retain its shape when the globe is opened by the creation of a surgical wound. It should be remembered that these agents need to be removed at the end of the surgery because they have been implicated in causing raised intraocular pressure postoperatively (Berson et al., cited in Noecker and Golightly 1999).

Some cytotoxic agents may also be used during ophthalmic surgery such as trabeculectomy to alter the healing process and reduce scar formation (see 'Nursing implications during glaucoma surgery' for more detail).

Further information is available in Foss (2001), Noecker and Golightly (1999) and McCoy (1992). Nurses should follow their own hospital protocols and the Nursing and Midwifery Council's *Guidelines for the Administration of Medicines* (NMC 2000).

Care and handling of microsurgical instruments

Microsurgical ophthalmic instruments have specific care requirements regarding their storage, handling, cleaning, inspection, testing and protection of delicate tips (ASORN 2002 for further details). Nursing considerations involve several safety measures. Cannulae should be checked as primed and patent before handing over. Luer-Lok connections are recommended to prevent accidental trauma. Avoid drawing up solutions until just before needed and use sterile sticky labels attached to each syringe to prevent misidentification of contents (Dobson 1991). During the case, instruments should not be wiped with gauze or towels because this may damage the instruments and leave fibres in the operative site.

Instruments should be passed with the working tips downwards and placed in the surgeon's hand ready for use, alleviating the need to look up from the microscope eyepieces. Extra care needs to be taken with tips and sharps because several ophthalmic procedures are carried out in a darkened room. Effective use of a tray system enables the scrub nurse quickly to locate the required instrument and maintain safety. Local protocols should be followed regarding the counting of instruments and swabs.

Specific nursing considerations of common ophthalmic surgical procedures

Cataract surgery

Phacoemulsification accounts for 77% of all cataract operations in the NHS (RCOphth 2001) and Foss (2001) states that it is now the preferred technique for cataract surgery. The Royal College also outlines the indications for cataract surgery, which includes lens opacity sufficient to compromise the patient's quality of life. There may be other indications for cataract surgery such as treating lens-induced ocular disease or facilitating treatment.

Phacoemulsification surgery uses ultrasonic waves delivered via a small needle vibrating at high speed to emulsify and aspirate the lens matter. This is combined with an irrigation system, which helps maintain the anterior chamber and cool the needle tip. This system allows for the removal of the cataract and replacement with an intraocular lens through a small incision, which means less leakage of irrigation fluid and increased anterior chamber stability. It also greatly reduces the incidence of postoperative astigmatism, because the wound is generally self-sealing.

Specific nursing implications during cataract surgery

Several phacoemulsification machines are available. All machines provide an irrigation, aspiration and emulsification facility, which needs to be regulated in order to maintain the anterior chamber. The nurse should understand the interrelationship of the following three factors and how they can be varied:

1. Infusion pressure
2. Vacuum setting
3. 'Phaco' tip size.

To achieve aspiration, vacuum is provided by either a peristaltic pump or a Venturi pump. These use different physical principles and have various pros and cons. Some modern machines combine the two types (for more detailed discussion, see Hope-Ross 2003). The nurse's role is to ensure that the machine is primed and ready for use when required and to be familiar with the various features of the machine being used in order to be able to troubleshoot in the event of a problem. The scrub nurse should also monitor the volume of fluid in the infusion bottle and arrange for this to be replaced when running low.

The aim of cataract surgery is to improve the patient's vision to within 0.9 D of the intended refractive outcome (RCOphth 2001). Several factors contribute to achieving this outcome, not least of which is that the correct intraocular lens (IOL) is implanted at the time of surgery. The scrub nurse should check the patient's notes for biometry results and confirm the chosen IOL with the surgeon immediately before the start of surgery and again before insertion. An understanding of refraction and what the intended refractive outcome is, will ensure that the correct IOLs are in stock. It will also ensure that the nurse understands the importance of making adjustments to the IOL power using a lens with a different A constant.

By being very familiar with the steps in the procedure the scrub nurse can contribute to reducing the length of the surgical procedure. This will benefit the patient's comfort and safety but also help prevent retinal toxicity from prolonged exposure to the microscope lights. The scrub nurse should also be familiar with the equipment needed if the procedure is converted to extracapsular cataract extraction or if anterior vitrectomy is required in the event of a rupture in the posterior capsule (for more detail, see Foss 2001, Wadood and Dhillon 2002).

Glaucoma procedures

Since the introduction of a more effective range of medical treatment, fewer glaucoma-filtering procedures are being performed. However, the ones that are performed are often more complex and patients are totally dependent on the success of the surgery. The nurse should have an understanding of the criteria used for individual assessment of the risk of failure and the strategies used to overcome these intraoperatively, including whether or not antimetabolites are to be used.

The procedure of trabeculectomy creates an internal drainage fistula for aqueous fluid. This is combined with the creation of a drainage bleb under the conjunctiva to provide resistance to the new aqueous exit route, and allowing for reabsorption back into the circulation. The purpose of the operation is to lower the intraocular pressure for patients with open-angle glaucoma.

Several techniques have been described. Wound-healing agents are commonly used in conjunction with this procedure to prevent the newly created drainage fistula from healing over. 5-Fluorouracil (5-FU) and mitomycin C are the two most common agents used in patients who have been identified as at high risk of failure from scarring. The usual precautions when handling cytotoxic drugs apply: masks, eye protection and gloves. Ideally these drugs should be pre-packed in a laminar flow set-up, but this is not always feasible because the dosage varies. Local policies should be drawn up for the safety of patients and staff. Particular care needs to be taken with counting swabs, where these are soaked in an antimetabolite and inserted over the sclera. These should be counted on insertion and removal and the application time monitored. The cytotoxics are always administered before the paracentesis and washed away with lots of fluid to ensure that none gets into the anterior chamber. The 'run-off' needs to be soaked up using a paper towel and disposed of in a cytotoxic bin. A separate trolley is necessary if cytotoxics are being used, in order to prevent accidental introduction of the cytotoxic into the anterior chamber after the paracentesis has occurred. This would be catastrophic, leading to destruction of cells inside the eye. Where possible, only disposable equipment should be used on this trolley. If any reusable items are used, they should be clearly labelled and handled accordingly during the decontamination and sterilization procedure.

Trabeculectomy surgery may be carried out in combination with cataract surgery as either a 'one-site' or 'two-site' procedure. The two conditions frequently coexist and fistulizing surgery can speed up the development of a cataract (Hitchings 2000).

Tube surgery may be carried out in a selected group of patients in whom trabeculectomy surgery is inadvisable. This involves the insertion of a silicone tube into the anterior chamber, which is connected to a plate anchored to the sclera under the conjunctiva. This allows for aqueous to pass down the tube and be reabsorbed into the circulation.

Finally, destruction of the ciliary body with a cyclodiode laser may be used for selected cases such as patients with little useful vision where previous medical therapy or filtering surgery has failed. Laser safety guidelines and postoperative management of pain are important nursing considerations. Migdal (cited in Hitchings 2000) suggests the use of steroid injection to control pain after treatment.

Squint

The main aim of squint surgery is to restore alignment of the visual axis, and if possible to restore binocular single vision and ensure that both eyes work together. Surgery will involve the repositioning of one or more of the extraocular muscles to straighten the eyes.

Surgery on the extraocular muscles may involve a variety of different techniques to alter the action of the muscles. Pfeifer and Scott (2002) suggest that the action of a muscle can be weakened, strengthened or transposed using different procedures according to the outcome required.

Weakening procedures

The most frequently performed procedure to reduce the action of a muscle is that of a recession, whereby the muscle is cut at its point of insertion and reattached with sutures at a measured distance posterior to the original insertion. This will reduce the tension of the muscle and may be documented in the notes as a minus sign in front of the distance in millimetres of the muscle recession.

Other weakening procedures include partial-thickness Z incisions on each side of the muscle tendon, without disinserting the muscle. This effectively lengthens the muscle, thereby reducing its action.

Strengthening procedures

The most common method of strengthening a muscle is a resection. The muscle is disinserted and shortened by excising a measured amount, and reattached with sutures back to its original point of insertion. This strengthens its action and is documented as a + sign in front of the amount to be resected. A muscle action can also be strengthened by advancing its point of insertion anteriorly, nearer to the limbus, thus strengthening it.

One other type of muscle surgery is to transpose the muscle in order to alter its field of action rather than a strengthening or weakening procedure. This shifts the muscle insertion up or down by half to one insertion width along the original axis. This procedure is used to correct A and V pattern deviations.

Specific nursing implications during squint surgery

Each patient must be assessed individually by the multiprofessional team beforehand and the theatre nurse must check that results are available from the different tests and investigations, i.e. by orthoptists, optometrists, paediatricians, neurologists and ophthalmologists. As it is estimated that up to 5% of all children have some degree of squint (Nickerson 2002), it is a relatively common paediatric ophthalmic procedure and requires a family-centred approach to planning care. The parents will need to be carefully prepared together with the child for a stress-free visit to the operating theatre. The surgery should be carefully explained and the family made aware that more than one operation may be necessary. Any allergies to medications or previous anaesthetic problems should be noted.

By being very familiar with the steps in the procedure the scrub nurse can be ready with the correct equipment to aid the smooth progress of the surgery and assist with holding muscle hooks, etc. The procedure may involve surgery on both eyes because the muscles work together in pairs to allow coordinated movement – so altering the action of one muscle will have an effect on the other. It is not necessary to have separate trolleys set up for a bilateral operation, because this is an extraocular procedure. Two drapes and bilateral skin preparation are required.

The most popular suture currently used is a double-ended, 6/0 Vicryl on a quarter circle spatulated needle, to control the depth of the suture. The scrub/assistant nurse will need to ensure that the suture is cut and mounted on the needleholder (one forehand and one backhand) before holding the squint hook, because this is a difficult single-handed manoeuvre. If an adjustable suture is used for an adult patient, the suture should not be cut but left double ended. This will be tied in a bow for alteration when the patient is awake enough to cooperate.

One final consideration during squint surgery is the oculocardiac reflex, which occurs when there is traction on orbital structures, the conjunctiva or the extraocular muscles. This reflex produces hypotension, which results in decreased cardiac output (Gavaghan 1998), leading to bradycardia and even asystole. This needs to be reported to the surgeon and the surgery halted until cardiac output is restored.

Vitrectomy

There are four main indications for vitrectomy surgery (Nunn 1996):

1. To clear the media, e.g. vitreous haemorrhage, inflammatory debris.
2. To gain access, e.g. to remove epiretinal membranes, foreign bodies or dropped nucleus.

3. To create a space, e.g. for gas, air or oil being used as tamponade.
4. To relieve traction, e.g. proliferative vitreoretinopathy/proliferative diabetic retinopathy (PVR/PDR).

Modern vitrectomy surgery uses the single-function, three-port, 20- or 25-gauge system. Access to the posterior segment via three sclerotomies is created with a 20- or 25-gauge blade. These ports allow access for the following:

• An infusion of either BSS or Hartmann's solution under the force of gravity and atmospheric pressure in order to maintain the intraocular pressure
• A fibreoptic light source to illuminate the surgical site
• Instrumentation, e.g. cutter, scissors, forceps, etc., depending on the requirement for the surgery.

A range of magnifying lenses is available, which are positioned on or over the cornea to improve the view. The scrub nurse may act in an assisting capacity to hold a contact lens in place during the procedure.

Specific nursing implications during vitreoretinal surgery

The nurse's role includes ensuring that the vitrectomy machine is primed and ready for use when required, and to be familiar with the various features of the machine being used, in order to be able to troubleshoot in the event of a problem. Training of new staff and regular updates will facilitate this.

Careful handling and positioning of the instruments, sharps, plugs and other equipment is particularly important because the surgery may be carried out in a darkened environment.

Monitoring intraocular fluid use, the types used, infection control (e.g. CJD), maintenance of intraocular pressure and addition of drugs – are important considerations for the nurse.

Health and safety issues relating to the use of ophthalmic lasers, cryotherapy equipment, and gas and heavy liquid also need careful consideration. The nurse needs to work within local and national policy guidelines, e.g. ensuring appropriate safety filters are in position on the microscope during laser use. The use of long-acting insoluble gas, e.g. sulphur hexafluoride (SF_6), as an internal tamponade, should be discussed with the anaesthetist, because there is a risk that nitrous oxide used as part of the anaesthetic will cause the gas bubble to expand and be detrimental to retinal circulation.

Lid surgery

The main function of the eyelids is to protect the globe from injury and excessive light (Snell and Lemp 1998). The lids also spread the tear film over the surface of the globe to lubricate it and they assist in the drainage of the tears through the puncta. Many different surgical techniques have been described to treat pathologies affecting the lids (see Collin 1989 for more detail). A good understanding of normal anatomy and physiology greatly assists understanding of the procedure being carried out and the intended outcome. Lid surgery also encompasses surgery to the lacrimal system and orbital structures. Therefore, the topic is too complex for detailed discussion in this chapter and only general nursing considerations are included.

Specific nursing implications during lid surgery

The anatomy of the eyelid is quite complex. Surgical 'identification of the landmarks' is made simpler if the patient is conscious during the surgery. Asking the patient to look up and down during the procedure helps identify structures and assists in predicting the final position of lids after the surgery. Therefore, most lid surgery is carried out on a conscious patient with sedation in certain circumstances and analgesia as required. See Table 11.2 for further detail.

Prepping generally involves cleaning the whole face with the selected antiseptic solution, followed by draping the patient's head and hair turban style. A separate drape is used to cover the patient's chin, neck and upper torso.

The reverse Trendelenburg or head-up position is commonly employed, while the surgical team stands throughout the procedure allowing flexibility in movement. This position has the added advantage of contributing towards haemostasis, although diathermy should also be set up and available at the start of the procedure. Lid surgery does not require the use of a microscope and so following the steps of the procedure on a video monitor is not routinely possible. The scrub nurse needs to ensure close positioning to the operating team in order to follow the procedure carefully and predict the surgical requirements.

Several types of suture material and needles may be required, e.g. for traction, muscle and skin closure, and it is recommended that the scrub nurse should discuss in advance what the surgeon's particular preference is. Careful counting of sharps and swabs is essential.

The eyelids have a rich blood supply from branches of the palpebral arteries (Collin 1989). As a result, surgery can cause swelling and bruising of the lid postoperatively. To minimize or prevent this a pressure bandage is usually applied at the end of surgery. The scrub nurse will require padding, e.g. gauze swabs for the dressing, and elasticated tape is preferable for increased tension. If bilateral lid surgery has been carried out, both eyes will be pressure bandaged leaving the patient sightless. Careful preoperative assessment and planning are required to ensure that the patient is fully aware of this and that coping measures are in place for the duration. In addition, if the procedure involves opening the orbital septum there is an increased risk of haemorrhage into the orbit, with the devastating possibility of blindness as a complication in 1:100 000 cases (Foss 2001).

Enucleation

This procedure may be carried out to remove a painful blind eye, for a malignant tumour or after severe trauma. It involves removal of the globe with a small portion of the optic nerve, leaving the conjunctiva and extraocular muscles behind. An orbital implant (hydroxyapatite) is usually inserted to restore lost volume in the socket and provide a good cosmetic appearance. The extraocular muscles are sutured to this and the conjunctiva closed. A retrobulbar injection of Marcain® (bupivacaine) is useful to control postoperative pain in the initial recovery period. A temporary conformer shell (size A–F) is inserted to maintain the shape of the eyelids, and a pressure dressing is applied.

For this group of patients a preoperative visit by the theatre nurse is recommended in order to reduce stress, allay anxiety, and provide patients with relevant information and reassurance that pain and nausea will be managed effectively in the postoperative period. One of the greatest fears many patients have, according to Hehir (2000), is that the wrong eye will be removed. For this procedure it is the doctor's responsibility to obtain informed consent and mark the eye carefully. The nurse will also carry out a number of checks before the patient arrives on the operating table.

There are two other different methods that may be used to remove an eye depending on the underlying pathology and individual circumstances. An evisceration procedure may be indicated after trauma, for a blind painful eye or in severe infection to prevent sympathetic ophthalmia. This technique involves scooping out the entire intraocular contents, leaving a scleral shell and the muscle attachments intact. Particular care is taken to ensure removal of all the uveal tissue. The surgeon may require an irrigation system for this. The postoperative management is the same as for an enucleation procedure.

An exenteration procedure, which is the most radical of all forms of eye removal, is generally indicated in the case of malignancy and therefore requires careful perioperative planning. An exenteration involves removing all the soft tissue of the orbit, including the eyeball, retrobulbar tissue and eyelids. In certain cases it may be possible to split the lids above the tarsal plate and retain sufficient skin to line the orbit. The patient may require further plastic reconstructive surgery.

The theatre nurse needs to ensure that any specimens taken are carefully labelled, recorded and sent to the appropriate department.

Keratoplasty

The replacement of a patient's cornea with donor corneal tissue is known as keratoplasty or corneal graft. This may be full thickness (penetrating keratoplasty) or partial thickness (lamellar keratoplasty). There are four main indications for a penetrating keratoplasty (Foss 2001):

1. To improve vision lost as a result of loss of corneal transparency
2. To relieve discomfort caused by a damaged corneal surface, e.g. bullous oedema
3. To eliminate infection (rare, e.g. fungal)
4. To seal a perforation.

Both types are preferably performed under general anaesthetic to provide a more controlled surgical environment, especially with penetrating keratoplasty where the eye is completely open for some of the procedure (open-sky technique).

Specific nursing implications during penetrating graft surgery

The nurse should check that donor cornea is available and has been cleared for use before sending for the patient. Clearance currently includes testing of the donor for human immunodeficiency virus (HIV) and hepatitis B and C. Careful review of the donor's history to reduce the risk of CJD transmission and an assessment of the suitability of the donor tissue should be completed. Careful documentation of donor and recipient is required.

Generally the patient's pupil should be constricted preoperatively to protect the intraocular structures. Structural support for the globe may be compromised when the whole cornea is removed, especially in aphakic and myopic patients. The surgeon may require a Flieringa ring. This is a stainless steel ring that can be sutured onto the sclera a few millimetres from the limbus, to prevent globe collapse or corneal edge distortion. Right- and left-sided scissors may be used (graft scissors) and a range of different sized trephines and Super Blades should be available, which are used to cut the surface layers of the patient's cornea and the corneal donor 'button' to size.

The scrub nurse should ensure that the donor material is positioned securely and safely on the scrub trolley until it is required. Handling of the donor material should be restricted to the surgeon only, to reduce the risk of accidental damage to the corneal endothelium.

References

Allen K, Golden LH, Izzo JL et al. (2001) Normalisation of hypertensive responses during ambulatory surgical stress by perioperative music. Psychosom Med 63: 487–92.

American Society of Ophthalmic Registered Nurses, Burlew J (2002) Care and Handling of Ophthalmic Microsurgical Instruments. Iowa: Kendal/Hunt Publishing Co.

Clarke P, Jones J (eds) (1998) Brigden's Operating Department Practice. Edinburgh: Churchill Livingstone.

Clouser S (2004) Toxic anterior segment syndrome: How one surgery center recognised and solved its problem. Insight XXIX(1): 4–7.

Collin JRO (1989) A Manual of Systematic Eyelid Surgery, 2nd edn. London: Churchill Livingstone.

Cooper J (1999) Teaching patient in post-operative eye care; the demands of day surgery. Nursing Stand 13(32): 42–6.

Crawford B (1999) Highlighting the role of the perioperative nurse – is preoperative assessment necessary? Br J Theatre Nursing 9: 309–12.

Department of Health (2001) Reference Guide to Consent for Examination or Treatment. London: DoH.

Dobson F (1991) Perioperative care of the visually impaired. Br J Theatre Nursing July: 4–9.

Duffy RE, Brown SE, Caldwell KL, Lubniewski A (2000) An epidemic of corneal destruction caused by plasma gas sterilization. Arch Ophthalmol 118: 1167–77.

Duguid IG, Claoue CM, Thamby-Rajah Y, Allan BD, Dart JK, Steele AD (1995) Topical anaesthesia for phacoemulsification surgery. Eye 9(part 4): 456–9.

Foss AJE (2001) Essential Ophthalmic Surgery. Oxford, Butterworth-Heinemann.

Gavaghan M (1998) Cardiac anatomy and physiology: a review. AORN Online 67: 802–22.

Gimbel HV, Pereira C (2002) Advances in phacoemulsification equipment. Curr Opin Ophthalmol 13: 30–2.

Hehir M (2000) Removal of an eye: Who cares? A nursing perspective. Ophthal Nursing 4(3): 8–11.

Hill PD (1992) Lasers and theatre nursing. Br J Theatre Nursing suppl: S18–19.

Hitchings R (ed.) (2000) Fundamentals in Clinical Ophthalmology: Glaucoma. London: BMJ Books.

Ho S-Y, French P (2002) Minimizing fire risk during eye surgery. Clin Nursing Res 11: 387–96.

Hope-Ross M (2003) Phakodynamics. Refractive Eye News August/September: 9–18.

Katz J, Feldman MA, Bass EB et al. (2001) Adverse intraoperative medical events and their association with anesthesia management strategies in cataract surgery. Ophthalmology 108: 1721–6.

Katzen J (2002) Management of anxiety in the refractive surgery patient. Insight XXVII: 103–7.

Kent S (2000) Antiseptic skin preparation revisited. Br J Periop Nursing 10: 364–9.

King R (1998) Anaesthetic practice. In: Clarke P, Jones J (eds), Brigden's Operating Department Practice. Edinburgh: Churchill Livingstone, pp. 93–145.

McCoy K (1992) Ophthalmic drug use in the OR. Insight XVIII(4): 10–21.

Michels M, Sternberg P Jr (1990) Operating microscope-induced retinal phototoxicity: pathophysiology, clinical manifestations and prevention. Surv Ophthalmol 34: 237–52.

Moon J, Cho K (2001) The effects of handholding on anxiety in cataract patients under local anaesthesia. J Adv Nursing 35: 407–15.

Murdock IE, Sze P (1994) Visual experience during cataract surgery. Eye 8: 666–7.

National Association of Theatre Nurses (1998) Safeguards for Invasive Procedures: The management of risks. Harrogate: NATN.

National Association of Theatre Nurses (2000) Back to Basics: Perioperative practice principles. Harrogate: NATN.

Newsom RSB, Wainwright WC, Canning CR (2001) Local anaesthesia for 1221 vitreoretinal procedures. Br J Ophthalmol 85: 225–7.

NHS Executive (2000) Action on Cataracts – Good practice guidance. London: DoH.

Nickerson B (2002) Nursing care of the paediatric patient following strabismus repair surgery. INSIGHT: J Am Soc Ophthal Registered Nurses XXVII(3): 64–5.

Noecker RJ, Golightly SF (1999) Pharmacology of ocular surgery. J Ophthal Nursing Technol May–June: 101–8.

Nordlund ML, Marques DV, Marques FF, Cionni RJ, Osher RH (2003) Techniques for managing common complications of cataract surgery. Curr Opin Ophthalmol 14(1): 7–19.

Nunn G (1996) Technical aspects of vitreoretinal surgery (unpublished lecture notes). London: Moorfields Eye Hospital NHS Foundation Trust.

Nursing and Midwifery Council (2000) Guidelines for the Administration of Medicines. London: NMC.

Pfeifer WL, Scott WE (2002) Strabismus surgery. INSIGHT: J Am Soc Ophthal Registered Nurses XXVII(3): 73–7.

Phillips C (1991) An eye-opening experience. Br J Theatre Nursing July: 14–15.

Reeves W (1993) Surgical experience of the ophthalmic patient. Insight XVIII(1): 16–22.

Roach VG (1989) Endophthalmitis: an ocular emergency. J Ophthal Nursing Technol 8(5): 203–5.

Royal College of Ophthalmologists (2001) Cataract Surgery Guidelines. London: RCOphth.

Royal College of Ophthalmologists (2002) Creutzfeldt–Jakob Disease (CJD) and Ophthalmology. London: RCOphth.

Royal College of Ophthalmologists and Royal College of Anaesthetists (2001) Local Anaesthetic in Ophthalmology Guidelines. London: RCOphth/RCA.

Royal National Institute for the Blind (2002). Changing the Way We Think About Blindness – Myths and reality. London: RNIB.

Schroeter K (2000) Advocacy in perioperative nursing practice. Assn Operating Room Nurses J (AORN J) 71: 1207–22.

Smith CA, Khoury JM, Shield SM et al. (2000) Unexpected corneal endothelial cell decompensation after intraocular surgery with instruments sterilized by plasma gas. Ophthalmology 107: 1561–6.

Snell RS, Lemp MA (1998) Clinical Anatomy of the Eye, 2nd edn. Oxford: Blackwell Scientific.

Southampton University (2002) Pre-operative Assessment: Setting a standard through learning. Southampton, University of Southampton.

Stanford-Kelly P (1997). Povidone iodine – microbial efficacy prior to cataract surgery. Ophthal Nursing 1(2).

Wadood AC, Dhillon B (2002). The role of the ophthalmic theatre nurse in phacoemulsification surgery. Ophthal Nursing 6(3): 25–7.

Waterman H, Grabham J (1995) Ophthalmic theatre nursing. Part 1: frameworks for practice. Br J Theatre Nursing 5(2): 26–9.

Waterman H, Mayer S, Lavin MJ, Spencer AF, Waterman NC (2002) An evaluation of the administration of sub-Tenon local anaesthetic by a nurse practitioner. Br J Ophthalmol 86: 524–6.

Williams M (2002) Preoperative visiting – an urban myth? Br J Periop Nursing 12(5): 168.

CHAPTER TWELVE

The care of patients presenting with acute problems

JANET MARSDEN

This chapter discusses the assessment, investigation, treatment and care of patients presenting with acute eye problems. As acute presentations may include almost all ophthalmic systems, many of the problems described here are also dealt with more fully in other chapters; only the more immediate needs of the patient are included here.

The clinician involved in the care of patients presenting acutely will vary depending on particular circumstances. In some areas, ophthalmic nurses undertake all the initial assessment and management of this group of patients. In other areas, the clinician is primarily an ophthalmologist, and optometry-led services continue to develop, particularly in primary care. General practitioners are still responsible for much of the eye care for patients presenting acutely as are emergency clinicians in general emergency units. This chapter aims to describe signs and symptoms displayed by patients who may present in acute settings and discusses management and care without attributing particular roles to different clinicians. It is irrelevant who cares for the patient, as long as the clinician who does is competent to undertake the role, understands the parameters of the role and is able and willing to refer when necessary to more appropriate care, and that care of the patient as well as the presenting problem is paramount.

Triage

In many acute settings, patients do not attend one by one, with plenty of time to assess and treat each person before the next arrives. It is essential to have some way of discriminating between all those who present and to have a system in place to ensure that patients are seen in order of their clinical need rather than the order in which they attend.

Triage is a method of prioritization of 'casualties', which emerged initially in the Napoleonic wars. The method then was the opposite of priorities now, in that the least injured soldiers were treated first to ensure that the fighting force remained strong. Those not likely to survive were not treated. Triage emerged in the form that we see now much later and was refined in the Korean and Vietnam actions. Triage involves identifying and giving a high priority to those people who have the most urgent clinical need. There are many ways of achieving this and many systems in place in acute ophthalmic areas, ranging from simple 'urgent', 'soon' and 'delayed' categories, to more complex methods. When undertaken most effectively, triage involves a decision about clinical priority based on presentation rather than diagnosis. Effective clinical management of the patient and efficient departmental management depend on accurate allocation of the clinical priority in the triage encounter. The triage encounter is not long enough to make a diagnosis and diagnosis may not be a good indication of clinical priority as a result of, for example, levels of pain.

Whatever system is in place, it must be systematic and rigorous and capable of being audited. It must also be seen to be fair in order that patients do not feel that there is discrimination involved in who is seen next.

One such method is that designed by the Manchester Triage Group (Mackway-Jones et al. 2005). This method, known as 'emergency triage' or more commonly 'Manchester triage', was designed for use in general emergency departments and has been adopted by most emergency departments in the UK and as a national triage system by a number of countries in Europe and further afield. It provides a standard to which ophthalmic acute or emergency settings must aspire and for that reason is discussed in detail here. Manchester triage uses a series of presentations and a limited number of signs and symptoms at each level of clinical priority. This ensures consistency between triagers and transparency of the decision to allocate a clinical priority. Traditionally, the clinician triaging a patient tends to have a feeling about what might be wrong with the patient and then seeks signs and symptoms from the history to prove or disprove his or her ideas. The tendency is to consider the common and easy possibilities first and move upwards to consider more severe possibilities only if the patient mentions other symptoms. Manchester triage is reductive – the method starts with the most severe possibilities and works downwards. A patient must be allocated a higher triage category if a discriminator in that category cannot be ruled out. The system therefore defaults to a safe priority. From a general emergency department perspective, there are 52 presentations and the triage practitioner must decide which to use. From an ophthalmic perspective, there is only one commonly used presentation and that is 'Eye problems' (Mackway-Jones et al. 2005). In the UK, the times allocated to areas of the national triage scale are as shown in Table 12.1.

Table 12.1 Times allocated to areas of the national triage scale

Colour	Name	Target time (minutes)
Red	Immediate	0
Orange	Very urgent	10
Yellow	Urgent	60
Green	Standard	120
Blue	Non-urgent	240

This 'blue' target has since been modified, in line with UK government targets that aim for all patients to be discharged from emergency care within 4 hours (Figure 12.1).

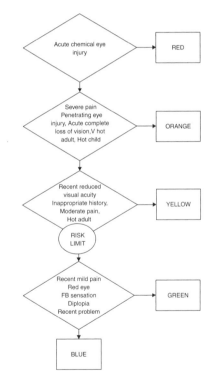

Figure 12.1 Manchester triage system – eye problems. (From Mackway-Jones et al. 2005.)

Triage is designed to be a very fast initial assessment of the patient to decide on a clinical priority. Visual acuity is a key component in the decision but, otherwise, all that is required is a brief history, bearing in mind the discriminator and the recording of the chosen discriminator and triage category (see box).

Triage example

A patient presents with a red, sore eye for 2 days without trauma and no reduction in vision:

- Red? Chemical eye injury can be ruled out
- The level of pain should be discussed; severe pain is 7–10 on a 10-point scale, moderate pain 4–6 and mild pain 1–5
- There is no history of trauma so penetrating trauma can be ruled out as can sudden complete loss of vision
- Further questioning and visual acuity will lead to a decision whether the patient falls into the yellow or green category based on the level of pain
- All that need be documented from this triage encounter is, in this case, **red eye, green**

Management of the workload with an effective triage system will ensure that all patients are cared for in a timely and appropriate fashion, bearing in mind their clinical priority, in a manner that is transparent and reproducible.

Telephone triage

A major expansion of the triage process has been the recognition and development of telephone triage. Giving advice by telephone has always been an integral part of the nurse's role, although not one that has been recognized as having a distinct identity and therefore a hidden part of the workload. Formalized advice giving by telephone has the potential to be a valuable tool in many settings – a fact that has been recognized in the development of NHS Direct, the telephone advice and helpline covering England.

Telephone triage was first described as a useful tool in the emergency care setting in the UK by Buckles and Carew-McColl in 1991. Various benefits have been attributed to the strategy by a number of different authors including reduced attendance as a result of explanations and self-care advice, redirection of patients to more appropriate agencies, identification of problems before the patient attends the department, cost-effectiveness due to a potentially reduced workload and pre-attendance patient empowerment.

Telephone triage also has its difficulties, however. The patient is not visible so many of the cues that experienced nurses take from the patient's appearance and behaviour are not available. The nurse may not even be able to gain information from the patient but may be talking to an intermediary such as a relative or neighbour or another health professional, all of whom may know the patient to a greater or lesser degree.

The demarcation line between telephone advice and telephone triage is debatable, but it is suggested that it occurs when a formalized process of decision-making takes place allowing identification of clinical priority and allocation to predetermined categories of urgency of need for medical evaluation and care. The decisions made in the telephone triage encounter may be that the patient needs to be seen now, that he or she needs to be seen within a number of days or perhaps that advice and self-care are all that is required in his episode. These decisions may be more formalized in terms of the areas to which patients are referred and timescales available, and will depend on local services. What is clear, however, is that it is even more difficult to make a decision about diagnosis by telephone, advice must be given in the light of the signs and symptoms elicited from the telephone call, which would be aided if a similar framework was employed to that used in face-to-face triage and, most importantly, that the conversation including information from the caller, and decisions made by the clinician, are recorded in detail.

Telephone triage, like triage, should be undertaken only by experienced practitioners. The availability of any protocols and charts does not remove the need for expert clinical knowledge. The decisions made in telephone triage arguably call for a higher level of skill and knowledge than when the patient is present and, certainly, the questioning skills of the practitioner must be very highly developed in order to gain the most useful information from a worried caller, quickly and effectively.

Like triage, telephone triage works well when it is carried out correctly and less well when corners are cut, or aspects, such as pain, are ignored. All triage systems must be auditable and this relies on good training of competent practitioners using their skills and knowledge, and the tools available to them, to best effect.

The patient's story

What the clinician needs to know is what has actually happened to the patient and what has prompted him or her to present today. Has something new happened or have symptoms have been going on for some time but the patient has become sufficiently worried to attend? Perhaps the patient has been prompted to attend by another person's intervention. It is important, as in all scenarios, to remain non-judgemental because, if the patient feels that perhaps he or she should not be attending because the problem is not particularly acute, he or she may include new symptoms, in order to legitimize attendance and these can confuse any decisions about the condition to a considerable degree. The art of questioning the patient is therefore to make the 'story' rather more specific and tease out signs and symptoms that the patient may not have considered pertinent, without prompting the patient into responses that are not true for them but are those that they think the clinician is looking for.

Minor trauma

The majority of (eye) injuries are superficial in nature and transient in their effects but place considerable demands on A&E services.

MacEwan (1989, p. 888)

The vast majority of eye injuries are, as MacEwan (1989) suggests, 'trivial' in terms of other presentations to general emergency care settings, but form a large proportion of those patients presenting acutely to ophthalmic services. It is always important to remember that, however 'trivial' or 'run of the mill' the patient's problem is to ophthalmic professionals, to the patient no injury is trivial; it is likely to be a major life event, causing pain, distress and anxiety.

Traumatic subconjunctival haemorrhage

This is common after a variety of injuries and is, in itself, self-limiting, requiring no treatment. Fluorescein should be instilled and the eye examined using a cobalt blue light on a pen-torch, ophthalmoscope or, ideally, a slit-lamp to rule out a conjunctival laceration. The patient should be reassured that the haemorrhage will resolve, usually over a period of weeks.

A traumatic subconjunctival haemorrhage that extends backwards so that the posterior border is not visible may be an indication of significant orbital trauma and may need further investigation if the history, and other signs and symptoms are indicative of this.

Identifying the extent of surface ocular trauma

A light source and single-use fluorescein minims or impregnated strips are the crucial elements in identifying the extent of corneal trauma (Figures 12.2 and 12.3). Both white- and cobalt blue-filtered light are necessary and magnification enables much more comprehensive assessment. The tools used may therefore range from a pen-torch or ophthalmoscope, a head loupe or ring light with integral magnification or, in the best case, to a slit-lamp and a clinician with the skills to use it!

Fluorescein stains damaged epithelial cells and shows a bright green/ yellow stain under cobalt blue light. It is therefore used to show the extent of both conjunctival and corneal epithelial loss. It is relatively non-toxic to ocular tissue so it may be used even where there is a suspicion of perforation. The two main components of the corneal injury are extent and depth and both must be assessed. The extent may be assessed using simple direct illumination from a pen-torch or ophthalmoscope. Depth is better assessed using a slit-lamp, but may be considered by using a slightly angled view of

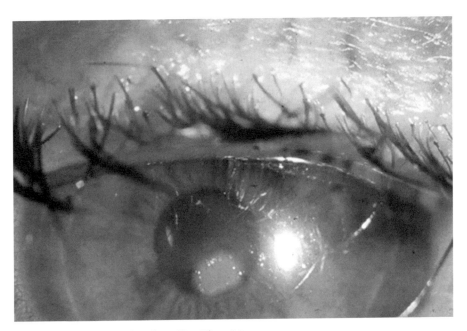

Figure 12.2 Corneal abrasion. (See Plate 1.)

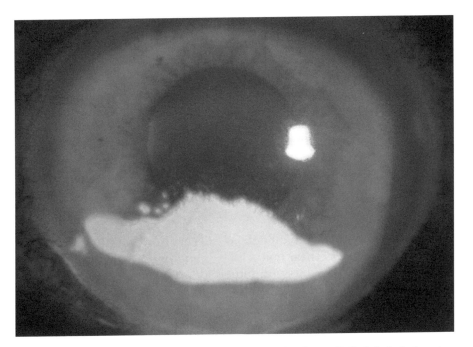

Figure 12.3 Exposure keratitis. (By courtesy of Angela Chappell, Ophthalmic Imaging Department, Flinders Medical Centre, Adelaide, South Australia.) (See Plate 2.)

the cornea, rather than considering the injury just from a 'straight-on' view (Marsden 2001). The degree of epithelial loss is not a good indicator of the severity of injury and, because pain is associated with epithelial loss, a high level of pain may not indicate a severe injury. It is always important to consider the depth of corneal foreign bodies before removal. Occasionally, foreign bodies may perforate the cornea and extend into the anterior chamber, and this must be identified so that appropriate measures may be taken for removal – perhaps in a theatre environment.

Findings should be documented, generally by illustrating the location and extent of the injury on a diagram. It is possible, when using a slit-lamp, to measure the extent of injury but, otherwise, as accurate an interpretation as possible should be drawn. This is useful for identifying the progress of healing at any subsequent review visits.

Fluorescein may be used in the identification of perforation of the cornea (or sclera) in cases where the eye appears to be intact but there is suspicion of deep penetration. A drop of fluorescein instilled into the lower fornix will spread over the cornea as the patient blinks. If there is corneal or scleral perforation, aqueous fluid will tend to leak out of the perforation and wash away the fluorescein film. If the eye is illuminated by a cobalt blue light, the observer will see black streaks appearing in the fluorescein film under the site of the injury. This will indicate an aqueous leak and is confirmation of perforation.

Treatment of surface ocular trauma

Having identified the extent of trauma there are a number of decisions to be made about treatment. Treatment decisions will affect patient comfort and the patient's experience of trauma. It is important therefore that care is optimized for each patient.

The three main areas that need consideration are the prevention of infection, the treatment of pain, and the optimization of healing.

Prevention of infection

One of the eye's major innate defence mechanisms against pathogens is the integrity of the corneal epithelium. The eye normally has a population of commensal bacteria (diphtheroids, staphylococci, streptococci), which prevent colonization with pathogenic bacteria (Forrester et al. 1996, Newell 1996). Disruption of the corneal epithelium allows penetration of the outer coat of the eye by these and any other opportunistic pathogens, which can result in infection of the cornea itself (infective keratitis) or infection of the interior structures of the eye (endophthalmitis), which can be catastrophic to ocular tissues and any prognosis for useful vision.

It can be seen therefore that any breach in the corneal epithelium requires treatment with topical prophylactic antibiotic until the epithelium is healed. Conjunctival epithelial loss is less likely to lead to ocular infection as a result of the nature of the specialized conjunctival immune system and its proximity to the globe rather than being part of it. Antibiotic prophylaxis is generally given after conjunctival injury.

As antibiotics are for prophylaxis, the choice should be one with a broad spectrum of activity and, in practice, in acute care settings, this is likely to mean either chloramphenicol or fusidic acid preparations (Fucidin). Short courses of topical chloramphenicol do not appear to cause systemic side effects (Besamusca and Bastiensen 1986, Gardiner 1991, Consumers' Association 1997) and it is considered to be a very safe drug, widely used throughout ophthalmology in the UK. Chloramphenicol is available in both drop and ointment form and fusidic acid as a viscous drop, which becomes clear and liquid on hitting the tear film of the eye. Chloramphenicol is usually prescribed four times daily and fusidic acid twice daily; this regimen should be continued until the epithelium is healed. Often, a 5-day course is prescribed but the reasons for this are traditional rather than evidence based. It can be left to the patient's discretion to stop the antibiotic once any pain has resolved, i.e. the epithelium has healed and the risk of infection has passed.

The choice of antibiotic treatment is often limited by what is available, but consideration must also be given to the vehicle – whether a drop or an ointment form is preferable. Fechner and Teichmann (1998) prefer ointment and Rhee and Pyfer (1999) suggest that both are as effective. Practitioner experience suggests, however, that ointment provides much more comfort, as a greasy surface between injured conjunctiva or cornea and lids, and certainly, if an eyepad is used, ointment should be used because the antibiotic will be present on the eye for much longer than a drop, underneath the eyepad. Ointment does tend to blur vision for a few minutes but this can be minimized by advising the patient to instil only a couple of millimetres rather than any more of the ointment. Patients should be informed that chloramphenicol has an unpleasant taste and, as the lacrimal drainage system eventually drains down the back of the throat, chloramphenicol drops or ointment will be tasted for some while after instillation.

If perforation of the cornea is suspected or confirmed, a single drop of unpreserved, single-dose chloramphenicol (in minim form) may be instilled before further assessment. Both preservatives and ointment are toxic to ocular tissues and should not be used.

Dealing with pain

Any breach in the corneal epithelium will cause a degree of discomfort or pain as corneal nerves are damaged and exposed and the extent of epithelial loss is likely to be related to the degree of pain experienced by the patient. Corneal pain is difficult to treat, but a number of strategies can be used and accurate assessment of the degree of pain is required. Conjunctival trauma causes much less pain and foreign body sites, whether conjunctival or corneal, are usually described as being irritable rather than painful.

Topical anaesthesia

For examination purposes only and to obtain an accurate visual acuity assessment, topical anaesthesia may be used. Repeated instillation will result in dose-related toxicity to the corneal epithelium and delay in healing caused by inhibition of cell division (Fechner and Teichmann 1998). This means in practice that, if patients are given topical anaesthetic drops to take home, their pain will be relieved but the corneal epithelial loss will not recover and may get worse.

Pupil dilatation

A component of the pain experienced is likely to be a result of ciliary spasm where there is more than a very small area of corneal epithelial loss. This can be seen because the pupil of the affected eye reacts more slowly than that of the uninjured eye. Relief of the spasm and a component of the pain may be achieved through instillation of drops such as tropicamide or cyclopentolate 1% to dilate the pupil. Of these, cyclopentolate 1% lasts the longer. The patient should be warned that these drops paralyse the ciliary muscle and so accommodation and the patient's near vision will be blurred because focusing is impossible. Atropine should never be used because it is completely irreversible and lasts from 10 to 14 days.

Topical analgesia

Prostaglandins play a major role in pain sensation and non-steroidal anti-inflammatory drugs (NSAIDs) are used systemically as analgesics to inhibit the enzyme cyclo-oxygenase and therefore decrease the synthesis of prostaglandins (Fechner and Teichmann 1998). Topical NSAIDs have been evaluated for use in corneal pain (Brahma et al. 1996) and found to be extremely useful. Their use does not appear to delay healing and no adverse effects have been found where the cornea is not otherwise compromised and the NSAID is used only for a short time. For patients with corneal pain, therefore, topical NSAIDs provide a significant degree of effective pain relief and are usually prescribed four times daily (Brahma et al. 1996, Fechner and Teichmann 1998, Rhee and Pyfer 1999).

Three NSAIDs are available in eye drop form: diclofenac sodium (Voltarol ophtha) and flurbiprofen sodium (Ocufen) in single-dose units and ketorolac trometamol (Acular) as a 5-ml bottle, which may be more cost-effective.

Systemic analgesia

Use of topical analgesia should almost remove the need for systemic analgesia. Pain associated with other branches of the trigeminal nerve is notoriously difficult to treat. Practitioner experience suggests that many common analgesics provide little relief for corneal pain and other strategies, such as those discussed, have a rather better effect. If systemic analgesia is suggested, the analgesic that the patient normally takes is as likely to be effective as anything else, although NSAIDs have been reported to work well.

Padding for corneal abrasion

To pad or not to pad, that is the question. A number of studies have been undertaken that address the question of eyepads and there have been equivocal results, ranging from faster to slower healing and suggesting, over a large sample, little effect on pain. Interpretation of these results suggests that there will be a number of patients below and a number above this mean conclusion. It is clear therefore that for some patients padding will make their situation better, whereas for some there is no doubt that their level of pain will increase. If the decision is to pad nobody, a significant number of patients will be denied effective pain relief. A strategy might therefore be devised to pad those patients who have significant pain while telling them that this is for comfort only and that, if the pad makes the pain worse, they should remove it.

A double eyepad should always be used, one pad folded over the closed lids and the other open on top of it (Figure 12.4). The whole is taped firmly to the face so that the patient cannot open the eye underneath the pad.

Medication (dilating drops, analgesia, antibiotic) should be instilled before patching and antibiotic ointment should be used because it will be present on the cornea for longer than in drop form. If comfortable, the pad should be left intact for 24 hours, then removed and instillation of medication started. If the pad is uncomfortable, it may be removed and medication started.

Do not pad the eye of patients who are driving home. If they leave the pad on and drive anyway, they are probably breaking the law, and certainly invalidating their insurance and driving extremely dangerously. If they take it off to drive, time, materials and effort have been wasted. Patients are much more likely to comply with advice if they are allowed to drive home and advised how to apply the eyepad when they arrive. A drop of local anaesthetic will facilitate a safe drive home.

Patients should never have both eyes padded at once because this is extremely disorienting and disabling. If both eyes are affected, the worst should be padded and pads given for use at home for the other eye if necessary.

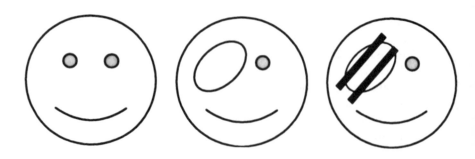

Figure 12.4 Eye padding: one pad is folded and placed over the closed lid, the other open over the top and taped down.

Optimization of healing

Education is needed to persuade the patient of the importance of continuing to use prescribed medication to avoid corneal infection.

Decisions whether to review simple corneal abrasions depend very much on the individual clinician. It is useful to review large abrasions to ensure that healing is taking place and that there is no loose epithelium that needs débriding.

Recurrent erosion syndrome

Recurrent erosion syndrome is a distinct possibility for those patients who have an animal or vegetable cause for their corneal trauma (e.g. plant or fingernail). The filaments that anchor the epithelium to Bowman's membrane may take even longer to heal and, until this happens, the epithelium is unstable and easily damaged. It is helpful to explain this to the patient and also that the time that they are most vulnerable to epithelial loss is at night because the epithelium sticks to the conjunctiva of the eyelid rather than to its basement membrane while the eye is relatively dry, overnight, and may be peeled off by the mechanical action of the lid opening on waking. This can be prevented until the epithelium is stable by using ointment at night before sleeping to keep the eye lubricated. 'Simple' ointment, or Lubri-Tears or Lacri-Lube (ointment base without drugs), should be used for a period of up to 3 months to prevent this happening.

Foreign bodies

Subtarsal foreign body

The patient often presents with a foreign body sensation and a history of something falling or blowing into the eye. Management involves everting the upper lid using a moistened cotton-tipped swab. Any foreign material trapped underneath the lid may be wiped off with the swab. Unless severe pain prevents lid eversion, no local anaesthetic should be instilled. The patient can confirm that all foreign bodies have been removed as the previously gritty pain disappears (Cheng et al. 1997). The eye should then be stained with fluorescein to rule out any corneal abrasion. If corneal abrasions are present, they are often linear and superficial.

If the corneal injury is minimal, a 'stat' instillation of antibiotic ointment is usually sufficient. If larger abrasions are present, they should be treated as corneal abrasions.

Conjunctival foreign body

Foreign bodies do not often penetrate the conjunctiva and are therefore easily wiped off using a moistened cotton bud after instillation of local anaesthetic. The resultant abrasion and any concurrent abrasion may be treated with antibiotic ointment. A pad is not usually necessary and the degree of pain experienced is much less than with corneal trauma.

Corneal foreign body

Corneal foreign bodies (Figure 12.5) are very common, from grinding wheels and other industrial machines, DIY and wind-borne foreign bodies. Superficial foreign bodies are often easily removed with a moistened cotton bud after instillation of local anaesthetic and the resultant small abrasion treated with antibiotic ointment.

Impacted corneal foreign bodies need to be removed using the edge of a 21-gauge hypodermic needle held tangentially to the cornea, with the hand resting on the patient's cheek or nose. The needle may be mounted on a cotton-tipped applicator or syringe for easier manipulation. After the initial removal of the foreign body, a rust ring often remains. This must be removed completely, but this is easier after 24–48 hours of treatment with antibiotic ointment.

Removal of a corneal foreign body with a needle is a procedure that must be carried out with extreme care. Although the cornea is tough, it is quite possible to penetrate it with a needle and, if the foreign body is 'dug' out too enthusiastically and the deeper layers of the cornea damaged, a corneal scar will result. This might cause major visual problems if it involves the visual axis. It is therefore important that, if the area possesses a slit-lamp, it is used during the removal of corneal foreign bodies, so that a high degree of magnification and support for the patient's head is possible. After removal of a foreign body, treatment is as for a corneal abrasion, although, because little corneal epithelium is lost and pain is minimal, a

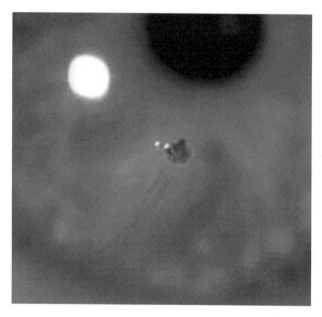

Figure 12.5 Foreign body. (See Plate 3.)

pad is not usually required. Many patients have repeat visits for removal of a corneal foreign body and treat them as an occupational hazard. Opportunities should be taken for health education about eye protection.

X-ray examination is indicated only if there is a definite history of a high-speed foreign body hitting the eye (e.g. hammer and chisel) and no foreign body can be found. It is most unlikely that one foreign body would penetrate the eye while another stayed on the cornea.

Superglue injuries

Cyanoacrylate glue is usually instilled into the eye by accident because the container may resemble an eyedrop or ointment applicator. The patient usually presents with eyelids stuck together and there is often a degree of pain. The tear film usually prevents adhesion of the glue to the globe and the pain is often caused by a corneal abrasion resulting from a plaque of glue that is inside the lids and is rubbing on the cornea.

Treatment consists of separating the lids and removing any pieces of glue from the fornices. The lids are usually separated by cutting the lashes very close to the lid margin because these are often what is holding the lids together. The dried glue must be picked off the lid margins. The procedure may be painful and lengthy. Extreme care must be taken not to injure the lid margin. Instillation of topical anaesthetic drop through any

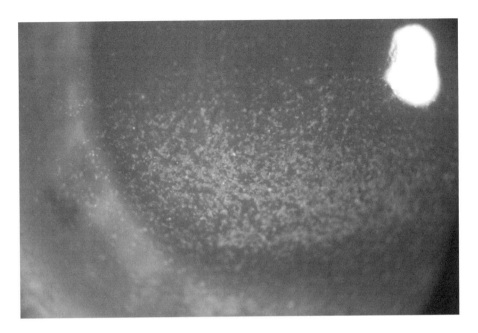

Figure 12.6 Punctate epithelial erosions (By courtesy of Angela Chappell, Ophthalmic Imaging Department, Flinders Medical Centre, Adelaide, South Australia.) (See Plate 4.)

gap in the lids will facilitate cooperation. Children may need a general anaesthetic. Any corneal damage is treated as an abrasion.

Blunt trauma

Blunt trauma occurs when the globe is hit with force. The globe may distort as a result of the pressure placed on it and this distortion may cause damage to any or all of the structures within it. As the force is removed, the globe springs back into shape. The force that this places on tissues within the eye may again cause disruption to them. A history of blunt ocular trauma (squash ball, shuttlecock, elbow to the eye, etc.) should give a high index of suspicion of this type of injury. Children in particular are likely to feel ill and drowsy, symptoms of head injury for which parents and carers will need advice.

Anterior segment contusion injuries

Hyphaema (Figure 12.7)

Traumatic hyphaema may be detected only with a slit-lamp (red blood cells floating in the anterior chamber) or may be visible with the naked eye, to the extent of filling the whole of the anterior chamber. Any hyphaema is likely to result in loss of vision. In cases where the hyphaema is large, red blood cells may block the trabecular meshwork, resulting in raised intraocular pressure (IOP) and severe pain. The pupil may be irregular or sluggish. Treatment of hyphaema may include bedrest in very severe cases, where the IOP is raised, or in children, but patients are most likely to be encouraged to rest at home. Sitting and sleeping upright should be encouraged in order to allow the blood cells to settle and absorb away from the visual axis. Red blood cells that are haemolysed while free in the anterior chamber or settled on the corneal endothelium may stain the corneal endothelium with haem pigment, which may affect vision. This stain takes some months to clear and reabsorbs from the periphery inwards. Central staining will cause visual disability and perhaps deprivation amblyopia in a young child (Eagling and Roper-Hall 1986). Regular review is undertaken to monitor IOP and treat any rise in pressure with appropriate agents such as acetazolamide. Hyphaemas may re-bleed, most often between 3 and 5 days after the initial trauma; the second bleed is invariably worse than the first and patients should be warned of what to do should this occur. The patient will need to have a posterior segment examination, generally when the hyphaema has settled and the eye is less tender, in order to assess retinal integrity.

Traumatic uveitis

This is a common effect of blunt trauma and may be the only sign of it. Treatment is as for any uveitis, with pupil dilatation and topical steroids.

Iris and pupil abnormalities

Traumatic mydriasis or miosis may occur as a consequence of blunt trauma and the pupil may be irregular when compared with the fellow eye as a result of partial or complete rupture of the iris sphincter. Disinsertion of the iris base from the ciliary body may cause what appears to be a 'hole' in the iris at its base (iridodialysis) and is often associated with hyphaema. No treatment is immediately necessary and surgery is unlikely to be undertaken unless the visual axis is compromised.

Lens abnormalities

The impact of the iris on the lens as the eye changes shape may leave a circle of iris pigment which can be seen after dilatation (Vossius' ring). Traumatic rupture of the zonules may occur. If 25% or more are ruptured, the lens is no longer held securely behind the iris. Luxation or subluxation

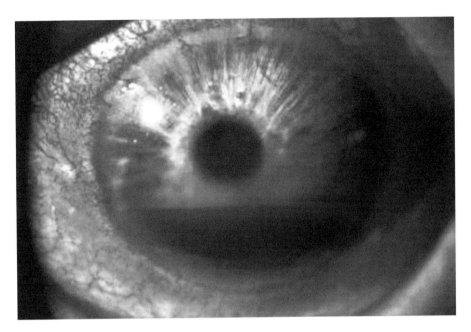

Figure 12.7 Hyphaema. (See Plate 5.)

of the lens may take place. There may be deepening of the anterior chamber caused by tilting of the lens posteriorly, or it may appear shallow as a result of anterior displacement. Pupil block and raised IOP may occur if the lens blocks the pupil. Iridodonesis (iris tremble) may be visible. Treatment may be required urgently if IOP rises or if the lens is dislocated anteriorly because it can compromise the corneal endothelium and cause corneal oedema; posterior dislocation into the vitreous is likely to be dealt with less urgently and a secondary intraocular lens implanted.

Concussion or contusion cataract may appear as an immediate or long-term consequence of blunt trauma. More rarely, the lens capsule may rupture, releasing soft lens matter into the anterior chamber, and this requires early intervention.

The angle

Angle recession is a term used to describe tears into the anterior face of the ciliary body, which alter the appearance of the drainage angle (Eagling and Roper-Hall 1986). This type of injury (seen with the aid of a gonioscopy lens) is seen in almost all patients who present with a hyphaema and varies in severity. Angle recession may be associated with permanent damage to the aqueous outflow pathways and this leads, in the long term, to fibrosis of the affected trabecular meshwork and glaucoma of the affected eye. This may develop some years after the initial injury so patients with this type of injury should be encouraged to have regular optometric examinations in order that the IOP may be checked if they are not to be followed up by an ophthalmologist.

Posterior segment damage

Macular oedema

Macular oedema after blunt trauma may settle quickly or persist for some time. Where it persists for more than a few days, pigment scarring of the retina may develop as the oedema settles and the reduction in vision may be profound. Cystic degeneration of the retina may develop after macular oedema, which may result in a macular hole that needs surgical repair.

Choroidal rupture

Distortion of the globe may stretch the tissues around their attachment at the optic disc. This stretching may cause splits or ruptures in the choroid that are usually arcuate in shape and may occur anywhere in the posterior segment, concentric with the optic disc. They may be associated with haemorrhage. The retina shows a crescent-shaped white area as the underlying sclera is exposed. If peripheral, the impact on the patient's vision may be minor – a peripheral scotoma. If the choroidal rupture occurs within the posterior pole, and particularly in the macular area, central vision may be profoundly affected.

Retinal injury

Commotio retinae results in reduced visual acuity and is the result of damage to the nerve fibre layer. It often resolves over a period of time.

Retinal tears, holes and dialysis

Retinal holes may be a late complication of blunt trauma caused by atrophy of damaged areas of retina. Retinal dialysis (detachment of the retina at the ora serrata) usually follows impact. Retinal detachment may follow in time, so often dialyses are treated with cryotherapy or laser treatment to prevent this.

Severe blunt trauma to the globe may result in avulsion of the optic nerve. The patient is likely to present with complete loss of vision. Preretinal or vitreous haemorrhage may obscure the optic disc and there is likely to be a complete afferent pupillary defect. There is complete disruption of the retinal circulation, which will not recover. (Table 12.2 on pages 228–9 lists decision-making in treating minor ocular trauma.)

Major trauma

Orbital injury

Both facial and skull trauma can result in orbital injury. The orbits are each composed of seven bones, the thinnest of which are the lamina papyracea over the ethmoid sinuses (along the medial wall) and the maxillary bone on the orbital floor (see also Chapter 22).

Medial orbital fractures

The lacrimal secretory system (especially the nasolacrimal duct) may be damaged and the medial rectus muscle may be trapped within fractures of the lamina papyracea. Dacryocystorhinostomy may be required if the nasolacrimal duct is obstructed. Surgical exploration of the medial orbit may be necessary if mechanical restriction of ocular motility is present.

Orbital floor fractures

These are often referred to as blow-out fractures because they are produced by transmission of forces through the bones and soft tissues of the orbit by a non-penetrating object such as a fist or ball. These fractures may be complicated by the entrapment of muscles and orbital fat, which limit ocular motility. Surgery is not always indicated because, often, oedematous tissues settle, freeing muscles and allowing correct motility.

Signs and symptoms

These include diplopia, enophthalmos, emphysema and infraorbital anaesthesia, and a classic presentation involves an injured patient, perhaps who would not have presented to A&E otherwise, blowing his or her nose and then attending because the eyelids have swollen alarmingly as air from the sinus has been driven into the tissues of the lid.

The patient should be given advice about the avoidance of Valsalva's manoeuvre, such as blowing the nose or straining at stool. Investigations should include orthoptic assessment accurately to assess the effect to the trauma on extraocular movement. Computerised tomography (CT) will be undertaken to identify the extent of trauma and plan repair. Broad-spectrum antibiotics are likely to be prescribed to prevent orbital cellulitis.

Table 12.2 Decision-making: treating surface ocular trauma

	Traumatic subconjunctival haemorrhage (superficial trauma)	Conjunctival abrasion	Conjunctival foreign body	Subtarsal foreign body	Corneal foreign body	Corneal abrasion	Corneal laceration	Conjunctival laceration
Likely degree of pain	Mild	Mild	Mild	Mild to moderate	Mild – irritation	Mild to severe	Mild to severe	Mild to moderate
Dealing with the pain	Ointment for lubrication of irregular ocular surface	Ointment for lubrication between conjunctiva and lid	Ointment as a single dose or depending on the extent of epithelial loss	Ointment as a single dose or depending on the extent of corneal and conjunctival epithelial loss	? dilate Ointment if not a deep cavity	? dilate Ointment Non-steroidal systemic ? pad	? dilate ? non-steroidal systemic	ointment
Stopping infection	No need, no break in integrity	Antibiotic ointment until feeling back to normal (conjunctiva healed)	Antibiotic ointment until feeling back to normal (conjunctiva healed)	Antibiotic ointment until feeling back to normal (conjunctiva healed)	Ointment or drops until feeling back to normal (cornea healed) Ensure all rust removed	Ointment or drops until feeling back to normal (cornea healed) Prevent recurrence by ointment at night	Drops until feeling back to normal (cornea healed) May need corneal contact lens	Ointment until feeling back to normal (cornea healed)

Table 12.2 continued

	Traumatic subconjunctival haemorrhage (superficial trauma)	Conjunctival abrasion	Conjunctival foreign body	Subtarsal foreign body	Corneal foreign body	Corneal abrasion	Corneal laceration	Conjunctival laceration
Review	Not normally	No need	No need	No need	For rust removal	If large, loose conjunctiva, not healing	Yes	If large
Other							If other than very small and shallow – refer	

Orbital apex trauma

Fractures of the orbital apex may result from direct, non-penetrating, blunt trauma or from penetrating trauma such as with large orbital foreign bodies. Orbital apex fractures present differently depending on the degree of injury to the vascular and neural structures within the orbital apex, and various syndromes have been defined to describe different presentations (Patel and Taylor 2002).

Optic nerve injury may occur, commonly as a result of traumatic optic neuropathy from indirect trauma (e.g. fractures of the base of the skull). Haematoma may compress the nerve or it may be damaged by foreign body or a fracture, which can result in a spectrum of injury from minor trauma to the nerve to complete transection. Injury to the cranial nerves present in the orbit (III, IV and VI) may present as extraocular muscle palsy with diplopia, and injury to the trigeminal nerve (V) as sensory disturbance to areas that it supplies.

It is most likely that patients with this type of injury will present first to general A&E, and clinicians there must be alerted to the possibility of ocular involvement from indirect trauma such as base of skull fractures, as well as from more direct trauma where the eyes themselves do not appear to be involved. Collaboration of ophthalmic units with A&E is necessary to ensure that patients with this type of injury do not lose vision unnecessarily. Patient complaints of loss of or reduction in vision must be taken very seriously; in order to quantify this, visual acuity must be checked regularly in this group of patients and ophthalmological opinion obtained immediately if vision is involved.

Retrobulbar haemorrhage

This may occur from direct or indirect trauma to the orbit and progress rapidly resulting in pain, proptosis of the globe, lid and conjunctival swelling, and congested conjunctival vessels. Subconjunctival haemorrhage may be dense and extend beyond the visible conjunctiva. If the globe begins to proptose after trauma, an ophthalmologist should be involved immediately. CT or magnetic resonance imaging (MRI) may be required urgently and the patient's visual acuity should be checked very frequently (perhaps every 10 minutes). If visual acuity reduces, emergency decompression by lateral canthotomy (a horizontal incision at the lateral canthus, through skin and conjunctiva, and then through the lateral canthal tendon, under local anaesthetic) will be required to relieve pressure on the optic nerve. Equipment for this procedure will not be needed very often but should be readily available in any area in which this group of patients is likely to present, so that avoidable loss of vision may be prevented. Wherever the patient presents, regular observation of the appearance of the patient accompanied by measurement of visual acuity and encouragement of the patient to report new symptoms where they are able will help to minimize complications of the injury.

Open trauma

An open eye requires immediate assessment. If any retained materials protrude from the globe, no attempt should be made to remove them. The material should be stabilized as far as possible, perhaps by taping it to the cheek if this seems appropriate or by covering the whole area with a plastic shield or small gallipot or receiver.

No pressure should be put on to an eye with a full-thickness injury and, although it might seem appropriate to cover the area with a pad, this should be done only if no other method of covering the eye exists, and should be undertaken only with extreme care. The pad must be loose and taped well away from the globe.

Patients with even very severe eye trauma may not have much pain if there is little corneal epithelial loss. The control of any pain and nausea must be a priority, however, because vomiting with an open eye is likely to lead to loss of the ocular contents. A rise in IOP may be minimized by caring for the patient with him or her either lying flat or sitting up at around a 30° angle.

Unless both eyes are extensively damaged, there should never be an occasion when both eyes are covered. A patient with one damaged eye is unlikely to be comforted, reassured or relaxed by having both eyes occluded and being unable to see anything going on around him or her or the person who is talking to him or her.

Lid trauma

For the eyes to be protected, the lids must be intact, in the correct position and without any disruption to their structure and function. Repair of lid trauma may be delayed as a result of the extremely good vascularization of the lids and associated structures, and may therefore be a planned activity rather than an emergency one, leading to the best possible functional and cosmetic result for the patient.

Ocular burns

Burns to the eye and surrounding structures present to the acute setting from a variety of domestic and industrial sources. Ocular burns may be divided most commonly into chemical, thermal and radiation, and chemical burns in particular can be quite devastating to the eye and to the patient's potential for vision. The degree of injury is dependent on the type of substance involved, but, most importantly, on the length of contact time. Patients with burns from heat or radiation have been separated from the source of the injury by the time they reach A&E or the ophthalmic unit. Patients with chemical injury are likely to have residual chemical in and around their eye and therefore need immediate treatment (irrigation) in order to minimize the injury. If the chemical injury is recent (3–4 hours) they will be triaged red – immediate – and all assessment, including visual acuity should be delayed until irrigation has taken place. A prompt and effective response to a chemical injury is vital to minimize tissue damage.

Chemical burns

These are the most urgent category of ocular burns and are usually caused by alkalis, acids or solvents. Alkaline chemicals include calcium hydroxide (lime), found in plaster and mortar, sodium or potassium hydroxide, which are used as cleaning agents (e.g. drain cleaner), ammonia, which is again used as a cleaning agent, and ammonium hydroxide which is found in fertilizer. Alkalis penetrate rapidly through corneal tissue, combining with cell membrane lipids, and result in cell disruption and tissue softening. A rapid rise in the pH in the anterior chamber may cause damage to the iris, ciliary body and lens. Damage to vascular channels leads to ischaemia.

Acids are less penetrating, and most damage is done during and soon after initial exposure. Acid substances precipitate tissue proteins, forming barriers against deeper penetration and localizing damage to the point of contact. Most commonly, domestic acid injuries are the result of car battery (sulphuric) acid. Most acids are used in dilute form; however, given sufficient concentration or volume, acids may cause severe ocular injury. Acid substances include hydrochloric, sulphuric and acetic acids, and also complex organic and inorganic compounds. Hydrofluoric acid (used particularly by stonemasons) is exceptional in that it causes progressive damage similar to an alkaline substance.

Solvents such as petrol, perfume, alcohol and volatile cleaning fluids, although very painful initially, tend to cause only minor and transient injury. Thermal and/or contusion injuries caused by the temperature or pressure of the chemical may be superimposed on the chemical injury.

Sequelae of ophthalmic chemical injury

Minor chemical burns of the eye are likely to heal rapidly without residual scarring. More severe burns result in an acute inflammatory response during which the corneal tissue is at risk of perforation as a result of the release of proteolytic enzymes from the white blood cells. As the eye heals, formation of scar tissue may cause vascularization and opacification of the cornea. Symblepharon – or adhesions between the conjunctiva which lines the lid and the conjunctiva covering the globe – may form and limit lid closure and eye movement, a problem that will necessitate major reconstructive surgery. The lids may be damaged and this can result in trichiasis where the lashes grow inwards and rub and irritate the eye. The lid itself may roll inwards (entropion) or outwards (ectropion) as a result of scarring and, again, cause problems with lid closure and exposure of the globe. Dry eyes often follow a chemical injury and are the result of damage to lacrimal ducts and secretory cells, causing reduced tear secretion. It is therefore most important that appropriate treatment starts as rapidly as possible, to minimize long-term problems and maximize visual potential.

Initial management

Irrigation
The initial treatment of any chemical eye injury involves copious irrigation to dilute the chemical and remove particulate matter. Irrigation should start immediately, using whatever source is available. Herr et al. (1991) found no difference in the efficacy of irrigation fluids and, therefore, the irrigating fluid of choice is physiological saline (0.9%) via a giving set to provide a directable and controllable jet. Sterile water may be used as long as appropriate equipment is available to ensure a controllable, directable flow of fluid. Failing the immediate availability of fluid and a giving set, a running tap may be used to irrigate the eye in the interim. Buffer solutions, which neutralize both acid and alkaline chemicals, are available in some areas but are expensive and therefore not widely used.

A drop of local anaesthetic (such as oxybuprocaine [Minims Benoxinate] 0.4%, amethocaine 1% or proxymetacaine 0.5%) should be instilled before irrigation to assist in patient compliance and to minimize pain. This may need to be repeated during the irrigation. Although repeated instillation of topical anaesthetic is not generally recommended, in order to facilitate effective irrigation and subsequent examination of the patient's eye, repeated instillation may be necessary to relieve pain and is therefore desirable.

During the procedure, the patient needs frequent information, explanations and reassurance. He or she may be encouraged to hold a container to collect the irrigation fluid and clothes should be protected with waterproof covering such as a cape or plastic sheet. Irrigation should take place with the patient sitting upright in a comfortable chair with his or her head supported and inclined to the side of the eye to be irrigated. Irrigating patients' eyes while they are lying down ensures only that they will get extremely wet and are less likely to be able to cooperate in the procedure as they strive to prevent themselves from what may feel like 'drowning'.

Contact lenses should be removed before irrigation. If left in place, a contact lens will ensure that a reservoir of chemical remains on the surface of the eye. The eyelids should be held open, manually or using a speculum, and all aspects of the cornea and conjunctiva irrigated, including the conjunctiva exposed by everting the upper lid. All particles of chemical matter should be removed, by wiping with a cotton-tipped applicator if necessary. Particles may lodge under the everted upper lid, in the upper fornix. This is usually impossible to visualize but may be reached by sweeping a wet cotton-tipped applicator under the edge of the everted upper lid and up into the upper fornix. Double eversion of the lid may be possible but this is a very uncomfortable procedure and full explanation, reassurance and perhaps another drop of topical anaesthetic will be required to ensure that the procedure is tolerated.

Any delay caused by attempting to identify the chemical or an appropriate neutralizing solution adds to the contact time and increases the risk of more severe injury. It is best to assume that previous irrigation, outside the ophthalmic setting, is inadequate and therefore effective irrigation is carried out. It is impossible to specify an exact time for irrigation or a volume of fluid that should be used because this depends on the nature of the chemical and its physical state as well as the patient's condition. Wagoner (1997) suggests that it is impossible to over-irrigate a chemically injured eye, and recommends irrigation for 15–30 minutes. At some point, however, irrigation must be stopped so that assessment, examination and treatment can commence.

The use of pH paper to check for adequate irrigation may be debatable. In alkaline injury, in particular, the chemical will leach out of the eye for a number of hours after injury, thus altering the pH of the tear film. Delay in therapy of a number of hours until the pH is back to normal (neutral = pH 7, the conjunctival sac normal pH is around 7.4 – Forrester et al. 1996) will delay healing and irrigation for this length of time and is not practicable or desirable. There is little in the literature to suggest when the pH of the tear film should be tested but, unless a number of minutes are left to elapse without irrigation before testing, it is possible that the irrigation fluid is being tested instead and this may lead to inappropriate cessation of irrigation. If this time is allowed to elapse before testing the pH of the tear film with indicator paper and the pH then proves to be abnormal, the eye has had a long period without irrigation in which further damage may take place. Ultimately, indicator paper is no substitute for prompt, adequate and thorough irrigation, and the clinical decision-making capabilities of the nurse coupled with a strong knowledge base will ensure that the decision to stop irrigation is taken appropriately.

After irrigation, the patient's visual acuity should be checked to provide a baseline. Cheng et al. (1997) suggest that patients with epithelial damage including less than one-third of the corneal epithelium or a similar area of conjunctival epithelium may be treated in the same way as a patient with a corneal abrasion; however, the eye may look deceptively normal as a result of tissue blanching and ischaemia which needs urgent assessment and treatment – a totally white eye after chemical injury may be a sign of severe ischaemia with a poor prognosis for vision. Accurate assessment of the condition of the eye is therefore vital.

Ophthalmic management usually includes:

• Topical steroids: to reduce and control inflammation.
• Topical antibiotics: prophylactic use to prevent secondary infection.
• Ointment: keeping burned surfaces apart with a layer of ointment will stop aberrant healing (symblepharon) and ointment also enhances patient comfort.
• Mydriatics, such as cyclopentolate 1%, to dilate the pupil, reduce pain caused by ciliary spasm and prevent adhesions between the iris and the lens (posterior synechiae) resulting from intraocular inflammation.
• Potassium ascorbate drops or systemic ascorbic acid: after alkali injury, ascorbate levels become depressed. This substance is believed to be necessary for the synthesis of collagen, so it may therefore be prescribed in order to maximize healing, although there is no evidence that it has any effect in humans (Mackway-Jones and Marsden 2003). Instilling a weak acid into a damaged eye is not pleasant for the patient and therefore admission to hospital may be required.

Rodding is a technique involving use of a glass rod and antibiotic ointment. The ointment is instilled into the eye and the rod is used, after instillation of topical anaesthetic, to spread the ointment over all surfaces of the conjunctiva, particularly in the upper and lower fornices, to keep the surfaces of conjunctiva apart and prevent the formation of symblepharon. This may need to be done regularly in a badly burned eye.

Solvent injury

After injury with a solvent, the patient often experiences acute and severe pain and 'stinging' in the eye, which may have settled somewhat by the time he or she presents to the clinical area. On examination, the eye is likely to be generally 'red' and punctate stains are seen on the cornea after instillation of fluorescein. Treatment of solvent injury is generally with antibiotic ointment to prevent infection and aid comfort. Pupil dilatation may help to minimize pain. The patient should be reassured that this type of injury resolves very quickly and is not likely to have any permanent effects.

Thermal burns

These usually involve damage to the lids, although any other external eye structures may be injured. Treatment of burns to lid skin is similar to that of thermal burns elsewhere on the body. Thermal burns range from very mild, such as those caused by tobacco ash, which may be treated as an abrasion – with dilatation of the pupil and chloramphenicol ointment – to the very severe caused by molten metal and glass, which may require reconstruction of the globe and surrounding structures. Thermal burns involving the lids can heal aberrantly, with scarring and tethering of lid skin and conjunctiva leading to lid closure and mobility problems. The eye should not be padded if lid burns are present (Onofrey et al. 1998).

Children in particular may sustain thermal burns to the cornea as a result of accidental exposure to a cigarette end, which if held by an adult is often at just the right height for a child to run into. Thermal corneal burns from this source are generally superficial (as a result of the child's immediate reaction and the wetness of the cornea) and may be treated as an abrasion. It would seem unlikely that corneal burns from cigarettes, in children, could be non-accidental as a result of the fast reaction to close the eyelids if something was seen coming towards the eye. Lid burns from cigarettes, however, should evoke suspicion in the clinician and urgent referral to a child protection specialist is advised. The child should be examined for burns elsewhere, but this should take place in an appropriate setting, not necessarily in A&E or the ophthalmic unit.

Radiation burns

Although all radiation can cause eye injury, ultraviolet radiation is the most common source of injury and, when caused by welding, is often known as 'arc eye'. 'Arc eye' is the result of injury by ultraviolet (UV) radiation, most commonly after exposure to welding arcs, but also after exposure to UV 'sunlamps' (sunbeds do not generally cause a problem because the intensity of the UV light is lower) (Figure 12.6). The UV radiation is absorbed by the corneal epithelial cells, and results in local cell death. There is a latent period before symptoms are experienced of 6–12 hours depending on the amount of exposure – this explains the traditional midnight to 2am presentation of these patients. The damaged epithelial cells slough off exposing the nerve fibres underneath. The patient will then present with a gritty, sometimes intensely painful eye(s) with photophobia, watering and blurring of vision. Lid erythema and oedema may be present. The patient is likely to need topical anaesthetic drops before assessment of visual acuity and examination of the eye. On staining with fluorescein, punctate staining is seen over the surface of the cornea where some cells have been destroyed.

Treatment is as for a corneal abrasion, with a mydriatic drop and antibiotic ointment as prophylaxis and for comfort. Oral analgesia may be necessary. Padding may help, but as both eyes are often affected, the worst eye only should be padded and the other treated with frequent applications of ointment. Complete recovery is usually within 24–36 hours. Metal inert gas (MIG) welding equipment uses high intensity white light which can burn the retina (in the same way as looking at the sun). Retinal examination may be required for patients whose vision does not return to normal after epithelial healing.

The non-traumatic red eye

Patients often present acutely with red eyes that are not associated with any trauma. It is important that all clinicians in contact with these patients are able to recognize signs and symptoms of common 'red eye' presentations so that appropriate and timely treatment can be facilitated. Many of the presentations discussed here are also discussed within other appropriate chapters. The presentation matrix is designed to remind clinicians of the presenting signs and symptoms of red eye so that appropriate decisions may be made about treatment and referral.

Subconjunctival haemorrhage

Patients may present with a spontaneous subconjunctival haemorrhage (Figure 12.8). Often, the patient has not noticed any irritation but has been prompted to attend by others noticing the haemorrhage. This presents as a deep red patch of blood under the conjunctiva, which may be quite small and circumscribed or may be severe enough for the conjunctiva to appear like a 'bag of blood'. Provided that there is no history of trauma, no treatment is needed. Subconjunctival haemorrhage may occasionally be associated with hypertension so blood pressure might be measured and recorded; however, the worry of the condition and 'white coat syndrome' may raise the patient's BP from normal levels. Patients with clotting disorders or those on anticoagulants including aspirin may be prone to repeat episodes and they should therefore be warned about this. As the patient's eye appears much worse than it is, a lot of reassurance may be needed.

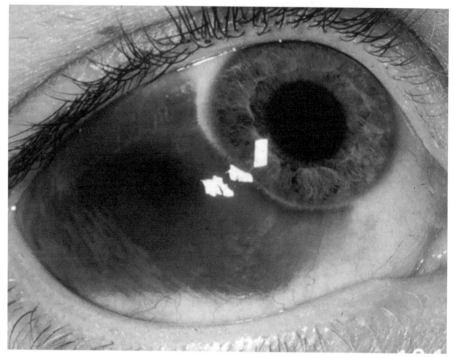

Figure 12.8 Subconjunctival haemorrhage. (See Plate 6.)

Subconjunctival haemorrhages will take up to 3 weeks to resolve and, because the conjunctiva is an elastic membrane, the blood may spread under it and actually appear worse, before it begins to resolve. The eye may feel irritable as the conjunctiva is moved from its normal place and may be irregular. Artificial tears may be useful in minimizing irritation while the haemorrhage settles. If there is a large amount of blood under the conjunctiva, uneven wetting of the cornea may occur as a result of the lid moving over misplaced conjunctiva rather than corneal epithelium. Corneal exposure may result, including dellen (a local area of corneal dryness). This can be treated if necessary and further damage prevented if the patient is encouraged to use frequent applications of lubricating ointment.

Infective conjunctivitis

Inflammation of the conjunctiva is by far the most common cause of red eyes. Organisms involved in infective conjunctivitis include bacteria and viruses. Other causes of infective conjunctivitis are much less common. Bacterial conjunctivitis in adults is, in itself, much less common than often thought (Tullo and Donnelly 1995), and most conjunctivitis in adults is caused by a virus, often a type of adenovirus. Conjunctivitis in children is more likely to be bacterial. Eyepads should never be suggested for patients with conjunctivitis. The warm, damp atmosphere underneath an eyepad will allow further organism growth and exacerbate the condition. Clinicians should have a high index of suspicion that a patient presenting with a uniocular, chronic conjunctivitis (one that may have been persisting for some weeks, without the other eye becoming involved and with minor irritation and discomfort only) may have a chlamydial infection, and appropriate swabs should be taken with referral to an appropriate genitourinary medicine specialist if a positive swab result is received. Generally, there is little point in taking conjunctival swabs in adults unless this condition is suspected, because a positive result of bacterial or viral conjunctivitis is most unlikely to change the treatment given to the patient. As conjunctivitis is highly infectious, patients should not generally be offered a review appointment because all viral and bacterial conjunctivitis is self-limiting. If blurring of vision becomes a problem, however, the patient should be encouraged to return because keratitis caused by adenovirus may occasionally, if severe, be treated with steroid drops (see Chapter 15).

Allergic conjunctivitis

This is very common and presents acutely in two distinct ways: first, red eyes with itching and watering and an appearance of large bumps (papillae) on the subtarsal conjunctiva (Figure 12.9). This presentation is particularly common during the 'hay fever season' and may therefore be associated with a runny nose, sneezing, etc. Systemic antihistamine treatment is effective as are antihistamine drops such as azelastine (Optilast), emedastine (Emadine) and levocabastine (Livostin Direct). Mast cell-stabilizing drops such as sodium cromoglicate help to stabilize the mast cell membranes and therefore prevent an allergic response They are useful if used by sufferers of allergic eye symptoms before the symptoms start, continuing them throughout the season, until the allergens are no longer present. Using them for an acute episode is unlikely be helpful because it takes between a week and 10 days for the mast cell membranes to stabilize so that the drops can begin to work. Olopatadine (Opatanol) has both an antihistamine and a mast cell-stabilizing effect and can therefore be used in an acute episode, and then carried on as a preventive measure.

The second presentation is by an acute and frightening atopic reaction, which involves massive chemosis or swelling of the conjunctiva that the patient often describes as 'jelly' on the eye. This is usually the result of the patient rubbing the eye with an allergen present on the hand or finger. Common allergens include some plant juices, pollen and animal dander or hairs. This condition is completely self-limiting and requires no treatment unless the chemosis is severe and protruding from the closed lids. In

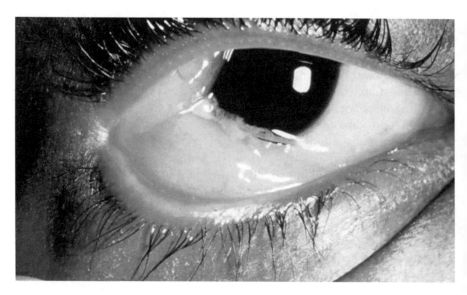

Figure 12.9 Chemosis. (See Plate 7.)

this case, lubricant drops might be necessary. Reassurance about the condition is likely to be necessary and, if the reaction is severe, the patient may need to be monitored for systemic effects of the allergen.

Anterior uveitis

Uveitis is an inflammatory condition that may be associated with systemic disease such as ankylosing spondylitis but is often idiopathic. It may also occur secondary to trauma. The most common presenting symptoms are photophobia, pain caused by iris and ciliary spasm, conjunctival redness (injection), which may be more marked around the corneoscleral junction (limbus), and decreased visual acuity. The reduction in vision is the result of protein and white blood cells that are part of the inflammatory reaction in the anterior chamber. The pupil, because of spasm and inflammation, is likely to be small (miosed) compared with the unaffected eye, and may react sluggishly. There will be a clear reflection of light when the cornea is illuminated, demonstrating the lack of corneal involvement, and there will be no staining with fluorescein (see Chapter 19).

Acute glaucoma (angle-closure glaucoma)

In acute glaucoma, the outflow of aqueous in the eye is obstructed by the peripheral iris covering the trabecular meshwork. As aqueous continues to be produced, the pressure inside the eye increases rapidly. This results in the sudden onset of severe pain (as a result of the increased IOP) and blurred vision (caused by corneal oedema). Haloes may be seen around lights. The pain is not likely to be localized in the eye, but may involve the whole head and may be accompanied by nausea, vomiting and abdominal pain caused by vagal stimulation. Patients are usually elderly and are likely to be hypermetropic (long-sighted). On examination, the patient's eye will be red and the reflection of light from the cornea will be very diffuse – showing that the cornea is oedematous. The pupil will be semidilated, oval and fixed. A great deal of explanation, reassurance and care is needed by these ill and often terrified patients (see Chapter 20).

Table 12.3 Differential diagnosis of the red eye

	Conjunctivitis	Uveitis	Glaucoma	Corneal ulcers
Lids	? swollen Follicles, papillae if allergic	Normal	Normal	May be swollen
Conjunctiva	Injected	Injected	Injected	Injected
Cornea	? punctate staining	Normal, bright reaction	Very hazy	Opacity/ stains with fluorescein
Anterior chamber	Deep	Deep	Shallow or flat	Deep
Iris	Normal	May look 'muddy'	May be difficult to see	Normal
Pupil	Normal	Slight miosis (compared with fellow) Sluggish	Fixed, oval, semidilated	Usually normal, may be slightly sluggish
Pain	Gritty	Deep pain in eye	Severe pain in and around eye and head	Gritty
Discharge	Pus/watery/ sticky in morning	May water	No	May water
Photophobia	If severe	Yes	No	Not usually
Systemically	? flu-like symptoms (urticaria)	Well	Nausea Vomiting Severe abdominal pain Dehydration	Well

Corneal ulcers

There are three main types of corneal ulcer that are likely to be seen as acute presentations. Differentiation between the different types of corneal ulcer is sometimes difficult, and the treatment is completely different:

- Bacterial ulcers occur as 'fluffy' white demarcated areas on the cornea that stain with fluorescein.
- Marginal ulcers appear as ulcerated areas that stain with fluorescein and are usually close to the limbus. They are part of a hypersensitivity response by the eye to staphylococcal exotoxins and are usually treated with steroid eyedrops.
- Ulcers caused by herpes simplex virus are known as 'dendritic' ulcers because of their branching, tree-like shape when stained with fluorescein. They are treated with aciclovir eye ointment primarily (see Chapter 16).

Painless loss of vision

There are many causes of painless loss of vision and many patients present with loss of vision acutely. It is often very difficult to differentiate between

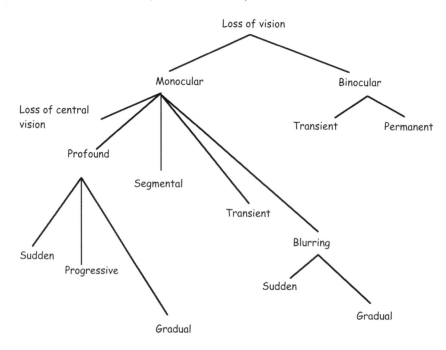

Figure 12.10 Classification of loss of vision (Marsden 1999).

causes that need immediate care by an ophthalmic service and those that will cope with a delayed referral, and indeed need referral to other specialists.

Classification of loss of vision is also problematic with a tendency to consider diagnoses rather than presentations. This section uses the diagram in Figure 12.10 as a schematic to divide loss of vision into different sections depending on the patient's presenting problem.

History

From the point of view of vision loss, it is important to ascertain the parameters of the problem:

- Was it sudden or gradual loss of vision? If sudden, is it possible that it has been there for a while but the patient has only just noticed (e.g. did the patient notice the loss of vision when he or she covered an eye – if that was the case, it may have been present for some considerable time)? If the loss was gradual, over what period of time has it occurred (days, weeks or even months)?
- Are there patches or areas of actual vision loss or is the vision generally blurred?
- Does the loss of vision involve some or all of the vision? Are there sectors of the field of vision that are missing? Is the loss worse centrally or peripherally?
- Was the loss transient? Has it come back now or is it recovering (for how long was vision affected?) or does it seem to be permanent?
- Is the vision now getting better, or worse, or is it staying the same?
- Are there any other symptoms that the patient is experiencing? Often, the patient may not consider other symptoms because the eye problem is the issue that worries him or her. If the patient is questioned, however, other symptoms may be ascertained that the patient does not readily associate with the eye problem, such as headache, weakness or pain elsewhere.

This information will help to categorize vision loss in order immediately to rule out some possibilities while leaving some avenues open for further investigation. Depending on the situation, most of these patients will be examined by an ophthalmologist, but there are many situations where the decision of what to do most appropriately for the patient must be made by another clinician, in primary care, in areas remote from ophthalmic medical services or in other areas such as emergency care settings.

Monocular versus binocular loss of vision

Ocular pathology, or optic nerve problems, will cause monocular loss of vision. A problem at or posterior to the optic chiasma, in the brain, will cause binocular loss of vision. It is most unusual for a patient to suffer from bilateral simultaneous eye disease causing loss of vision. The only exception to this would be in the case of bilateral blurring of vision that has appeared over a number of days. This is characteristic of papilloedema.

A generalization, but one that almost always works in practice, is that, if a patient complains of binocular loss of vision, the problem is likely to be of neurological rather than ophthalmic origin.

Binocular loss of vision

Migraine

One of the most common causes of transient, bilateral loss of vision is classic migraine. The patient is likely to complain of transient loss of vision and flashing lights, and scintillating images may appear, as may fortification spectra. The patient may experience the loss of large parts or sectors of the visual field. This aura usually lasts for 20–30 min and then resolves, followed by a severe headache. In a first episode of migraine, the patient may be very frightened by the visual symptoms and may not associate the headache with the loss of vision. Another migraine type is known as acephalgic migraine. The patient experiences the aura, but does not go on to develop the headache. It may be quite difficult to explain to the patient that these symptoms do not actually constitute an eye problem.

Homonymous hemianopia (Figure 12.11)

Hemianopia – loss of half of the visual field, homonymous – on the same side.

The patient may complain that he or she is unaware of things approaching from the side of the field defect. The patient may also have trouble with reading because he or she may not be able to follow a line of print. Visual acuity may be only mildly reduced in each eye because part of the macular function on each side is likely to be intact. Distance visual acuity testing may demonstrate that the patient is unable to see the letters on the Snellen chart on the side of the field defect.

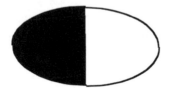 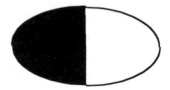

Figure 12.11 Field loss in homonymous hemianopia.

The most common areas of damage are in the optic radiation and the occipital cortex. The hemianopia may be incomplete and temporal lobe lesions cause predominantly upper field loss.

Causes of homonymous hemianopia include vascular lesions such as embolus or haemorrhage, tumours and inflammatory lesions in these specific areas of the brain. This type of field defect may accompany obvious systemic symptoms such as hemiparesis or hemiplegia. Referral to settings other than ophthalmology would be most appropriate and the patient needs a neurological assessment.

Bitemporal hemianopia (Figure 12.12)

Loss of the field of vision on the temporal side in each eye.

Bitemporal field loss usually indicates a lesion in or around the optic chiasma. Most chiasmal lesions result from compression by tumours arising from structures around the chiasma such as pituitary adenoma, meningioma, craniopharyngiomas or aneurysm (Cheng et al. 1997). The patient may complain of blurring of the temporal field. Cranial nerve palsies may also occur as a result of compression by a tumour and the patient should be asked about symptoms of double vision. Evaluation by a neurologist is urgently required for patients presenting in this way.

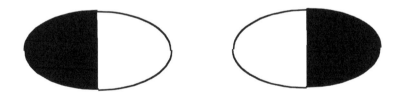

Figure 12.12 Field loss in bitemporal hemianopia.

Monocular loss of vision

Profound loss of vision

This is characterized by complete or severely diminished vision affecting the whole of the visual field. This may occur suddenly or gradually over a period of days.

Sudden, profound loss of vision suggests a vascular cause and the most likely causes of this are central retinal artery occlusion and vitreous haemorrhage (see Chapter 21, p. 461).

Vitreous haemorrhage

This is the most likely cause if there is an associated history of diabetes. The patient may not be aware of eye changes related to the diabetes, especially if no regular eye screening takes place. The patient may be aware of the haemorrhage occurring and may describe a cloud of floaters (the first blood) which becomes more dense over a short period, resulting in a profound loss of vision. Any attempt by the clinician to visualize the back of the eye will be unsuccessful as a result of the blood in the vitreous cavity. Laser is usually the treatment of choice once the retina can be visualized. The patient may need a great deal of support and explanation in order to understand the lack of apparent urgency in treating debilitating loss of vision.

Central retinal artery occlusion

In this condition, the patient may describe the vision disappearing 'like someone switching the light off'. The loss may be absolute and is, at best, likely to be 'count fingers' or less. Some patients retain a degree of central vision as a result of the presence of a cilioretinal artery, an anatomical anomaly. The retina is likely to be pale as a result of swelling within the retina, and the foveal (macular) area is seen as a 'cherry red spot' because the retina is very thin and the choroid is seen underneath the retina, without swelling to mask the colour. An embolus in the central retinal artery may be seen. This condition is an ophthalmic emergency and although investigations about the cause of the condition are necessary (urgent erythrocyte sedimentation rate or ESR and C-reactive protein or CRP because giant cell arteritis may be a factor, lipid profiles, full blood count – to rule out coagulopathies and ultrasonography of the coronary arteries and echocardiography – in order to identify the site of the embolus), immediate treatment can start wherever the patient presents, even before the patient sees an ophthalmologist. Treatment is aimed at allowing increased perfusion of the retina by reducing the IOP. It includes the administration of intravenous acetazolamide 500 mg to reduce IOP, ocular massage, to encourage the outflow of aqueous, and often the patient is asked to rebreathe exhaled air by breathing into a paper bag. This increases the carbon dioxide concentration in the body, thus dilating blood vessels and possibly allowing the embolus to move further into the retinal circulation. If this occurs, a sector of visual loss, rather than profound loss, may be a good outcome for the patient. An anoxic retina is irreversibly damaged in 90 minutes (Pavan-Langston 2002) and for a patient who wakes up with this condition, or who does not attend immediately – the vast majority of patients – the visual outcome of this condition is usually poor.

In some conditions, vision loss may become progressively more profound over the whole field of vision over a number of days. The most likely cause of this is optic neuritis, which is described under 'Blurring of vision'.

Profound loss of vision that appears gradually, starting with a segment of the visual field and enlarging to cover the whole of it, is likely to be the result of a retinal detachment. This is described under 'Segmental loss of vision' below and in Chapter 21.

Segmental loss of vision

The most likely causes of the loss of an area of the visual field in one eye are vascular causes such as occlusions of branches of the retinal artery or vein, or retinal detachments. If the onset is sudden and stays the same, the cause is likely to be vascular. If the area of visual loss changes over time, the cause is more likely to be a retinal detachment.

Branch retinal artery and vein occlusions (see Chapter 21)

These may be seen with an ophthalmoscope; the branch artery occlusion will lead to a segment of retina being paler than the rest, all the vessels will appear in the correct location and an embolus may be seen in one of the vessels. There may be multiple retinal haemorrhages seen if the cause of the loss of vision is a branch retinal vein occlusion. The haemorrhages will be in the area of retina that is served by the blocked vein. Retinal oedema may be seen and an occlusion may be visible. There is no immediate treatment for either of these conditions although follow-up by an ophthalmologist will be necessary.

Retinal detachment (see Chapter 21)

Spontaneous retinal detachment affects around 1 in 10 000 of the population each year. It is more common in males and in short-sighted (myopic) eyes (Pavan-Langston 2002). It usually occurs in middle age as a result of collapse of the vitreous gel, causing traction on a weak area of retina which produces a hole (rhegmatogenous retinal detachment). Other causes include traction on the retina in conditions where fibrovascular tissue has developed between the retina and vitreous, such as in diabetic retinopathy (traction retinal detachment) and subretinal disorders such as tumours or inflammation that allows passage of fluid behind the retina, which pushes it off its basement membrane (exudative retinal detachment).

Symptoms characteristic of retinal detachment include the following:

- Flashing lights, which are the result of traction on the retina or of areas of the retina moving. The only way that the brain can interpret movement of the retina is in terms of light so, as the retina moves, the brain interprets and the patient 'sees' flashes of light.
- Floaters: the appearance of a large circular floater is the result of the detachment of the vitreous gel from its attachment at the optic disc. A

shower of tiny floaters is likely to be caused by haemorrhage into the vitreous because a small retinal blood vessel is involved in the retinal tear.
- A sector of loss of vision may be noticed that tends to enlarge over a period of hours or days. The patient may complain of seeing a 'shadow' that tends to move, or a curtain or cobweb descending over the eye. This is the result of an area of retina that is detached and may be enlarging or moving within the patient's field of vision.
- Central vision may be lost as a result of macular detachment.

The detached retina will appear grey and may seem slightly wrinkled. If central vision is present, the macula is still attached and it is likely that surgery will be immediate in order to preserve this situation. If central vision is affected, it is likely that the macula is detached. If this has happened within a matter of hours, surgery is likely to be immediate in order to attempt to reattach it and preserve some of its function. If the macula has been detached for some time, it is likely that surgical delay of a few days will not adversely affect the outcome for vision because macular function is not likely to be restored (Cheng et al. 1997).

Loss of central vision

Common causes of loss of central vision include age-related macular degeneration (AMD), optic neuritis, central serous retinopathy and macular burns.

Age-related macular degeneration

Age-related macular degeneration refers to a gradual degeneration of the macula. It is the most common cause of visual loss in those aged over 75, and affects around 20% of individuals. There is usually a very gradual loss of central vision. The patient may have noticed that they have to use a bright light to read by and that words fade after a few minutes. Although this is not an acute problem, elderly patients may present to acute settings because they have reached a point where they can no longer manage the problems alone. There is little effective treatment for this condition. Patients retain navigating vision – their peripheral visual field is not affected. Registration as visually impaired may enable the patient to access appropriate services, although this is a purely voluntary registration. Registration as visually impaired in England may be undertaken by any clinician, and AMD confirmed by an optometrist, for example, is enough to mobilize Social Services involvement. Involvement of Social Services can lead to benefits for the patients in terms of rehabilitation. AMD may also present acutely in younger patients and any loss of vision that involves distortion of central vision should have an early assessment because the 'wet' form of AMD may respond to treatment (see Chapter 21).

Optic neuritis (see Chapter 23)

This refers to inflammation of the optic nerve. Episodes are usually monocular, although they may be binocular. It is most common in adults between the ages of 20 and 40 and is more common in women. Optic neuritis is the presenting feature in 25% of patients with multiple sclerosis (MS) and occurs in 70% of established cases. Many patients with idiopathic optic neuritis will go on to develop MS. Various texts suggest figures of 50% (Pavan-Langston 2002), 60% (Onofrey et al. 1998) and 'most' (Cheng et al. 1997).

The patient is likely to present with loss of central vision, which may progress to a generalized loss of vision and can become severe. It is maximal after about 2 weeks and tends to recover after 4–6 weeks. Over a period of months, most patients recover 6/12 vision or better.

Other symptoms include pain around or behind the eye which is worse on ocular movement (as a result of the inflamed optic nerve moving as the eye moves). Perception of colour in the affected eye is likely to be reduced. This can be tested using the top of a red pen and comparing the perception of red in each eye. The pupil reactions will be abnormal and the optic nerve head may appear normal or be swollen. Steroids may be prescribed if vision loss becomes profound. Referral to a neurologist or neuro-ophthalmologist for further assessment and possible treatment is the preferred course of action. A possible diagnosis of MS should not be discussed immediately because, even with a confirmed diagnosis of optic neuritis, MS is still only a possibility and the acute setting has neither the time nor the resources for the counselling that may be necessary in this situation.

Central serous retinopathy

Central serous retinopathy (CSR) occurs usually in young adult males and has an unknown cause. Symptoms commonly include a unilateral blurring of central vision and a generalized darkening of the visual field with some distortion. Visual acuity is usually only mildly reduced. It is rare for it to be less than 6/18, but it may reduce to 6/60 (Cheng et al. 1997). Although referral to an ophthalmologist is necessary, most episodes of CSR resolve within 3–6 months. Treatment is not usually indicated although laser treatment has been shown to assist resolution in some cases where the CSR episode persists.

Macular burns

These may be caused by MIG welding equipment as described earlier. Although very rarely experienced, looking at the sun, for example, during a solar eclipse can result in macular burns and indeed the last such eclipse in the UK resulted in a number of patients with irreversible retinal damage. The opportunity for appropriate health education before a solar eclipse is great – they are extremely predictable. Health education information that that there are no sunglasses strong enough to prevent eye damage as a result of looking at the sun may, however, be something that ophthalmic professionals do not generally consider.

Blurring of vision

Blurring of vision may be the result of problems anywhere from the cornea to the optic nerve and the brain. Many patients will have problems in differentiating between generalized blurring and loss of central vision, and therefore careful questioning is again needed to obtain a full picture of the problem.

Sudden onset blurring of vision may be caused by vitreous haemorrhage or vascular occlusions. These have been dealt with elsewhere. Other causes of blurring of vision tend to develop more gradually and may include CSR and optic neuritis. Again, these have been dealt with earlier in this chapter and in other chapters. Patients with papilloedema often present with blurring of vision. This may be worse in one eye and may be exacerbated by, for example, standing up (Cheng et al. 1997). Concurrent symptoms may be ignored by the patient in favour of the eye problem. Patients with bilateral swollen optic discs need urgent neurological referral.

Patients occasionally present with refractive errors that they have not noticed previously. It may be that they have covered one eye and noticed that the vision in the remaining eye is not good. This may provoke much anxiety and encourage them to self-refer. Visual acuity should be checked using pinholes to negate the effect of any refractive error. If vision improves dramatically with pinholes, a large significant proportion of the blurring is likely to be caused by refractive error and, in the absence of any other findings, the patient may be referred to an optometrist.

Opacities in any of the clear structures of the eye will result in blurring of vision because less light is allowed to reach the retina. The most common opacity is the result of cataract (see Chapter 18). Again, the patient may just have noticed the loss of vision, possibly by closing one eye, or worry about the symptoms may have prompted self-referral. A more worrying presentation is if the lens opacity has occurred after trauma, or is in a younger person, and further investigations may be appropriate.

Corneal problems also result in blurring of vision (see Chapter 16).

Transient loss of vision

Transient loss of vision may be caused by a vast range of conditions. A number of these such as papilloedema and migraine have been dealt with earlier. Other, common causes of transient loss include carotid artery disease and giant cell arteritis. Intermittent angle-closure glaucoma is a rare but possible cause of these symptoms.

Carotid artery disease

Retinal emboli from carotid artery disease often produce transient visual loss known as amaurosis fugax. This may be described as a curtain being lowered and then lifted over the vision. It is likely to last seconds to minutes rather than hours. It may be a sign of impending cerebrovascular accident and so cardiovascular investigations are appropriate. Turning the head may precipitate an attack and this is characteristic of carotid artery disease.

Giant cell arteritis

Patients with giant cell arteritis often complain of headache and tenderness over the scalp. This may be obvious when they comb their hair. They may also notice jaw claudication and pain on chewing. An urgent ESR is indicated and may be more than 80 mm. Treatment is with high doses of steroids, definitive diagnosis is by temporal artery biopsy and frequent monitoring of the patient's condition will be required.

Intermittent angle-closure glaucoma

Patients may present with symptoms of pain in and around the eye and blurring of vision that begins, usually at night, when the pupil becomes larger as a result of the reduced light levels, and may last a number of hours, It may have resolved by the time the patient presents. If the anterior chamber appears shallow, and the symptoms are as described, intermittent angle-closure glaucoma may be suspected and urgent prophylactic laser treatment can be undertaken to prevent further attacks.

References

Besamusca F, Bastiensen L (1986) Blood dyscrasis and topically applied chloramphenicol in ophthalmology. Docu Ophthalmol 64: 87–95.

Brahma AK, Shah S, Hillier VF et al. (1996) Topical analgesia for superficial corneal injuries. J Accid Emerg Med 13: 186–8.

Buckles E, Carew-McColl M (1991) Triage by telephone. Nursing Times 87(6): 26–8.

Cheng H, Burdon MA, Buckley SA, Moorman C (1997) Emergency Ophthalmology. London: BMJ Publishing Group.

Consumers' Association (1997) Drugs and Therapeutics Bulletin 35(7): 49–52.

Eagling EM, Roper-Hall MJ (1986) Eye Injuries: An illustrated guide. London: Gower.

Fechner PU, Teichmann KD (1998) Ocular Therapeutics. Thorofare, NJ: Slack.

Forrester J, Dick A, McMenamin P, Lee W (1996) The Eye: Basic sciences in practice. London: Saunders

Herr RD, White GL Jr, Bernhisel K et al. (1991) Clinical comparisons of ocular irrigation fluids following chemical injury. Am J Emerg Med 9: 228–31.

MacEwan CJ (1989) Eye injuries: a prospective survey of 5671 cases. Br J Ophthalmol 73: 888–94.

Mackway-Jones K, Marsden J (2003) Ascorbate for alkali burns to the eye. J Emerg Med 20: 465–6.

Mackway-Jones K, Marsden J, Windle J (2005) Emergency Triage, 2nd edn. London: BMJ Books.

Marsden J (1999) Painless loss of vision. Emerg Nurse 6(9): 13–18.

Marsden J (2001) Treating corneal trauma. Emerg Nurse 9(8): 17–20.

Newell FW (1996) Ophthalmology: Principles and concepts, 8th edn. St Louis, MO: Mosby.

Onofrey BE, Skorin L Jr, Holdeman NR (1998) Ocular Therapeutics Handbook. Philadelphia, PA: Lippincott-Raven.

Patel B, Taylor S (2002) Orbital fracture, apex: www.emedicine.com/oph (last accessed 4 April 2005).

Pavan-Langston D (2002) Manual of Ocular Diagnosis and Therapy. Philadelphia, PA: Lippincott, Williams & Wilkins.

Rhee DJ, Pyfer MF (eds) (1999) The Wills Eye Manual, 3rd edn. Philadelphia, PA: Lippincott, Williams & Wilkins.

Tullo AB, Donnelly D (1995) Conjunctiva. In: Perry JP, Tullo AB (eds), Care of the Ophthalmic Patient, 2nd edn. London: Chapman & Hall.

Wagoner MD (1997) Chemical injuries of the eye: current concepts in pathophysiology and therapy. Surv Ophthalmol 41: 275–313.

CHAPTER THIRTEEN

The challenge of eye health care in developing countries

SUE STEVENS, INGRID COX AND ANDREW R POTTER

This chapter aims to give an overview of ophthalmic problems in the developing world. The reader will recognize the different challenges in the approach to eye care delivery in areas with limited resources and the considerations needed for working in a developing country.

Introduction – world blindness

The World Health Organization estimates that there are around 37 million blind people worldwide and around 124 million with low vision, comprising a total of over 161 million people with some degree of visual impairment (Table 13.1). Ninety per cent live in developing countries and the real tragedy is that 80% of this blindness is avoidable, i.e. preventable or treatable. It is estimated that 7 million people become blind each year. Most live in the poor countries of Africa and Asia where eye care services and trained

Table 13.1 Global causes of blindness as a percentage of total blindness (data for 2002)

Condition	Percentage
Cataract	47.8
Glaucoma	12.3
Age-related macular degeneration	8.7
Corneal opacities	5.1
Diabetic retinopathy	4.8
Childhood blindness	3.9
Trachoma	3.6
Onchocerciasis	0.8
Others*	13.0

* e.g. trauma, leprosy, refractive error
From World Health Organization (2004).

eye health workers are a scarce resource. Half the burden of blindness is caused by blinding cataract simply because there are not enough ophthalmologists in developing countries. The ophthalmologists who do exist work in the major cities whereas most of the population live in rural communities. Furthermore, poor people cannot afford the fees charged by many ophthalmologists, some of whom also do not perform surgery. Many causes of blindness affect old people who fear going to hospital or who believe that deteriorating vision is an inevitable part of growing old.

Prevention and cure of blindness are among the most successful and cost-effective interventions in health-care delivery. The challenge for the ophthalmic community worldwide is to bring affordable and accessible quality eye care to the developing world. The aim must be to reduce the intolerable burden of unnecessary blindness that affects millions in poor countries.

VISION 2020: The Right to Sight

This global initiative, a collaborative effort by the WHO and the International Agency for the Prevention of Blindness (IAPB), aims to eliminate the main preventable and treatable causes of blindness by the year 2020 (WHO 1997). This requires many people to work together in global partnership to achieve this goal. It involves the active participation of UN agencies, governments, international non-governmental development organizations, health professionals, philanthropic institutions and individuals. The main focus of the initiative is threefold:

1. Control of the major causes of blindness
2. Human resource development
3. Creation of infrastructure and technology.

Eye problems in developing countries

Cataract (Figure 13.1)

Cataract accounts for at least half of all blindness worldwide. In industrialized nations age-related cataract is common in the increasing over 65-age group, and cataract surgery is the most frequently performed surgical procedure.

In the developing world, where there are insufficient ophthalmologists and where city eye clinics are inaccessible to the huge and increasing rural population, cataract blindness has become a burden on the community.

How to tackle the 'backlog problem' of blinding cataract in developing countries is much debated. Should the latest western technology be

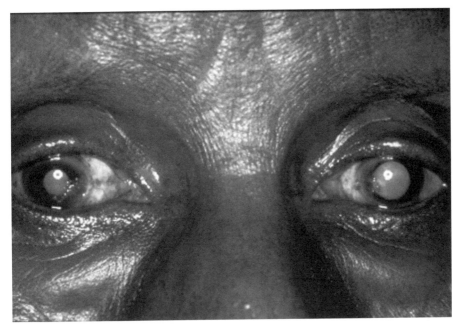

Figure 13.1 Bilateral blinding cataract and solar keratopathy. (Courtesy of GJ Johnson.)

transferred to rural Africa or Asia? Or should much simpler techniques be employed? Who will pay for eye surgery for the world's poorest citizens? How can highly trained surgeons and nurses be motivated to work in isolated and uncomfortable communities in order to reach the rural blind? However, it is possible to perform high-quality, high-volume and low-cost cataract surgery in remote tropical communities by:

- raising awareness in communities about cataract and its treatment
- training existing health-care personnel to perform cataract surgery
- using a 'standard list' for bulk buying of equipment (operating light, operating microscope, etc.) and consumables (sutures, viscoelastic, antibiotics, steroid drops and injections, etc.)
- ensuring a high through-put of patients to reduce costs.

In such circumstances modern cataract surgery can be costed at between $US30 and $US50 per patient.

Some developing countries, recognizing that there will not be enough ophthalmologists within the foreseeable future to address the cataract problem, have trained medical assistants and specialist nurses to perform cataract surgery. Periodic supervision by a visiting ophthalmologist can help to ensure that standards are maintained.

Climatic droplet keratopathy (Figure 13.1)

Prolonged exposure to bright sunlight can cause the formation of a horizontal band of translucent protein material, which looks like 'droplets' in the superficial corneal stroma and affect the interpalpebral exposed cornea. At the early stages there is little visual loss. However, this may progress in time to yellow deposits across the band and vision is then markedly reduced.

The wearing of sunglasses may protect against this solar keratopathy.

Diabetes

Diabetes is on the increase and is now also recognized as a problem in developing countries. It is no longer a disease affecting those with an affluent lifestyle. There is a need to improve awareness, among communities and eye health workers, that this serious condition can, untreated, cause multisystem disease. Sophisticated screening methods are not readily available in the developing world, but all health professionals need to be fully aware of diabetes particularly if it is a public health problem in their region. Patients with diabetes need regular ophthalmoscopy and referral for expert opinion, but it is not easy to provide this in many developing countries.

Glaucoma

Glaucoma may account for almost 15% of world blindness. Open-angle glaucoma, so common in Africa, is a 'silent' disease. There are no symptoms until it is very advanced. In industrialized nations many patients are diagnosed at routine examination by optometrists. In many tropical countries, especially on the African continent, optometrists are rare. Therefore, inevitably, many patients with glaucoma present late when blindness in one or both eyes has occurred. Furthermore, tests to confirm the diagnosis of glaucoma, such as visual fields and gonioscopy, may not be easily accessible in the tropics.

Another difficulty is that drugs to lower intraocular pressure (pilocarpine, α and β blockers, carbonic anhydrase inhibitors, etc.) are relatively expensive for those on low incomes in poor countries. They may be unavailable in rural districts. All this makes the treatment of glaucoma a real challenge. Although it is a common disease, the diagnosis is often made late when the disease has progressed. Further, its treatment with drugs is very expensive.

Specialist nurses can be taught to perform fundoscopy routinely and note and record the cup:disc ratio of the optic nerve head. Where slit-lamp applanation tonometry is not available, a hand-held Schiötz tonometer (Figure 13.9) is still used with reliable accuracy. Realistically, the treatment of primary open-angle glaucoma in poor countries is surgical, i.e. trabeculectomy. Once performed there is usually no further need for expensive pressure-lowering eyedrops. Regular follow-up of operated patients is advised and, of course, the patient must be warned that no surgery is without risk. The alternative, in many cases, is to prescribe timolol or pilocarpine, but it is likely that the patient will not be able to afford these eyedrops for the rest of his or her life or they will not be readily available. Primary closed-angle glaucoma is more commonly found in races of Mongoloid origin – in east Asia and among the Inuit (Eskimos).

HIV/AIDS

Ninety-five per cent of the 42 million people with HIV/AIDS live in developing countries where the disease manifests itself very differently from the industrialized west. The mortality is higher and earlier in the course of the disease, as it was in the industrialized world before the advent of drug therapies that are now widely available.

Herpes zoster ophthalmicus has long been a marker for HIV infection in Africa and Kaposi's sarcoma and squamous cell carcinoma of the conjunctiva are also well recognized. The reported incidence of cytomegalovirus (CMV) retinitis is relatively low in Africa. This is thought to be a result of the lack of treatment and consequent early death before this complication arises. The added tragedy for Africa is that eye health workers are also falling victim to HIV/AIDS, thus reducing, even more, the availability of a trained workforce. Encouragingly, a few large companies have started to supply anti-HIV drugs in Africa.

Leprosy (Hansen's disease) (Figure 13.2)

Although leprosy is becoming a rare disease, there are upwards of 10 million people who have had the disease and still suffer from its complications. New cases continue to be discovered in some parts of the tropics.

Leprosy is caused by the acid-fast bacillus *Mycobacterium leprae*. It predominantly affects the skin, superficial nerves, nose and throat. Infection is by droplet infection or skin contact. It is, however, possible to live in close contact with an infected person without acquiring the disease.

There are two classic forms of leprosy:

1. Lepromatous leprosy, where there are millions of bacilli in the skin lesions and the nose.
2. Tuberculoid leprosy, where there are few bacilli in the skin lesions.

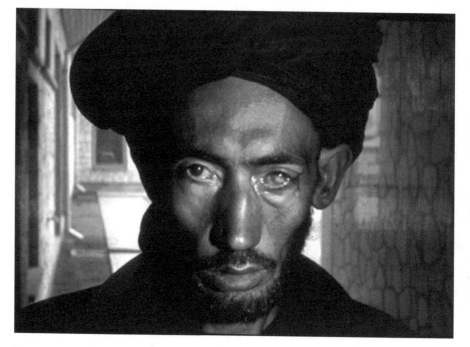

Figure 13.2 The face of leprosy. (Courtesy of JDC Anderson.) (See Plate 8.)

Where peripheral nerves are involved the skin becomes anaesthetic. Skin infection and ulceration may follow. Fingers and toes may be lost through repeated open wounds after unfelt trauma or burns.

Nerve palsies can occur, notably of the ulnar nerve of the forearm causing a 'claw-hand' and of the peroneal nerve in the leg causing foot drop. Facial nerve palsy causes lagophthalmos, leaving the eye exposed. Repeated trauma from the wind, dust, foreign bodies, flies, etc. causes exposure keratitis and corneal ulceration. In the long term, the cornea becomes scarred and opaque. There may also be ectropion.

Chronic uveitis causes miosis and posterior synechiae. Secondary cataract and glaucoma lead to loss of vision and blindness. Involvement of the skin of the eyebrows causes the hairs to fall out (madarosis).

Modern triple drug therapy can swiftly eliminate the leprosy bacilli. Rifampicin, dapsone and clofazimine are the first-line drugs used in combination. Second-line treatment may include ofloxacin, minocycline and clarithromycin. Some patients experience treatment 'reversal reactions' that need emergency treatment with high doses of oral steroids.

Uveitis in leprosy should be treated with atropine to keep the pupil well dilated to prevent the formation of posterior synechiae. Lagophthalmos may be corrected by a surgical tarsorrhaphy to reduce the corneal exposure.

Loa-loa

Loa-loa is a filarial disease found only in west and central Africa. The vector fly *Chrysops* sp. bites an infected person, ingests the microfilariae found in the human skin and transmits these to another person. The microfilariae develop into adult worms that migrate around the body. The eye may be affected in two ways:

1. The adult worm may be seen under the bulbar conjunctiva making snake-like movements. This causes pain and ocular irritation. Treatment, under a local anaesthetic, enables removal of the worm.
2. A 'calabar' swelling is an oedematous inflammatory swelling that may occur around the orbit and eyelids. The swelling usually resolves in a few days.

Low vision and refractive error

Low vision services have historically been inadequately provided for in eye care delivery. This, unsurprisingly, has been even more marked in developing countries. This is largely a result of lack of awareness and skilled personnel, and the high cost of optical devices. An estimated 68 million worldwide require low vision care and are likely to benefit if services were made available to them.

Uncorrected refractive error is an important cause of visual impairment in many countries. An estimated 2.3 billion worldwide have refractive error, the vast majority of whom could be helped by spectacles, but only 1.8 billion have access to eye examination and affordable correction. The remainder – one-third of whom live in Africa, many of them children – live with uncorrected error and visual impairment. In developing countries it is often difficult to provide an efficient refraction service.

Onchocerciasis (river blindness) (Figure 13.3)

Onchocerciasis is a chronic infection caused by the filarial nematode *Onchocerca volvulus*. It occurs predominantly in west and central Africa, with foci in Central America and parts of east Africa. It is estimated that it affects more than 40 million people and may have blinded up to half a million.

The infection is transmitted by bites of the black fly, *Simulium* sp., which breeds in fast-flowing rivers (hence 'river blindness'). The fly takes a blood meal from an infected person, ingesting microfilariae from the skin. These microfilariae can be transferred to the skin of an uninfected person. Once in a new host, some of the microfilariae develop into adult worms that live in nodules under the skin, often over the bony prominences of the iliac crest, rib cage, shoulders, knees or forehead. Each female adult worm can

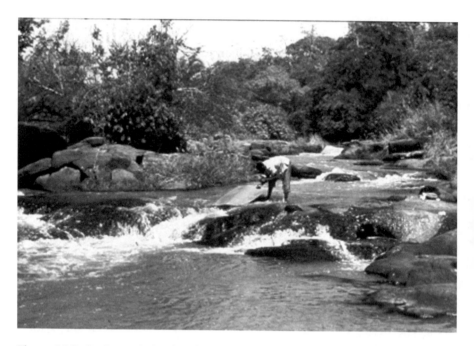

Figure 13.3 Onchocerciasis (river blindness): the Simulium fly breeds in fast-flowing water. (Courtesy of J Stilma.)

produce thousands of microfilariae that lodge in the skin, joints and the eye. They may be seen in the aqueous humour and in the cornea of heavily infected individuals. Ocular lesions include a sclerosing keratitis (a brown–white opacification of the mostly peripheral cornea), uveitis, chorioretinitis, retinal pigmentary disturbance and optic nerve atrophy.

Treatment of infected individuals is with ivermectin, one dose annually for 10–15 years, which is the estimated lifespan of the adult worms. Ivermectin is a very safe drug and is being used to treat whole communities in endemic areas of west and central Africa. Ivermectin has been generously donated by Merck Inc.

In the past, spraying with insecticide of breeding sites in well-oxygenated waters of free-flowing rivers reduced the vector fly population. This reduced transmission of the parasite.

From 1974 to 2002 the Onchocerciasis Control Programme in west Africa was responsible for vector control (spraying rivers) and the distribution of ivermectin. Since 2002 each country concerned has taken over control of its national programme and will continue ivermectin distribution. There should now be no new cases of onchocerciasis and, within a generation, all those blind or with low vision caused by the disease will have died. The disease may therefore become extinct.

Pterygium

Pterygium is a common condition in hot climates especially in semi-desert areas with a prolonged dry season, hot dry winds, dust in the atmosphere (e.g. the 'harmattan' of west Africa) and exposure to the sun from an outdoor occupation or lifestyle. In some areas in the tropics, considerable stigma is attached to this condition.

Pterygia usually develop in the region of the nasal limbus, but can also occur at the temporal limbus. Pterygium can grow so large as to cover the central cornea and hide the pupil. The eye is then blind. Treatment is surgical excision, but recurrence is frequent.

Trachoma

Trachoma is a chronic infection of the conjunctiva, both tarsal and bulbar, caused by *Chlamydia trachomatis* (Figure 13.4). The infection thrives in conditions of poverty where hygiene standards are low. It especially affects children and the women who look after them. Repeated infections cause the conjunctiva to become scarred. Scarred conjunctiva contracts and pulls the eyelid edge inwards. The eyelashes begin to rub against the cornea, eventually causing ulceration and vascular corneal scarring. The patient endures constant ocular discomfort and the opaque cornea makes the eye blind.

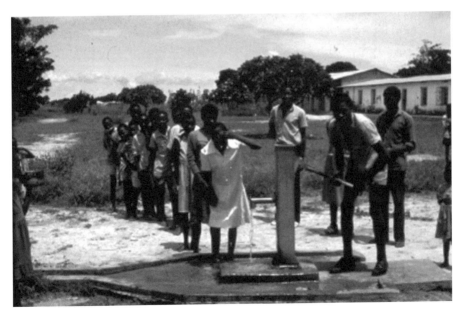

Figure 13.4 Availability of water affects the prevalence of trachoma in a community. (Courtesy of Hans Limburg.)

Secretions from the chronically infected eyes provide the source of transmission from person to person, via flies, hands, clothes, towels, etc. Re-infection is common within households where:

- there is insufficient water for regular washing
- there is absence of toilets/latrines, leaving excreta in the open air to attract flies
- animals are kept close to the home.

The clinical diagnosis of trachoma is made by inspecting the tarsal conjunctiva of the upper eyelid. The WHO has produced a simplified classification for the grading of clinical trachoma, shown in the box.

WHO classification of trachoma (Figure 13.5)

TF	trachomatous inflammation with follicles
TI	trachomatous inflammation – intense
TS	trachomatous scarring
TT	trachomatous trichiasis
CO	corneal opacity

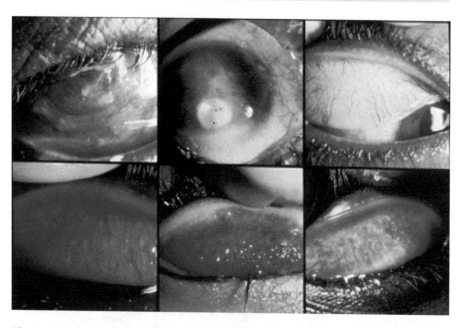

Figure 13.5 Trachoma grading (anti-clockwise from top right as grading classification): everted eyelid, normal healthy eye; corneal opacity (CO); trachomatous trichiasis (TT); trachomatous inflammation – follicular (TF); trachomatous inflammation – intense (TI); trachomatous scarring (TS). (By courtesy of the International Centre for Eye Health – ICEH.) (See Plate 9.)

Since 1996 the WHO and other organizations working to eliminate trachoma as a public health problem have adopted the 'SAFE' strategy to deal with the problem.

'SAFE' strategy

S = Surgery to correct entropion and trichiasis
A = Antibiotics to treat the chlamydial infection
F = Facial cleanliness to reduce transmission of the infected secretions in the community
E = Environmental improvements, e.g. improved access to clean water, construction of latrines, disposal of domestic waste

Many operations have been devised to correct entropion and trichiasis. The WHO recommends a procedure called bilamellar tarsal rotation (Bailey and Lietman 2001). As trachoma affects predominantly isolated communities, surgery should be offered at minimal cost to the patient and within his or her locality. However, even if surgery is offered without payment, only half of those who could benefit actually accept surgery.

For many years tetracycline ointment 1%, usually twice daily for 6 weeks, has been the standard treatment. No resistance has been reported to tetracycline, an inexpensive antibiotic.

More recently a single dose of azithromycin has been shown to be as effective. Compliance is better than with a course of local tetracycline ointment. Pfizer Inc. is donating azithromycin for mass distribution in endemic communities.

In the long term, trachoma will be eradicated only with a general improvement in standards of living, most notably in the provision of clean water and the hygienic use of toilets. Consequently, the efforts of water engineers will make as much impact on the elimination of trachoma as health-care personnel.

Trauma

An estimated 1.6 million people worldwide are blind as a result of eye injuries. Many people in developing countries never seek eye care after an accident and later suffer major consequences for which there is often no source of treatment. Even when warnings are given of the danger of eye injury, often vulnerable people do not heed advice. Children are commonly victims of eye trauma, not only because of their innocence but because they lack elder supervision or are members of a workforce who are employed at a much younger age in developing countries and therefore prone to occupational injury.

Vitamin A deficiency (xerophthalmia) (Figure 13.6)

Vitamin A deficiency occurs in malnourished young children and may account for over 200 000 children becoming blind each year. A similar number will die from associated pathology, especially measles and malnutrition.

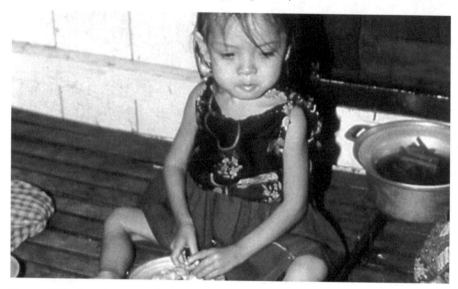

Figure 13.6 A malnourished child with bilateral corneal ulceration due to vitamin A deficiency. (Courtesy of DMM McGavin.)

Vitamin A is found in red/orange fruits and vegetables, e.g. mango, papaya, sweet potato, carrots, palm oil, dark-green leafy plants (spinach, cassava leaves, baobab leaves, etc.) and in animal foods such as fish liver oil, animal liver, eggs, butter, dairy products and meat.

The body needs vitamin A to maintain the integrity of the epithelial surfaces of the skin, mucous membranes, conjunctiva, cornea, digestive tract and lungs. In the eye the conjunctival goblet cells that secrete mucus are dependent on vitamin A for their function. Mucus acts as the wetting agent to maintain a tear film over the cornea and conjunctiva. In the retina, rod photoreceptors need vitamin A for their functioning. Vitamin A also helps maintain the body's immune status.

Measles attacks mucous membranes causing conjunctivitis, Koplik's oral ulcers, upper and lower respiratory tract infections, and diarrhoea. A child on the borderline of malnutrition may become clinically deficient in vitamin A because the child with measles is miserable and reluctant to eat. The combination of not eating and prolonged diarrhoea in a child may develop into marasmus or kwashiorkor and acute vitamin A deficiency. Mortality is high.

Ocular lesions in xerophthalmia

- Conjunctival and corneal dryness.
- The cornea loses its shiny appearance. The conjunctiva becomes thickened and may wrinkle.
- Bitot's spots (Figure 13.7): there is a white frothy appearance of the interpalpebral conjunctiva. Bitot's spots may outlast the acute deficiency and be seen later in healthy children.
- Corneal ulceration, which may be associated with bacterial or herpetic infection.
- Corneal softening (keratomalacia), usually of rapid onset.
- Corneal perforation.
- Night blindness caused by poor rod photoreceptor function.

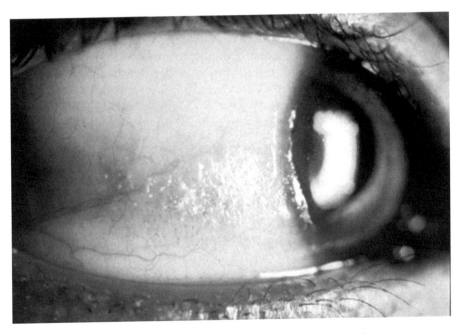

Figure 13.7 Bitot's spots. (See Plate 10.) (Courtesy of DMM McGavin.)

Treatment of vitamin A deficiency

For a child aged 1 year and over:

- 200 000 IU vitamin A – on presentation
- 200 000 IU vitamin A – the next day
- 200 000 IU vitamin A – within 1 or 2 weeks.

For a child under 1 year of age, half the above doses should be given.

All children in the tropics with measles should receive vitamin A on presentation, as should all children with corneal ulcers or any signs or symptoms of xerophthalmia. High doses of vitamin A must not be given to pregnant women because there is a danger of foetal malformation.

Children with corneal ulceration will also need antibiotic eyedrops or ointment and atropine 1% to dilate the pupil. Steroid eyedrops must never be used when there is an ulcerated cornea.

Mothers of children with xerophthalmia should be given advice on diets containing enough vitamin A and protein. However, communities in which vitamin A deficiency occurs are usually very poor and, in such circumstances, specific dietary advice may be unrealistic.

Traditional eye medicine

For centuries, before effective modern medicines became available, herbal medicines were used to treat many medical problems. Many of the first modern medicines were derived from plants (digitalis from the foxglove, quinine from tree bark and morphia from poppies).

Some traditional practices are harmful (Figure 13.8), and this is especially true in eye disease. It is easy to see why. A red, sore eye may have a

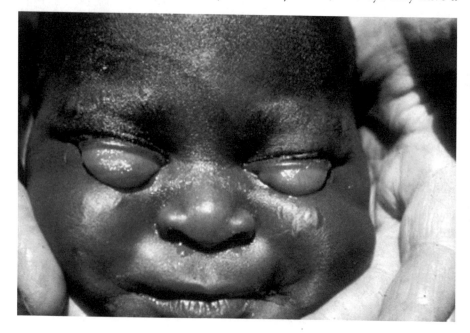

Figure 13.8 Severe chemosis – the result of traditional eye medicine. (By courtesy of E Sutter.) (See Plate 11.)

corneal ulcer and instilling a herbal and non-sterile concoction can only aggravate the ulceration and introduce fungi and bacteria. Some traditional remedies are caustic (onion or lemon juice). Breast milk or human urine has also been used to treat eye disease. Urine containing *Neisseria gonorrhoeae* can blind an eye within 24 hours.

Eye workers in the tropics often see patients who have first used 'traditional eye medicines' before presenting at an eye clinic. Direct questioning of the patient or an accompanying relative is often needed before this is admitted. However, this needs some sensitivity because information may be withheld if the patient or carer recognizes disapproval in the health worker.

In some countries efforts are being made to educate local traditional healers, and integrate them into primary eye care programmes, while discouraging the use of harmful substances in the eyes of those who consult them. Couching as treatment for blinding cataract is still practised by traditional healers in some parts of Africa and elsewhere. Three methods are reported:

1. A concoction of herbal juices is instilled into the eye. The effect of this is to loosen the zonule. The cataract may then slip backwards into the vitreous.
2. A fine needle, either metallic or a sharp thorn, is inserted through the cornea and, by manipulation, the dense cataract is dislodged, usually backwards into the vitreous.
3. A 'bolus' of sand or gravel impacts the eye when a spent cartridge, held against the closed eye, is struck by the healer. The lens may dislocate.

Sometimes couching achieves its purpose and the eye is rendered aphakic, improving the patient's vision. But it is just as likely to lead to intense intraocular inflammation, infection and endophthalmitis.

Community eye health

Community eye health, or community ophthalmology, is a population-oriented approach to eye health and disease. This approach is making eye care in developing countries more accessible, because it considers the eye problems and care of communities as a whole. Ophthalmologists are not seen as pivotal in meeting the needs of the community; rather, the role of nurses and other eye health workers is emphasized as being important in the development of eye care interventions.

Community eye health consists of the following four components:

1. Needs assessment in the community, e.g. blindness surveys and examination of communities.

2. Development of strategies for the control of blinding eye disease, e.g. vitamin A supplements for children and promoting face washing.
3. Planning, management and evaluation of prevention of blindness programmes.
4. Health education and health promotion.

The role of the ophthalmic nurse in developing countries

In the developing world, eye care teams have included eye care workers from a variety of training backgrounds. However, as a result of the VISION 2020 initiative (WHO 1997), human resource development for mid-level cadres of eye workers is beginning to bring encouraging changes. Qualified nurses in developing countries are rare and for such nurses to become specialists in the field of ophthalmology is quite a consideration because other specialities are often more attractive.

Current practice in eye care and standards needs to be maintained, and skills further developed, so that the work carried out by eye health workers continues to ensure positive results in reducing avoidable blindness.

Ophthalmic care is delivered at three levels in developing countries: primary, secondary and tertiary.

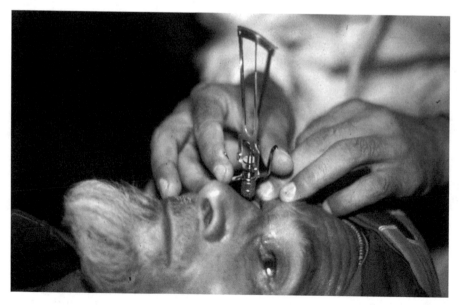

Figure 13.9 Schiötz tonometry remains a skill practised widely in developing countries. (Courtesy of DMM McGavin.)

Primary level (community eye health/primary eye care workers)

As stated in the previous section, community eye health is a population-oriented approach to eye health and disease that makes eye care more accessible to communities.

The governmental health budgets of developing countries are already overstretched. HIV/AIDS and its consequences, inappropriate use of resources (financial and human), poor infrastructure, lack of management to monitor and control, limited health budgets and increasing population growths largely contribute to this situation.

For many people, hospitals are seen as imposing and frightening places in large cities and are often visited only if the problem is considered potentially fatal. Many people cannot afford to visit hospitals and are often deterred from doing so following rumours about 'western' medicine offered there or the experiences of friends and relatives. Consequently, a vast amount of health care in the developing world takes place in the villages.

Raising awareness and delivery of primary eye care are not carried out by specialist ophthalmic nurses. At this primary level, the ophthalmic nurse acts as a teacher. Key people in the community are taught how to identify eye problems, recognize the health challenges that communities face, and how to accept and adapt to new ideas. In many parts of Africa, traditional healers have been trained to do this work. As well as being respected and trusted members of the community, their services are readily accepted. Once trained, they become community eye health/primary eye care workers responsible for eye care in one or more local villages. The training is very practical and village based where the constraints and difficulties of working in the community can easily be recognized.

The community eye health worker is taught practical ophthalmic skills. However, much of the teaching involves how the patient perceives the problem and how these problems are classified into three simple categories – urgent, immediate and routine – with a view to referral for treatment.

Urgent

Ophthalmia neonatorum and eye trauma are emphasized in this category – two conditions that cause unnecessary blindness to many in the developing world, especially children.

Immediate

Mature cataract, red eye, trichiasis, sudden and gradual loss of vision, and poor vision in children are considered as immediate referrals.

The eye care worker is taught how to recognize the symptoms and signs and helped to understand and become assertive about the need for speedy referral to the nearest secondary level (district hospital) facility where there is a more qualified eye specialist.

Routine

Routine conditions are those that, once trained, the eye worker will be able to treat without referral, such as conjunctivitis. In addition, he or she will be responsible for health education among the local community groups, e.g. schools and churches.

The community eye health/primary eye care worker role can become a skilled and strategic position, making a direct impact on village eye health.

Secondary level (district hospital/health units)

At this level the role of the ophthalmic nurse varies according to the health structure already in place and the initiatives that the country may have taken to develop the eye care team:

- In some parts of Africa, the ophthalmic clinical officer (OCO) or technicien supérieur en optalmologie (TSO) in Francophone Africa, with 2 or 3 years of training in ophthalmology, is able to perform cataract surgery and refraction. Ophthalmic nursing experience is often the basis for such training. In Africa, there are not enough ophthalmologists to work at the district level and so training for this cadre is essential (Ministre de la Santé, République de Rwandaise 2002).
- In other parts of Africa, the ophthalmic nurse may attend 1- or 2-year training courses in ophthalmology, resulting in more managerial experience than diagnostic skills. The nurse will have a good overview of the health-care system in the country, eye conditions and treatment available and experience in managing a clinical area, and may be responsible for biometry and simple refraction (Ministry of Health, United Republic of Tanzania undated).
- In east Africa, qualified general nurses may undertake a 3-month intensive ophthalmic course, resulting in skills such as a diagnosis of common eye conditions, basic refraction and minor surgical procedures, e.g. lid surgery and chalazion incision. This training is very practical and is certainly filling a gap in east Africa. However, it is currently under review as more OCOs are being trained at the district level and consideration is being given as to the need for the 3-month course.
- In Pakistan and India, ophthalmic nurse training is modular and includes diagnostic, treatment and referral skills. This forms the basis for further training in optometry and orthoptics, low vision management, ophthalmic technology and public health ophthalmology (Khyber Institute of Ophthalmic Medical Sciences, undated).

Tertiary level (teaching hospital)

At this level, Africa is better served with ophthalmologists and OCOs/TSOs, and the ophthalmic nurse plays much more of a traditional nursing role and acts as a link between all clinical services and nursing areas. The department of ophthalmology has a sister-in-charge who plays a recognized role in nursing management and is also part of the eye care management team. Each clinical area is led by a designated ophthalmic nurse (Ministry of Health, Kenya 2002a).

At the ophthalmic tertiary level, as with other specialities, work is beginning to be divided into subspeciality areas.

Diabetes

The increasing number of patients with diabetes in the developing world is a major cause of concern and has necessitated the development of 'diabetic ophthalmic nurse educators'. These ophthalmic nurses, once subspeciality trained, are responsible for running diabetes clinics that monitor the patient's diabetes control and provide health education, including an understanding of the principles of diabetic eye disease, for patients and relatives.

Glaucoma

Some tertiary units have set up specialist glaucoma clinics where the ophthalmic nurse is responsible for tonometry, optic disc assessment and visual fields. This is a very encouraging and positive move forward for ophthalmic nurses in developing countries. Training is provided by the ophthalmologist, and the nurse's aptitude and willingness to develop these skills are carefully considered. No formal training has yet been developed in this subspeciality.

Childhood blindness

Vision therapy is a fairly new concept within comprehensive eye care services (assessment, optical provision, rehabilitation and special education of the visually impaired). A 1-year course is under way in Africa preparing ophthalmic nurses to become vision therapists (Ministry of Health, Kenya 2002b). The therapist will work with an ophthalmologist and/or paediatric ophthalmologist and refractionist to assist in the assessment, prescription and training in the use of low vision devices for a child with low vision. The therapist also trains the vision support teachers and works closely with them in blind (and integrated) schools, to develop training programmes to assist teachers in developing skills and furthering the education of these children. In addition, the therapist will help to develop the community eye health/primary eye care worker's role in identifying school children who may have low vision.

Outreach services

The ophthalmic nurse may also be responsible for organizing outreach services from the district or tertiary level hospital to the community. These activities raise awareness about local primary eye care and health education services. This is an important role because patients, surprisingly, are willing to express their fears and anxieties to an outsider who comes with the eye care worker. The ophthalmic nurse, as the link between hospital and community, is vital.

Continuing education

Each ophthalmic nurse has a responsibility in the continuing education and training of all eye care workers. Tertiary level personnel take the lead in developing skills and knowledge throughout the eye care team, including the training of non-nursing staff and newly employed staff. On-going training is part of the sister's role in ensuring that standards are maintained and monitored. Consideration is always given to current practice and how this may be developed and improved.

Summary

The ophthalmic nurse, a multiskilled mid-level professional, works in the community and at district level as a diagnostician or assistant to the OCO/TSO – a comprehensive eye care worker, bridging the gap between the community eye health/primary eye care level and the secondary/district hospital level. At the tertiary level, the ophthalmic nurse concentrates on improving the skills of the nursing team in order to meet the challenges of VISION 2020.

Considerations for working as an expatriate nurse

Preparation

Eye health care is very different in developing countries and, as explained above, so is the role of the nurse. Preparation for working overseas is important; it is advisable to seek as much advice, personal and professional, as possible. Those who have already served overseas will be an excellent resource. Information about the country, its health-care status and its culture is vital.

Transfer of all skills and use of all previous experience, in a very unfamiliar setting, cannot be expected – nor should they be imposed on national staff. It is necessary to have certain skills but nobody will have the monopoly on these and some skills, perhaps long since lost by eye health professionals in the industrialized world, e.g. Schiötz tonometry, may have to be learned 'in the field' (Figure 13.9).

An appreciation of the community eye health approach to eye care delivery is necessary for adapting to work in a developing country. Working at the primary health-care level and providing basic health education are fundamental activities and a major challenge. It is important to ensure that all experiential learning is supported by the various components of ophthalmic nurse education, supported and complemented by topics specific to community eye health, which may be resourced through appropriate ophthalmic teaching materials and further education.

Expectation

All expatriates will witness limited resources – human, technological and financial. Consequently, professional roles may not be well defined. Attitudes towards working in a developing country as a health worker must be guarded; there will be professional and skilled workers already among the national staff who will have a wealth of knowledge and experience with very responsible, and sometimes influential, positions. Teaching plays a large part in the expatriate's new environment. Although it takes time to adapt and learn new skills (we must never think we arrive fully equipped!) before being able to be part of service delivery, teaching is a valuable and rewarding contribution, especially for those whose stay will be shorter. Longer term, there may be opportunities to extend one's role but it is wise to be wary about accepting invitations to learn how to perform cataract surgery, for example, when time in training national staff, thus transferring certain skills and experience, will more effectively enable such a service to be sustainable.

One of the hardest things to accept and adapt to, and perhaps witness on a daily basis, is the level of poverty and the value placed on human life which may not necessarily be the same as that of one's home country. This may reflect past traumatic experiences of loss and bereavement that have so impacted the lives of national health-care workers.

Contribution

Working in the developing world will provide even more appreciation of the complementary relationship of nursing and medicine. Team work is vital; everyone plays an equally important part and contributes to the multi-benefit effect of working in a different culture. This leads to an awareness of the extended role of health-care workers at any level. There is always a two-way benefit and the experience offers a unique mutual teaching and learning experience.

The extended role of the nurse has been established for many years in many developing countries. Confidence in examining and treating patients without any medical supervision or referral will be expected, e.g. refraction and low vision skills are sought by many agencies seeking eye health workers.

Good quality care, at reasonable cost, is a requirement of all communities and the aim of most governments. Nursing experience at management level is valuable. Maintaining standards is close to every good nurse's heart, and teaching basic nursing principles and management skills is among the most valuable of the contributions that the expatriate nurse can make.

Most nurses who return from service overseas will claim to have gained and learned probably more than they gave or taught. But whatever one's contribution, it is always vital in such poorly resourced areas.

Implication

Returning home, after living and working in such an environment, will inevitably have implications – the so-called 'reverse culture shock'.

There may be little interest shown by friends and colleagues in the experience gained and the resulting professional development, e.g. there may be little appreciation of primary eye care and its considerable development overseas over many years, whereas such 'new' initiatives in the home country may be considered something that the expatriate has missed out on. The resourcefulness, adaptability and humility, inevitably learned overseas, can benefit changing health-care services in the industrialized world.

There may be difficulty tolerating the materialism in today's society or the sophistication of the home country's health service – some even experience extreme frustration and, perhaps, a need to consider a redirection of career. Most, however, accept a representative role and become passionate about creating awareness of the needs of the developing world.

Acknowledgement

The authors wish to thank Dr Murray McGavin for reviewing this chapter.

References

Bailey R, Lietman T (2001) The SAFE strategy for the elimination of trachoma by 2020: will it work? Bull WHO 79: 233–6.

Khyber Institute of Ophthalmic Medical Sciences (undated) Manual for BSc in Ophthalmic Technology for Allied Health Care Personnel in Pakistan, Peshawar, Pakistan.

Ministre de la Santé, République de Rwandaise (2002) Plan National de Lutte Contre la Cecite.

Ministry of Health, Kenya (2002a) Higher Diploma in Ophthalmic Nursing. Department of Nursing, Kenya Medical Training College.

Ministry of Health, Kenya (2002b) Curriculum for Diploma in Vision Therapy Faculty of Rehabilitative Health Sciences. Department of Occupational Therapy, Kenya Medical Training College.

Ministry of Health, United Republic of Tanzania (undated) Curriculum for Advanced Diploma in Ophthalmic Nursing (ADON). Tanzania Department of Human Resource for Health Development.

World Health Organization (1997) Global Initiative for the Elimination of Avoidable Blindness. WHO/PBL/97.61 Rev.1. Geneva: WHO.

World Health Organization (2004) Magnitude and Causes of Visual Impairment. Factsheet 282. Geneva: WHO.

Recommended learning and information resources

All these publications are available from IRC/ICEH. See address below.

Community Eye Health Journal, edited by Victoria Francis, ISBN 0953-6833

Collaboration with African Traditional Healers for the Prevention of Blindness, edited by Paul Courtright et al., ISBN 981-02-4377-4

Directory of Teaching and Information Resources for Blindness Prevention and Rehabilitation, Sue Stevens, ISBN 1-902541-09-X

Epidemiology of Eye Disease, edited by GJ Johnson et al., ISBN 0-340-80892-6

Eye Care in Developing Nations, Larry Schwab, ISBN 1-56055-043-0

Eye Diseases in Hot Climates, John Sandford Smith, ISBN 81-8147-412-0

Eye Surgery in Hot Climates, John Sandford Smith, ISBN 1-8439-5796-5

Global Initiative for the Elimination of Avoidable Blindness, edited by World Health Organization, WHO/PBL/97.61

Hanyane: A Village Struggles for Eye Health, Erika Sutter, Allen Foster and Victoria Francis, ISBN 0-333-51092-5

Ophthalmic Operating Theatre Practice: A manual for developing countries, edited by Ingrid Cox and Sue Stevens, ISBN 1-902541-08-1

Address

International Resource Centre (IRC) and International Centre for Eye Health (ICEH), London School of Hygiene and Tropical Medicine, Keppel Street, London WC1E 7HT, UK. Website: www.iceh.org.uk, www.jceh.co.uk.

CHAPTER FOURTEEN

Eyelids and lacrimal drainage system

LES MCQUEEN

The eyelids are two pairs of easily underestimated structures that are often thought of more in terms of their cosmetic appearance than they are in terms of the important part that they play in protecting the eye, maintaining visual clarity and controlling ocular comfort (Figure 14.1).

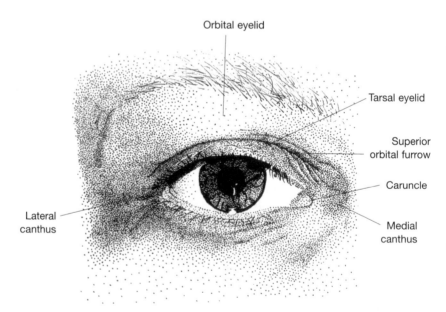

Figure 14.1 External view of the eye and lids.

Grossly, they appear fairly simple structures that function only to open and close, sometimes consciously, on demand, in response to excess light or to unwanted images, or when winking to attract attention. Often, however, lids function unconsciously while lubricating the eye during blinking or as experienced in that often uncontrollable response to tiredness.

Lid and associated conditions are often misdiagnosed by the non-ophthalmic specialist. Commonly blepharitis is confused with conjunctivitis, styes (hordeolum) diagnosed as chalazia (meibomian cysts) and the watering eye thought to be caused by blocked tear ducts.

If misdiagnosis occurs patients can easily become disheartened by the poor response that they get from topical eyedrops and treatments, so it is essential that ophthalmic clinicians have a sound knowledge of the structures and functions of the lids and that their part in maintaining ocular health and vision is not underestimated.

As the roles of ophthalmic nurses have continued to expand within the hospital eye service, and in response to the increasing number of patients being referred to the hospital eye services with a range of symptoms often vaguely attributed to 'lid problems', for many patients their first port of call for assessment is likely to be to a nurse-led service.

In nurse-led services ophthalmic nurses offer a wide range of both medical and surgical treatments and advice for patients with a range of symptoms commonly attributed to 'lid conditions'. Perhaps, more importantly, they have the clinical skills and ability to create the time within the nurse-led services to listen to patients, to make patients feel valued and as a result to 'tailor' treatments to assist compliance and ultimately achieve a successful outcome.

To assist in role development of practitioners and with the development of patient-focused services, in this chapter we look at the lids in more detail, and explore the normal anatomy, physiology and functions in order to highlight their importance.

A variety of lid conditions and associated pathologies is considered, and advice and good practice guidance for both treatable and chronic non-resolving lid conditions are included.

Functional anatomy and physiology of the lids (Figure 14.2)

The upper and lower lids are composed of essentially four layers of tissues: skin, muscles, tarsal plate and an inner lining of conjunctiva which is continuous with that of the conjunctiva that lines the fornices and covers the sclera up to its attachment with the cornea at the limbus.

Skin layer (and blood supply to the lids)

The eyelids are covered by a relatively thin layer of skin and folds of skin that contain sweat and sebaceous glands. The lids, and the muscles contained within them, have a rich blood supply which originates from the

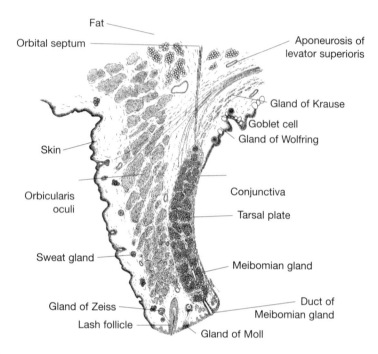

Figure 14.2 Section through the lid.

ophthalmic facial, superficial temporal and intraorbital arteries. The richness of this blood supply can be problematic, particularly if the lids are traumatized by blunt or lacerating injuries causing extensive bruising, swelling and bleeding, which can make a fuller ocular examination difficult. However, conversely, the richness of this blood supply helps to ensure that lid injuries, particularly lacerations, or planned lid surgical procedures, heal relatively quickly.

Muscle layers (and nerve supply)

There are three distinct muscle layers contained within the lids: orbicularis oculi, levator palpebrae and Müller's muscle.

Orbicularis oculi

The fibres from this muscle surround the lids in a concentric fashion and, when stimulated to function by the facial nerve, the lids close.

The levator palpebrae (superioris)

The fibres from the anterior edge of this muscle are attached to the skin of the upper lid, with some fibres attached to the lateral and medial lid margins and, when stimulated by the oculomotor nerve, result in the upper lid lifting and the eye opening.

Müller's muscle

This is a thin sheet of involuntary muscle fibres, which is stimulated by the sympathetic nervous system. When stimulated it provides additional elevation of the upper lid.

The upper lid receives its sensory nerve supply from the ophthalmic division of the trigeminal nerve, and the lower lid its sensory supply from the maxillary division of the trigeminal nerve.

The tarsal plates (tarsus)

These small 'D'-shaped structures within the eyelids are composed of dense fibrous tissue (almost cartilaginous), about 1 mm thick, 29 mm in length and 10 mm in vertical height centrally, in the upper lids. They have a protective function in addition to giving the lids structure and assisting in the mechanics of opening them. Within each of the upper and lower tarsus there are 25–30 sebaceous meibomian glands, the ducts of which open on to the lid margins. The sebaceous oils from these small glands form part of the tear film layer of the eye and the oils are spread across the surface of the eye during the blinking action of the lids.

The conjunctiva

The bulbar conjunctiva (covering the globe) continues into the fornices and then folds back on itself and continues to line the inside of the eyelids where it is referred to as the palpebral conjunctiva. It is a mucous membrane that contains goblet cells, which produce mucus secretions that, along with the meibomian secretions, form part of the tear film layer of the eye.

Other lid structures and landmarks

The lid margins and grey line

The lid margins are about 25–30 mm in length and 2 mm wide. They can be divided into anterior and posterior portions by the landmark known as the 'grey line'. Anterior to the grey line are the skin, orbicularis oculi muscle and lashes. Posterior to the grey line are the openings to the meibomian ducts, tarsus and conjunctiva. The grey line is of particular importance anatomically to surgeons specializing in lid surgical procedures and is relatively avascular, taking a long time to heal.

The lashes

There are two to three rows of lashes spaced along the anterior portion of the lid margins. They serve primarily a protective function, deflecting small air-borne foreign bodies away from the eye during the blinking process. They have small sebaceous glands (glands of Zeiss) within the follicle at their root, and the oils from these glands and from other small, modified sweat glands near the base of the lash (glands of Moll) keep the lashes soft and supple. The lashes, whether going through the natural processes of growing, falling out and being replaced, or during epilation (being plucked out) in the treatment of trichiasis (ingrowing lashes), will tend to regenerate every 4–6 weeks.

The meibomian glands

These are elongated sebaceous glands that are contained within the tarsal plate. There are about 25–30 of these glands per lid and the ducts from the glands open on to the posterior portion of the lid margin, behind the grey line. The sebaceous oils from these glands are spread across the surface of the eye during blinking, and serve to make up the oil layer of the tear film that assists in delaying tear evaporation.

The lacrimal punctae

These are two small raised openings found at the medial margins of the upper and lower lids. They form the openings to the channels of the

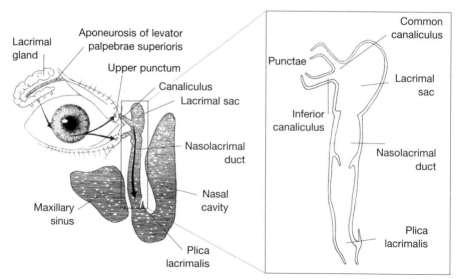

Figure 14.3 Lacrimal drainage system.

lacrimal drainage system (the canaliculi, lacrimal sac and nasolacrimal duct). Each punctum is surrounded by a small sphincter muscle, which gives the openings their raised appearance (Figure 14.3).

Lid examination

Before slit-lamp examination of the lids, some time should be taken to look at their general position and appearance. Simple observations of the lids in both the open and the closed positions can often give an indication of underlying, or associated, pathologies. This is also an opportunity to look at the mechanics of lid function: do they open and close smoothly, is there any evidence of lid lag (delayed movement of the lids on down-gaze associated with thyroid eye disease) or incomplete closure (which can lead to corneal exposure problems by the eye being exposed during sleep)?

The beginning of the examination should involve facing the patient and looking generally at the position of the lids and the size of the palpebral fissure (the distance between the upper and lower lid margins) and, in doing so, comparisons can be made between the right and left eyes. The lid margins should be examined along with the colour and nature of the skin of the lids. The clinician should observe for any 'lumps and bumps' or for any excess skin tissue in the upper and lower lids (dermatochalasia) and for the presence of any crusting or signs of discharge along the lid margins. The natural position of the lids should be considered and compared between the right and left eyes, this time in relation to the position of the lashes, lid margins and puncta.

The initial examination should also include gently touching the lids to feel for discrete 'lumps and bumps' that may not be obvious to the naked eye. Gently pinching the skin folds and tissue of the lids can also be useful in checking skin laxity and elasticity. Lid eversion (turning the lids) to look at the general appearance of the palpebral conjunctiva can also be performed at this point, although it may be more beneficial to do this during slit-lamp examination so that a more detailed look at the conjunctiva can be achieved, and discomfort for the patient can be minimized by having to evert the lids only once.

Lid conditions and disorders

This section of the chapter explores a variety of common lid conditions and abnormalities and where appropriate the management of each is discussed.

Much of the information in this section has been gained from 'hands-on' experience of, and involvement in, the assessment of lid disorders, while working with patients in a variety of clinical settings.

The treatment options detailed below are generally based on published evidence but, in addition, some options are based on practitioner and patient experiences and practices that they have found to work. All of the treatment options are based on the realization that listening to what patients tell the clinician, and gaining the patient's confidence, are essential to the successful management of lid problems.

Blepharitis

By far the most common lid disorder, blepharitis (Figure 14.4) is essentially an inflammatory condition of the lids that may occur with, or without, the presence of bacterial primary or secondary infection (commonly a staphylococcal infection). If left untreated other complications such as lid notching, chalazion (meibomian cyst), trichiasis (ingrowing lashes), conjunctivitis, punctate keratitis and corneal ulceration (particularly 'marginal' corneal ulcers) can develop.

This condition can be acute or chronic in nature (chronic more commonly) and is associated with signs such as crusting and thickening of the

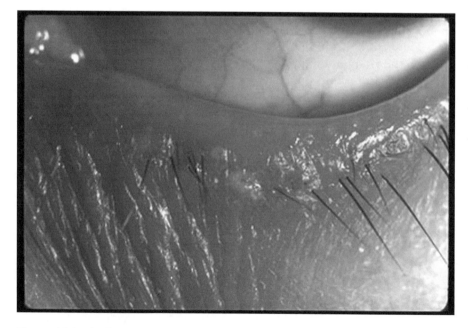

Figure 14.4 Blepharitis. (See Plate 12.)

lid margins, crusting and scaling along the bases of the lashes, causing the lashes to clump together, or madarosis where there are fewer lashes present than would normally be expected. In the more chronic types of blepharitis there is also the characteristic development of redness/ red-rimmed appearance of the lid margins, caused by increased numbers of small blood vessels encroaching on the lid margins (hyperaemia), as a result of the inflammatory response.

Patients will complain of a long history of problems and variety of symptoms including: excessive watering, burning, itching, foreign body sensation, dryness/grittiness, and sensitivity to sunlight and bright lights; most patients will be very distressed about the symptoms by the time they are referred for an ophthalmic specialist opinion. The severity of the symptoms with which people present often appears disproportionate to what is found on examination, and patients are frequently puzzled when only lid hygiene is offered as a treatment (if there is no presence of bacterial infection), when what they really want is eyedrops or ointment to 'make it better'.

It is important to consider all these factors, when explaining the nature of the condition to the patient, particularly given that the management may take some time and that it may never be resolved completely.

A good understanding of the condition and perseverance and compliance with treatment are the crucial factors in reducing discomfort, and the potential for other associated lid conditions and ocular complications.

Classification

There are many classifications/identifiers used to describe blepharitis, but for ease of understanding these can be commonly classified into anterior marginal blepharitis, in that the signs are more evident anterior to the grey line of the lid margin, or posterior marginal blepharitis in that the signs are more evident posterior to the grey line and often characterized by additional meibomian gland dysfunction (meibomitis). Posterior blepharitis is easy to miss because symptoms may be severe but the signs of blepharitis are mild (Kanski 2003).

Whether the blepharitis is anterior or posterior marginal, the symptoms experienced by the patient remain the same; the classification, however, is important from the examiner's point of view in that it will inform the best choice of treatment(s) suited to the management of the blepharitis.

Meibomitis (meibomianitis)

This is a chronic inflammatory condition affecting the meibomian glands, characterized by the presence of a 'whitish froth' sitting along the lid margins and the presence of large 'globules' of sebaceous oils at the openings of each of the meibomian gland ducts. It may be a stand-alone condition but more often is found in association with posterior marginal blepharitis. If left untreated it can lead to the development of chalazia (meibomian cysts).

The management of blepharitis (and associated conditions)

Blepharitis is a multifaceted condition, which may often require a variety of treatment approaches over a period of time in order to reach the point where the patient's symptoms are minimized to a tolerable level, and the clinical signs also cleared or reduced to a minimum.

In addition to an accurate diagnosis, patient compliance with treatments, and treatment regimens, designed around the patient's dexterity, lifestyle activities and functional visual acuity, are essential ingredients for success.

Lid hygiene

The term 'lid hygiene' often suggests to patients that to need 'hygiene' they must be somehow less than clean. With proper explanation of the condition, this can be overcome and the connection between hygiene and dirt in the context of blepharitis removed.

Lid hygiene is essentially the process involved in clearing away any discharge, crusting or flaking skin from the lid margins and lash roots, and there are a variety of solutions and techniques that can be used during the cleansing process.

Some time will have to be taken to describe in detail the physical process involved in cleaning the lids properly, so as to highlight the importance of a good lid hygiene technique in the often underestimated treatment of blepharitis, and as a safeguard against the development of other associated lid conditions.

There is much debate around the choice of, and dilution ratios of, solutions that are used for cleaning the lids. Some rationales behind the choices are based on evidence from clinical trials, and some simply based on the practitioner's preference in relation to feedback from patients and results obtained in practice. Solutions that can be used for lid cleaning range from dilute 'baby shampoo' (good for heavily crusted and dry flaking lid margins because it acts as a wetting agent), saline and bicarbonate of soda solutions (soothing in meibomitis and when symptoms include burning and itching), through to plain cooled boiled water (easiest to use because it is readily available for most and requires no mixing or calculation of dilution ratios) (Shaw 2002, Paranjpe and Foulks 2003).

There are also a few branded solutions that can be bought over the counter, but by far the best 'solution' to use is the one most tolerated by the patient, the one that gives the best result and essentially the one that is most convenient for the patient to use.

In addition to the method/solution most suited to the clinical signs/symptoms being treated, the solution and method that you choose will be influenced by the patient's vision and dexterity, tolerance of the cleansing solution and lifestyle activities, and is totally dependent on the patient's ability to comply, and understanding of the need for compliance during the early stages of treatment.

No matter which technique or solution is used, the outcome should, however, essentially be the same, in that the lids and lashes should be free of discharge, crusting and flaking skin.

Lid hygiene is usually performed twice a day as a minimum, but may be repeated as often as necessary and as convenient for the patient. During the initial treatment of blepharitis a sample regimen that is easy for patients to remember is: twice a day for 2 weeks, twice a day on alternate days for 2 weeks, then twice a day as and when they can, or feel they need to. Asking people to commit/comply to a twice-daily lid hygiene routine indefinitely is probably unreasonable, particularly as symptoms are resolved and in the absence of other associated ocular complications.

The issues around ongoing compliance need to be balanced against the possibility of recurrence by reinforcing the need to return to a more strict routine of twice-daily hygiene if symptoms begin to worsen and also by reinforcing the need for some form of ongoing lid hygiene activity in order to prevent symptom recurrence and development of associated ocular complications.

Method for use in patient information

This method is used if the patient has good dexterity and vision or if someone is performing the hygiene:

- Using your preferred solution and cotton buds dip the cotton bud into the solution and pull the lower lid down, and slightly away from the eye. Then, using the moistened cotton bud, firmly but gently wipe along the lid margin and base of the lashes. This process can be repeated two or three times until the lid margins and lashes are clear of crusting. You should use new cotton buds for each lid and for each eye.
- For heavily crusted lids you may find gently washing around the eyes or applying a well-soaked warm facecloth, or gauze pad (warm compress), to the lids for a few minutes, before using the cotton buds, helps to soften the crusting and make the cleaning easier.

- The upper lid needs to be gently pulled up so as to tilt the lid margin out slightly and away from the eye and then, using a new wetted cotton bud, wipe along the upper lid margins and lash roots in the same way that you did for the lower lid.
- Finally with the lids closed, using a well-soaked gauze pad or cotton-wool ball, clean gently along both sets of lashes and around the whole of the lid area to remove any dislodged crusting, and then 'pat dry' using a tissue.

If the patient is unable, either physically or visually, to use the cotton bud technique, a simpler method of cleaning the lids should be used. Using well-soaked gauze pads, a clean face cloth, cotton-wool balls or one of the over-the-counter lid wipes, and with the lids closed, encouraging a twice-daily cleaning routine will hopefully help to reduce crusting. Although this is a less effective way of cleaning the lids, because the lid margin is not specifically cleaned, it is better than no cleaning at all.

Warm compress and lid massage

In addition to lid hygiene, warm compress and lid massage can be of use to assist in the management of meibomitis, and to encourage the outflow of sebaceous oils through the meibomian ducts, minimizing the risk of chalazion development.

Warm compress, as it implies, is the use of a warm facecloth or gauze pad applied to closed eye lids for 2–3 min, before performing the lid massage. The warm compress has the dual effect of helping reduce inflammation and also increases the blood supply to the lid tissues. As in lid hygiene, lid massage should probably be done about twice daily; if repeated more frequently than this it may cause more irritation than good.

In its simplest form lid massage involves tightening the skin of the lower lid by gently pulling down with a finger from one hand. Using a finger from the other hand, and using a 'horizontal' rolling motion, the finger should be firmly but gently pressed upward towards the lid margin, so as to encourage the flow of sebum into the opening of the meibomian ducts and on to the lid margin where it can then be wiped away during the lid hygiene routine. The process should be repeated for the upper lid, but this time rolling in a downward motion towards the lid margin (Paranjpe and Foulks 2003).

For people with meibomitis, and those prone to recurrent chalazia, a combination of warm compress, lid massage and lid hygiene can be of benefit.

A more complicated but arguably more effective method of lid massage to encourage outflow involves the use of a thin rounded object such as a pencil or the like in a rolling motion, instead of a finger. Realistically for most, however, it can be difficult to manipulate the object and hold the lids, and great care needs to be taken not to damage the cornea or globe by accidentally rolling the pencil into the eye.

Topical or systemic antibiotics may be required where there is lid infection as well as inflammation and for meibomitis. Topical antibiotics should be applied after lid cleaning.

Chalazion (meibomian cyst)

A chalazion (Figures 14.5 and 14.6) is a cyst that results from blockage of one or more meibomian gland ducts. It usually starts as a small painless (lipogranulomatous) lump a few millimetres away from the lid margin, as a result of the anatomical position of the gland within the tarsal plate. Blockage of the ducts is usually secondary as a result of the presence of blepharitis or meibomitis.

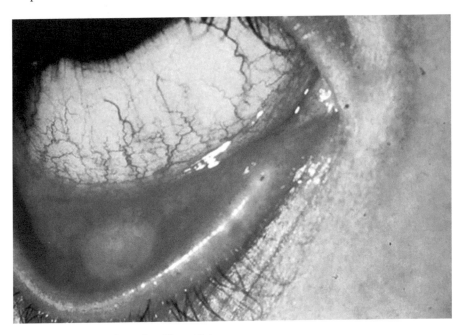

Figure 14.5 Chalazion. (See Plate 13.)

Small cysts may spontaneously resolve over a period of 3–6 months or leave a small residual lump that cosmetically goes unnoticed and does not cause any discomfort. However, in the presence of underlying blepharitis or meibomitis, chalazia do have a tendency to recur and often cause repeated discomfort for the patient during the more acute stages of development. Some chalazia do not resolve and can go on to become quite large, inflamed and infected, requiring medical and/or surgical intervention.

As a result of the inflammatory response a non-resolving cyst tends gradually to increase in size with time and, if secondary infection develops, the

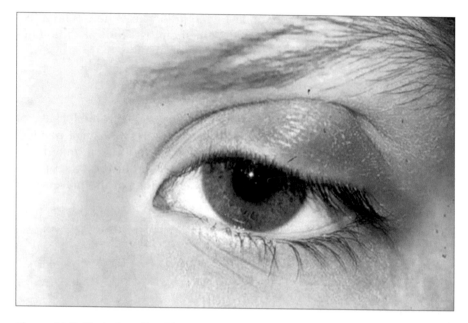

Figure 14.6 Chalazion. (See Plate 14.)

swelling may spread to involve the whole of the lid, causing increasing discomfort and the skin tissues around it to redden.

Cysts affecting the upper lid can cause blurring of vision (induced astigmatism), as a result of pressure on the cornea from the swelling, or can reduce vision by the gravitational/mechanical drooping of the lid during the acute inflammatory/infected stage (Kanski 2003).

Initial treatment during the early acute stages with warm compress, lid massage, lid hygiene and topical antibiotics (such as chloramphenicol 1% four times daily for up to 2 weeks) should be used if the chalazion is infected. If the cyst does not resolve, or the patient has discomfort or is unhappy with the cosmetic appearance of the lid, surgical intervention may be required. Surgical intervention should not take place if the chalazion is infected because the infection may spread to other structures in the lid.

Incision and curettage are the surgical procedure used for non-resolving chalazia, usually performed under a local anaesthetic injection (e.g. xylocaine 2%) with a drop of topical anaesthetic, and involve everting the lid, incising the cyst, expressing the contents and curetting (scraping out) the cyst wall to break down granulation tissue and prevent recurrence. It may also be necessary, as part of the procedure, to excise any redundant/excess granulomatous conjunctival tissue occasionally found on lid eversion.

A firm eyepad should be applied until any bleeding has stopped and the patient started on a topical antibiotic (fusidic acid twice daily or chloromycetin four times daily) for 1 week after the procedure. Bruising is a common complication of the procedure because the lids are very vascular and the injection, clamp or procedure may damage blood vessels in the lid. Advice must be given that it may take a week or two for any bruising or inflammation to resolve completely, and options should be discussed for ongoing management of any underlying pathologies that could prevent the development of more cysts in the future.

An alternative to surgery is injection of triamcinolone diacetate aqueous suspension, diluted with lidocaine (lignocaine) to a concentration of 5 mg/ml, through the conjunctiva into the chalazion. The success rate on first injection is around 80% (Kanski 2003). Steroid injection is contraindicated in patients with dark skin because the steroid may cause temporary or permanent depigmentation of skin (www.revoptom.com/handbook/sect1d.htm).

Hordeolum (stye)

This is a small abscess caused by a staphylococcal infection of a gland of Zeiss or Moll that opens into the eyelash follicle. It is differentiated from a chalazion in that it will be located much nearer the lid margin and cause localized swelling around the base of the affected lash(es).

Although styes usually resolve on their own, warm compress and topical antibiotics may be necessary, and epilating affected lashes can help release retained fluid within the abscess.

Infestation of lashes – phthiriasis palpebrum

The louse phithiris pubis is adapted to live in pubic hair but may be transmitted to other hair covered areas, particularly the eyelashes. They are the only louse likely to be found in this area. They cause irritation and itching and are often found in children. Although sexual abuse should be considered, transmission from vectors such as pillows and sheets is most likely as well as indirect contact from infested carers (Lopez Garcia et al. 2003). The lice must not be merely pulled from lashes. They tend to bury their heads in the skin of the lid and body parts such as the head or legs may be left behind. Kanski (2003) suggests trimming lashes at their base or the use of mercuric oxide 1% ointment (not available in the UK), anticholinesterase agents, laser or cryotherapy as treatment options. Lopez Garcia et al. (2003) consider these treatments and others, many of which are very toxic to the eye (e.g. chemicals in alcohol), do not kill the louse eggs (e.g. fluorescein 20%) or would not be possible in children (e.g. lash cutting, laser or cryotherapy). They recommend malathion, an anticholinesterase, in a water rather than an alcohol base, applied to the lid margin in a single application by a health professional, and left unwashed for 24 hours, to kill both lice and eggs. The British National Formulary (September 2004) also suggests aqueous malathion (e.g. Derbac M) for lice on eyelashes.

Concretions

These are small, yellow/white calcium deposits found within the tiny blood vessels of the palpebral conjunctiva. With time and as blood flows through these tiny vessels, calcium deposits can accumulate and lead to the development of small 'crystal-like' structures, which because of their 'jagged' and irregular edges rupture through the vessel walls and conjunctiva, causing grittiness and irritation.

They are fairly simple to remove (pick out) using an orange or green needle under topical anaesthetic, such as benoxinate or amethocaine. Some patients have multiple concretions and it is difficult sometimes to tell which has eroded through the conjunctiva and is causing problems. Staining the eye with fluorescein will stain exposed concretions only and they can then be removed.

Trichiasis

This is the name given to ingrowing, or inturning, eyelashes. If left untreated the offending lash(es) can cause irritation and watering, and eventually lead to corneal damage and ulceration from repetitive abrading of the corneal surface. The exact mechanism of why lashes may grow inwards is not known, although for some patients it may occur as a result of chronic blepharitis or damage and scarring after lid trauma and lacerations, particularly lacerations involving the lid margins and after surgery or radiotherapy.

Epilation

Epilation (plucking/pulling out) of the offending lash(es) is the first choice of treatment for most patients. Using a good pair of epilating forceps (Bennet's or similar) grab the lash at its base and swiftly and firmly pull out the lash, taking care to remove the whole lash and avoid breaking it.

Epilated lashes will usually grow again over a 4- to 6-week period and the lash may grow back into its normal position, away from the eye. If the lash continues to turn inward when it regrows, the patient or relatives can be taught how to epilate it themselves, or return to the department every 4–6 weeks, or as and when any irritation is felt, for repeat epilation.

Electrolysis

This procedure is of use for patients with trichiasis when commitment to repeated epilation is not an option, for whatever reason. It is performed as a local anaesthetic procedure, e.g. using benoxinate 0.5% drops into the eye and a xylocaine 2% injection into the skin at the base of the offending lashes. An electrolysis needle is inserted into the lash follicle to the root of the lash and a small electric current passed along the length of the needle to ablate the lash root and prevent it from regrowing.

In performing electrolysis, as the electric current is passed into the lash follicle, the skin around the lash root may blanch slightly, and the achievement of a good result is indicated by the treated lash almost 'falling out' when epilated as opposed to having to be forcibly pulled out.

Electrolysis is not always successful (about 60% success rate) and, although it can be repeated, for some patients further interventions such as cryotherapy (to freeze the lash root via a skin approach) or surgical lid split and cryotherapy (to freeze the lash root by direct contact with the lash follicle) may be necessary.

Entropion and ectropion

Entropion (Figure 14.7)

Three types of entropion can be identified: involutional or age related, cicatricial and congenital.

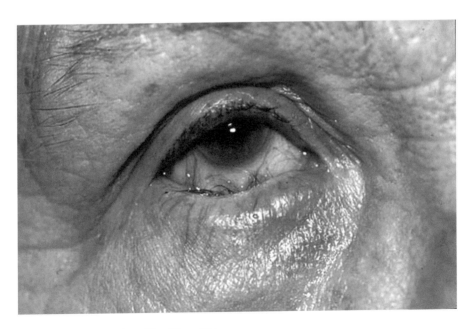

Figure 14.7 Entropion. (See Plate 15.)

Sometimes known as 'senile entropion', involutional entropion is a condition involving age-related tissue laxity, resulting in horizontal lid laxity and vertical lid instability caused by weakness or damage to the lower lid retractors. This allows the preseptal part of the orbicularis muscle to override the pretarsal part and to tip the lid inwards (Kanski 2003). If left untreated, it will undoubtedly cause irritation and corneal damage, and increase the risks of developing corneal ulceration. Initially, the entropion may be intermittent, and the patient may complain of only occasional watering and discomfort but, with time, the lid usually becomes permanently inverted.

This condition can be observed, in its early stages, in elderly patients who have 'squeezed' their eyes shut after the instillation of eyedrops as part of routine assessment. This also reinforces the point that there is more to instilling eyedrops than just putting the drop in and that assessment of the patient is a continuous function of any ophthalmic clinician.

Short-term management of entropion involving lid taping is often prescribed. Lid taping is carried out by placing a small piece of tape under the lashes at the lid margin and gently pulling the affected lid outward and away from the eye, taping it down onto the cheek and entrapping any excess skin folds. This can stop the lashes rubbing on the cornea but care must be taken to ensure that the lid is not under too much tension and that the patient can still close the eye. A wound closure strip is often perfect for this role because it is narrow, strong and sticky enough to hold the lid in place, as well as easy to remove without causing damage to fragile skin.

An alternative to lid taping, or when lid taping is not indicated (i.e. when the power of the inturned lid is likely to pull the tape into contact with the eye, or the patient cannot manage to change and reapply the tape), is to encourage the patient to get into the habit of frequently pulling the lid down and out away from the eye. This can be effective and a good routine that is easy for patients to remember is gently to pull the lid down every hour on the hour.

Long-term management will require surgical correction to evert the lid back into its normal position. This may involve everting sutures to prevent overriding of the preseptal orbicularis. If this is not effective, other procedures such as the Weiss procedure (full-thickness horizontal lid split with everting sutures) or the Quickert procedure (transverse lid split with everting sutures and lid shortening) are available (Collin 1989).

Cicatricial entropion, where scarring of the palpebral conjunctiva causes contraction and pulls the upper or lower lid margin inwards, may follow, for example, trachoma, trauma (heat, chemical or mechanical) and ocular cicatricial pemphigoid. Treatment may be medical, using a bandage lens to prevent lashed rubbing on the cornea, or surgical, involving lid rotation and mucosal grafts.

Congenital entropion is rare but more common in Oriental races (Kemp 2001) where skin folds tend to make the lower lid roll inward. This often settles with time but, if not, excess tissue in the anterior part of the lid can be removed.

Ectropion

Ectropion may be classified as congenital or acquired, the acquired causes being involutional, mechanical, cicatricial and paralytic (Beaconsfield 2001). It is a condition where the lower lid everts outwards and away from the globe; it is therefore the opposite of entropion. It is commonly associated with epiphora (excessive watering) caused by the malpositioning of the lid and punctum, or by scarring and closure of the punctum depending on the chronicity of the condition:

- Congenital ectropion may be the result of spasm of orbicularis in the newborn or caused by skin shortage in some cases of children with Down's syndrome. Spasm is managed by gently repositioning the lid and using ointment to lubricate exposed conjunctiva. Lubricants or eventually skin grafting is used to manage skin shortage.
- Mechanical ectropion is caused by lid lesions that mechanically evert the lid. Management is by removal of the cause.
- Involutional ectropion mainly affects the lower lid and is a result of tissue laxity. It is associated with epiphora caused by malposition of the punctum and irritation, chronic conjunctivitis, exposure keratitis (caused by abnormal lid position and incomplete closure of the lids during sleep), conjunctival scarring and hypertrophy resulting from prolonged exposure of the palpebral conjunctiva. Treatment is surgical and depends on the extent of lid ectropion and lid laxity, and medial and lateral canthal tendon laxity. Procedures include lid shortening with or without removal of excess skin and correction of tendon laxity.
- Cicatricial ectropion is caused by scarring of surrounding tissues that pull the lid away from the eye. Treatment includes excision of scar tissue with treatment of the skin deficiency by 'Z'-plasty or skin graft.
- Paralytic ectropion is caused by a facial nerve palsy. As the nerve palsy may recover, treatment initially is aimed at keeping the eye moist and preventing damage by exposure. A longer-term solution, if exposure is not well managed, is temporary tarsorrhaphy where the lateral aspects of the upper and lower lid are sutured together. If the palsy does not resolve, permanent surgical treatment may be required.

In all cases, initial treatment will consist of ocular lubricants and, in the case of facial nerve palsy, taping the lids closed at night will protect the cornea of patients with a poor Bell phenomenon. Before surgical correction the patency of the puncta and lacrimal drainage should be investigated to see whether or not surgical correction of the lids will also resolve the accompanying epiphora.

Ptosis

Ptosis is the name given to an abnormal drooping position of the upper lid. It can be a simple mechanical drooping associated with weight and the effects of gravity, e.g. in the presence of upper lid cysts, tumours and lid oedema/bruising after blunt trauma.

It can also, however, have a 'neurogenic' origin (associated with third nerve palsy and Horner's syndrome), a myogenic origin (either simple congenital or acquired as in myasthenia gravis) or aponeurotic origin (senile age related, occurring postoperatively or in the presence of blepharochalasis).

Patients with ptosis tend to develop a characteristic backward head tilt to improve vision, particularly if the lid drops to a level covering the pupil. Mechanical ptosis is simply treated by removing the cause or waiting until any tissue swelling has subsided. Other forms of ptosis obviously require thorough medical investigation and/or surgical management.

Miscellaneous 'lid lesions'

The diagnosis of lid lesions is a skill that can be easily developed, if knowledge of the anatomical position and physiology of the structures within the lids is sound.

If there is any doubt, whatsoever, about the nature or histology of the lesion being assessed or treated, a second opinion should always be obtained and, if appropriate, a biopsy of the lesion, or the excised lesion itself, sent for histological analysis.

Sebaceous cyst

This, as its name suggests, is a cyst involving one of the sebaceous glands in the skin of the lids. It can appear anywhere on the lids and usually starts off as a small, painless, yellowish/white lump that slowly increases in size with time.

Treatment is by surgical excision under local anaesthetic and is primarily done for cosmetic reasons. Care must be taken to ensure that the contents of the cyst and the capsule that surrounds it are removed during excision to prevent recurrence.

Sometimes long-standing cysts can become keratinized, leading to the development of a 'cutaneous horn' which appears as a brownish and crusted protrusion arising from the base of the cyst. This can be excised under local anaesthetic, again ensuring that the main body of the cyst and cyst capsule are also removed.

Cysts of Zeis and Moll

These are small cystic lesions that usually occur as a result of blockage of one or more of the sweat glands in the skin of the lids.

Cysts of Moll

These contain clear fluid and are translucent, often resembling small water-filled 'blisters' near the anterior lid margin. They can be simply punctured with an orange hypodermic needle and the fluid expressed using a cotton bud. Excess skin tissue left, after expression of the contents of the cyst, usually flattens with time leaving no visible signs of its presence.

Cysts of Zeiss

These contain sebum, and are yellowish in colour; again they are found near the anterior lid margin. These, too, can be punctured with an orange hypodermic needle and the contents expressed with a cotton bud. However, they can re-form if the gland becomes blocked off again and may need a fuller surgical excision, under local anaesthetic.

Provided that the procedure is explained and informed consent is gained and documented in patients' notes, as with any other surgical procedure, patients can often tolerate the simpler 'puncture and express' procedure at the slit-lamp, without the need for local anaesthetic infiltration. They are usually extremely happy that the procedure is so simple and that the lesion is resolved. A small puncture is made in the skin of the lid so antibiotic ointment might be supplied to be used on the skin, to prevent infection, until healing has taken place.

Papillomatous lesions

These are small 'warty' looking skin tag lesions found on the skin tissue of the lids. From their base attachment at the skin, they elongate and flatten out, and have an almost 'mushroom'-like appearance. They can be simply lifted and, using either a blade or cautery, excised under local anaesthetic.

Xanthelasma

Xanthelasmas are yellowish, flattened and slightly elevated lipid deposits visible at the medial (inner canthal) portions of the skin tissues of the lids.

More common in women and in the upper lids, they tend to develop and spread into the lid tissues slowly with time. 'Historically' they were thought to be associated with high systemic lipid levels, but there is little evidence to support the theory. Some practitioners might still check blood lipid levels as a routine, particularly in the presence of other risk factors. Treatment by surgical excision under local anaesthetic is mainly instigated to improve cosmetic appearance.

Basal cell carcinoma (rodent ulcer)

Basal cell carcinoma (BCC) (Figure 14.8) is a malignant tumour affecting the skin tissues and accounts for about 90% of malignant lid tumours. In the lids it is more commonly found at the medial canthal portion of the lower lid, and initially presents as a very slow-growing, painless, slightly raised, crusted lesion. Initially, a pearly lesion with growth, the edges of the lesion appear rolled inwards with a crater-like depression at its centre. It is a vascularized lesion that has a tendency to bleed if 'picked at' or bumped, and is not tender. Although malignant, it does not metastasize but will tend slowly to invade the skin tissues surrounding it. Surgical excision is recommended on a 'sooner rather than later' basis, particularly for tumours located near the punctal or canalicular areas of the lids, so as to

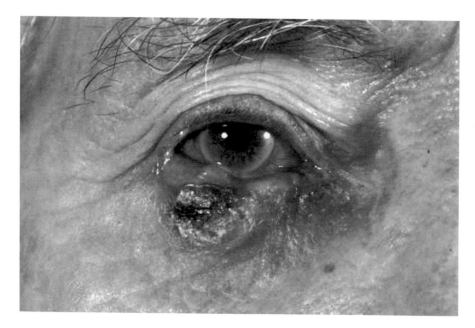

Figure 14.8 Basal cell carcinoma. (By courtesy of the Ophthalmic Imaging Department, Manchester Royal Eye Hospital.) (See Plate 16.)

prevent further spread and involvement of the lacrimal drainage structures and the need for more complicated reconstructive surgery.

Squamous cell carcinoma

Less common than basal cell tumours, squamous cell carcinomas (SCCs) develop more rapidly, and can metastasize to involve nearby lymph nodes. Although, in the early stages, the tumours can be similar in appearance to that of a papillomatous lesion or BCC, they progress more rapidly to become larger nodular lesions with scaly surfaces that may ulcerate. Treatment is usually by wide surgical excision (a much more radical excision of tissues than that involved in BCC excision – Kanski 2003), some form of lid reconstruction surgery and/or radiotherapy.

Mohs' micrographic surgery

For both BCCs and SCCs, Mohs' micrographic surgery is considered to be the gold standard management technique. Where it is not available, no defect after tumour removal should be reconstructed without formal histopathological advice of complete tumour removal (Leatherbarrow 2001).

Mohs' micrographic surgery allows a three-dimensional assessment of tumour margins, and is generally performed by a dermatological surgeon with special training in tumour excision and margin mapping. It removes the tumour in a sequence of horizontal layers, examining each as a frozen section. Residual cancer can be mapped and further horizontal layers are removed in the areas where cancer has been identified, until cancer-free layers are obtained. In this way, a minimum of normal tissue is removed while removing all of the cancer-bearing tissue. Although this technique is time-consuming, it has been shown to give the highest rate of cure for malignancies growing on various body surfaces (Leatherbarrow 2001) and has removed the need to remove large areas of normal tissue around the margins of the tumour to ensure that all has been removed.

The lacrimal system (tear film production and drainage)

The lacrimal system is the collective name given to the structures responsible for the production, flow and drainage of the aqueous layer of the tear film across the eye. The continued flow of tears across the eye is essential for corneal lubrication (including corneal oxygenation), ocular comfort and maintenance of visual clarity.

For the lacrimal apparatus to function effectively the structure, integrity, position and normal functions of the lids are essential. The aqueous layer of the tear film (99% water) is produced by the lacrimal gland, which lies in a small indentation (fossa) in the lateral aspect of the bone below the eyebrow. The fluid travels down through the lacrimal ducts, which open into the upper fornix. It is then spread across the surface of the globe.

The blinking motion of the lids, and a little help from gravity (or the occasional unintentional 'sniff'), encourages any excess tear fluids downwards and inwards in the direction of the lid margins and towards the puncta. The fluid is pushed into the upper and lower puncta (70% into the lower punctum), where it flows along the upper and lower canaliculi, into the common canaliculus. The fluid then drains into the lacrimal sac and finally exits via the nasolacrimal duct where it empties down into the back of nasal cavity and the throat.

The anatomy of tear outflow and drainage explains why patients often 'taste' topical eyedrops after instillation. It also explains the rationale for punctal occlusion in the treatment of dry eyes, and the rationale behind occluding the lower punctum to enhance the therapeutic effect of eyedrops used in the treatment of other ocular conditions such as glaucoma, both these techniques reducing drainage from the eye.

Epiphora

This is the more appropriate term given to excessive watering of the eyes resulting from obstruction/blockage within some part of the lacrimal drainage system. Epiphora is different from the excessive lacrimation (watering) that occurs in response to ocular irritation, or when emotionally upset in that it is caused by a drainage, rather than an over-production, problem.

Epiphora may be present in one or both eyes and blockages can occur at the punctum (punctal stenosis) or within the canalicular passageways (often caused by an inflammatory response causing a narrowing of the lumen of the canalicular vessels), or result from blockages within the lacrimal sac or nasolacrimal duct.

Dacryocystitis

Dacryocystitis is an inflammatory and often painful condition affecting the lacrimal sac, which can be acute or chronic in nature. As a result of the inflammatory response the sac or nasolacrimal duct can become obstructed and the passage of tear fluids blocked. If secondary infection occurs it can lead to lacrimal abscess formation.

Broad-spectrum systemic antibiotics and a warm compress may have some benefit in the early stages, but painful abscess formation may require a stab incision, through the skin, to release any pus. Once any acute infection has been treated patients usually progress to being listed for a dacryocystorhinostomy (DCR), which is the surgical creation of new drainage channels into the nasal cavity.

In investigating the cause of epiphora and after having excluded any other mechanical causes for drainage problems, e.g. as a result of malpositioning of the lids and/or puncta, such as in ectropion or some lid cysts, a 'sac washout' procedure should be performed to assess the patency of the drainage system.

Sac washout

To most ophthalmic specialists (particularly those working in the outpatient setting), this is a fairly simple and routine procedure that is carried out regularly.

If the technique is good and knowledge of the lacrimal drainage pathways sound, the clinician can provide much more in the way of 'useful' information other than 'patent or blocked' to aid the decision process around the ongoing management of lacrimal drainage problems and epiphora.

Patients often look horrified and sound terrified when the procedure is explained, but this is where simple diagrams and skills, confidence and reassuring manner will come into play, helping the patient to relax, trust the clinician and ultimately give his or her cooperation. Practically, a quiet, well-lit environment also helps as does having the patient comfortably seated/positioned for the procedure.

The procedure is not painful but most patients will experience a little discomfort and, although a topical anaesthetic drop is often instilled before the procedure, it really has little effect in anaesthetizing the canalicular pathways, so it serves more to reduce any blinking that would normally occur when the surface of the eye is touched, or as a result of working so near to the eye itself.

The technique
After instilling a topical anaesthetic eyedrop, if this is felt to be helpful, the punctum can be dilated, if required, with a Nettleship's dilator, because insertion of the cannula can be difficult if there is punctal stenosis. Often, however, the bore of the cannula is smaller than the tip of the dilator and therefore easier to insert, so this step is often ignored.

A lacrimal cannula (attached to a 2-ml saline-filled syringe) is gently inserted into the lower punctum in a downward and horizontal direction inwards towards the nose, following the natural pathway of the canaliculus. The cannula should be pushed, very gently, a little further along and into the lacrimal sac, until the tip of the cannula touches the medial wall of the lacrimal sac and lacrimal bone (known as the 'hard stop'). At this point, the cannula should be pulled back slightly, away from the hard stop, and the saline can be injected slowly.

If there is no resistance felt during this process, and the drainage pathways are obstruction free, the patient will almost straight away feel the saline as it flows through the drainage channels into the back of the throat.

Partial obstructions (in the canaliculi) may be felt as a slight 'resistance' as you are passing the cannula along into the lacrimal sac; for partial blockages lower down in the drainage channels, resistance may be felt while syringing in the saline and usually result in a delayed swallow reflex. Total blockages result in no saline/swallow reflex occurring at all, and are often accompanied by much resistance while trying to insert the cannula or syringe the saline through it.

If a blockage occurs at the common canalicular level, and prevents you from getting the cannula into the sac and feeling the 'hard stop', the spongy resistance that you feel is often referred to as the 'soft stop' and indicates the likely site of the blockage to be at that level within the drainage channels. If the blockage occurs below the level of the common canaliculus the saline is often seen to regurgitate via the upper punctum.

The more skilled the clinician becomes at this procedure, the more descriptive and useful the finding may become in locating and describing the location of any blockages, which will influence ongoing care management decisions. The particular findings of the procedure can be explained to the patient along with explanations about possible 'next steps' and treatment options.

Dry eyes

In addition to the production, flow and drainage of tears, the quantity, quality and composition of the tear film are key factors in maintaining ocular comfort, ocular health and visual clarity. In addition tear film quality also relies on the additional secretions from the accessory glands of Krause and Wolfring (found in the fornices), on the sebaceous oils from the meibomian glands and mucin (the mucus secretions) from the goblet cells in the conjunctiva.

The outer lipid layer of the tear film helps to prevent evaporation of the aqueous layer as the eye is exposed to air. It also lowers the surface tension of the tear film, allowing water to be drawn into it, and acts as a lubricant between the lids and the surface of the globe.

The middle, aqueous layer supplies atmospheric oxygen to the corneal epithelium, washes away debris from the eye and facilitates leukocyte action after injury. It has an important antibacterial action as a result of the presence of lysozyme, immunoglobulin IgA and lactoferrin, and fills any minute irregularities of the corneal surface, allowing more accurate refraction of light.

The inner mucin layer aids in wetting of the corneal surface by the aqueous layer, turning the anterior corneal surface from a hydrophobic to a hydrophilic state (Kanski 2003). Deficiencies in any of these layers can give rise to types of dry eye and dry eye symptoms. The complexities and mechanisms of the systemic and ocular causes associated with dry eyes probably warrant much more discussion than can be given here, but from the patient's perspective, no matter the cause, the symptoms of 'dryness', grittiness, burning sensations and ocular discomfort will undoubtedly be the same.

As in blepharitis the severity of the symptoms and discomfort experienced by the patient often appear disproportionate to what would be expected from clinical findings (Rhee and Pyfer 1999). This can be complicated by serious underlying systemic or ocular conditions that need investigation, explanation and treatment, in addition to managing the dry eye symptoms. Those who work with patients with dry eyes often find that the dry eye symptoms can take over the lives of those who have them and an enormous amount of support, education and empathy is required to enable patients with dry eye to manage and live with their symptoms. The basic principles of management are:

• to establish the cause of the dry eyes
• to treat any underlying causes
• to assess the quality and quantity of the tear film
• to find the best treatment options that aid compliance and give maximum comfort and resolution of symptoms.

Quantity and quality of tear film are both important and lead to different options for treatment.

Quantity

Quantity is measured by using Schirmer's test (Figure 14.9). The tip of a predesigned small strip of blotting paper is placed into the lateral portion of the lower canthus (to avoid irritation and trauma to the cornea). The patient is asked to keep the eye open and blink normally and after 5 minutes the amount of tear secretions that have soaked onto the strip is measured. Obviously, a piece of paper in the lower fornix may produce some irritation, so this test may be undertaken after topical use of anaesthetic drops to obtain a reading without eye irritation and this is known as Schirmer's test 2. The normal amount of tears that would be expected in this 5-minute period without anaesthetic is 15 mm or more, and slightly less with anaesthetic. Less than 6 mm indicates impaired tear secretion whereas 6–10 mm is borderline (Kanski 2003).

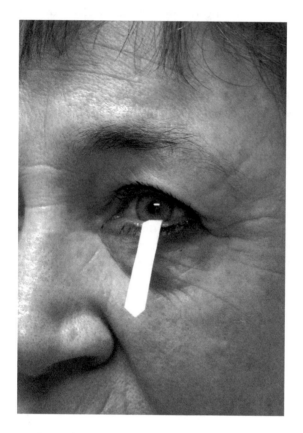

Figure 14.9 Schirmer's test.
(By courtesy of Angela
Chappell, Ophthalmic
Imaging Department,
Flinders Medical Centre,
Adelaide, South Australia.)

Quantity can also be observed during slit-lamp examination because there should be a 2- to 3-mm 'pool' of tears sitting on and above the lower lid margin.

Quality

Tear film break-up time (Figure 14.10) is an indication of tear film stability and therefore of quality of the tear film. Using a slit-lamp, the tear film is observed after instilling a drop of fluorescein 2%. The tear film is examined using a wide beam of light and a cobalt blue filter. The patient should be asked to blink and the time recorded between this and the moment when black spots or lines begin to appear in the tear film as it starts to dry. A tear break-up time of less than 10 seconds is abnormal (Rhee and Pyfer 1999).

The tear film should also be studied closely and clarity, debris and mucus strands should be noted. During examination, the conjunctiva, lid margins and openings of the meibomian ducts should also be considered for any contributing meibomitis, blepharitis or conjunctivitis that could impact on the quality of the tears.

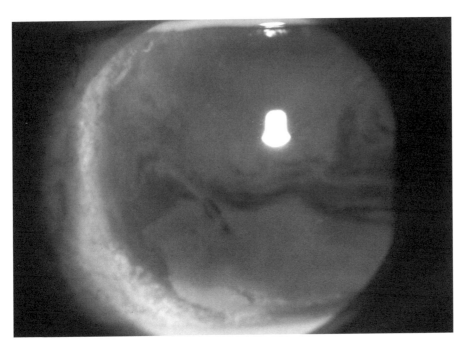

Figure 14.10 Tear film break-up time. (By courtesy of Angela Chappell, Ophthalmic Imaging Department, Flinders Medical Centre, Adelaide, South Australia.) (See Plate 17.)

Dysfunction of the lipid layer of the tear film can lead to evaporative dry eye and this may be the result of meibomitis or obstructed meibomian glands causing oil deficiency. Deficiency of the aqueous layer leads to a hyposecretive dry eye (which may result, for example, from age changes in the lacrimal gland or from Sjögren's syndrome) and the two may coexist (Kanski 2003).

Treatment and practical guidance

The first line of treatment for most patients with dry eyes will be some form of ocular lubricant, and there are a multitude of drops and ointments designed for this purpose. The plethora of lubricants available all have a commonality in that they add lubrication to the eyes, although, pharmacologically, they may well have been designed to work on different parts of the tear film layer, depending on any underlying ocular pathology and the nature of the resultant tear film deficiency.

Finding the right ocular lubricant(s) for the patient can often be a time-consuming exercise, and can involve a process of trial and error until one (or combination of lubricants) is identified that is best tolerated by the patient, the easiest for them to use and, from a compliance point of view, fits in with the patient's lifestyle needs of being put in as frequently, or preferably as infrequently, as possible to manage the symptoms.

A simple practical and effective way of achieving a good result, in a relatively short period of time, involves giving the patient a variety of two or three different kinds of ocular lubricants with which to experiment.

Each one can be tried at first a minimum of three or four times a day and, in addition, as often as the patient feels the need. It should be explained that there are no drugs in these drops so they may be used extremely frequently if necessary. If symptoms are not resolving the drops can be tried in combinations. During this process and over a period of time, say 4–6 weeks, it may be helpful for patients to keep a diary of which one(s) they used, how often they had to put them in and the therapeutic effect they had on controlling their symptoms. This engages patients in their treatment and enables them to feel that active management of their symptoms is in progress rather than their just being given a bottle of drops. Patients expect the treatment that they are given to work and, if the first bottle of artificial tears does not work, they may lose faith in the clinician and the system. If drops were being used very frequently, provision of preservative-free drops would be appropriate to prevent preservative toxicity.

Punctal occlusion

For patients who have severe dry eyes and those who get little symptomatic relief from the use of topical lubricants alone, the insertion of punctal plugs may be considered, to assist in keeping the lubricants/tear film on the surface of the eye for as long as possible (Figure 14.11).

Often, temporary collagen plugs can be inserted through all four puncta into the canaliculi, initially to start to see if there is any effect on the control of symptoms.

Collagen plugs dissolve over a period of a few weeks and if symptoms have resolved or at least been reduced to a tolerable level, then more permanent occlusion using silicone plugs would follow. Some silicone plugs are designed to fit into the puncta (Figure 14.11) whilst others are designed to fit into the canaliculus. Even with the insertion of silicone plugs, most patients, particularly with severe dry eye symptoms, will have to continue with additional topical lubricant drops. Very occasionally, epiphora can result following insertion of the more permanent plugs and the resultant watering can be as distressing for the patients as their dry eye symptoms. If necessary, punctal plugs can simply be removed (canalicular ones using a sac washout technique), but then treatment options will have to be reconsidered for the management of the dry eye symptoms.

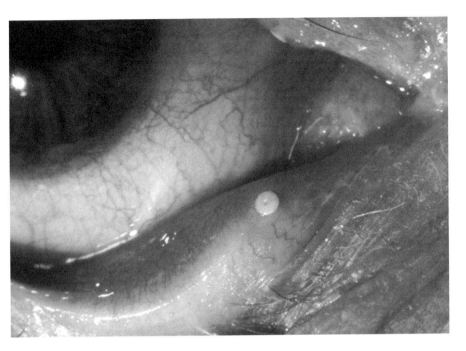

Figure 14.11 Punctal plugs. (By courtesy of Angela Chappell, Ophthalmic Imaging Department, Flinders Medical Centre, Adelaide, South Australia.) (See Plate 18.)

There is a need for continuing education and information about the the treatment options for dry eyes so that patients understand that it is manageable rather than curable, and that much of the management is in their hands.

For this process to work, the cause of the dry eye must have been identified, any pre-existing pathology such as meibomitis or blepharitis must have been treated and the tear film examined so that the clinician can be selective and ensure that the lubricants offered to the patient are the ones most appropriate for the management of the dry eyes.

References

Beaconsfield M (2001) Ectropion. In: Collin R, Rose G (eds), Plastic and Orbital Surgery. London: BMJ Books.

British Medical Association, Royal Pharmaceutical Society of Great Britain (2004) BNF 48. London: BMA/RPSGB.

Collin JRO (1989) A Manual of Systematic Eyelid Surgery, 2nd edn. London: Churchill Livingstone.

Kanski JJ (2003) Clinical Ophthalmology, 5th edn. London: Butterworth-Heinemann.

Kemp E (2001) Entropion. In: Collin R, Rose G (eds), Plastic and Orbital Surgery. London: BMJ Books, pp. 24–31.

Leatherbarrow B (2001) Tumour management and repair after tumour excision. In: Collin R, Rose G (eds), Plastic and Orbital Surgery. London: BMJ Books, pp. 44–66.

Lopez Garcia JS, Garcia Lozano J, Matrinez Garclintonena J (2003) Phthiriasis Palpebrum: Diagnosis and treatment. Archivos de la Sociedad Española de Oftalmologica 78(7): 365–74.

Paranjpe DR, Foulks GN (2003) Therapy for meibomian gland disease. Ophthalmol Clinics N Am 16: 37–42.

Rhee DJ, Pyfer MF (1999) The Wills Eye Manual, 3rd edn. Philadelphia, PA: Lippincott, Williams & Wilkins.

Shaw ME (2002) Recognising and managing blepharitis. Ophthalmic Nursing: Int J Ophthal Nursing 6: 22–5.

CHAPTER FIFTEEN

The conjunctiva

AGNES LEE

Anatomy and physiology of the conjunctiva

The conjunctiva is a thin transparent mucous membrane that derived its name from the Greek 'conjo' (as in conjoined) because it is attached to the eyelids and the eyeball. The conjunctiva:

- lines the upper and lower lids (palpebral conjunctiva)
- is reflected at the superior and inferior fornices on to the sclera (bulbar conjunctiva) up to the limbus where it becomes continuous as the first layer of the corneal epithelium.

Therefore, it is divided into three parts:

1. Palpebral conjunctiva
2. Bulbar conjunctiva
3. Conjunctiva in the fornices.

The conjunctiva's upper layers consist of stratified columnar epithelium and vary from two layers thick over the tarsal plate to five to seven at the corneoscleral limbus. Lymphocytes and melanocytes are scattered throughout the basal layers of the conjunctiva. The conjunctival stroma consists of loosely arranged bundles of collagenous tissues containing fibroblasts. Conjunctiva also contains macrophages, mast cells and leukocytes, all of which play a part in any inflammatory response (Newell 1996).

Palpebral conjunctiva

The palpebral conjunctiva is slightly thicker than the bulbar conjunctiva, is firmly attached to the tarsal plate, and lines the upper and lower lids. The palpebral conjunctiva is extremely thin and transparent and the yellowish tarsal glands can easily be visualized in the posterior surface of the tarsal plate by eversion of the lids. Blood vessels are also clearly visible. The palpebral conjunctiva is divided into three zones:

1. Marginal zone: this extends from right across the border of the lid to the back of the eyelid. The tarsal glands and lacrimal punctum can be seen emerging from this point. It is important to note that, as the conjunctival epithelium is continuous with the lining of the inferior meatus of the nasal cavity, the infection can easily be spread between these two structures (Forrester et al. 1996).
2. Tarsal zone: this zone is thin, vascular and light red in colour.
3. Orbital zone: this contains cylindrical and cuboidal cells. In addition, the accessory lacrimal glands (of Krause and Wolfring) are situated here.

On the posterior edge of the lid margin, along the posterior edge of the openings of the tarsal glands, the conjunctiva joins the skin of the lid. Here, the non-keratinized squamous epithelium of the conjunctiva is continuous with the keratinized stratified squamous epithelium of the skin.

Bulbar conjunctiva

The bulbar conjunctiva is very thin and lines the anterior portion of the eyeball (including the insertions of the extraocular muscles and Tenon's capsule) and is loosely attached to the sclera, except near the limbus where it increases in thickness. It moves over the sclera easily and, as it is transparent, blood vessels are clearly visible.

The plica semilunaris, which is a crescent-shaped fold in the inner canthus, can be seen in the medial fornix of the conjunctiva. It is richly supplied with goblet cells, which secrete mucin, an important component of the pre-corneal tear film that protects and nourishes the cornea. Lying within the medial side of the plica is the lacrimal caruncle (small, pinkish, ovoid body of modified skin possessing a few fine colourless hairs) containing sweat and sebaceous glands.

At the corneoscleral limbus, the cells of the conjunctiva change to stratified squamous non-keratinized epithelium which is continuous with the epithelium of the cornea.

Conjunctiva in the fornices

This lines the upper and lower lids and is loosely attached to the underlying fascial expansions of the sheaths of the levator and rectus muscles. Contraction of these muscles can pull on the conjunctiva so that it moves with the eyelid and eyebrow (Snell and Lemp 1998).

Conjunctival glands

- Goblet cells: responsible for secreting the mucus part of the tear film and scattered throughout the conjunctiva.
- Glands of Krause and Wolfring: also known as the accessory lacrimal glands which secrete some of the watery part of the tear film.

These glands have no nervous control.

Conjunctival blood vessels

The arterial supply of the conjunctiva arises from the palpebral and anterior ciliary arteries. The peripheral arterial arch supplies the inferior and superior conjunctival fornices and the bulbar conjunctiva whereas the marginal arterial arch supplies the palpebral arteries.

Lymph drainage

The conjunctival lymph vessels are arranged as a deep and superficial plexus in the submucosa of the conjunctiva. Those vessels on the lateral side of the eye drain into superficial parotid nodes and those from the medial side into the submandibular nodes.

Nerve supply of the conjunctiva

The innervation of the bulbar conjunctiva is from the long ciliary nerves, branches of the nasociliary nerve, which in turn is a branch of the ophthalmic division of the trigeminal nerve. The superior bulbar conjunctiva and superior fornix conjunctiva are supplied by the frontal and lacrimal branches of the ophthalmic division. The inferior fornix is from the lacrimal branch of the ophthalmic division and the infraorbital nerve from the maxillary division of the trigeminal nerve (Snell and Lemp 1998).

Functions of the conjunctiva

The conjunctiva is responsible for production of the mucus component of the tear film (from goblet cells) (Forrester et al. 1996) and its accessory glands help to ensure a continually moist environment. It also has a protective function – evaporation of tears lowers the temperature in the conjunctival sac, effectively inhibiting microbial growth. This is assisted by the junctions of hemidesmosomes to their basement membrane, which may prevent or limit bacterial colonization. It acts as a physical barrier, preventing foreign bodies from entering the orbit and providing a moist environment so that a clear cornea is maintained.

Abnormal physiology seen in infectious and inflammatory disorders of the conjunctiva

The clinical features that must be considered in the diagnosis of any conjunctival infection or disorder in conjunctival infections and inflammatory disorders include the following:

- Papillae: this is a non-specific response of the conjunctival tissue to many acute and chronic inflammatory disorders. The various types of inflammatory cells such as lymphocytes, plasma cells and eosinophils are seen to invade the conjunctival stroma. This is seen mainly in bacterial and allergic eye conditions.
- Follicles are milky, translucent and lobular and contain lymphocytes and macrophages.
- Discharges can be different types, textures and colours depending on causative organisms and aetiology:
  - mucopurulent discharge is usually a sign of bacterial infection varying in colour from cream to yellowish to green
  - serous, watery discharge is usually a sign of viral or allergic-type disorder
  - ropey and stringy serous discharge with mucus thread is associated with vernal conjunctivitis.
- Injection/hyperaemia – congestion of conjunctival blood vessels: the distribution of congestion is important in the diagnosis. Diffuse injection in the fornices is normally found in conjunctivitis, sectoral injection indicates episcleritis and ciliary injection might indicate iritis.
- Petechial haemorrhages: pinpoint haemorrhages found in the palpebral or bulbar conjunctiva.
- Conjunctival chemosis: swelling of the bulbar conjunctiva in response to infection or inflammation.
- Conjunctival staining: breakdown of the conjunctival epithelial cells resulting in 'stain' (with fluorescein) which represents missing epithelial cells. Staining can be any size or shape depending on what has damaged or killed the epithelium.
- Conjunctival scarring: the end result of a wide variety of severe inflammation found in conditions of severe dry eyes, entropion, trichiasis, chemical injury and trachoma.
- Symblepharon: adhesions between the palpebral and bulbar conjunctiva after trauma, burns and infections.
- Pseudomembrane: this is seen in severe infection resulting in conjunctival epithelial hyperplasia and may be peeled off the palpebral conjunctiva. True membrane is fibrin cellular debris which indicates a more severe inflammatory response and can cause significant bleeding when peeled.

- Preauricular lymph nodes: enlargement can indicate acute or severe infection. These glands are often a swollen and tender area just in front of the ear.

Conditions of the conjunctiva

Conjunctivitis

Infective conjunctivitis is extremely common and accounts for many of the cases of 'red eye' presenting to both primary and secondary care. Although a first response to red eye is often topical antibiotics, bacterial conjunctivitis is uncommon in adults. An accurate history and examination reveal that the vast majority of conjunctivitis is viral in origin (Tullo and Donnelly 1995) and that explanation and supportive measures are much more effective than antibiotics which will not resolve the problem and leave the patient feeling let down, because the clinician has promised and failed to cure him or her. Bacterial conjunctivitis is common in children, however. Conjunctivitis can be acute, hyperacute, recurrent or chronic depending on for how long the conditions persist. It is easily transmitted especially when there is close physical contact.

Bacterial conjunctivitis

This is inflammation of the conjunctiva with diffuse injection of the superficial episcleral vessels, bulbar conjunctiva and occasionally papillae of the palpebral conjunctiva of the upper and lower lid. The eye is sticky throughout the day and yellow or green pus is evident. The condition is common in children and normally starts off in one eye before transmitting itself to the other eye. Unilateral conjunctivitis is uncommon. Even if it starts as unilateral, it usually spreads to the other eye, so advice must be about treatment of the fellow eye. The severity of conjunctivitis is dependent on the causative organism.

Pathophysiology
To protect itself the eye has a number of defence mechanisms, e.g. the tear film contains immunoglobulin (IgA), the blink reflex moves pathogens away from the eye into the canaliculi, the immune system tolerates general and non-pathogenic bacteria that normally colonize the eye but excludes external organisms that try to enter the eye. In the event of any of these defence mechanisms breaking down, pathogenic bacterial infection is possible. In addition pre-existing eye conditions such as blepharitis, dry eyes, poor contact lens hygiene, chronic infection of the lacrimal sac and the prolonged use of ophthalmic medications can cause conjunctival inflammation.

Causative organisms

The main causative organisms are *Streptococcus pneumoniae*, *Staphylococcus aureus*, *Haemophilus influenzae*, *Pseudomonas aeruginosa* and gonococci.

Signs and symptoms

The individual is likely to present with a red, irritable eye, describing the sensation as 'gritty' rather than painful. The lid margin and lashes are usually crusty and the eyes wet. Eyelids are stuck together particularly on waking up as a result of discharge during the night. Discharge is likely to be purulent and profuse, and the lashes may be coated. The patient may be mildly photophobic and the lids may be oedematous. The conjunctiva is diffusely injected but there will be no conjunctival staining with fluorescein.

Management of acute bacterial conjunctivitis

Requesting cultures and sensitivity tests may be useful for accurate diagnosis but are not necessary in order to give effective treatment and are expensive. Swabs should be taken, however, in the case of very young babies (infection in a child aged under 28 days is notifiable in the UK as ophthalmia neonatorum), or adults with very profuse discharge where gonococcal infection might be suspected. Bacterial conjunctivitis responds very well to a broad-spectrum antibiotic.

The eye examination must take into account the following:

* Upper and lower lids for any signs of oedema and discharge.
* Upper and lower lashes for signs of blepharitis.
* Everting the upper and lower lids and examination of the tarsal plate for any signs of follicles which could indicate a viral rather than a bacterial infection.
* Everting the tarsal plate can also sometimes reveal a non-adherent pseudomembrane found in severe conjunctivitis.
* Pattern of hyperaemia in the tarsal and bulbar conjunctiva.
* Corneal integrity: marginal corneal infiltrate can be found in staphylococcal and haemophilus infection.

Treatment

Although acute bacterial conjunctivitis is usually self-limiting and does not cause any serious damage, patients presenting with acute bacterial conjunctivitis should be treated in order to shorten the course of the disease, thereby reducing the spread of the disease and most importantly reducing the risk of more widespread extraocular disease.

Broad-spectrum antibiotics such as topical chloramphenicol are very effective in treating bacterial conjunctivitis and are usually prescribed four times a day and, if warranted, as an ointment at night for a period of 5–7/10 days. Chloramphenicol should also be used with caution in any pregnant women and an alternative should be used in breast-feeding women.

Children with acute bacterial conjunctivitis are normally prescribed fusidic acid (Fucithalmic) because this necessitates only a twice-daily drop regimen.

In cases of severe bacterial conjunctivitis, a pseudomembrane can sometimes be seen loosely adherent to the palpebral conjunctiva. Pseudomembranes consist of coagulated exudate that adheres loosely to the inflamed conjunctiva and is a response to severe inflammation or infection. They are typically not integrated with the conjunctival epithelium (unlike the true membrane, which is fibrin cellular debris, becoming interdigitated with the vascularity of the conjunctival epithelium). It is important that the pseudomembrane be removed from the conjunctival epithelium by peeling it with a forceps. A little bleeding may be encountered.

It is important never to pad the eye in any acute eye infection. If mild photophobia is present, encourage the use of dark glasses instead.

Care

Health education information, particularly on how to control the spread of infection, should be given. Regular handwashing should take place especially before and after drop instillation and, if discharge is profuse, it might be wise to change pillowcases daily. Face cloths and towels should not be shared, and make-up should be discarded. Attention to hygiene should be reiterated where there are children. The use of disposable tissues to wipe the eye should be encouraged.

The clinician must ensure that the patient understands how to use the medication before leaving the department: chloramphenicol drops should be kept in a cool place, preferably in a fridge. Drops and ointment should never be shared and should be discarded at the end of the treatment period.

Information on how to keep the lids clean and free from discharge may be needed (cooled, boiled water and cotton wool or tissues), especially by parents of small children who may also need extra help instilling the prescribed medication effectively.

If a patient wears contact lenses, the use of these should be discontinued until the infection has cleared up. Disposable lenses should be discarded. Where possible, any information given should be reinforced with written information.

It is often not necessary to review these patients again because they respond very well to topical antibiotics. Before discharge, patients must be told to come back if there is no resolution of symptoms within 72 hours, if there has been a change in visual acuity, the development of new symptoms, or if there is moderate or severe eye pain.

Gonococcal conjunctivitis

Gonococcal conjunctivitis (Figure 15.1) is a sexually transmitted infection (STI) known sometimes as hyperacute conjunctivitis. Again the normal

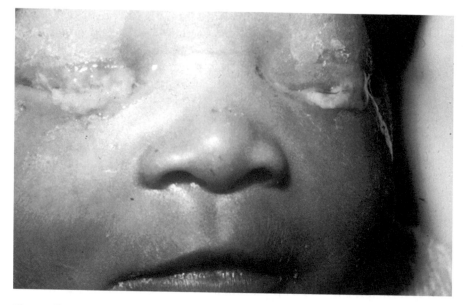

Figure 15.1 Gonococcal conjunctivitis (baby). (See Plate 19.)

mode of transmission is through sexual contact, genital/ocular or hand/ocular transmission, but casual interaction with infected individuals has also been reported as a cause. The organism responsible is *Neisseria gonorrhoea*. Systemically, gonococcal infections are associated with infection of the rectum, urethra and cervix.

Symptoms
- Sudden onset – becoming severe in less than 12 hours
- Pain
- Signs
- Severe purulent discharge
- Acute red eye
- Conjunctival papillae and chemosis: papillae are a common nonspecific response of the conjunctival tissue to inflammation and consist of tiny elevations of various types of inflammatory cells (lymphocytes, plasma cells, eosinophils) which are tightly packed together, with a vascular core (Ragge and Easty 1990)
- Corneal epithelial haze and defect
- Possible peripheral ulcers
- Severe cases of perforation.

Management
Eye swabs and conjunctival scrapings should be performed for Gram staining. With Gram stain, epithelial parasitism by Gram-negative diplococci is seen (Mandava et al. 1999), which confirms the diagnosis.

Treatment

Hourly penicillin is usually the treatment of choice for 24 hours and then it is tapered according to clinical response. If there is no clinical response, hourly cefuroxime may be used, again over 24 hours and the dose tapered according to clinical response. As the infection is systemic as well as ocular, referral to a genitourinary clinic is required where systemic treatment (injections of benzyl penicillin 50 000 units IM twice a day for 7 days) and contact tracing can commence.

Care

Extreme sensitivity is required in dealing with the sexual connotations of this infection within the ophthalmic department. Partners may accompany the patient but the patient may not, as yet, wish for this diagnosis to be shared. Compliance with all forms of treatment is needed in order to prevent transmission of the infection, and full and frank discussion about the connotations of the infection may need to take place to ensure concordance and compliance with treatment.

Ophthalmia neonatorum

Ophthalmia neonatorum or conjunctivitis of the newborn is the term used by the World Health Organization (WHO) for any conjunctivitis with discharge occurring during the first 28 days of life. It is a notifiable disease in the UK and is caused by various agents. The chief culprit used to be *Neisseria gonococcus* but, although it is still seen occasionally and appears to be increasing, *Chlamydia trachomatis* is by far the most common cause. Both organisms cause infection to the baby's eyes during delivery through the birth canal. The incubation period of *Neisseria* sp. is 2–3 days. If left untreated, gonococcal neonatal conjunctivitis can cause corneal ulceration, leading to endophthalmitis and blindness. It is prudent to treat all purulent discharge in the newborn as gonococcal until proved otherwise. The transmission rate for gonorrhoea from an infected mother to her newborn is 30–50% (Hammerschlag 1993, O'Hara 1993).

Chlamydial neonatal conjunctivitis is, however, less destructive although it can last months if left untreated and may be followed by pneumonia (Vaughan et al. 1992). The incubation period is 5–12 days. Other causes of infections may include staphylococci, pneumococci, *Haemophilus* spp. and herpes simplex virus.

The risk factors associated with ophthalmia neonatorum are premature rupture of the membranes, resulting in ascending infection from the cervix and vagina, documented or suspected STI, postpartum contact and local eye injury during delivery (Yetman and Cody 1997).

Signs and symptoms
- Lid oedema
- Purulent discharge (much more purulent and profuse in gonococcal conjunctivitis), sometimes blood-stained
- Chemosis.

Management of ophthalmia neonatorum
Ophthalmia neonatorum caused by chlamydial infection is diagnosed through laboratory investigation and when a positive eye swab is made. The baby is treated with topical tetracycline or erythromycin and, as this condition can be associated with otitis media and respiratory and gastrointestinal tract infections, such infants are treated with oral erythromycin ethyl succinate suspension 12.5 mg/kg four times daily for 14 days.

Nursing care
The condition must be clearly and carefully explained to both parents (if available). Both parents should be told the baby's diagnosis, how the baby came to acquire the infection and the recommended treatment. As the infection is transmitted by the mother during delivery, it is vital that both parents are screened and examined for genital infection. Tact and sensitivity are required when the parents are told to attend the genitourinary clinic and what problems could arise if they do not receive treatment.

If the baby's eyes are sticky, the carers should be shown how to clean the eyes using clean cotton wool and warm water. They should also be shown the correct method to instil the drops.

The importance of any follow-up care in the hospital or community must be stressed.

Viral conjunctivitis

Definition and description of adenovirus conjunctivitis
Adenoviruses are small infectious agents (DNA viruses) and 47 different types have been identified. These viruses often cause upper respiratory tract infection, conjunctivitis (Figure 15.2) and other infections such as colds or flu. Adenoviruses are responsible for 3–5% of acute respiratory infections in children and 2% of respiratory illnesses in adults. The virus is extremely contagious and the usual mode of transmission of this virus can be through contaminated fingers and vectors such as medical instruments (e.g. applanation tonometers). Inhalation of air-borne viruses may also lead to systemic illness with eye involvement. Viral conjunctivitis is by far the most common conjunctivitis in adults. Although it usually begins in one eye, the best intentions of the patient are unlikely to stop it spreading to the fellow eye within days.

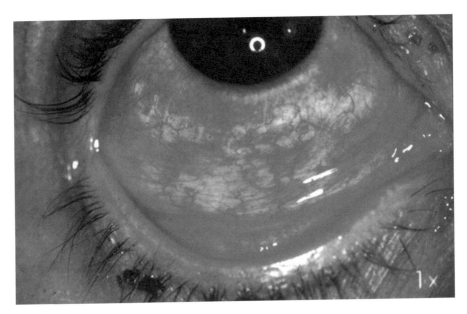

Figure 15.2 Viral conjunctivitis. (See Plate 20.)

Signs and symptoms of adenovirus conjunctivitis
Symptoms
- Foreign body sensation
- Feeling of dryness
- Mild photophobia in some cases
- The lids are likely to be stuck together in the morning as a result of dried secretions
- Vision may be affected as a result of corneal involvement
- Corneal involvement may cause pain
- Sore throat may be present
- Other upper respiratory tract symptoms such as a recent history of a cold.

Signs (Ragge and Easty 1990)
- Diffuse hyperaemia
- Lid oedema may be present
- Profuse watering
- Conjunctiva may be chemosed
- May have subconjunctival haemorrhage or petechial haemorrhages on lid conjunctiva
- Tender preauricular node – unilateral or bilateral
- Follicles (multiple tiny translucent swellings) on lid conjunctiva and often at the limbus; follicles are seen on the slit-lamp as rounded, avascular

white or grey structures containing lymphocytes surrounded by small vessels arising at the border and encircling it (Vaughan et al. 1992); they are inflamed lymphoid tissue

- Marked papillary response may also be present on the tarsal plate
- Lesions may be seen on the corneal epithelium, which may be punctate or nummular; they may spread to stroma producing punctate scarring (subepithelial opacities), which may compromise vision initially and last for some months before resolving spontaneously
- The tear film is likely to be poor with a break-up time that may be instantaneous.

Management

There is no effective drug therapy for adenoviral conjunctivitis. Eye swabs are not therefore necessary unless diagnosis is uncertain (and are expensive and can be painful) (Ragge and Easty 1990).

It is essential that patients are given a full explanation of their condition because the primary function of the management of this condition is patient awareness and reducing discomfort through education and decreasing symptomatology. Adenoviral conjunctivitis often has symptoms out of all proportion to its importance and can be an intensely distressing condition. Advice and information should include the following:

- The roughness of the conjunctiva (follicles – Figure 15.3) is what makes the eyes feel so gritty and irritable.
- The patient with viral conjunctivitis often complains of dryness, along with a watery eye. The tears, although profuse, are inadequate in quality and dry up very quickly; the eye responds to the irritation and dryness by producing more.
- Topical antibiotics are ineffective with adenovirus conjunctivitis and secondary bacterial infection is uncommon.
- Artificial tears may help to control the feeling of dryness and irritation and these may be used frequently (e.g. half-hourly or more often).
- A bland ointment such as simple eye ointment may also be helpful.
- The treatment contains no drugs and can therefore be used as required to ensure comfort.
- Cold compresses on the lids may ease the irritation of this very distressing condition.

The patient should be aware that viral conjunctivitis may persist for 3–6 weeks and the symptoms of dryness may last much longer, necessitating the use of artificial tears, sometimes for months or even years.

Adenovirus is contagious until the symptoms have peaked. It could be argued that patients should be advised to avoid work until the symptoms have peaked. However, this would not normally be advised for any other viral infection, such as a cold, so advice should be based on symptoms and

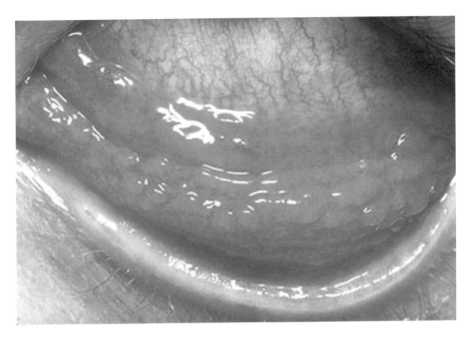

Figure 15.3 Follicles. (See Plate 21.)

the person's role. Certainly, contact in the workplace with food and children should be discouraged. Schools and nurseries are unlikely to be happy about children attending with red eyes, but, as the red eye can persist after the condition has peaked and is no longer contagious, information may need to be given to the parents to pass on to the school about the nature of the infection.

Chlamydial infection must be considered if clinically indicated such as in the case of subacute onset, delayed resolution and uniocular infection.

Infection control
Adenovirus is highly infectious and infection control is of paramount importance, both for patients – they should use their own towels and facecloths and be encouraged to wash their hands after touching their eyes or instilling drops – and for the department. Handwashing is the first line of defence in control of any infection and is vital to stop the spread of viral conjunctivitis (Gleavy 1990). Many major epidemics of viral conjunctivitis associated with ophthalmic units have been linked with poor handwashing techniques and inadequate disinfection of equipment (Tullo 1980, Jernigan et al. 1993). Adenovirus has the capacity to survive in the desiccated state on various surfaces.

Examination equipment should be cleaned between each patient, including, for example, switches and pens which act as vectors but are often not considered. Sodium hypochlorite solution (500 parts per million) is effective against many organisms and infection control departments should be involved to ensure effective procedures. Handwashing should be supplemented by alcohol gels or wipes to ensure compliance by health-care workers.

Epidemic keratoconjunctivitis

The onset of epidemic keratoconjunctivitis (EKC) is caused by adenovirus types 8, 19 and 37, with an acute onset, occurring first in one eye and then both; as a rule the first eye is more severely affected. The patient complains of general discomfort and, on slit-lamp examination, follicles, petechial haemorrhages, chemosis (may be gross), and oedema of the caruncle and pseudomembrane may be seen. This type of adenoviral infection is particularly severe.

Corneal involvement is usually seen (as described earlier). The management of EKC is as already described. The use of steroids to treat infiltrate is usually thought to be unhelpful.

Pharyngoconjunctival fever

This is another adenoviral infection presenting with conjunctival findings similar to simple adenoviral infection and caused by adenovirus 3 and occasionally adenovirus 4. It is characterized by a temperature of 38.3–40°C, sore throat, conjunctival injection, giant follicular conjunctivitis that begins unilaterally with the fellow eye being involved in 2–5 days. Outbreaks may be epidemic and have been linked to contamination from swimming pools. The illness is generally self-limiting, although fairly debilitating, and supportive therapy is all that is needed.

Chlamydial/adult inclusion conjunctivitis

Definition and description

Chlamydial conjunctivitis should be considered if conjunctivitis is unilateral and chronic and large follicles are seen subtarsally.

Chlamydial (inclusion) conjunctivitis is caused by *C. trachomatis* serotypes D–K and is usually sexually transmitted (Mandava et al. 1998). Women seem to be more susceptible than men to systemic infection, although men are more likely to notice symptoms than women. Eye lesions may present about 1 week after sexual contact. There may be systemic signs and symptoms of vaginitis, cervicitis or urethritis. Diagnosis of inclusion conjunctivitis may be difficult even with laboratory investigation. Infants whose mothers have untreated chlamydial infections have a 30–40%

chance of developing neonatal chlamydial conjunctivitis (ophthalmia neonatorum).

Pathophysiology

Chlamydia trachomatis is an intracellular parasite and has its own DNA and RNA; as a result it is more closely related to bacteria than to viruses. It is known that subgroup A causes chlamydial infections, serotypes A, B, Ba and C cause trachoma and serotypes D–K produce adult inclusion conjunctivitis (Mandava et al. 1998). The incubation period is usually 2–7 days. The usual mode of transmission is through sexual exposure, hand contact from a site of genital infection to the eye, sharing infected eye make-up or towels and mother infecting the neonate during delivery.

Signs and symptoms

Symptoms
• Subacute red eye, which was never acute and is not settling
• Foreign body sensation
• Drooping of upper lid
• Photophobia.

Signs
• Watery discharge
• Lid swelling
• Palpable preauricular node may be present
• Superficial punctate keratitis
• Micropannus
• Large follicles in upper and lower fornices
• Possibility of formation of pseudomembrane and haemorrhage.

Management

As a result of its implications, *suspicion* of chlamydial infection should not trigger discussions about STIs. Introducing the subject before an accurate diagnosis can be made may induce suspicion and tension into relationships. Although informed consent should be given for the swab, as for any investigation, it might be thought sufficient to explain that this is for one of the infective agents that is treatable and not mention its possible nature of transmission.

The treatment for chlamydial infection is simple and effective once it has been diagnosed by a positive eye swab. Results are usually available in 3 days, although rapid results may be possible in urgent cases. Tetracycline hydrochloride, chlortetracycline or erythromycin ointment four times a day for 3 weeks is the first line of treatment. Oral antibiotics will need to be prescribed and might include regimens such as tetracycline 250–500 mg four times a day for 3 weeks, or amoxicillin and erythromycin 250–500 mg four times a day for 3 weeks.

Sensitivity and tact must be shown to the patients and their partners when a diagnosis of chlamydial infection is made. Patients and their partners must be fully informed of the circumstances surrounding the disease as an STI and the importance of treating the partners who may be asymptomatic because they will be at risk. Appointments must be made for the patients and their partners at a genitourinary medicine clinic.

It is important that patients finish any course of treatment and attend all their appointments to avoid systemic complications. Untreated chlamydial infection can result in pelvic inflammatory disease, leading to infertility or long-term pelvic pain. If a woman has chlamydial infection when she is pregnant, she is at a higher risk of having an ectopic pregnancy or a premature birth. In addition to giving her newborn baby an eye infection, lung infection is also a possibility. For men, although the complications are rare, inflammation of the testicles causing infertility is a possibility. For both men and women, Reiter's syndrome and appendicitis are added complications.

Herpes simplex virus conjunctivitis

Herpes simplex virus (HSV) is usually seen before or simultaneous with the appearance of vesicular lesions on the eyelids. It occurs during primary infection (HSV-1 and also possibly HSV-2) or during recurrent episodes of ocular herpes (Vaughan et al. 1992). The disease course usually runs for 3–4 weeks, begins unilaterally, with the fellow eye involved within a week. Slit-lamp examination may reveal pseudomembrane and conjunctival ulceration, and there is usually tenderness of the preauricular lymph nodes. The cornea is frequently involved because of its association with herpes simplex keratitis with superficial punctate staining, and formation of dendrites is common. Occasionally, uveitis may be present. Recurrence is common, with 50% of patients having a second episode within 2 years.

Early treatment is required and antiviral agents such as aciclovir 3% ointment, idoxuridine 0.1% or trifluorothymidine (F_3T) are prescribed. The use of steroids is absolutely prohibited because these will aggravate the herpes simplex infections and make the condition worse.

Molluscum contagiosum

This is a viral infection of the skin affecting mainly children. If a molluscum lesion is located on the eyelid margin, a secondary follicular conjunctivitis may develop as an immune reaction to the poxvirus particles being shed into the eye. The usual management is excision of the lid lesion and the follicular reaction will resolve.

Axenfield conjunctivitis

This is usually mild and asymptomatic with upper large palpebral follicles. It usually runs a chronic course and treatment is unnecessary.

Measles, mumps and rubella conjunctivitis

These three conditions may be accompanied by a mild bilateral follicular conjunctivitis, which appears similar to simple adenoviral infection; therapy is usually supportive.

Toxic and irritating follicular conjunctivitis

This can be caused by long-term use of certain ocular medications, heavy make-up, environmental irritants, sensitivity to soap, etc. as a result of hypersensitivity reaction. Slit-lamp examination may reveal a mixture of papillae and follicles. The condition is usually unilateral, depending on cause. Management consists of replacement ocular medications, encouraging better hygiene and where possible isolating and removing irritants. Artificial lubricants may be helpful.

Trachoma (see also Chapter 13)

Trachoma, by definition (also known as granular conjunctivitis or Egyptian ophthalmia), is a contagious, chronic inflammation of the mucous membranes of the eye caused by an organism called *Chlamydia trachomatis*, a parasite closely related to bacteria. The spread of trachoma is either through discharge from an infected child's eyes passing on to hands, on clothing, hand-to-eye contact or by flies that land on the faces of infected children. The infection is highly contagious in its early stages.

Trachoma occurs world wide but most often in poor rural communities. It is widespread in the Middle East, parts of the Indian subcontinent, south Asia and China. Pockets of blinding trachoma are also found in Australia (among native Australians), the Pacific Islands and Latin America. It is the world's leading cause of preventable blindness and problems occur in areas where there is overcrowding and poor sanitation. Infection usually occurs in childhood and the early symptoms of trachoma include the development of follicles on the conjunctiva of the upper eyelids. The patient also experiences oedematous eyelids, discharge, pain and photophobia. Repeated attacks will cause scarring of the inner eyelids, leading to entropion. The continuous rubbing of the inturning lashes (trichiasis) on the cornea as the result of the entropion eventually will lead to severe cornea scarring resulting in severe loss of vision and blindness. In addition, blindness is also caused through repeated secondary bacterial keratitis.

Diagnosis is based on the patient's history and slit-lamp examination of the eye. Small samples of cells can be taken from the conjunctiva and stained (Giemsa staining) to confirm diagnosis.

Treatment of early stage trachoma consists of giving antibiotic treatment of tetracyclines, erythromycin or sulphonamides for 4–6 weeks. Treatment should start immediately without waiting for the lab results. Some medical personnel combine oral medication with topical antibiotic ointment. However, tetracycline should not be given to pregnant women or children aged less than 7 years. Patients presenting with ocular complications as a result of end-stage trachoma may be treated surgically, either a corneal graft or an entropion repair. Prognosis is often excellent in the early stages. However, if the patient's ocular presentation includes follicular formation, prevention of blindness depends very much on the severity of follicles, the development of scarring, the degree of eyelid deformity and corneal involvement, and the episodes of additional recurrent bacterial infection.

The WHO estimates that 6 million worldwide are blind as a result of trachoma and more than 150 million people are in need of treatment. Primary intervention advocated by the WHO for preventing trachoma infection includes improved sanitation, reduction of fly-breeding sites, proper disposal of human and animal waste, and increased facial cleanliness (with clean water) among children at risk of disease (WHO 2001).

The WHO, along with an alliance of interested parties, have adopted the 'SAFE' strategy to combat trachoma by the year 2020. The four components of strategy include:

(1) surgery
(2) antibiotic treatment
(3) facial cleanliness
(4) environmental changes.

Other types of conjunctivitis

Allergic conjunctivitis

Allergic conjunctivitis affects 6 out of 10 allergy patients and is usually associated with hay fever. Allergic conjunctivitis occurs when the eye comes into contact with a substance to which the sufferers are sensitive. This is a common but not a serious condition and it is more of a nuisance than anything else. There are many types of allergens or substance to which the eyes can become sensitive such as the following:

- Pollen: flowers, trees and grasses and weeds all release pollen into the air and this is carried by the wind. When the pollen count is high, especially in spring and summer, the patient may experience allergies.
- Pets: hairs from pets particularly cats can cause allergies. The tiny dandruff-like scales that household animals shed can become trapped in furniture and carpets.
- Other common allergens: cosmetics, house mites and pollution.

Pathophysiology

Allergy may occur to normally harmless antigens (known as allergens) or to infectious agents. The allergic response is known as type 1 hypersensitivity and exists in two phases: the sensitization and effector phase.

A harmless antigen causes the production of an antibody (IgE) on first exposure. This then comes into contact with mast cells and basophils, which have receptors for IgE antibody (sensitization). The patient will experience no symptoms after initial binding; however, introduction of the allergen stimulates the production of more IgE and increases the possibility of cross-linking with existing antibodies on the mast cell surface, causing the mast cell to degranulate. Degranulation releases a large number of inflammatory mediators such as histamine, prostaglandins and bradykinin. Histamine causes the itchy symptoms experienced by patients and induces vasodilatation and mucus secretion by goblet cells.

Prostaglandins directly stimulate nerve endings to produce sensations of itching and pain and also increase vascular permeability and vasodilatation.

Acute allergic conjunctivitis

Allergic conjunctivitis presents acutely in two distinct ways.

The first is by an acute and frightening atopic reaction that involves massive chemosis or swelling of the conjunctiva, which the patient often describes as 'jelly' on the eye (Figure 15.4). The cornea appears to have sunk backwards as the conjunctiva protrudes beyond it. This is an alarming but self-limiting condition that often occurs in children. The chemosis usually resolves spontaneously within a couple of hours, often more quickly, so there is little need for intervention with drugs or drops and, as the eye is sensitized to allergen at this stage, reaction to drops or preservative may be potentiated. Reassurance is required and supportive treatments such as cold compresses may be soothing.

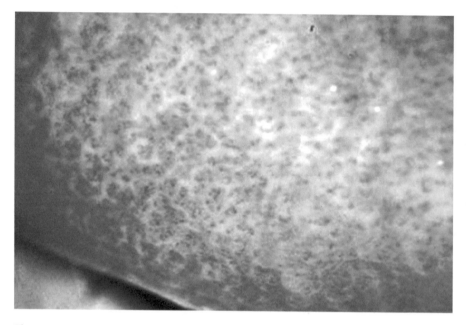

Figure 15.4 Papillae. (See Plate 22.)

The second is more common and less dramatic.

Signs and symptoms

- Itching that may be severe
- Hyperaemia
- Eyelid chemosis and erythema
- Watery discharge
- Foreign body sensation
- Burning of the eye
- Papillae
- History of seasonal or other allergies
- Lack of palpable preauricular lymph nodes
- Other systemic conditions such as rhinitis and asthma.

Treatment

The primary aim of management is alleviating the symptoms and support of the patient. The most effective but perhaps least practical is to prevent exposure to any known allergen. As this is not always possible, mast cell stabilizers such as lodoxamide and sodium cromoglicate are applied four times daily. These drops prevent the onset of allergic reaction by blocking the adherence of the IgE-allergen compound to the mast cell. Side effects of these drops may include transient burning and stinging. Once degranulation of the mast cell membrane has occurred (and histamine has been released), it will take 7–10 days for the membrane to restabilize. Mast cell-stabilizing drops will therefore have no apparent effect for 7–10 days. Once an allergic reaction has occurred, antihistamine drops will be useful (ketotifen, levocabastine, emedastine) and may be used in combination with a mast cell stabilizer. A drug that combines both properties is olopatadine.

Care

Patients presenting with allergic conjunctivitis are usually aware of what to avoid in order to minimize their symptoms. Patients, especially those with a history of seasonal allergic conjunctivitis, should be told to avoid where possible exposure to any substances that precipitate symptoms and recommended prophylactic treatment with a mast cell stabilizer, which should be used for the duration of the season to prevent symptoms.

Cold compresses, artificial tears or gel can be used together for relieving symptoms. In addition, topical decongestants that cause vasoconstriction and thereby retard the release of the chemical mediators into the tissues from the bloodstream can be used. The use of antihistamine systemically can also be beneficial.

Vernal conjunctivitis

This is a more serious seasonal disorder affecting children and young adults. The prevalence of vernal conjunctivitis is higher in warmer climates. The onset is typically between the ages of 3 and 25 years and males are more affected than females.

Signs and symptoms

Symptoms
• Itching
• Blepharospasm
• Photophobia
• Copious mucoid discharge
• Blurred vision.

Signs
• Giant cobblestone papillae (palpebral form of vernal conjunctivitis)
• Areas of superficial punctate keratitis
• Diffuse papillary hypertrophy on the palpebral conjunctiva especially on superior tarsal plate

- Hyperaemia
- Chemosis
- Severe cases have superiorly located corneal shield ulcers
- Horner–Trantas dots (gelatinous, white clumps of degenerated eosinophils at the superior limbus, known as limbal form of vernal conjunctivitis).

Treatment and care

Treatment and care are as for allergic conjunctivitis. If a shield ulcer is present, topical steroids should be given four to six times a day with a prophylactic antibiotic and cycloplegic agent in addition to mast cell stabilizer and cold compresses (Mandava et al. 1998).

Giant papillary conjunctivitis

This is often associated with a soft or gas-permeable lens wearer and is seen as a local allergic reaction. Sometimes this condition can occur in patients with ocular prostheses and sutures. The tear levels of IgE, IgG and IgM are elevated, as in vernal conjunctivitis, in which the mast cells are activated (Pavan-Langston 2002).

Signs and symptoms

- Decreased contact lens tolerance
- Superficial punctate staining, especially superiorly
- Photophobia
- Giant cobblestone papillae
- Mucus discharge
- Hyperaemia
- Fine papillae in lower tarsal plate.

Management and nursing care

Patients are advised to stop their contact lens wear for a couple of weeks until all the inflammation and superficial punctate staining are gone. It is also advisable that patients see an optician for their contact lens check in relation to the fit, the continued suitability of their current contact lenses, and contact lens hygiene including preservative-free solutions. If symptoms persist, it may be necessary to change to a different type contact lens or discontinue permanently.

Superior limbic keratoconjunctivitis

This condition primarily affects the upper tarsus and superior bulbar conjunctiva, especially at the limbus, and is usually bilateral. This affects females more than males.

Pathophysiology

The aetiology and pathogenesis are unclear and numerous causative agents have been implicated. Infectious agents such as bacteria, viruses and fungi have been implicated. An autoimmune aetiology has also been considered, based on the course of the disease with periods of exacerbations and remissions. There has also been an association with thyroid disease and other autoimmune disease. One theory that is widely regarded is that during blinking the loose conjunctival tissue rubs against the limbus, causing a mechanical irritation. Predisposing factors such as prominent globe in cases of thyroid disease or tight lids have been implicated as causes of the condition. A newer theory suggests that these patients have a degree of tear deficiency to the superior keratoconjunctiva, resulting in significantly reduced levels of vital tear-based nutrients to the affected region as well as friction from the upper lid.

Signs and symptoms

- Burning, foreign body sensation
- Red eye
- Mild photophobia
- Nondescript pain
- Papillae on the superior palpebral conjunctiva
- Sectoral injection on the superior bulbar conjunctiva
- Fine punctate staining on superior cornea, limbus
- Superior corneal micropannus and filament.

Management

This is a chronic and recurrent disorder and there is no 100% effective treatment. The treatment of choice has been 0.5–1.0% silver nitrate solution applied topically to the superior bulbar and tarsal conjunctiva to cauterize the irregular tissue, thereby promoting growth of new healthy epithelium. Other treatment, such as pressure patching as well as bandage hydrogel lenses to alleviate mechanical irritation, has been employed. Surgical intervention such as surgical recession or resection of the superior bulbar conjunctiva has been employed. Vitamin A eyedrops have also been somewhat effective in treating this condition. All patients presenting with superior limbic keratoconjunctivitis should have a systemic work-up.

Miscellaneous disorders of the conjunctiva

Phlyctenulosis

There are two forms of phlyctenulosis: conjunctival and corneal. There is always the appearance of a focal, staining nodule of limbal tissue on the conjunctiva, usually as a response to staphylococcal exotoxins and blepharitis. Treating the blepharitis with eyelid hygiene instructions usually causes the disappearance of phlyctenulosis. If phlyctenulosis is severe, antibiotic drops alone are effective, although a combination with steroid drops may be used.

Subconjunctival haemorrhage

Rupture of the superficial conjunctival vessels (not caused by trauma) can occur spontaneously and is usually unilateral. Sometimes the cause can be attributed to vomiting, severe eye rubbing, coughing, heavy lifting or sneezing. The possibility of blood dyscrasias cannot be ruled out in cases of recurrent or bilateral subconjunctival haemorrhage. The onset is usually sudden and it is extremely alarming for the patient to see an extremely red eye. The eye is examined on the slit-lamp and sometimes, in severe subconjunctival haemorrhage, a dark red mass of the bulbar conjunctiva can be seen which spills over the lower lid margin. Depending on the extent of the subconjunctival haemorrhage, this condition normally settles within 2 weeks.

It is important to reassure patients and inform them that the haemorrhage will subside and that they will often notice a yellowish discoloration as the haemorrhage fades. It is important, if a patient is on anticoagulant, that an international normalized ratio (INR) is performed or advice is sought from the anticoagulant lab. Similarly, if patients are on aspirin, they are advised to see their GPs. Artificial lubricant may be prescribed to soothe any minor discomfort. It is also advisable to check the patient's blood pressure to detect any underlying hypertensive state or monitor cases of known hypertension.

Pinguecula

These are yellowish, slightly raised, lipid-like nodules commonly found in the nasal and temporal limbal bulbar conjunctiva. The base of the pinguecula abuts on to the limbus but never crosses the corneoscleral frontier. Pinguecula can become vascularized and inflamed and is a common presentation to the eye emergency department; it may be associated with corneal punctate epitheliopathy and corneal dellen (corneal thinning secondary to dryness).

Pinguecula is commonly found in patients who are middle-aged with a history of chronic exposure to sun or living in a hot, dry, dusty atmosphere. There is no predilection for sex or race and both eyes are usually affected.

Pathophysiology

As mentioned previously, this condition typically affects the older population and is a conjunctival degenerative process that is initiated by continuous exposure to ultraviolet (UV) light or other irritants. As a result, this alters the elastic and collagen tissue of the conjunctival stroma, leading to elastic tissue degeneration and deposition of abnormal elastic fibres in the conjunctival substantia propria.

Management

In general treatment is given only if the patient complains of acute irritation and if the pinguecula is inflamed. In cases of mild pingueculitis or when a dellen is present, suitable lubricating drops or ointment is prescribed. Patients are educated in the use of eye protection or sunwear to minimize eye exposure.

Where symptoms are severe, weak topical steroids such as prednisolone 0.12% may be given or a non-steroidal medication such as Acular (ketorolac trometamol) or Voltarol (diclofenac sodium) may be prescribed.

Pterygium

This is another degenerative condition of the conjunctival tissue. Slit-lamp examination reveals a raised, triangular, whitish wedge of fibrovascular tissue encroaching onto the nasal cornea. In some instances, the vascularized cornea may become red and inflamed and is a common presentation to the eye department. Surgery is usually indicated if it encroaches on the pupillary area.

Pathophysiology

There are potentially contributory factors to the formation of pterygium. These may include exposure to UV-A and UV-B, allergens, irritants such as wind, dirt, dust, air pollution, and in people who spend a great deal of time outdoors. Heredity may also be a factor.

Degeneration of the conjunctival stroma results in replacement by thickened, tortuous elastic tissue. Activated fibroblasts in the leading edge of the pterygium invade and fragment Bowman's layer as well as a variable amount of superficial corneal stroma.

Management

This is education of the patient, such as avoiding dusty and smoky environment and the use of sunwear to protect the eyes in mild cases of pterygium. Ocular lubrication is also helpful. If the pterygium is inflamed, treatment is usually a mild topical steroid four times daily to the affected eye.

Surgery usually consists of the removal of pterygium and a small portion of superficial clear cornea beyond the area of encroachment.

Conjunctival tumours

Tumours in the conjunctiva can be either benign or malignant. Benign tumours include:

- dermoids
- pigmented naevus
- granuloma
- papilloma.

Malignant tumours include:

- malignant papilloma
- epithelioma
- sarcoma (may originate from pigmented naevus)
- rodent ulcer (as direct extension from lids).

Other miscellaneous 'lumps' and 'bumps' include:

- concretions
- retention cysts.

Dermoids

A dermoid is a congenital benign tumour arising from the mesoderm and ectoderm which may involve the cornea and sclera; it is composed mainly of collagen and is commonly located in the inferotemporal limbal area. The lesions are white (limbal dermoid) or yellow (dermolipoma), solid and have hairs protruding from them. A dermoid tumour normally remains quiescent, although it can enlarge around puberty. Surgical intervention is indicated if the vision is threatened or if a cosmetic deformity is particularly significant.

Pigmented naevus

This is usually congenital and may develop in the early years. The lesion is normally smooth, flat with well-circumscribed edges, and is most commonly seen nasally within the bulbar conjunctiva. Cysts may be seen within the lesion and are a key diagnosis of its benign nature. However, a malignant melanoma may develop from a naevus and enlargement may be an early sign of malignancy (Cullom and Chang 1993). Management consists mainly of baseline colour photographs to document growth and these patients may be reviewed every 6 months or 1 year. If the lesion is enlarging, or patients exhibit signs of malignancy such as ulceration, change in pigmentation, haemorrhage and development of feeder vessels, such patients will require a biopsy.

Granuloma

This can occur at any age and is found predominantly on the tarsal conjunctiva. Granuloma inflammation usually occurs around a site of irritation such as foreign body or around a discharging chalazion and can be associated with systemic disease such as sarcoidosis and tuberculosis (Vaughan et al. 1992). Management involves incisional or excisional biopsy.

Papilloma

A papilloma can be either flat (sessile) or on a stalk (pedunculated) with an irregular surface. Papillomas are common in patients over the age of 40 years and can usually be seen in the fornix or caruncle. Two different forms can be distinguished:

1. Viral: recurrences are common with multiple lesions.
2. Non-viral: single lesions more common and may be pigmented, often thought to be pre-cancerous. Basal cell carcinoma of the conjunctiva is rare but can appear similar to a papilloma.

Malignant melanoma

Malignant melanoma of the conjunctiva is rare and presents itself as a raised, pigmented or non-pigmented lesion that appears in patients in their early 50s and is rarely seen in people younger than 20 years. It may resemble benign melanosis or naevus and may develop on its own (without any histological or clinical evidence of a pre-existing lesion in about 10% of cases) or in areas of previous pigmentation (about 20% of cases)

(Roque 2001). Both sexes are equally affected and it predominantly affects fair-skinned people. Lesions may be multiple.

It is crucial that a good history of growth characteristics of each lesion is elicited from patients who may be aware of subtle changes that may be helpful in identifying these lesions. It is also important for a good physical slit-lamp examination to be carried out. The clinical presentation can be variable. Conjunctival melanomas can extend onto the peripheral limbus with some growing circumferentially around the limbus (Roque 2001). It is rare to find a melanomatous nodule located on the central cornea.

The treatment for conjunctival melanoma is surgical excision. Exenteration of the orbit is sometimes necessary for a large melanoma that has invaded the orbit. However, this procedure does not improve the prognosis. The poor survival rate may somehow suggest that metastasis has already occurred at the time of treatment and confirmation of the extent of the disease at diagnosis is the most important factor to determine the outcome (Roque 2001).

Miscellaneous 'lumps' and 'bumps' of the conjunctiva

Concretions

Small white to yellowish calcium deposits usually 1–3 mm in size found in the lower or upper or both palpebral conjunctivae. The patient is usually asymptomatic unless it protrudes through the conjunctiva and causes irritation. These concretions can be seen singly or multiply. If irritation persists, it can be removed with a sterile green needle after a drop of local anaesthetic such as benoxinate or amethocaine. Prophylactic antibiotic ointment such as chloramphenicol four times a day for 3 days is prescribed to prevent any infection.

Retention cysts

These are clear filled cysts seen anywhere in the conjunctiva; they may be filled with lymphatic fluid or secretions from the glands of Krause or Wolfring (Figure 15.5). Patients are often asymptomatic; a large cyst causing irritation can be drained by piercing the conjunctiva with a sterile green needle after a drop of local anaesthetic. These cysts have the tendency to refill so it is important that patients perform ocular massage with topical lubricant after drainage. It is also a wise precaution to prescribe a topical antibiotic to minimize any infection.

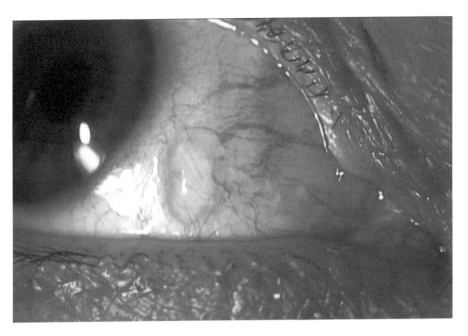

Figure 15.5 Conjunctival cyst. (See Plate 23.)

Conjunctivitis associated with systemic conditions

Ocular rosacea

This condition is seen in patients with acne rosacea and occurs in people who are light skinned. On physical examination, patients will exhibit signs of erythema, pustules, and papules of the forehead, cheek and nose. Patients' main symptoms are bilateral chronic ocular irritation, foreign body sensation, hyperaemia of the eyelids and recurrent episodes of chalazion. The inferior cornea is involved with superficial or deep vascularization and may extend into the stroma. The treatment consists of tetracycline 250 mg four times a day with the dose being tapered off once relief of symptoms is obtained.

Ocular cicatricial pemphigoid

This is thought to be a type of hypersensitivity reaction with a slowly progressive cicatrizing conjunctivitis. The course of the disease is characterized by periods of remissions and exacerbations usually occur in patients over the age of 55 years. On examination, there are signs of superficial punctate keratitis, inferior symblepharon, secondary bacterial conjunctivitis, entropion and trichiasis. Systemically, there are signs of scarring of the mucous membrane of the nose, mouth, pharynx, oesophagus and anus. Management consists of slit-lamp examination, work-up, conjunctival swabs, and mouth and nose examination. Treatment consists of systemic and local steroids and copious artificial lubricant. Surgical correction entropion and electrolysis of trichiasis may be considered.

Erythema multiforme major (Stevens–Johnson syndrome)

This is essentially a disease of the mucous membranes and skin as a result of acute hypersensitivity reaction. It may also be precipitated by drugs such as tetracyclines, phenytoin or penicillin, or infectious agents such as various bacteria, viruses, fungi and herpes. There is an acute onset of fever, red eye, rash and general malaise, and it is common in children and young adults. Signs include 'target' skin lesions (red-centred vesicles surrounded by a pale ring and then a red ring – Cullom and Chang 1993), bullous skin lesion on the hands and feet, and severe mucosal lesions on eyes and mouth. Again, corneal vascularization, scarring of the conjunctiva, dry eyes, symblepharon, eyelid deformities, corneal ulcers, corneal perforation and endophthalmitis may develop.

Taking a good history is essential in order to determine the precipitating factor. Slit-lamp examination should include lid examination and examination of the fornices. Conjunctiva and corneal scrapings are taken if infection is suspected. Blood tests such as electrolytes and a full blood count are essential. Treatment consists of topical and systemic steroids, topical antibiotic and artificial lubricant. Nursing care includes support for patients and relatives and frequent oral toilet and general care of the patient's skin.

Connective tissue disease

Reiter's syndrome

This is a triad of disease manifestations consisting of non-specific arthritis, conjunctivitis and urethritis. This is more common in men than women. There has been some success with treatment with oral tetracycline plus steroid for any systemic indications.

Systemic lupus erythematosus

This is a multisystem disorder thought to have an autoimmune aetiology, usually occurring in the third or fourth decade of life. Women are more susceptible than men. Signs and symptoms include butterfly rash on face, non-specific conjunctival findings such as hyperaemia, and fine papillae, keratitis and non-granulomatous inflammation. Treatment consists of aspirin, chloroquine and steroids. Uveitis is normally treated with topical steroids and cycloplegics.

Polyarteritis nodosa

This is arteritis of small and medium vessels caused by severe hypersensitivity occurring more frequently in men than women. There are many systemic findings such as nephritis, hypertension and pulmonary involvement. Ocular signs consist of episcleritis, scleritis and involvement of the retinal circulation (Snell and Lemp 1998).

References

Cullom R, Chang B (1993) The Wills Eye Manual: Office and emergency room. Diagnosis and treatment of eye disease, 2nd edn. Philadelphia, PA: JB Lippincott Co.

Forrester J, Dick A, McMenamin P, Lee W (1996) The Eye: Basic sciences in practice. London: WB Saunders Co.

Gleavy D (1990) The nursing role in epidemiology, risk management and patient-public education. J Ophthal Nursing Technol 9: 215–19.

Hammerschlag M (1993) Neonatal conjunctivitis. Paediatr Anal 22: 346–51.

Jernigan J, Lowry B, Hayden F (1993) Adenovirus type 8 epidemic keratoconjunctivitis in an eye clinic: risk factors and control. J Infect Dis 167: 1307–13.

Mandava S, Sweeney T, Guyer D (1998) Colour Atlas of Ophthalmology: The Manhattan Eye, Ear and Throat Hospital pocket guide. New York: Thième Medical.

Newell FW (1996) Ophthalmology: Principles and concepts, 8th edn. St Louis, MO: Mosby.

O'Hara M (1993) Ophthalmic neonatorum. Paediatr Clin N Am 40: 715–25.

Pavan-Langston D (ed.) (2002) Manual of Ocular Diagnosis and Therapy, 5th edn. Philadelphia, PA: Lippincott, Williams & Wilkins.

Ragge NK, Easty DL (1990) Immediate Eye Care. New York: Wolfe Publishing Ltd.

Roque M (2001) Conjunctival melanoma. J Emerg Med 2(5).

Snell R, Lemp M (1998) Clinical Anatomy of the Eye, 2nd edn. Oxford: Blackwell Scientific Publications.

Tullo AB (1980) Clinical and epidemiological features of adenoviral keratoconjunctivitis. Trans Ophthalmol Soc 100: 263–7.

Tullo AB, Donnelly D (1995) Conjunctiva. In: Perry JP, Tullo AB (eds), Care of the Ophthalmic Patient: A guide for nurses and health professionals. London: Chapman & Hall.

Vaughan D, Asbury T, Riordan-Eva P (1992) General Ophthalmology, 13th edn. New York: Prentice-Hall International Inc.

World Health Organization (2001) Disease Factsheet: Trachoma. World Water Day. Geneva: WHO.

Yetman R, Cody D (1997) Conjunctivitis: a practical guideline. J Paediatr Health Care 11: 238–41.

Chapter sixteen
The cornea

Bradley Kirkwood

The essential requirement of the cornea is to maintain its clarity because
it is the 'window' that allows light rays to enter the eye. Despite its highly
exposed position, the cornea along with the tear film acts as a robust
defence system between the eye and the environment. Optical properties
and refraction rely on the maintenance of corneal shape and clarity. Even
the smallest of corneal changes in the visual axis may result in visual distortion and disability for the patient.

Medical and surgical treatments of the cornea are geared towards the
restoration of corneal transparency and improving functional vision. This
chapter focuses on the areas such as the anatomy and physiology of the
cornea, some of the more common diseases, disorders and dystrophies,
some of the surgical procedures currently used in corneal transplantation
and diagnostic equipment for the cornea. The final section of this chapter provides the reader with a discussion around the various
keratorefractive procedures currently available.

Anatomy and physiology

Optical properties and macroscopic anatomy

The normal cornea is a transparent and avascular tissue. The anterior
corneal surface is covered by the tear film and the posterior surface is
directly bathed by the aqueous humour. The transitional zone between the
cornea and sclera is the richly vascularized limbus. The normal shape of
the anterior corneal surface is convex and aspherical.

Externally, the cornea may appear round in shape but is actually oval.
Horizontally, the normal cornea measures 11–12 mm compared with 9–11
mm vertically. This is the result of the sclera extending over the corneal
margin in the superior and inferior aspects. The central corneal thickness
is about 0.52 mm, and increases gradually towards the periphery where it

is about 0.7 mm thick. The radius of curvature is between 7.5 and 8.0 mm at the central 3-mm optical zone of the cornea, where the surface is at its steepest and is almost spherical, to a variably less steep cornea in the periphery, giving the cornea a prolate shape. The refractive power of the cornea is 40–44 D.

Microscopic anatomy and physiology

The tear film comprises three layers: lipid, aqueous and mucin. The cornea consists of three different cellular layers and two interfaces: epithelium, Bowman's layer, stroma, Descemet's membrane and endothelium. Components of the tear film and cornea, and within the layers of the cornea itself, interact with each other to maintain the integrity and function of the tissue. The individual layers are described below.

Tear film

The tear film covers the surface of the cornea. The thickness of the tear film is about 0.7 mm. The tear fluid consists of three layers: the most superficial layer is the lipid layer which is produced by the meibomian glands and the glands of Zeiss and Moll in the eyelids; the middle layer is the aqueous layer produced by accessory lacrimal tissue and the lacrimal gland; and the inferior layer is the mucin layer which is derived from the secretion of goblet cells within the conjunctiva. More than 98% of the total volume of the tear is water. The tear film contains many biologically important factors, including electrolytes, glucose, immunoglobulins, lysozyme, albumin and oxygen. Therefore, the tear film acts not only as a lubricant for the cornea but also as a source of nutrition, and it aids in the maintenance and repair of the corneal epithelium and is essential in providing an optical smooth surface for clear vision.

Cornea

The corneal epithelium is 50–60 μm thick and composed of two to three layers of superficial cells, two to three layers of 'wing' cells, and one layer of columnar basal cells. Only the basal cells have the ability to proliferate. The daughter cells gradually emerge to the anterior surface of the cornea, differentiating into wing cells and subsequently into superficial cells. This process can take up to 14 days before the superficial cells are desquamated into the tear film. The outer surface layer of the superficial cells comprises microplicae and microvilli, making their surface irregular. The tear film plays an important contribution in making the surface optically smooth by plugging the gaps.

Basal cells of corneal epithelium adhere to the basement membrane. The basement membrane is composed of the layers called lamina lucida and lamina densa, which add strength to the membrane. Hemidesmosomes are located on the underside of the basal cells and linked to anchoring fibrils. Anchoring fibrils penetrate the basement membrane and reach the stroma where they form anchoring plaques. The health of this adhesion complex is critical in the connection of epithelium to Bowman's layer and anterior stroma.

Bowman's layer is 12 μm thick and consists mainly of randomly arranged collagen fibres. It is considered the anterior portion of the corneal stroma and plays an important role in the maintenance of the epithelial structure. Bowman's layer does not regenerate after injury.

The stroma encompasses over 90% of the cornea and is crucial in the maintenance of shape, strength and transparency. The stroma consists primarily of collagen fibres, keratocytes and proteoglycans. Corneal transparency relies on the regular arrangement of collagen fibres. Any disarray in the uniformity of the fixed interfibre distance, as in the case of stromal oedema or scarring, will result in a loss of corneal transparency.

Descemet's membrane is composed largely of collagen and is 7 μm thick. It is firmly joined to the posterior surface of the stroma and does not regenerate after trauma.

The corneal endothelium comprises a single layer of cells that are hexagonal, uniform in shape and closely interdigitated. The most important physiological function of the endothelium is to regulate the water content of the stroma through active ion transport systems. Endothelial cells are unable to replicate, and rely on neighbouring cells to enlarge and spread to cover a defective area. When the endothelial cell count decreases considerably, the endothelial transport capability becomes overwhelmed and corneal oedema results.

Limbal stem cells

The centripetal movement of corneal epithelial cells during the healing phases has been well demonstrated. In the cornea, the localization of epithelial stem cells at the limbus has been postulated, along with the link between the cells assisting with corneal healing. However, there has been no direct evidence of the presence of limbal stem cells because of the lack of specific positive stem-cell markers (Boulton and Albon 2004).

Innervation

The cornea is one of the most innervated structures in the body. Sensory innervation of the cornea occurs primarily through the ophthalmic branch of the trigeminal nerve (cranial nerve V). Nerve fibres penetrate the cornea in the peripheral stroma. As the fibres travel towards the central cornea, the axons become finer. Fibres also branch anteriorly to create a terminal subepithelial plexus. The nerve fibres lose their myelination soon after entering the cornea. Clinically, the loss of superficial epithelium exposes the nerve endings, which results in severe ocular pain.

Healing phases of a corneal epithelial loss

The processes involved in the healing of corneal epithelial wounds can be described in three separate phases that are, in reality, part of a continuous process. These stages in epithelial healing can be described as the latent phase, where the movement of existing basal epithelial cells at the corneal wound margin occurs; cell migration and adhesion where the epithelial cells spread across the wound area before mitosis commences, and where extracellular matrix proteins such as fibronectin and laminin appear on the wound site surface to aid with epithelial adhesion; finally, there is cell proliferation until the normal epithelial thickness is restored. An important prerequisite for stability of regenerated corneal epithelium is tight adhesion to the underlying stroma. There are many factors that will affect the healing process, including the size and depth of the wound, tear film quality and the causative agent.

Examination of the cornea

Slit-lamp examination

By using a slit-lamp biomicroscope, pathological processes in the cornea can be directly observed. Furthermore, the cornea is conveniently placed for observation with a slit-lamp. Different lighting techniques can assist in the visualization of corneal pathology and these techniques are discussed elsewhere in the book.

Corneal diagnostic instruments

Corneal diagnostic instruments are specialized methods of examination to yield valuable information for the diagnosis and treatment of corneal disease. Techniques discussed here include keratometry, corneal topography, specular microscopy, confocal microscopy and pachymetry.

Keratometry measures the radius of corneal curvature within a 4-mm central optical zone. Such devices provide illuminated object mires that are reflected from the surface of the cornea acting as a convex mirror. The radius of curvature of the anterior corneal surface is determined from four reflected points that are evaluated as two pairs. The keratometer (Figure 16.1) determines the power and location of the steepest meridian and the power of the meridian 90° away, and is therefore useful in diagnosis and monitoring of corneal astigmatism. It is also useful in diagnosis of steep or flat corneas. The disadvantage of the keratometry readings is that it measures the central cornea only.

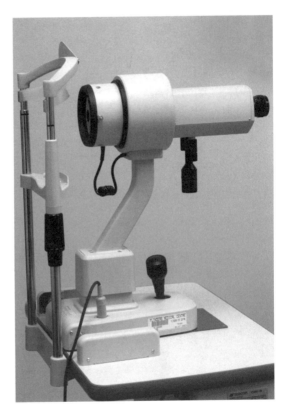

Figure 16.1 Keratometer. (All the photographs in this chapter are by courtesy of Angela Chappell, Ophthalmic Imaging Department, Flinders Medical Centre, Adelaide, South Australia.)

Videokeratoscopy, otherwise known as corneal topography, provides an overall mapping of the corneal shape through quantification and displays the map on a video screen. The videokeratoscope displays a colour-coded map for easy interpretation (Figure 16.2). The red or hot colours depict abnormal corneal steepening. This is useful for diagnosis of corneal disorders and monitoring of both regular and irregular corneal astigmatism. Corneal topography is also used in the preoperative and postoperative assessment for keratorefractive surgery.

Specular microscopy is the highly magnified photography of the corneal endothelium. The specular microscope enables visual observation,

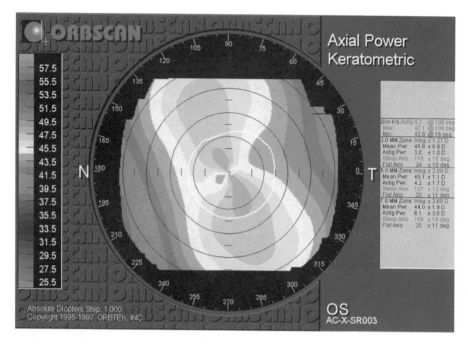

Figure 16.2 Corneal topography of astigmatism. (See Plate 24.)

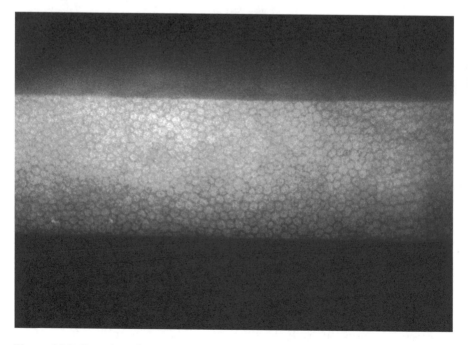

Figure 16.3 Specular micrograph of a normal endothelium. (See Plate 25.)

examination and analysis of the number, size, shape and density of the endothelial cells (Figure 16.3). Corneal disorders such as Fuchs' dystrophy can be monitored with specular microscopy.

Confocal microscopy is a non-invasive investigation that provides a level of high magnification and resolution and the opportunity to study the different layers of the cornea at a cellular level, allowing any corneal pathology to be observed, measured and analysed over time.

Pachymetry is the measurement of corneal thickness. Optical, ultrasonic and laser methods are now available. A pachometer is the name given to the instrument. Pachymetry is used in the preoperative assessment for keratorefractive surgery and can also be used in monitoring the function of the corneal endothelium.

Tear film disorders

When considering tear film disorders, the ocular surface microenvironment of the eyelids, conjunctiva, cornea and tear film needs to be evaluated. Any alteration in this environment has the potential to cause a tear film disturbance. In this section, the tear film, cornea and dry eye are focused on.

In simplistic terms, dry eye can be divided into two categories: aqueous tear-deficient dry eye and evaporative dry eye (Foulks 2003). Sjögren's syndrome is an example of aqueous tear deficiency and meibomian gland dysfunction is an example of evaporative dry eye. Patients with dry eyes can present with an assortment of symptoms, the most common of which include foreign body sensation, burning, itching, light sensitivity and transient blurry vision. Dry eye disease is a chronic disease. The symptoms are exacerbated by environmental factors, such as humidity and air movement, which lead to increased tear evaporation. Also the demands of certain visual tasks, such as driving, reading or using a computer for extended periods, reduce the blink reflex and aggravate dry eye symptoms. Ironically, patients can complain of excess tearing if the eye becomes so irritated that reflex tearing mechanisms are activated.

In diagnosis of a dry eye, the clinician relies on the patient history together with a decreased tear film break-up time and reduced Schirmer's test, along with a careful slit-lamp examination of the ocular surface and eyelids. Fluorescein dye stains punctate epithelial erosions particularly of the inferior cornea. The corneal epithelium may desquamate as filamentous threads (filamentary keratitis) (Figure 16.4). Rose Bengal is a diagnostic dye that stains dead or devitalized epithelial cells, mucus and corneal filaments, all of which are associated with dry eyes.

Medical treatment for dry eyes includes ocular surface lubrication in the form of drops, gels and ointments. These should be used on a frequent

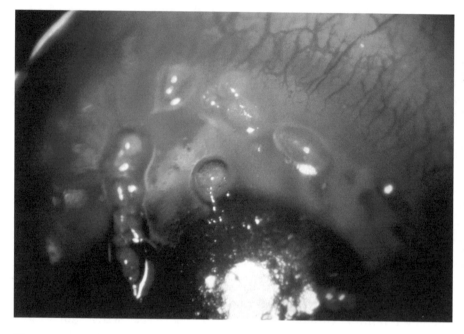

Figure 16.4 Filamentary keratitis. (See Plate 26.)

basis for them to be therapeutic. Surgical treatment is in the form of temporary or permanent punctal occlusion to assist with tear preservation.

Dry eye is a chronic condition that can often be controlled but not cured. Commonly, management of these patients is psychological. Nurses need to spend time counselling these patients with careful explanation of the problem to assist in reducing patient's complaints, frustrations and fears.

Corneal disorders

Microbial keratitis

Microbial keratitis is an ocular and sight-threatening condition and can present in a bacterial, fungal and protozoal form. Bacterial keratitis and fungal keratitis are discussed in this section. Acanthamoeba keratitis, a protozoal form of corneal infection, is discussed under 'Contact lens'. Commonly, microbial keratitis occurs in compromised corneas such as after trauma, contact lens wear and dry eyes. Clinical signs of corneal ulceration and stromal inflammation (infiltrate) are considered corneal infection until proved otherwise by negative microbial investigations.

Bacterial keratitis (Figure 16.5) can be caused by a wide variety of bacteria, although common organisms include staphylococci, streptococci,

Pseudomonas aeruginosa, *Moraxella* spp. and *Haemophilus influenzae* (Coster 2002).

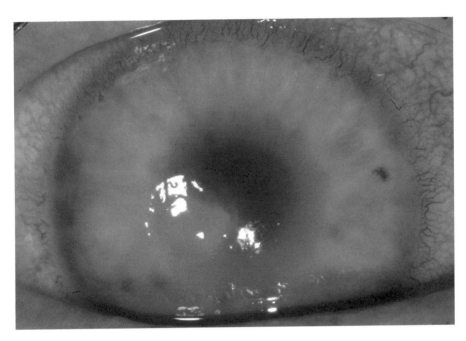

Figure 16.5 Bacterial keratitis. (See Plate 27.)

When there is sufficient evidence based on clinical examination to raise suspicion of a possible infectious aetiology, laboratory studies are required to identify the specific causative organism. Based on the features of clinical examination, results from laboratory investigation and knowledge of the potential corneal pathogens, a therapeutic plan is then initiated.

The selection of an antibiotic for a patient with a corneal ulceration is based on the preference of the ophthalmologist. A combination of a topical aminoglycoside (e.g. gentamicin) and a second-generation cephalosporin (e.g. cephalothin) or monotherapy with a fluoroquinolone (e.g. ofloxacin) is possible. The fluoroquinolones are more convenient to use but are not so effective against streptococci. Initially, topical antibiotics should be given frequently for the first 2–3 days and the clinical response evaluated daily for the first week, and then according to the clinical picture.

Fungal keratitis is less common than bacterial keratitis but should be considered a differential diagnosis of any corneal infection. Fungal keratitis has a tendency to be more common in hotter and tropical regions. Fungi from both filamentous and yeast organisms have been implicated in corneal infections. For the onset of filamentous fungal keratitis, commonly with *Fusarium solani* or *Aspergillus* spp., trauma most often occurs outdoors and involves plant matter (Kanski 1999). The yeast organism, *Candida albicans*, tends to occur in patients with chronic corneal disorders and immunosuppression (Kanski 1999). Clinically, ulcers have a feathery border with the infiltrate extending beyond the epithelial defect but, because clinically it is difficult to establish a diagnosis of fungal keratitis, the use of microbial investigations is of extreme importance.

Fungal ulcers are less responsive to medical therapy than bacterial ulcers because topical antifungal preparations are relatively non-specific and drug penetration is limited. Natamycin or miconazole drops are the drug of choice. Topical corticosteroids are contraindicated in fungal keratitis. Débridement of the corneal epithelium can assist with the penetration of topical medication. As corneal perforations are common with fungal keratitis, when progression of the keratitis is noted, penetrating keratoplasty should be performed.

Very frequent drops hourly or even half-hourly, perhaps overnight, can be a major burden for the patient. A significant amount of education and support is necessary to ensure that patients understand the reason for the therapy and are able to comply with its requirements. It should not be assumed that, because the clinician says that a particular drug regimen should happen, it will, and many factors such as concurrent medical conditions, age and ability to use the therapy, and the care needs of other members of the family may conspire against the requirements of therapy. Early intervention by asking about home circumstances may help strategies to be put in place to ensure effective treatment.

Herpes simplex keratitis

Herpes simplex keratitis is a common condition affecting the cornea. After primary infection, the virus travels up the sensory nerve to the trigeminal ganglion where it resides in a latent state, retaining the ability to become active at any time. Reactivation triggers the virus particles to travel down the trigeminal nerves and shed onto the mucosal surface and then enter epithelial cells and create recurrent infection.

The most common presentation of herpes simplex keratitis is the dendritic ulcer (Figure 16.6). The features of a dendritic ulcer include a branching, linear lesion with terminal bulbs and swollen epithelial borders, which contain live virus. Although the diagnosis of primary and recurrent ocular herpes simplex virus (HSV) infection relies on a thorough ophthalmic examination, viral culture can help make a definitive diagnosis.

An enlarged dendritic ulcer that is no longer linear is referred to as a geographic ulcer (Figure 16.7). This lesion can be thought of as a widened

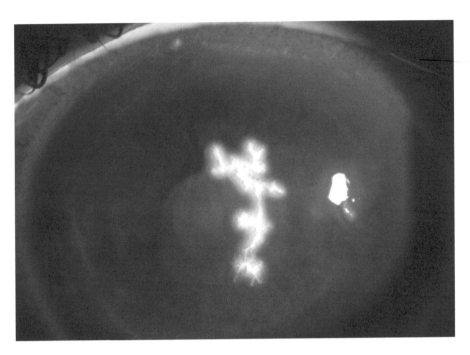

Figure 16.6 Dendritic ulcer caused by herpes simplex virus. (See Plate 28.)

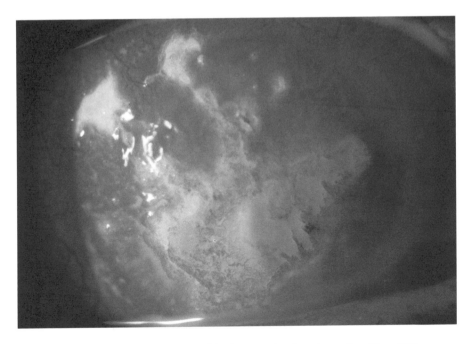

Figure 16.7 Geographic ulcer caused by herpes simplex virus. (See Plate 29.)

dendritic ulcer. Similar to a dendritic ulcer, it is a true ulcer in that it is an epithelial lesion extending through the basement membrane. Also similar to a dendritic ulcer, it has swollen epithelial borders, which contain live virus.

The treatment of herpetic keratitis is with antiviral agents that impair viral replication. Aciclovir is one of the topical preparations available and is effective in treating epithelial conditions. The treatment of corneal stromal disease caused by herpetic keratitis is aimed at reducing the stromal inflammation. This is done effectively with topical corticosteroids but often together with an antiviral because topical steroids enhance viral replication in the epithelium.

Peripheral corneal disease

Dellen

Dellen (Figure 16.8) may occur as an age-related change or secondary to other ocular abnormalities. Clinically dellen are saucer-like depressions in the corneal surface. Although they may be idiopathic, they are more commonly adjacent to elevated areas of conjunctiva or conjunctival chemosis, leading to 'shadowing' of an area of cornea and drying and epithelial breakdown. Treatment with ocular lubricants or perhaps pressure patching to ensure corneal lubrication will accelerate the healing process.

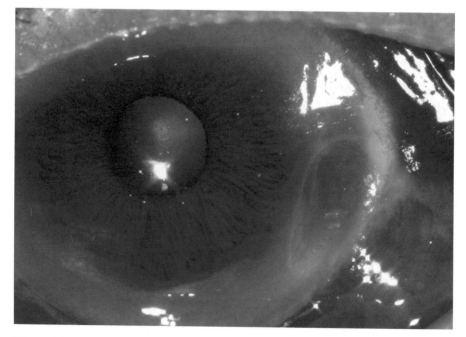

Figure 16.8 Corneal dellen. (See Plate 30.)

Marginal keratitis/phlyctenular keratitis

Marginal keratitis is most commonly caused by staphylococci, usually as a result of chronic blepharitis/blepharoconjunctivitis, and is secondary to the host's antibody response to the staphylococcal antigen (Mozayeni and Lam 1998). Staphylococcal marginal keratitis begins with localized peripheral stromal infiltrates, which tend to occur along the oblique meridians (i.e. 2-, 4-, 8-, 10-o'clock positions). The infiltrates are typically separated from the limbus by a thin strip of clear cornea measuring 1–2 mm in width. They may be single or multiple and tend to spread, in parallel with the contour of the limbus. Topical corticosteroids in combination with an antibiotic are the mainstay in treatment of marginal keratitis. Warm compresses, eyelid hygiene and a topical antibiotic applied to the eyelid margin are helpful in the control of eyelid inflammation.

Phlyctenular keratitis is commonly reported as a disease of children and young adults. It is known as an inflammatory disorder, leading to corneal nodules, most commonly at the limbus (Figure 16.9). It is believed to be a form of T-cell–mediated (i.e. type IV) hypersensitivity caused by an antigen located in the microbe (Robin et al. 1998). Eyelid hygiene with a topical antibiotic or antibiotic–corticosteroid ointment is the management regimen. The association between phlyctenular disease and tuberculous and chlamydial infection has also been described.

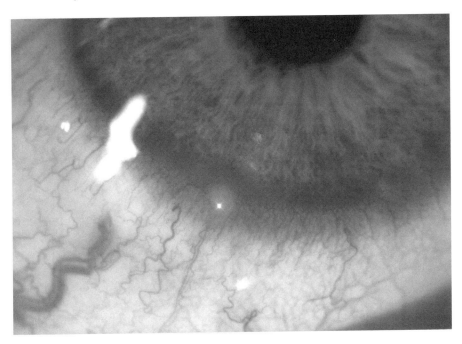

Figure 16.9 Phlycten. (See Plate 31.)

Corneal degenerations

Arcus senilis

Corneal arcus senilis is a degenerative change involving lipid deposition in the peripheral cornea. The lipid deposition starts clinically as a grey to yellow arc, first in the inferior cornea and then in the superior cornea. As the deposition progresses, the arcs meet, forming a complete ring. Corneal arcus has no visual significance and so no treatment is necessary. However, patients under the age of 40 with corneal arcus have an increased risk of coronary artery disease and should be evaluated for hyperlipidaemia.

Lipid keratopathy

Lipid keratopathy is a collection of yellow or cream-coloured lipids containing cholesterol, neutral fats and glycoproteins deposited in the superficial cornea, usually in areas of vascularized corneal scars.

Band keratopathy

Band keratopathy is a corneal disorder characterized by the deposition of calcium salts in both Bowman's layer and the subepithelium. Clinically, it usually begins at the corneal periphery in the 3- and 9-o'clock positions, and then a complete band from limbus to limbus may form in later stages. As the calcific deposition progresses it becomes white and chalky and can break through the epithelium, causing ocular irritation. Treatment includes chelation with application of EDTA (ethylenediaminetetra-acetic acid) and excimer laser phototherapeutic keratectomy (PTK) to clear the visual axis and improve the patient's vision. This may have to be repeated at intervals as the keratopathy returns. Patients need to be aware of this possibility so that they can re-present as required.

Corneal dystrophies

Corneal dystrophies can be present in any layer of the cornea. In general, corneal dystrophies are categorized into epithelial, Bowman's layer, stromal and endothelial. Diagnosis can be made with examination, clinical appearance and familial tendencies.

Anterior basement membrane dystrophy, also known as map–dot–fingerprint dystrophy, is the most common epithelial corneal dystrophy. It is a bilateral, autosomal dominant dystrophy. On examination with the slit-lamp, grey patches, microcysts and/or fine lines are seen in the central epithelial layer. It is an abnormality of epithelial basement membrane anchoring itself to Bowman's layer. As a result patients are prone to spontaneous recurrent corneal erosions.

The treatment is the same for recurrent corneal erosion, whether traumatic or dystrophic. First it consists of simple lubricating ointment at bedtime for at least 2 months. Failing this, a bandage contact lens may be used to help protect the corneal epithelium from the lids while healing; anterior stromal puncture may be instigated as a form of tacking down the abnormal area, and mechanical débridement of the loosened epithelium and excimer laser PTK may also be used to aid in the management of these patients. Corneal abrasion is painful – recurrent corneal abrasion is painful and often frequent, and patients are likely to need support in understanding the condition so that they are able to manage it effectively.

Reis–Bückler corneal dystrophy is an autosomal dominant hereditary disorder of Bowman's layer. The disorder presents during early childhood and affects both eyes equally. Clinical findings include opacification of the central cornea surface, which can have a honeycomb or a geographical configuration. In later stages of the disorder, scarring can occur which reduces the vision significantly; patients may have a predisposition to recurrent corneal erosions. Treatment options include excimer laser PTK or may require corneal transplantation to restore vision.

Granular dystrophy is a bilateral corneal disorder characterized by the deposition of small, discrete, sharply demarcated, greyish-white opacities in the anterior central stroma (Figure 16.10). It is transmitted as an autosomal dominant trait that appears in the first or second decade of life.

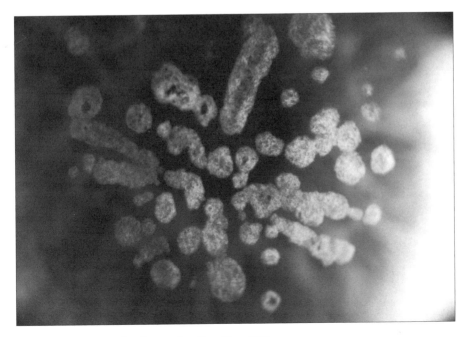

Figure 16.10 Granular dystrophy. (See Plate 32.)

Visual impairment is rare before the fifth decade and usually occurs secondary to the opacification of the intervening stroma. Most patients with granular dystrophy do not require treatment. If vision is markedly reduced, surgical intervention can be considered. Surgical management varies based on the depth and extent of the stromal lesions. The traditional surgical approach has been penetrating keratoplasty.

Macular corneal dystrophy is characterized by bilateral corneal opacities resulting from intracellular and extracellular deposits within the corneal stroma. It is inherited as an autosomal recessive trait. Vision is usually severely affected by the time patients reach their 20s or 30s. In the early stages of the disease, slit-lamp examination demonstrates a ground-glass-like haze in the central and superficial stroma. With progression of the dystrophy, small, multiple, white opacities with irregular borders are seen. These opacities are more superficial and prominent in the central cornea and are deeper and more discrete in the periphery. Penetrating keratoplasty is the surgical modality of choice.

Lattice dystrophy is a bilateral condition that commonly appears in the first decade of life. It is inherited as an autosomal dominant trait. Early features of lattice dystrophy include discrete ovoid or round subepithelial opacities, anterior stromal white dots and small refractile filamentary lines. With time, patients may also develop a diffuse central anterior stromal haze that reduces patients' visual acuity. With further progression, the

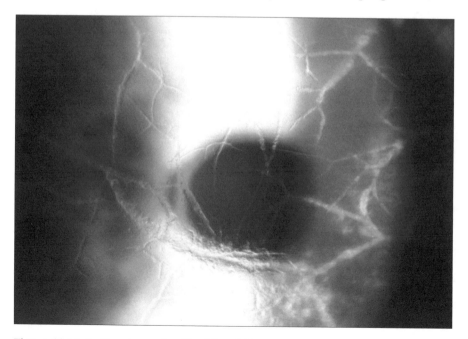

Figure 16.11 Lattice dystrophy. (See Plate 33.)

lesions can appear as thicker, radially oriented branching lines, giving a lattice appearance (Figure 16.11). Penetrating keratoplasty has a high rate of success in these patients.

Fuchs' endothelial dystrophy has an autosomal dominant inheritance pattern with a late onset and slow progression, rarely becoming symptomatic before the age of 50 years. It is a bilateral process but may be markedly asymmetrical. The initial manifestation of Fuchs' dystrophy is central corneal guttata. The guttata appear as dark spots on the posterior corneal surface by direct illumination. Pigment dusting is also commonly present on the endothelium. Specular microscopy may be helpful in diagnosing this condition (Figure 16.12). Patients in an early stage of disease are not symptomatic. Progressive stromal oedema results in a ground-glass opacification with marked thickening of the central cornea. Early medical management may include topical hypertonic saline drops, which may assist with reducing corneal oedema. Penetrating keratoplasty is the treatment of choice for patients with reduction in vision sufficient to impair their normal activities.

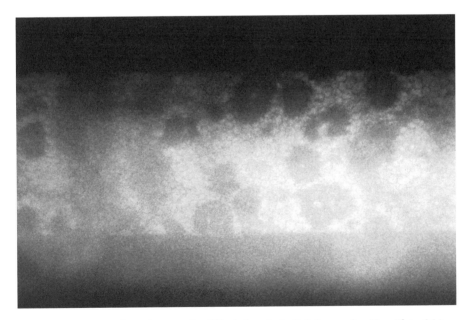

Figure 16.12 Specular micrograph of Fuchs' endothelial dystrophy. (See Plate 34.)

Corneal ectasia

The non-inflammatory ectatic diseases of the cornea discussed in this section are keratoconus, pellucid marginal degeneration and keratoglobus.

Keratoconus is the most common corneal ectasia. Corneal thinning is a hallmark of these ectatic diseases.

Keratoconus is a clinical term used to describe a condition in which the cornea assumes a conical shape because of thinning of the stroma and subsequent protrusion with irregular astigmatism. Keratoconus usually occurs bilaterally, but can be asymmetrical. The onset of keratoconus occurs at about the age of puberty and typically progresses in a variable fashion over a period of 10–20 years. Keratoconus is associated with systemic conditions such as Down's syndrome and atopy, but most cases of keratoconus are sporadic. The aetiological role of heredity in the development of keratoconus has not been clearly established and genetic studies are currently being conducted.

Clinically, patients have a progression of myopia with associated irregular astigmatism. The measurement of corneal topography is valuable in the diagnosis and monitoring of this condition (Figure 16.13). Munson's sign is visible, bulging of the lower lid when the patient looks down, and is indicative of keratoconus in the later stages (Figure 16.14). Slit-lamp signs include a deposition of iron in Bowman's layer around the base of the cone called Fleischer's ring. Also at the level of Bowman's layer, a series of fine, vertical, parallel 'stress' lines at the apex of the cone may be noted, called Vogt's striae. In very advanced cases of keratoconus a condition called corneal hydrops may occur. This is the result of a tear in Descemet's membrane, allowing fluid into the stroma creating an opaque cornea. Early management of keratoconus involves spectacles for the correction of myopia and astigmatism. Gas-permeable or semi-rigid contact lenses are used when spectacles become ineffective. Corneal transplantation is reserved until contact lens management is unsatisfactory.

Pellucid marginal degeneration is a bilateral, inferior, peripheral, corneal disorder characterized by a band of thinning extending from the 4- to the 8-o'clock position. The area of thinning is usually found 1–2 mm central to the inferior limbus. Patients with this condition usually come for treatment between the second and fifth decades of life, with complaints of blurred vision resulting from irregular astigmatism. The abnormal corneal contour induces a gross shift in the axis of astigmatism. Management is similar to keratoconus, with contact lenses or corneal surgery.

Keratoglobus is a rare, congenital, bilateral disorder characterized by the entire cornea protruding from generalized thinning, most marked in the periphery. The cornea tends to be of normal or slightly increased diameter. Management of keratoglobus follows the same principles as keratoconus, although as a result of the extreme shape and thinning of the cornea, this provides extreme challenges for both the contact lens fitter and surgeon.

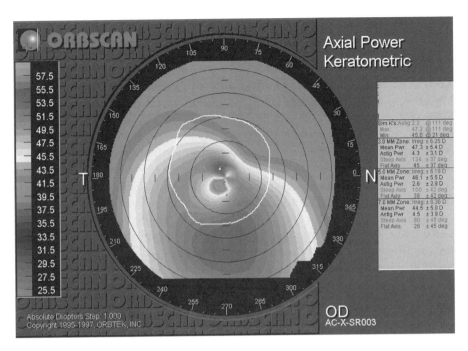

Figure 16.13 Orbscan of keratoconus. (See Plate 35.)

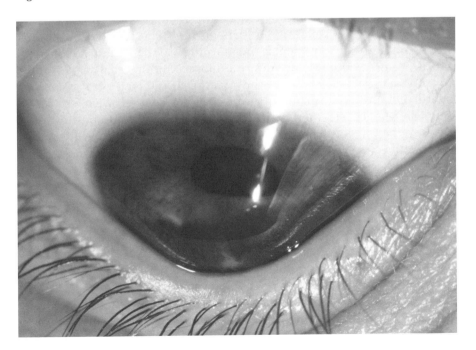

Figure 16.14 Munson's sign. (See Plate 36.)

Miscellaneous keratopathies

Recurrent corneal erosion

Recurrent corneal erosion is invariably caused when a sudden, sharp, abrading injury from a fingernail, vegetable matter or a paper cut causes a corneal abrasion. The injury heals clinically leaving no evidence of damage. Secondary breakdown can occur at any time after the injury when the basal cell of the epithelium loses its adhesion to the basement membrane, which detaches and becomes loose and unstable. Some other causes of recurrent corneal erosions are anterior corneal dystrophies, patients with diabetes, tear film abnormalities and after excimer laser PTK.

Classically, recurrent corneal erosion occurs at the time of awakening. During the night the pressure of the eyelid on the dry epithelium produces adhesion to the epithelium, which is stronger than the adhesion of the epithelium to the basement membrane. So, on awakening, opening of the eyelid separates away the epithelium. Each episode causes a variable amount of ocular pain, tearing and photophobia.

Treatment of corneal erosion is aimed at promoting epithelial regeneration and maintaining an intact ocular surface for a sufficient time to allow re-formation of the normal basement membrane complexes responsible for tight adhesion. Application of a lubricating ointment at night for at least 2 months may help to reduce the friction between the corneal epithelium and the eyelids. Often patients find that the single night that they do not instil the ointment is the morning where the recurrent erosion returns. Many people therefore use a lubricating ointment as a routine measure before bed to stop this painful condition from recurring. Débridement of abnormal epithelium may be required when it is loose. Bandage contact lens therapy is designed to relieve pain and to protect loosely adherent epithelium from the abrasive action of the eyelids so that epithelial healing can occur. Surgical treatment includes anterior stromal puncture, superficial keratectomy and excimer laser PTK. Good education helps patients to manage this condition effectively.

Bullous keratopathy

Bullous keratopathy occurs when the cornea decompensates as a result of a reducing number of endothelial cells. This can be the result of trauma, corneal endothelial dystrophy, or after cataract surgery and artificial lens implantation, known as pseudophakic bullous keratopathy. As the endothelial cells reduce, the cornea swells and affects the patient's vision. This swelling is also painful. Commonly, patients with bullous keratopathy experience vision symptoms that are worse in the morning but improve as the day progresses. This occurs because the excess fluid evaporates into the air along with the tears.

The main goals in the management of bullous keratopathy are to reduce swelling, provide comfort and restore useful vision. Saline eye drops can assist with reducing some corneal swelling. A contact lens may be used temporarily for comfort, but it will not improve vision. The mainstay treatment is corneal transplantation.

Wilson's disease

Wilson's disease is an autosomal recessive disorder characterized by the generalized accumulation of copper in the blood and urine. The Kayser–Fleischer ring is a valuable diagnostic sign. The ring is golden brown to blue–green, situated in Descemet's membrane with characteristic progression first superiorly and inferiorly, then extending the full circumference in the peripheral cornea. This can be best appreciated by standard slit-lamp biomicroscopy.

Vortex keratopathy

Certain systemic medication can cause corneal epithelial changes. Deposits are bilateral, golden or grey in colour, and appear in a whorl-like pattern (Figure 16.15). These changes, known as vortex keratopathy, seldom

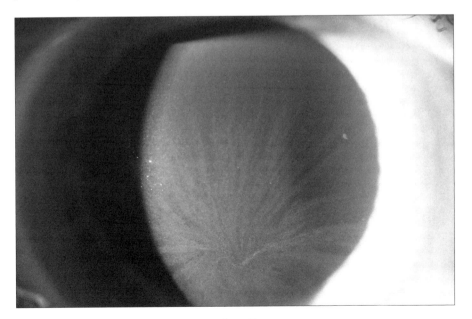

Figure 16.15 Vortex keratopathy. (See Plate 37.)

affect the patient's vision and enter the corneal epithelium via the peril-imbal vasculature. Amiodarone and chloroquine are examples of systemic medication causing vortex keratopathy.

Exposure keratopathy

Exposure keratopathy often results after a seventh nerve palsy or associ-ated with dysthyroid ophthalmopathy, leading to exposure of the inferior third of the cornea and localized drying. Small-to-moderate epithelial defects develop and increase the risk of corneal infection. Nocturnal lagophthalmos may also occur when the patient sleeps with the eyelids open resulting in corneal exposure.

Management for exposure keratopathy includes artificial tears and lubricating ointments, occlusive patches and shields, and lid taping as temporary solutions. Partial or complete tarsorrhaphies should be con-sidered if prolonged insult to the ocular surface is evident or anticipated.

Neurotrophic keratopathy

Neurotrophic keratopathy occurs in the absence of corneal sensitivity. The most common causes for corneal anaesthesia are after herpes simplex or herpes zoster corneal infections and damage to the trigeminal nerve through surgery or tumour. The trophic corneal defects can vary in sever-ity, ranging from punctate epithelial staining to larger recalcitrant epithelial defects characterized by heaped, rolled edges of grey epithelial cells. These epithelial defects increase the risk of corneal infection and potential stromal melting. Although not fully understood, it appears that corneal sensation is essential for maintaining healthy epithelial cells.

Management of neurotrophic keratopathy is directed towards preserv-ing corneal integrity with artificial tears, lubricating ointments, occlusive patches and lid taping as temporary solutions. Partial or complete lid tar-sorrhaphy is considered if prolonged insult to the ocular surface is evident.

Contact lens

Various contact lenses are available for patients including rigid gas-permeable (RGP), soft, extended wear and disposable contact lenses. Patients who wear contact lenses are routinely placing foreign bodies on their corneas and altering the normal anatomy and physiology. In most circumstances, any complications from contact lenses resolve with discon-tinuation. Two of the more common corneal complications from contact lenses are toxic and hypoxic changes. Fortunately microbial keratitis is not as common, but nevertheless potentially sight threatening.

Toxic

Chemicals used in disinfection systems, and to a lesser degree preservatives used in cleaning solutions, can produce subepithelial opacification similar to that seen in adenoviral keratoconjunctivitis. Inadvertent instillation of cleaning and disinfection solutions can damage the epithelium, producing diffuse epithelial staining. Typically, lenses are placed in the eye with cleaning or disinfecting solution still on the lens. This causes immediate pain, redness, tearing and photophobia. Diffuse punctate staining defects, conjunctival injection and irritative symptoms usually resolve with 1 or 2 days of lens removal. Subepithelial opacities are treated with topical corticosteroids or, commonly, left to resolve spontaneously.

Hypoxic

Contact lens wear decreases the oxygen reaching the cornea. The resulting hypoxia can have the acute effect of epithelial cell death or may cause chronic changes to the superficial cornea. If acute hypoxia compromises epithelial metabolism, the epithelium becomes oedematous (Figure 16.16) and eventually desquamates. In early stages, oedema causes blurred vision;

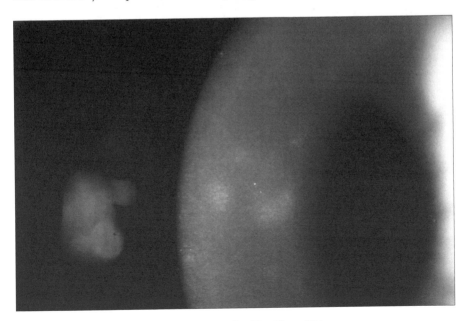

Figure 16.16 Contact lens-induced hypoxia. (See Plate 38.)

this is followed by pain, redness and photophobia. Subepithelial opacities are also seen in chronic corneal hypoxia that comprises clumps of polymorphonuclear leukocytes and mononuclear cells. Soft lenses in particular are prone to causing superficial, peripheral corneal neovascularization called pannus.

Corneal infection

Corneal infection is potentially the most devastating of the complications of contact lens wear. When clinical suspicion of corneal infection is high, the lesion should be scraped promptly for stains and cultures, and treatment should be initiated without delay. The mainstay of treatment is frequent dosage with topical broad-spectrum fortified antibiotics, modified by the results of the smears and cultures. Two potentially sight-threatening pathogens should be considered until proved otherwise by microbial culture. The first is *Pseudomonas aeruginosa* (Figure 16.17), an aggressive Gram-negative pathogen that has the potential to progress from a corneal ulcer to an abscess and corneal perforation within 48 hours if not treated properly. The second is acanthamoeba keratitis, caused by a ubiquitous protozoa *Acanthamoeba* sp. found in water, soil and air samples. The organism exists in two forms: a motile trophozoite and a double-walled

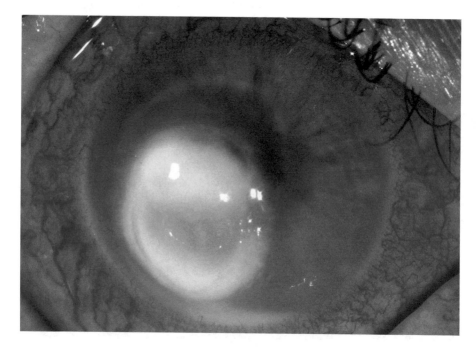

Figure 16.17 Bacterial keratitis caused by pseudomonas aeruginosa. (See Plate 39.)

cyst form, making eradication of this organism difficult. Acanthamoeba cysts are resistant to anti-amoebic eye drops such as Brolene (propamidine isethionate) and can lie dormant for months and possibly years. The clinician should have a high degree of suspicion for *Acanthamoeba* spp. in any contact lens wearer with a keratitis and should culture appropriately.

Counselling and fully educating patients who wear contact lenses is imperative. This includes personal hygiene, correct cleaning/disinfecting techniques and wearing specific lenses according to the product recommendations. Triaging skills may be utilized to give a high priority ophthalmology appointment to patients with contact lens complications.

Corneal surgery

Corneal transplantation has been around for many years with the first corneal transplant being performed in 1906 by Dr Eduard Zirm. Since then instrumentation and eye banking techniques have improved dramatically, along with the success of corneal transplantation. The principal indications in order of why corneal transplantation is performed are optical (to improve vision), therapeutic (to relieve pain), structural (in the management of corneal thinning or perforation) and cosmetic (to restore

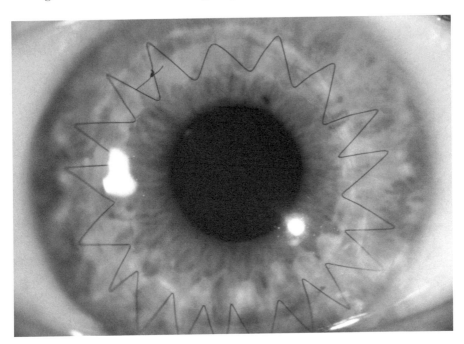

Figure 16.18 Penetrating keratoplasty.

a normal appearance) (Kanski 1999). Keratoconus is the most common reason for corneal transplantation, followed by bullous keratopathy and Fuchs' dystrophy (Coster 2002).

Penetrating keratoplasty is the most common from of corneal transplantation. This refers to the surgical replacement of a full-thickness 'button' of the host cornea with a donor cornea, then sutured in place (Figure 16.18). The prognosis of a successful penetrating keratoplasty reduces if there is corneal vascularization, glaucoma, active anterior uveitis and previous graft failures.

Postoperative care includes educating the patient to recognize any signs or symptoms of graft complications and the importance of seeking specialist medical assistance promptly. Long-term topical corticosteroids are maintained to assist in reducing any immune response.

Complications include a wound leak that may require re-suturing, loose or broken sutures requiring removal because they may precipitate a rejection episode (Figure 16.19), or glaucoma. Recurrence of original disease may also occur. Corneal graft rejection can occur at any stage after penetrating keratoplasty. It presents as an increase in ocular inflammation with increasing corneal oedema. Treatment of graft rejection comprises increasing the dosage of topical corticosteroids and then, as the process reverses, the frequency can be reduced. Primary graft failure can also occur when the

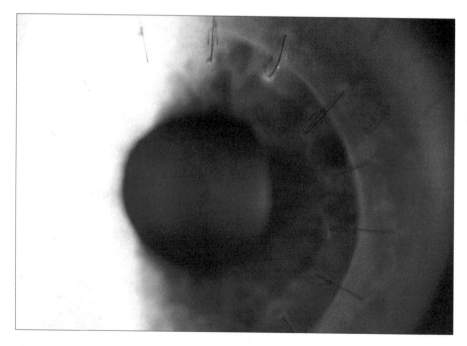

Figure 16.19 Loose corneal suture. (See Plate 40.)

endothelium of the graft is not functioning. The graft is replaced if it does not clear within the first 2 weeks after surgery. Postoperative graft astigmatism is the frequent complication after penetrating keratoplasty. Regular astigmatism < 5 D can be corrected with spectacles or contact lenses. Higher degrees of astigmatism cause severe image degradation and can be reduced with incisional surgery.

Lamellar keratoplasty is a corneal transplantation procedure of a partial-thickness donor tissue implanted onto a recipient's corneal bed with an intact Descemet's membrane. Two general indications for lamellar keratoplasty are optical and structural. Although the surgery is technically more difficult, it does propose some distinct advantages over penetrating keratoplasty. First, it is an extraocular procedure and so avoids the potential complication of endophthalmitis and, second, as the endothelium is not transplanted, graft rejection is significantly decreased.

Postoperative care includes protecting the eye from trauma and infection. Topical corticosteroids are tapered and ceased sooner than after penetrating keratoplasty.

Complications include opacification and vascularization of the interface occurring despite topical corticosteroid therapy. Epithelial, subepithelial and stromal rejection can occur occasionally, but respond well to topical corticosteroid therapy.

Although not all ophthalmologists perform corneal transplantation, nurses should be familiar with the different techniques and postoperative complications because patients do not always return to their corneal surgeons when problems arise and many of these problems require immediate intervention to save the graft. Nurses may also be called on to provide preoperative and postoperative counselling and education to patients.

Keratorefractive surgery

As the cornea is responsible for two-thirds of the refraction of light rays in the eye, a number of surgical procedures have been introduced to reduce or eliminate refractive errors by altering the shape of the cornea. The basis of keratorefractive procedures comprises flattening or shortening a myopic eye, steepening or lengthening a hypermetropic eye, and flattening or neutralizing the steep meridian of astigmatism. Different procedures are able to correct varying amounts of myopia, hypermetropia and astigmatism. In general, the further the amount of correction a patient requires away from the ideal range, the less likelihood there is of a highly accurate final refractive outcome. Incisional, photoablative and photothermal surgical procedures are briefly described in this section, and include a short discussion on wavefront technology and its role in photoablative surgery.

A comprehensive discussion of the procedures, the exact theory and bio-mechanics behind incisional and laser–tissue interactions is beyond the scope of this chapter.

Incisional

Radial keratotomy (RK) is a refractive procedure to reduce a small amount of myopia. Creation of radial incisions of about 90% thickness in the peripheral cornea with a specially designed diamond blade flattens the central cornea and reduces myopia (Figure 16.20). Advantages of RK compared with other refractive procedures include inexpensive instrumentation and a relatively quick recovery of vision with minimal discomfort. Disadvantages include permanent corneal weakening, fluctuating vision, glare and progressive hypermetropic shift. This procedure has largely been replaced by other methods to correct myopia.

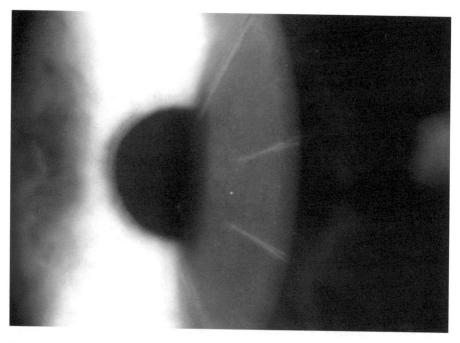

Figure 16.20 Radial keratotomy. (See Plate 41.)

Astigmatic keratotomy (AK) is a surgical procedure to correct astigma-tism. Corneal incisions of 85% depth are placed in the steep meridian of the astigmatism with the aim of flattening this meridian. Straight trans-verse or arcuate incisions can be used and are usually placed in the 7–8 mm diameter optical zone. This procedure has the same advantages as RK and is used during cataract surgery to reduce astigmatism and for post-cataract and corneal graft astigmatism.

Intrastromal corneal ring (ICR) is a procedure in which a polymethyl-methacrylate (PMMA) ring or ring segments are implanted into the peripheral corneal stroma to correct myopia. The ring or ring segments, available in different ring thickness relative to the amount of myopia correction, flatten the anterior corneal curvature with no removal of tissue from the central optical zone. The surgical technique involves making a small radial incision at the 6-mm diameter optical zone; a stromal dissector creates a channel for the rings to be inserted, and then an 11/0 nylon suture is required to close the incision which is removed when the wound is healed. A significant advantage of the ICR is that it is a reversible procedure.

Photoablative

The use of the excimer laser to remove cornea with microscopic precision has been a major advancement in the field of keratorefractive surgery. Photorefractive keratectomy (PRK) is a procedure where the epithelium is mechanically removed by the surgeon before the laser is applied to reshape the cornea. This procedure received good refractive outcomes in low-to-moderate myopic correction and is technically easy to perform; however, it has lost its appeal as a result of unpleasant side effects. Severe pain, light sensitivity and tearing for the first few days while the epithelium heals are unavoidable. Visually significant corneal haze as a result of the healing phase can occur in some patients causing reduced visual acuity. Recurrent corneal erosion is also common after PRK. Refractive stability can take up to 6 months and regression can occur particularly in higher myopic and hypermetropic patients.

Laser in situ keratomileusis (LASIK) has become more popular than PRK because of the rapid visual recovery and reduced postoperative pain. This procedure combines creating a lamellar flap, about 180 μm thick and 10 mm in diameter, with a specially designed microkeratome, lifting the flap, applying the laser and then replacing the flap. Complications include microkeratome malfunction and flap abnormalities such as thin or incomplete flaps and buttonholes. Epithelial ingrowth can occur when epithelial cells are lodged between the undersurface of the flap and stromal bed. These cells often regress with time or, if they involve the visual axis, can be mechanically removed by lifting the flap and debriding the cells. Diffuse lamellar keratitis (DLK) is a non-specific inflammatory response causing diffuse interface haze and reduced vision. This condition responds well to topical corticosteroids. Dry eyes occur as a result of reduced corneal sensation in the area of flap. This returns to normal between 6 and 12 months and regular artificial tears are required during this time. Keratectasia after LASIK has occurred when there is less than 250 μm of stroma remaining and the cornea becomes structurally unsound and bulges forward. Gas-permeable contact lenses or corneal transplantation may be required for treatment.

Laser subepithelial keratomileusis (LASEK) is a newer procedure and provides an alternative method of manually creating and removing the epithelial flap. This eliminates the microkeratome-related complications in LASIK. The epithelium is carefully trephined, devitalized with diluted alcohol and then gently peeled back. After the application of laser the epithelial flap is repositioned and a bandage contact lens applied until the epithelium is healed. The visual recovery is not as rapid as after LASIK and there is more patient discomfort, although not as severe as postoperative PRK. Corneal haze can also occur to a lesser degree than in PRK.

Treatment of certain corneal disorders with excimer laser has also been advocated in the procedure called PTK. By photoablating the corneal surface on corneal disorders such as recurrent corneal erosion, band keratopathy and anterior corneal dystrophies, visual function is improved by reducing or eliminating corneal opacities and smoothing the anterior corneal surface. It also delays the need for corneal transplantation. The surgical technique is the same as PRK.

Photothermal

Thermal keratoplasty (TK) uses heat to shrink corneal collagen, thus producing corneal steepening and the correction of mild hypermetropia. A non-contact holmium:YAG (yttrium–aluminium–garnet) laser is currently used for this procedure and eight laser treatment spots are applied to the cornea at a 6-mm optical zone and then an additional eight spots at the 7-mm optical zone. The major advantage is the ability to correct hypermetropia without operating over the central optical zone. Regression, however, remains a significant disadvantage. Conductive keratoplasty (CK), a similar procedure, uses radiofrequency waves instead of laser to induce collagen shrinkage and correction of hypermetropia.

Wavefront technology reveals higher-order aberrations or a distortion of a light ray in a patient's optical system not detected with corneal topography. It is being utilized together with LASIK for a procedure called 'customized' ablation. With the production of advanced eye tracking devices, a small spot scanning laser in combination with wavefront analysis, the potential for treating all corneal aberrations at the time of surgery and achieving the best possible visual outcome for the patient seem theoretically possible. However, application of this theory to clinical practice is proving to be more challenging than at first thought and further work is required to study these possibilities.

Ophthalmic nurses are being exposed to patients who have had keratorefractive procedures or are being asked about the procedures and whether they are suitable candidates for a procedure. Nurses may also be called on to provide preoperative and postoperative counselling and education to patients. Changes in the cornea caused by photorefractive techniques, in particular, can lead to misleading biometry before cataract surgery, with the consequent problems caused by the implantation of an inappropriate lens. Patients undergoing such procedures should know that this can be a problem and have a full set of keratometry readings taken before surgery, which should be recorded in the notes and given to them to keep safely in case they need cataract surgery in the future.

Acknowledgement

Clinical photographs were supplied by Angela Chappell, Ophthalmic Imaging Department, Flinders Medical Centre, Adelaide, South Australia.

References

Boulton M, Albon J (2004) Stem cells in the eye. Int J Biochem Cell Biol 36: 643–57.

Coster D (2002) Fundamentals of Clinical Ophthalmology. Cornea. London: BMJ Publishing Group.

Foulks G (2003) Challenges and pitfalls in clinical trials of treatments for dry eye. Ocular Surface 1: 20–30.

Kanski J (1999) Clinical Ophthalmology, 4th edn. Oxford: Butterworth-Heinemann.

Mozayeni R, Lam S (1998) Phlyctenular keratoconjunctivitis and marginal staphylococcal keratitis. In: Krachmer J, Mannis M, Holland E, Palay D (eds), Cornea Text and Color Atlas. CD-ROM. Mosby CD online. Chapter 109.

Robin J, Dugel R, Robin S (1998) Immunologic disorders of the cornea and conjunctiva. In Kaufman H, Barron B, McDonald M (eds), The Cornea, 2nd edn. Boston, MA: Butterworth-Heinemann, Chapter 23.

CHAPTER SEVENTEEN

The sclera

AGNES LEE

Anatomy and physiology of the sclera

The sclera is a white tough fibrous tissue that covers five-sixths of the eyeball and provides structural integrity to the globe. It is the eye's protective coat and it is thickest posteriorly (1 mm) and thinner (0.6 mm) near the junction with the cornea and where the rectus muscles are inserted (0.3 mm). The outer surface of the sclera is normally smooth except at the muscle insertions.

The colour of the sclera varies from white with a bluish tinge in children, because the sclera is normally thinner and the pigment cells of the choroid show through, to white with a yellowish tinge in elderly people as result of deposition of fat. The sclera is for the most part avascular much like the cornea, but, unlike the cornea, the sclera is opaque preventing light from entering the eye other than through the cornea.

Above the sclera is the episclera, which is of similar composition to the sclera but contains blood vessels. It is the episclera that in part provides some of the nutritional requirements of the sclera. The functions of the sclera are:

- to provide a rigid insertion for the extraocular muscles
- to protect the inner structures of the eye
- to maintain the shape of the eyeball and maintain the exact position of the different parts of the optic system (Snell and Lemp 1998)
- To prevent the entry of light.

The sclera is subdivided into three layers:

1. Episclera
2. Scleral stroma
3. Lamina fusca.

Episclera

This external layer is made out of loose connective tissue that is connected to the fascial sheath of the eyeball (Tenon's capsule) by fine strands of tissues. The episclera has a rich blood supply from the anterior ciliary arteries. The anterior ciliary arteries normally lie quite deep in the conjunctiva and are conspicuous only in the presence of inflammation.

Scleral stroma

This layer consists of dense fibrous tissue that is intermingled with fine elastic fibres. The fibres run in concentric rings around the limbus and around the opening of the optic nerve whereas elsewhere the fibres run in interlacing loops. The irregular arrangement of collagen fibrils, forming a mat-like structure, is responsible for the opaqueness of the sclera, in contrast to the cornea where the fibrils run parallel with the surface, resulting in transparency. The sclera is elastic and responds to deforming forces by lengthening (elastic response) and then stretching (viscid response) (Snell and Lemp 1998).

Lamina fusca

This is the inner aspect of the sclera located adjacent to the choroid, separated from it by the perichoroidal space; it contains star-shaped pigment cells and thinner collagen fibres. The collagen fibres provide a weak attachment between the sclera and choroid. The lamina fusca also contains many grooves caused by the passage of blood vessels and nerves.

The limbus

This is the name given to an area about 1 mm wide at the periphery of the cornea. It marks the junction between the cornea epithelium and the conjunctiva (conjunctival limbus) on one surface and the corneal and sclera on the other (corneal junction).

Just posterior to the limbus is a circular canal (canal of Schlemm), lying within and therefore forming a groove in the sclera. Posterior to the canal is a ridge of tissue, the scleral spur, which forms the attachment for the ciliary muscle.

Tenon's capsule (fascia bulbi)

This is made out of fibrous membrane consisting of compact collagen fibres and forms the fascial sheath of the globe. It envelops the globe and separates it from the orbital fat forming a socket. Its inner surface is smooth and separated from the outer surface of the sclera by an episcleral space. Attaching it to the sclera are bands of connective tissue. The tendons of the extraocular muscles pierce Tenon's capsule which forms a tubular sleeve over each tendon. Tenon's capsule is attached to the sclera 1.5 mm posterior to the corneoscleral junction. Posteriorly, it fuses with the meninges around the optic nerve. It is pierced by the ciliary nerves and vessels, and the vortex veins. The globe and its fascial sheath move together on orbital fat.

Scleral apertures

The optic nerve exits the globe medial to the posterior pole. This perforation of the sclera is called the posterior scleral foramen (Snell and Lemp 1998) and the sclera is fused here with the dura and arachnoid coverings of the optic nerve. Where the sclera is pierced by the optic nerve, it has a sieve-like appearance (lamina cribrosa) and is a weakened area. (If it bulges outwards as a result of raised intraocular pressure, it produces a cupped disc.)

- Four vortex veins – one in each quadrant – pierce the sclera posterior to the equator of the eye.
- Smaller perforations result from the anterior ciliary arteries and veins as well as aqueous veins from the Schlemm's canal.
- The long and short ciliary nerves also perforate the sclera.
- Anteriorly, there is a large aperture in the sclera where the cornea is located.

Scleral blood supply

The sclera is a relatively avascular structure. The posterior part of the sclera is supplied by the long and short posterior ciliary arteries. The episclera has a rich blood supply arising from the episcleral plexus.

Nerve supply

The nerve supply is via the short ciliary nerves, which supply the posterior portion of the sclera, and the ciliary nerve, which pierces the sclera around the optic nerve. The anterior portion of the sclera is supplied by the two long ciliary nerves.

Abnormal physiology seen in inflammatory disorders of the sclera

Ciliary flush

The episcleral plexus, which is formed by branches of the anterior ciliary arteries, exists beneath the conjunctiva. In cases of inflammation involving the cornea, iris or ciliary body, marked vasodilatation may occur especially in the limbal area surrounding the cornea (Snell and Lemp 1998).

Localized/sectoral hyperaemia

Scleral vessels are significantly dilated as are the overlying vessels of the episcleral and bulbar conjunctiva, as seen in cases of episcleritis and scleritis.

Dull aching pain

Dull aching pain in cases of scleritis is a result of profuse nerve innervation. In addition, the pain is made worse on extraocular movement as a result of muscle insertion in the sclera.

Diseases of the sclera

Episcleritis

Episcleritis (Figure 17.1) is a self-limiting inflammatory condition of the episcleral connective tissue, which lies between the conjunctiva and sclera.

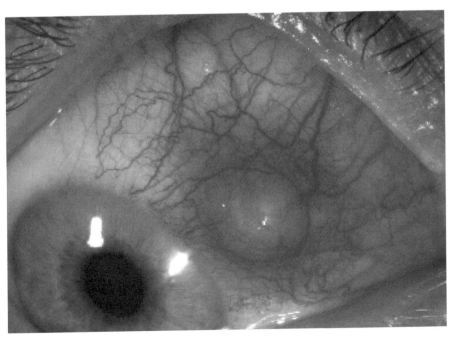

Figure 17.1 Episcleritis. (By courtesy of Angela Chappell, Ophthalmic Imaging Department, Flinders Medical Centre, Adelaide, South Australia.) (See Plate 42.)

Episcleritis presents as a relatively asymptomatic acute onset of a sectoral red eye. On examination, there is sectoral injection of the episcleral and overlying conjunctival vessels. The eye's red appearance is often mistaken for conjunctivitis but there is no discharge, foreign body section or the presence of any follicles. It typically looks worse than it is.

Pathophysiology

The pathophysiology is not clearly understood but this benign inflammatory condition is commonly seen in young adults. It is usually a mild, self-limiting, recurrent disease. The inflammatory response is localized to the superficial episcleral vascular network (Hampton 2001). Women are more affected than men and in most cases the disorder is idiopathic although one-third have an underlying systemic condition such as rheumatoid arthritis, gout, systemic lupus erythematosus (SLE), inflammatory bowel disease, sarcoidosis, herpes zoster virus (HZV) or herpes.

Two different clinical types may be found (Ragge and Easty 1990):

1. Simple: the congestion is diffuse.
2. Nodular: there is localized hyperaemia and swelling which is mobile over the surface of the globe.

Simple episcleritis can recur at 1- to 3-monthly intervals and usually lasts 7–10 days; most resolve after 2–3 weeks, although prolonged episodes may be more common in patients with associated systemic conditions (Hampton 2001). Some patients may have an attack of episcleritis during spring or autumn. Stress and hormonal changes have also been implicated.

Patients with nodular episcleritis have prolonged attacks of inflammation that are painful. The cornea is unaffected although long-standing or recurrent episcleritis may lead to dellen formation. The anterior chamber is deep and quiet.

Signs and symptoms

- Localized sectoral injection of episcleral vessels with perhaps some overlying conjunctival injection
- Mild-to-moderate discomfort or tenderness
- Nodules in nodular episcleritis
- In cases where the diagnosis is difficult, blanching the conjunctiva and episclera vessels with phenylephrine 2.5% will allow for better evaluation of the underlying sclera
- History of systemic disease listed above
- Vision is not usually affected.

Management

All patients should have a thorough history taken. Most cases are self-limiting, with little or no permanent damage to the eye even without treatment. Therefore, many of these patients will not require any treatment. The use of artificial tears can be beneficial in cases of discomfort. Non-steroidal drugs such as diclofenac (Voltarol) can be prescribed for persistent discomfort. If patients present with more than three episodes of episcleritis, a referral to a medical physician is recommended. Steroid drops are still the treatment of choice for some clinicians.

Scleritis

This is more serious than episcleritis and patients presenting with scleritis complain of severe ocular pain that can involve the adjacent head and facial regions (Figure 17.2). The scleral vessels are involved with vessel dilatation, including the overlying vessels of the episcleral and bulbar conjunctiva. The inflammation has a slightly bluish hue as a result of deeper vessel involvement.

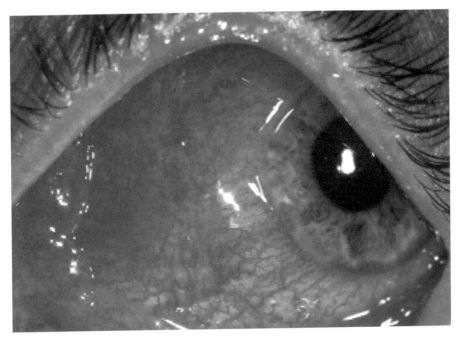

Figure 17.2 Scleritis. (By courtesy of Angela Chappell, Ophthalmic Imaging Department, Flinders Medical Centre, Adelaide, South Australia.) (See Plate 43.)

Pathophysiology

Over 50% of the scleritis has an underlying systemic cause. The common related disorders are ankylosing spondylitis, rheumatoid arthritis, systemic lupus erythematosus (SLE), Wegener's granulomatosis, polyarteritis, gout, syphilis and herpes zoster virus (HZV). Scleritis may follow ocular surgery, typically presenting within 6 months postoperatively, with necrosis adjacent to the site of surgery. The cause is unknown. Scleritis may also be caused by infective spread from a corneal ulcer or from trauma (Kanski 2003).

Left untreated, scleritis has the potential to spread to the anterior and posterior segment of the eye, causing proptosis, cataract, secondary glaucoma, cystoid macular oedema, choroidal effusion, exudative retinal detachment and optic atrophy. It is therefore imperative to distinguish this disorder from episcleritis and that treatment be started as early as possible after diagnosis.

Signs and symptoms

- Gradual onset of redness and pain
- Vision may be decreased
- Photophobia
- Scleral nodules
- Peripheral keratitis
- Secondary uveitis
- In cases of necrotizing scleritis, the sclera takes on a bluish hue where the sclera has become thinned, revealing the underlying choroids; in necrotizing scleritis, an ischaemic area is visible; where there is no evidence of inflammation the condition is known as scleromalacia perforans.

It is important always to consider the underlying cause to be systemic unless proved otherwise. Patients should always be referred for a comprehensive medical examination and investigations such as full blood count (FBC), erythrocyte sedimentation rate (ESR), antinuclear antibody (ANA), HLA-B27, rheumatoid factor, angiotensin-converting enzyme (ACE), Lyme titre and chest radiograph are performed.

Generally, topical steroids alone are insufficient to treat scleritis. Systemic treatment such as an oral non-steroidal anti-inflammatory drug, e.g. ibuprofen 600 mg four times a day or indometacin 25 mg, has a proven effect. However, if the inflammation is severe or necrotizing, a systemic steroid such as oral prednisolone may be prescribed. In rare cases, the patient may require immunosuppressive agents and should be managed by a rheumatologist. The treatment of scleritis can be complex and so the disease process must be clearly documented at each stage.

Anterior necrotizing scleritis with inflammation

This is the most severe form of scleritis and is bilateral, although not necessarily simultaneous in 60% of cases. The mortality rate is 25% within 5 years of the onset of scleritis as a result of systemic vascular disease (Kanski 2003). Perforation may occur and inflammation may spread to the uveal tract. This is an intensely painful and distressing condition and patients will need a lot of support, in terms of both their eye condition and the systemic problems associated with severe vascular disease. Treatment includes oral or intravenous prednisolone along with immunosuppressive agents such as cyclophosphamide or ciclosporin.

References

Hampton R (2001) Episcleritis. J Emerg Med 2(7).
Kanski JJ (2003) Clinical Ophthalmology, 5th edn. London: Butterworth-Heinemann.
Ragge NK, Easty DL (1990) Immediate Eye Care. New York: Wolfe Publishing Ltd.
Snell R, Lemp M (1998) Clinical Anatomy of the Eye, 2nd edn. Oxford: Blackwell Scientific Publications.

CHAPTER EIGHTEEN

The lens

LES MCQUEEN

Anatomy

The lens (Figure 18.1) is a fairly small anatomical structure within the eye measuring (in adults) about 9–10 mm in diameter and 4.75–5 mm at its thickest point between the anterior and posterior poles. It is a clear biconvex avascular structure, which lies immediately behind the iris and pupil.

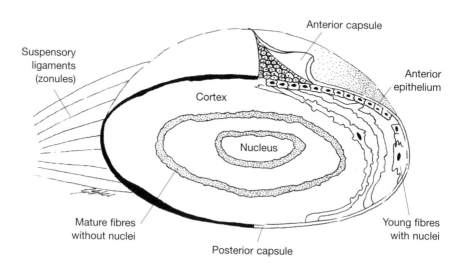

Figure 18.1 Section through the lens.

The lens also lies in front of the anterior vitreous face and is supported in place by the suspensory ligaments (zonules), which arise from the ciliary processes and attach themselves to the lens capsule. Although small in size it has amazing refractive powers and its function is to help focus light rays on to the retina during accommodation.

Structure and physiology of the lens

The lens capsule

The capsule is a semipermeable elastic basement membrane, which surrounds the cortex and the nucleus of the lens. It is composed of a number of lamellae (fibrils) stacked on top of each other. The capsule varies in thickness from 4 μm (at the posterior pole) to 23 μm close to the equator on both anterior and posterior surfaces. The lens capsule is an elastic membrane by nature, which facilitates changes in the shape of the lens during the process of accommodation. The capsule is highly resistant to chemical and toxic influences, but it does, however, allow water and electrolytes from the aqueous fluid to pass through it.

The lens substance (cortex and nucleus)

The lens substance is composed of a single layer of cuboidal epithelial cells (lying immediately beneath the anterior capsule) and of soft, densely packed, lens fibre cells. Within the substance of the lens there is very little extracellular space. The cells within the lens are nourished by the diffusion of proteins, minerals and enzymes, passing into and out of the aqueous fluid through the lens capsule.

Together with the unique structure of the lens cells, it is the selective permeability of the capsule that maintains the transparency of the lens. The cortex of the lens accounts for about 16% of the lens substance and is histologically indistinct from the nucleus of the lens which accounts for the remaining 84% of the lens substance. The thickness of the cortex gradually increases throughout life, whereas the thickness of the lens nucleus decreases with age.

Functions of the lens (refraction and accommodation)

Refraction may be defined as the change in direction of light when it passes from one transparent medium into another of a different optical density: the denser the medium the slower the light is able to pass through it (see Chapter 2).

A crude example of this process may be seen if a 30-cm (12-inch) ruler is submerged half-way into a basin of water. As the ruler moves from air into water it appears to bend slightly in the middle at the point where it passes into the water.

The transparent media of the eye, namely the cornea, aqueous, lens and vitreous, refract light rays travelling through to the retina. Each of these media has a different optical density and assists in the refraction of light rays on to the retina. The lens, however, is the main refractive structure within the eye possessing about 19 D of refractive power.

If the refractive power of a normal (emmetropic) eye were fixed and unable to be changed, only objects at infinity (in reality, more than 6 m away) would be clearly seen. To focus the light rays from objects nearer than infinity on to the retina, the lens must be able to increase its refractive power by changing its shape. This process is known as accommodation and is enabled by contraction of the ciliary muscle, which in turn releases the tension on the suspensory ligaments, allowing the lens to become more spherical in shape.

In addition to the lens becoming more spherical in shape, the pupils also constrict slightly when looking at near objects, and in order to maintain binocular single vision the eyes converge. When looking at distant objects the eyes come back to the midline, the pupils enlarge slightly and the lens becomes more elliptical in shape.

This whole process of focused vision is dependent on each component mentioned above happening, but primarily in relation to this chapter it is reliant on:
- the clarity of the lens
- the elasticity of the lens capsule and zonules
- the selective permeability of the lens capsule
- the ability of the lens to change its shape during accommodation.

Developmental abnormalities of the lens

Congenital aphakia

This is total absence of the lens, and is an extremely rare condition associated with severe abnormal fetal ocular development.

Spherophakia and microphakia

In these conditions the lens is smaller and more spherical in shape and the zonular fibres fail to exert traction on the lens capsule. This is associated with connective tissue disorders such as Marfan's syndrome, where the defects or weaknesses in the zonular fibres result in dislocation of the lens.

Lenticonus

This is a developmental abnormality of the lens, characterized by a localized cone-shaped protrusion of the axial portions of the anterior and posterior lens surfaces. It is usually associated with a high degree of axial lens-induced myopia.

Degenerative changes in the lens (cataract formation)

The lens is normally a transparent colourless structure, but if it loses its transparency cataract results and, although this may be for many reasons, age is by far the most common with 95% of people aged over 65 years having some degree of lens opacity (Gregory and Talamo 1996). Reidy et al. (1998) found cataract in 30% of people aged over 65 in a UK-based study. Cataract is responsible for 17 million cases of treatable blindness in the world – the major cause of treatable blindness (Gregory and Talamo 1996). Cataracts are usually present in both eyes, but are often more evident in one eye than the other.

As part of the normal ageing process the lens loses its transparency. It increasingly absorbs more ultraviolet (UV) and visible light and changes in colour from pale yellow through an amber discoloration to brown. This progressive discoloration is thought to arise from degenerative changes in the lens proteins, and from abnormal protein metabolism within the nucleus of the lens.

Cataracts are slow in their progression, and as such are more commonly seen in elderly people or in the later years of life. However, cataracts may also be classified as:

- congenital
- traumatic (blunt or penetrating injuries)
- secondary as a result of pre-existing ocular conditions, e.g. glaucoma, choroiditis and uveitis
- secondary as a result of pre-existing systemic diseases, e.g. diabetes and severe eczema, and metabolic disorders such as galactosaemia
- toxic as a result of radiation or the side effects of certain medications, the most common being the prolonged use of oral steroids.

As the cataract develops the lens loses its ability to accommodate for near vision (presbyopia). The lens also thickens and, as it does, it leads to increasing short-sightedness (index myopia). Any opacification of the lens, with or without presbyopia or index myopia will influence the passage of light through it to the retina, and will therefore affect the vision in some way.

Rapidly developing cataracts, and in particular the sudden onset of a mature uniocular cataract, should be treated with suspicion because this may indicate the presence of ocular malignancy or underlying retinal detachment. In general, however, the following are common symptoms that patients complain about in relation to the development of cataract:

- An overall gradual reduction in vision.
- Glare while driving at night or in bright light/sunlight, and difficulty seeing objects outdoors in bright sunlight, known as reduced contrast sensitivity (mainly associated with posterior subcapsular lens opacities).
- Difficulties in reading small print.
- A difficulty in seeing distant objects or, for example, people's faces on the other side of the street or bus numbers.
- Colour shift: there is poor appreciation of colours; as the cataract develops the lens becomes more absorbent at the blue end of the spectrum (mainly associated with nuclear sclerotic cataract).
- Monocular diplopia (particularly associated with cortical spoke opacities).
- Visual field loss, depending on the position and density of the lens opacity.
- Probably most commonly not being able to find a pair of spectacles that enables the patient to see as well as he or she would like to.

In assessing the effects of cataracts, it is important not only to look at the level of visual impairment caused, but also more importantly to look at the impact the visual impairment has on the patient's lifestyle.

Examination in relation to cataract assessment

The presence of cataract is one of the most common reasons that patients are referred to the eye department by their GP. Often, patients have also attended their optician for a routine eye test, and as part of the ocular examination their optician has noted the presence of lens opacities.

Most optometry referrals give a really detailed account of the ocular examination, and identify other ocular pathologies that may be pre-existing. Some optometry referrals may also relate their findings to the impact that any visual impairment has on the patient's lifestyle.

Once referred, patients may be screened through the traditional, medically led outpatient clinic, and then perhaps referred on to some form of preoperative assessment clinic before surgery. However, patients may also be screened via nurse-led cataract services in which the ocular examination as well as the more psychosocial aspects of assessment are undertaken by nurse practitioners.

Recent developments, cataract re-design projects and the introduction of one-stop services, have led to nursing roles featuring much more in the overall assessment – the decision to proceed and preparation of patients for cataract surgery.

Before examining the lens and other related ocular structures, it is essential to have knowledge of any other long-standing pre-existing or underlying ocular pathologies, which may influence decision-making in the management of the cataract.

Optometry referrals for assessment of cataract usually identify any pre-existing ocular pathology, e.g. amblyopia (lazy eye), strabismus (squint), any retinal disorders, e.g. age-related macular degeneration (ARMD), and any abnormalities of the optic nerve, intraocular pressures and visual fields. However, in addition to this information, it is essential that the immediate preoperative assessment of a patient's suitability for cataract surgery excludes the presence of other ocular conditions that would compromise surgical intervention.

Specifically, in relation to the lens itself, slit-lamp examination is essential to identify any other pre-existing ocular pathologies.

Examination of the lens and cataract

For general examination purposes, the lens may be subdivided into three key areas: the capsule (anterior and posterior), the cortex and the nucleus (Figure 18.2). Using the slit-lamp it is possible to examine in fine detail

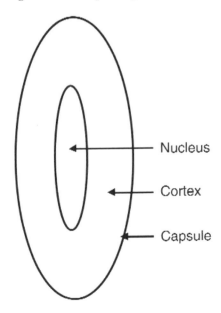

— Nucleus

— Cortex

— Capsule

Figure 18.2 Simplified diagram of a section through the lens.

each of these structures, and to observe the amount and position of any lens opacification.

In addition to noting the position of the lens itself, it is advisable to examine the lens in a systematic fashion, starting with the anterior lens capsule and working through the cortex and nucleus to the posterior capsular surface.

Anterior lens capsule

Tiny pigmented adhesions, small fragments of iris tissue visible on the anterior capsular surface or the presence of posterior synechiae (iris adhesions to the anterior lens capsule) often indicate previous or pre-existing inflammatory disease such as iritis.

The more serious pseudoexfoliation syndrome is also recognized by the white/grey flake-like deposits adherent to the anterior capsular surface. In addition to the flake-like deposits around the pupillary margin of the iris, a characteristic circular pattern of flake-like deposits can be seen, corresponding to the position of the iris pupillary margin as it moves across the anterior capsular surface. The flakes may also deposit on the trabecular meshwork and cause glaucoma. Cataract extraction in this case may be associated with any complications such as severe inflammation (Newell 1996).

Slit-lamp examination gives the most detailed exploration of the lens, but direct ophthalmoscopy is also useful in determining whether the opacification is affecting the visual axis. By shining the ophthalmoscope light through the pupil to obtain a red reflex, opacities can be seen as shadows, and their position can be determined in relation to the visual axis, enabling a judgement to be made of their impact on visual acuity.

As well as classifications of cataract, there are many different types – blue dot, Christmas tree, lamellar (found in children), snowflake, cuneiform and stellate to name but a few. Although cataracts may develop in many forms the three most common types are (1) cortical, (2) nuclear sclerotic and (3) posterior subcapsular.

Cortical cataract

Cortical cataracts are opacities confined to the lens cortex. They are commonly white in colour and may be present in either the anterior or the posterior lens cortex. It is not specifically the amount of cortical opacification that causes visual disturbance, but more importantly the position of the cortical cataract that will determine the effect on the patient's vision, e.g. an abundance of radial (spoke-like) cortical opacities may cause little in the way of visual disturbance, whereas small central cortical opacities obstructing the visual axis may cause significant visual problems.

As cortical cataracts develop the whole of the lens cortex ultimately becomes white (known as a mature cataract) which can totally obstruct the passage of light through to the retina. Mature cataracts need to be removed, because, if left they may progress to become hypermature and cause severe intraocular inflammatory changes as a result of lens proteins escaping through the lens capsule. The intraocular pressure may rise rapidly if this happens.

Nuclear sclerotic cataract (senile cataract)

Nuclear cataracts (Figure 18.3) develop very slowly over a period of years and often the patient is unaware that they have visual difficulties until the cataract is quite advanced. Indeed, many older people simply associate reduced vision with being a natural part of the ageing process. Visual disturbance is very gradual and is more often than not associated with reduced distance visual acuity and diminished colour perception.

The lens nucleus moves from being colourless and transparent to pale yellow through to a darker amber or brown discoloration. This discoloration is confined to the lens nucleus and can be seen on slit-lamp examination by directing the light beam obliquely through the lens.

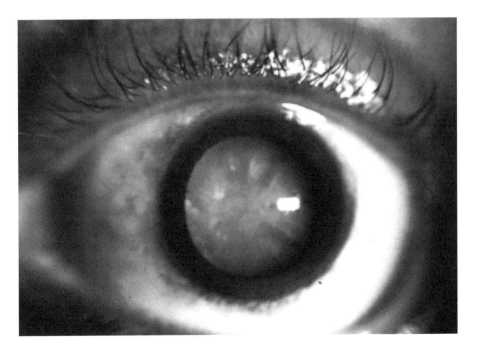

Figure 18.3 Cataract. (See Plate 44.)

Posterior subcapsular cataract

As its name suggests this type of cataract is caused by opacification of the inner surface of the posterior lens capsule. It tends to progress fairly quickly over a period of months, and it is predominantly associated with glare in addition to reducing the visual acuity.

On slit-lamp examination it can be seen as a fine white mesh (almost spider web like) spreading across the inner surface of the posterior lens capsule; as it develops it can sometimes spread to involve the inner surface of the anterior lens capsule.

As with cortical cataracts it is not just the amount of opacification that causes visual problems; small central areas of opacification along the visual axis (known as axial plaques) can cause significant visual impairment.

The management of cataract

As the cataract develops it may be possible for the patient's optometrist to manage any early index myopia with changes in the spectacle prescription. In assessing a patient's need for surgery a common misconception held by most patients is that, if they have cataracts, they must be removed.

With the exception of mature or hypermature cataracts, and cataracts that prevent a clear examination of the fundus in the management of retinal disorders and diabetes mellitus, this is not the case. The level of vision in relation to the patient's lifestyle and functional capabilities is really the only determining factor that indicates whether or not surgery is necessary.

Even patients with a lot of cataract may be managing well enough to be independent and are happy with the vision that they have (albeit reduced). It may not be appropriate for them to progress to surgery with its inherent risks. If people with cataracts decide to proceed to surgery, a number of investigations must be undertaken to obtain the best possible outcome for vision, as part of a preoperative assessment.

Preoperative assessment

A comprehensive preoperative assessment is required and this may take place on the same day as an ophthalmologist consultation, thus saving a patient visit to the hospital (Prasad et al. 1998, Rose et al. 1999, NHS Executive 2000). This usually consists of:

• a medical evaluation, including recording details of current medication and history of allergies
• biometry

• the identification of social problems, which may require support so that services may be arranged and surgery is not delayed.

In addition to this information it is essential, in order that it can be dealt with before surgery, that the immediate preoperative assessment of a patient's suitability for cataract surgery excludes the presence of:

• conjunctivitis
• infective corneal ulceration
• episcleritis/scleritis (inflammation of the episcleral or scleral blood vessels)
• blepharitis (chronic inflammatory lid disease ± lid infection)
• infective lid lesions, e.g. chalazion (meibomian cyst)
• entropion/ectropion (outward or inward turning of the lids)
• trichiasis (ingrowing lashes)
• excessive lacrimation of unknown cause.

A large part of the preoperative assessment visit is concerned with information and education so that patients have all the knowledge that they need to consent to surgery.

Biometry (IOL calculation)

Preoperatively it is essential to estimate the power of the lens implant to be used during surgery, in order to achieve either normal vision (emmetropia) or the desired refractive error postoperatively. This involves a series of measurements of the eye, including assessment of the corneal curvature and the axial length of the globe so that calculations can be made of the intraocular lens (IOL) power needed at surgery.

The desired refractive error postoperatively relates to the surgeon implanting an IOL that will give the patient the best usable visual acuity depending on his or her previous refracted visual acuity. The most common example of this would be to keep a very short-sighted person (a high myope) slightly short-sighted (myopic) after surgery because he or she would tolerate this better having been myopic all his or her life. Discussions about lifestyle may also influence the decision, e.g. if the patient spends a great deal of time reading or undertaking close work, particularly if not mobile, IOL power may be calculated to enable good near vision without spectacles.

The calculation of the power of the IOL implant used during cataract surgery is therefore probably the most critical component of the preoperative assessment process. Although the technicalities of the biometry equipment used in the calculation of IOL power may differ between ophthalmic units, the principles of measurement are essentially the same.

There are various mathematical formulae used in the calculation of IOL powers, a common example being the SRK 11, developed in 1988 by Sanders et al. In general, however, most biometry machines come supplied with a range of pre-programmed IOL formulae already installed. These can usually be adapted or indeed additional formulae installed depending on the surgeon's preferences.

Each IOL also carries what is known as an 'A' constant value that relates to the position of the IOL as it sits within the eye. The 'A' constant value is also pre-programmed into the biometry machine because this value is needed in the IOL power calculations. In addition to the formulae and the 'A' constant values there are two further sets of measurements needed in the calculation of IOL power, namely:

1. Keratometry (measurements of corneal curvature)
2. Measurement of the axial length of the eye.

Keratometry

This involves measuring the curvatures of the cornea, known as taking K readings. Nowadays automated keratometers make this task simple. Other manual forms of keratometer such as the Schiötz keratometer, need some degree of training and expertise in their use if you are to obtain accurate measurements from them.

K1 and K2 readings are taken and fed into the biometry machine. K1 and K2 correspond to measurements of the vertical and horizontal curvatures of the cornea. They are usually represented in millimetres but they may also be represented in dioptres.

Axial length measurements

These are taken using A-scan ultrasound techniques. As the ultrasound waves pass through the eye, the pulsed echoes from the structures within the eye are reflected and stored within the biometry machine, enabling highly accurate calculation of the axial length measurement.

There really is little room for any margin of error when performing biometry. Inaccurate measurements will lead to unexpected, if not unacceptable, postoperative refractive errors, and in some cases may necessitate removal of the implanted IOL and replacement with an IOL of more appropriate/tolerable power. It is therefore essential to gain the fullest cooperation of the patient while performing biometry readings.

The final product after biometry readings is a printout detailing a range of IOL powers and corresponding refractive errors, enabling the surgeon accurately to predict and select the IOL that would give the best visual acuity (or refractive results postoperatively) suited to individual patient needs.

Cataract surgery

Advances in cataract surgery

'Couching', a technique that involved pushing the cataractous lens back into the vitreous and therefore away from the visual axis, was the initial method of choice in ancient Indian and Arabian medicine and is still used to improve vision in parts of the world today (see Chapter 13). The first successful removal of cataractous lens was undertaken in 1750 by Jacques Davial (Albert and Edwards 1996).

Cataract surgery has come a long way since then. Intracapsular surgery was very successful for many years and has been superseded by extracapsular surgery. Extracapsular lens extraction has also been superseded in most areas by phacoemulsification techniques. It is necessary to understand all these techniques because there are still many people seen in clinical practice who have undergone these types of cataract operations and they are still practised.

Intracapsular lens extraction

In this procedure the whole of the lens (including the lens capsule) is removed using a cryoprobe through a large corneal or limbal incision. The zonules are often weakened first using chemical agents (such as Zonulysin) and then the cryoprobe is held next to the lens capsule. The cryotherapy machine is then switched on so as to freeze the probe tip; this causes the capsule and the lens to adhere to the probe and the whole lens is simply removed.

This technique for lens extraction is quite clumsy compared with more modern techniques, and it carries with it high rates of retinal detachment resulting from shifting and displacement of the vitreous gel of the eye into the space left by removal of the whole lens. Removal of the whole lens led to a large refractive error and correction after this type of surgery was obtained by using spectacles (aphakic/cataract glasses) of +10 D power. Patients need to have both eyes operated on within a short timescale in order to be fitted with their corrective spectacles, and many experienced problems related to the high magnification associated with their spectacles.

Early developments in the use of intraocular lenses eased this and patients can either be fitted with iris clip or anterior chamber lens implants, and spectacle prescriptions of more acceptable powers can be used. The corneal section is usually sutured with five sutures, leading to the possibility of iris prolapse through a slipped or broken suture and long-standing astigmatism until the section is stabilized. Tight sutures might add to astigmatic problems. Suture sites have the potential to become infected.

Extracapsular lens extraction

This is a much safer technique that is still used extensively. This procedure still needs a large corneal or limbal incision with the potential problems discussed above. However, instead of removing the whole lens, the soft lens matter (cortex) and the nucleus of the lens are expressed through an opening created in the anterior capsule. The use of a viscoelastic substance introduced into the anterior chamber helps it to retain its shape and to protect the corneal endothelium. By applying a gently tilting pressure on the cornea with a squint hook (or similar instrument) and vectis (loop) placed under the lens nucleus itself, the contents of the lens can be removed, leaving the capsule in place. After expression of the lens nucleus any remaining soft lens matter (cortex) can be removed by irrigation and aspiration techniques. Variations in the technique for creating the capsular opening in order to facilitate removal of the lens contents are common.

During this procedure the surgeon requires great skill and dexterity and, although the incidence of retinal detachment is greatly reduced, it still occurs after this type of lens extraction. Other common complications are retention of the soft lens matter and accompanying surgically induced uveitis, rupture of the lens capsule and forward shifting of the vitreous gel and disruption/dislocation of the zonules during lens expression.

Refractive correction for this type of surgery is more likely to involve the use of posterior chamber lens implants, whereby the lens implant is inserted into the remaining capsular bag. Subsequent correction by the optometrist is much easier, and patients can be fitted with more acceptable spectacle prescriptions after their surgery. The sutures remain in place for some months or years until they absorb or are removed intentionally because they break and cause irritation to the patient.

This is still the procedure of choice in many areas of the world because the instrumentation associated with it is much less complex and expensive than for phacoemulsification surgery. Its results are comparable with phakoemulsification techniques. The eye does not recover as quickly as a result of the large incision; removal of the sutures can change the contour of the eye and induce astigmatism which will need to be corrected so that the patient can see well.

Phakoemulsification

This technique, pioneered by Kelman in the late 1960s (Stein et al. 1994), involves using ultrasonic vibrations to sculpt and break up the lens cortex and nucleus before irrigation and aspiration of the lens contents. Phacoemulsification is undertaken through a small incision (about 3 mm). A single continuous circular tear is made in the anterior capsule (capsulorrhexis), and then, using hydrodissection (again under a blanket of viscoelastic substance), the nucleus and cortex are separated. Sculpting of the lens follows which breaks up the nucleus into four quadrants; each segment is then aspirated until the nucleus is removed. Irrigation and aspiration remove the remaining soft lens matter (cortex), and the initial 3-mm incision may be enlarged to about 5.5 mm, to facilitate insertion of the lens implant. Recent developments and use of folding lenses negate the need for the wound enlargement stage of this procedure.

As a technique for cataract extraction phakoemulsification has many advantages over the more traditional surgical techniques. It is a fast technique and, often, no sutures need to be used. The small incision lessens the possibility of wound leaks and iris tissue prolapse. Sculpting of the lens nucleus before removal makes it a much more refined technique with reduced incidence of capsular rupture. Surgically (or suture) induced astigmatism is less, and generally the wound into the eye heals much more quickly, making it easier for patients to return to normal day-to-day activities within a relatively short time frame.

There are disadvantages to this technique, however, including a longer learning period for practitioners (Stein et al. 1994) and the fact that the procedure is entirely dependent on expensive equipment.

Cool laser

Another technique that is beginning to be used in some areas is that of the 'cool laser'. The cataract removal system uses a laser to generate shockwaves by striking a titanium target at the end of an aspirating hand piece (O'hEineachain 2002). The procedure takes place in a similar way to phakoemulsification, through a very small incision (1.4 mm) but the laser does not generate heat, which prevents the burning of the cornea and heating of tissues that may occur with phakoemulsification.

Intraocular lenses

The first lens for implantation within the eye was introduced by Ridley in 1949 (Stein et al 1994). Continuing development of IOLs has improved the visual outcomes of cataract surgery and reduced magnification and distortion of images to zero. Intraocular lenses may be placed in a variety of positions within the eye as already discussed, with the preferred position being in the capsular 'bag' which remains after extracapsular cataract extraction because it is the most anatomically correct. Most IOLs are simple lenses (the optic) with fixation devices attached, often curved loops (the haptic). The haptic may be compressed; the lens is implanted into the capsular bag and then acts as a 'spring' to keep the lens in position. Lenses may be rigid or compressed so that they 'unfold' over a number of hours when in position inside the eye.

A single vision lens can correct vision for either distance or near, but not for both, so it is likely that the patient will still need spectacle correction after surgery. Continued developments in surgical techniques and the use of multifocal IOL implants in younger patients have the additional benefit of no longer needing to rely on spectacles for reading or distance postoperatively. The use of multifocal lenses does require surgery to be performed on both eyes within a short time frame, but clinically this does not appear to be a problem.

Although some patients report the presence of glare when night driving after the insertion of a multifocal lens (caused by the design shape of the IOL itself), the problem is usually tolerated by most within time. Accommodating lenses, where the lens position changes as the person changes focus, are also in use and development of new and better IOLs continues.

Complications of cataract surgery

No surgery is simple and straightforward until it is completed. Possible complications during and after cataract surgery include the following:

- Raised intraocular pressure resulting from blockage of aqueous outflow channels with the viscoelastic substance used. The pressure may also rise as a reaction to the surgery or as a result of inflammation. The patient is likely to experience pain and new blurring of vision, which occurs some hours after surgery.
- Rupture of the posterior capsule during surgery may result in the nucleus dropping back into the vitreous, necessitating vitrectomy either during surgery or later. Posterior capsule rupture may also result in the need to insert a different type of IOL.
- A shallow anterior chamber may be caused by inhibition of aqueous production, a wound leak resulting from surgery or postoperative trauma, or raised pressure. If the chamber becomes very shallow, the corneal endothelium may be damaged by touching the iris and this may result in permanent corneal oedema.
- Uveitis occurs as an inflammatory response to surgery. It is a normal consequence of surgery and so patients will be treated postoperatively, with eyedrops containing a steroid, to reduce and control this inflammation. Increased pain and redness of the eye may occur if the

inflammation increases and modification of the drop therapy may be required.

- Displacement of the IOL may occur after surgery and will necessitate further surgical intervention to replace it or correct its position.
- Infection is always a possible complication of surgery and for this reason, prophylactic antibiotic drops will also be prescribed after cataract extraction.
- Retinal detachment may occur after cataract surgery in a very small number of cases.
- Oedema of the retina at the macula (cystoid macular oedema) is also recognized as a complication of cataract extraction and is likely to cause some disturbance of central vision. It often disappears over time (see also Chapter 21).

Posterior capsular opacification is the most frequent long-term complication of surgery, and is reported in between 10 and 50% of all cases (Apple et al. 2001). The posterior portion of the remaining lens capsule becomes opacified and the patient reports reduction in vision. Posterior capsular opacities are easily dealt with in a painless and fast outpatient procedure, using a laser to burn a hole in the capsule (YAG or yttrium–aluminium–garnet capsulotomy) (Figure 18.4).

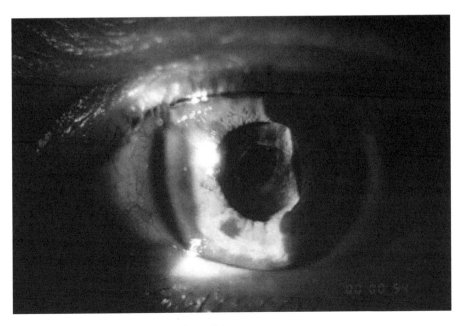

Figure 18.4 Capsulotomy. (See Plate 45.)

Approaches to care of the cataract patient

Cataract is a common cause of visual impairment affecting about 30% of the population over the age of 65 years. In parallel with the improvements in the anaesthetic and surgical techniques used in cataract extraction, trends towards day-case care have developed.

Changes in attitudes, roles and the working relationships between ophthalmic health-care professionals have greatly influenced the development of day-case care. Probably one of the most influential factors is the increasing expanded role work undertaken by ophthalmic nurses in the preoperative assessment and postoperative management of cataract patients.

It is the nursing role, from the initial screening of GP or optometrist referrals, through to increased nursing input into patient care in preoperative assessment clinics, that has created flexibility in the coordinating of theatre lists, transport arrangements and admission routines, which have influenced the rapid development of day-case care.

The preoperative (surgical) assessment clinic facilitates better opportunities to provide more detailed information in relation to the perioperative management of cataract for patients. Increased patient involvement and subsequent cooperation in care planning lead to the negotiation of much more flexible approaches to perioperative care.

In the postoperative management of cataract patients, the increased use of local anaesthesia, whether by facial blocks or sub-Tenon's or subconjunctival injections, or the more recent use of topical anaesthetic drops, negates the need to keep patients in hospital overnight.

Small incision phacoemulsification and the subsequent shortening of the recovery time that patients need postoperatively after cataract surgery have also assisted in shortening the length of hospital stay for patients.

Surgical (wound) healing rates are much faster and the delicate nature of the surgical techniques used usually result in much less disruption to the anterior chamber and fewer postoperative complications.

In addition to the above helping in the development of one-stop cataract services, this has influenced the development of nurse-led postoperative ocular examination (also known as first dressing) in both the hospital and the community settings.

References

Albert DM, Edwards DD (1996) The History of Ophthalmology. Oxford: Blackwell Science.

Apple DJ, Peng Q, Visessook N et al. (2001) Eradication of posterior capsule opacification: documentation of a marked decrease in Nd:YAG laser posterior capsulotomy rates noted in an analysis of 5416 pseudophakic human eyes obtained postmortem. Ophthalmology 108: 505–18.

Gregory JK, Talamo JH (1996) The crystalline lens and cataract. In: Pavan-Langston D (ed.), Manual of Ocular Diagnosis and Therapy, 4th edn. Boston, MA: Little, Brown.

National Health Service Executive (2000) Action on Cataracts. London: DoH .

Newell F (1996) Ophthalmology: Principles and concepts, 8th edn. St Louis, MO: Mosby.

O'hEineachain R (2002) Cool laser blasts way to micro-incision cataract surgery. Eurotimes: www.escrs.org/eurotimes/December2002/cool.asp (accessed 15 October 2003).

Prasad S, Tanner V, Patel CK, Rosen P (1998) Optimisation of outpatient resource utilisation in cataract management. Eye 12: 403–6.

Reidy A, Minassian DC, Vafidis G et al. (1998). Prevalence of serious eye disease and visual impairment in a north London population: population based, cross sectional study. BMJ 316: 1643–6.

Rose K, Waterman H, Toon L, McLeod D, Tullo A (1999) Management of day-surgery patients with cataract attending a peripheral ophthalmic clinic. Eye 13: 71–5.

Stein HA, Slatt BJ, Stein RM (1994) The Ophthalmic Assistant, 7th edn. St Louis, MO: Mosby.

CHAPTER NINETEEN

The uveal tract

BRONWYN WARD, SUSANNE RAYNEL AND GAYLE CATT

Anatomy and physiology

The uveal tract makes up the middle layer of the globe and is protected by the cornea and sclera. Although it is a continuous layer it has three distinct parts: the choroid, ciliary body and iris, which differ in location and structure. The term 'uvea' is derived from the Italian *uva*, a grape, because the uveal tract is the vascular layer of the globe and so, when it is examined, it looks like the inside of a dusky grape skin. The choroid has cells containing melanin pigment, which also contribute towards the 'grape-like' colour.

The choroid

The choroid is a vascular layer situated between the retina and sclera; it is about 0.22 mm thick posteriorly thinning to 0.1 mm at the periphery; it is firmly attached to the margins of the optic nerve posteriorly and anteriorly joins the ciliary body. Blood is supplied to the choroid by the short posterior ciliary artery and drainage is via the choroidal and vortex veins; the nerve supply comes from the oculomotor nerve via the posterior ciliary artery. The choroid extends from the optic nerve towards the ora serrata and is continuous with the ciliary body and iris.

The choroid can be divided into three distinct layers: basal lamina, blood vessels and lamina fusca. The basal lamina, more commonly called Bruch's membrane, is very thin (2–3 μm); it is the inner layer of the choroid and is situated between the retinal pigment epithelium and the choriocapillaris. It consists of two layers, the outer made up of collagen and the inner being the basement membrane of the pigment epithelium.

The middle layer of the choroid is a meshwork of blood vessels where the arteries and veins are external, whereas a dense network layer of capillaries, the choriocapillaris, is internal. This meshwork of blood vessels is sandwiched between the basal lamina and lamina fusca. The lamina fusca is the outer layer of the choroid and, as the name suggests, is a supporting structure between the blood vessel layer and the sclera.

The primary function of the choroid is to provide nourishment to the outer layer of the retina but it also has a role in reducing internal reflection of stray light rays via pigment cells (melanin) and aids in the dispersal of heat that may collect in the retina.

The ciliary body

The ciliary body (Figure 19.1) is between 4 and 6 mm wide, roughly triangular in shape, and situated between the anterior choroid and the root of the iris. It is adherent to the sclera just behind the limbus, continuous with the iris and extends from the scleral spur to the ora serrata. Blood is supplied to the ciliary body by the anterior ciliary arteries and long posterior ciliary arteries, and drainage is via the anterior ciliary veins, long posterior ciliary veins and vortex vein. The nerve supply comes from the oculomotor nerve via the short ciliary nerve.

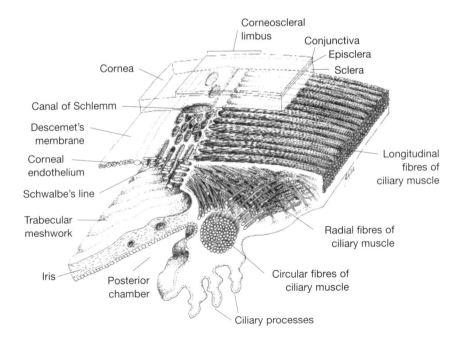

Figure 19.1 The ciliary body and angle.

The ciliary body can be divided into three distinct sections: the pars plicata, pars plana and ciliary muscles. The pars plicata is the anterior part of the ciliary body and lies between the pars plana and iris. It appears corrugated and is about 2 mm long. It is from the pars plicata that the ciliary processes arise. There are about 70 ciliary processes and these are composed of vascular tissue, mainly capillaries and veins, covered by epithelium. The ciliary processes can be divided into two layers: the outer layer is an extension of the pigment epithelium of the retina and the inner layer is unpigmented and continuous with the neural retina. The ciliary processes are responsible for the formation and secretion of aqueous: first into the posterior chamber and then via the pupil to the anterior chamber. The lens is also held *in situ* by fine suspensory ligaments that arise in the ciliary processes and valleys, known as zonular fibres (zonules of Zinn).

The pars plana is the posterior part of the ciliary body; it is about 4.5 mm long and lies next to the ora serrata. Whereas the pars plicata appears corrugated, the pars plana is generally flat and it is via the pars plana that vitreoretinal surgery is undertaken. There is also some attachment of zonular fibres from the lens to the pars plana.

The ciliary muscles form the bulk of the ciliary body, and lie adjacent to the sclera; they are made up of a combination of longitudinal, circular and radial fibres, which are controlled by the oculomotor nerve. It is the ciliary muscles, specifically the circular fibres, that are responsible for accommodation. The circular fibres contract and relax the ciliary processes, thus allowing the lens to become more convex and allowing light rays to be focused on the retina when looking at objects nearer than 'infinity'. The longitudinal fibres are responsible for influencing the microscopic channels of the trabecular meshwork, facilitating the outflow of aqueous and thereby assisting with the regulation of intraocular pressure.

The iris

The iris is the most anterior structure of the uveal tract arising from the ciliary body; it is situated behind the cornea and in front of the lens. It is a coloured diaphragm separating the anterior and posterior chambers of the globe and has a central hole, the pupil, through which aqueous passes between the two chambers and light rays enter the globe. Although the iris appears rigid, it is in fact 'floppy' and is supported, to remain in place, by the lens. Without this support it trembles (iridodonesis). The iris is made up of a vascular stroma located anteriorly and pigmented epithelium located posteriorly. The stroma is divided into an anterior border (loose collagen tissues with densely packed pigmented or non-pigmented cells) and a deeper stroma. The anterior border forms the pupillary zone of about 1.5 mm width. The remaining, wider area of iris is the ciliary zone with iris crypts formed by irregular atrophy. The border of the anterior area is known as the collarette, which is a circular ridge and the site of the minor vascular circle of the iris.

The sphincter and dilator muscles of the iris are found within the stroma. The sphincter muscle is about 1 mm wide and surrounds the pupil, facilitating constriction of the pupil; it is innervated by the parasympathetic fibres of the third cranial nerve. The dilator muscle consists of multiple radial fibres in the periphery facilitating pupil dilatation innervated by sympathetic fibres. The sphincter muscle is stronger than the dilator muscles and, if the normal functioning of the muscles is interrupted, the sphincter muscle will overpower the dilator muscle, which is demonstrated in patients presenting with iritis when the pupil is small.

The stroma of the iris also contains melanin-containing pigment cells and the density of these cells determines the colour of the iris. At birth pigment is absent from the iris but by the age of 1 year the pigment is laid down and this is why caucasian babies all appear to have blue eyes at birth; this may change by the time they are aged 1 year but iris colour will not change after this. In brown eyes, the surface of the iris is smooth and heavily pigmented; in blue eyes it is irregular with multiple crypts.

The iris receives its blood supply from the long posterior ciliary artery and the anterior ciliary artery. These join to form the major circle of the iris which lies in the pars plicata and sends branches posteriorly into the ciliary body, as well as forward into the iris; this then forms the minor circle of the iris. The venous return of the iris is via the vortex veins.

Uveitis

Uveitis refers to inflammation of the uveal tract and is the third most common cause of blindness in developed countries, generally affecting people aged 20–50 years with children making up about 5% of cases. Uveitis may be classified in many ways but a simple classification is on the basis of anatomy, clinical features and aetiology (Kanski 2003).

Anatomical classification: inflammation of the structure

- Iritis: iris
- Cyclitis: ciliary body and anterior vitreous
- Iridocyclitis: iris, ciliary body and anterior vitreous
- Choroiditis: choroid.

However, retinitis, vitritis or optic neuritis may be included in the diagnosis if the retina, vitreous or optic nerve is involved. The conditions are more commonly referred to as:

- anterior uveitis: inflammation of the iris (iritis) or iris and ciliary body (iridocyclitis)
- intermediate uveitis: chronic inflammation of the pars plana, the extreme periphery of the retina and choroid

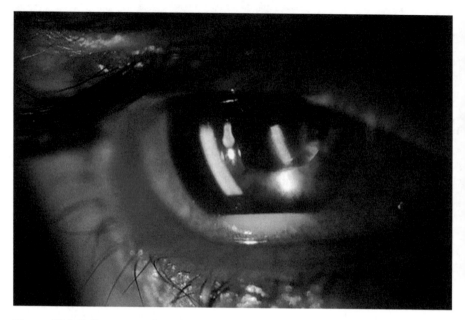

Figure 19.2 Inflammatory hypopyon. (See Plate 46.)

- posterior uveitis: inflammation of the choroid and retina
- panuveitis: diffuse uveitis involving both anterior and posterior ocular structures.

Clinical classification

Uveitis may be classified as acute (with a sudden, acute onset lasting for up to 3 months) and chronic (persisting for less than 3 months with a frequently insidious onset which may be asymptomatic).

Aetiology

Exogenous uveitis is caused by either external injury or invasion of micro-organisms or other agents external to the patient. Endogenous uveitis is caused by micro-organisms or other agents from within the patient. Kanski (2003) suggests five main types of endogenous uveitis:

1. Associated with systemic disease
2. Infections with micro-organisms such as bacteria (tuberculosis [TB] or Lyme disease), viruses (herpes zoster, herpes simplex or HIV) or fungi (*Histoplasma* spp., *Candida* spp.)
3. Infestations such as with *Pneumocystis carinii* or *Toxoplasma canis*

4. Idiopathic specific uveitis entities, which are a group of disorders associated with systemic disease but with specific features of their own (Fuchs' heterochromic cyclitis)
5. Idiopathic uveitis (which makes up around 25% of cases).

Other endogenous causes include a response to soft lens matter in hypermature cataract, or scleritis as well as sympathetic ophthalmia. Some diseases that primarily affect other structures (such as toxoplasmosis, which primarily affects the retina) may cause an overspill of inflammation into the choroid and vitreous (American Academy of Ophthalmology – AAO 2003).

Anterior uveitis

Anterior uveitis is the inflammation of the iris and/or ciliary body (anterior uvea). This is the most common form of uveitis and is often unilateral and acute in onset. It may also be referred to as iritis (inflammation of the iris) or iridocyclitis, if the iris and ciliary body are involved.

Causes

There is a wide range of causes of uveitis as described above, but description may also be based on the type of inflammation (Table 19.1).

Granulomatous uveitis is generally initiated by invasive organisms causing an inflammatory response. Clinically, the keratic precipitates (KPs)

Table 19.1 Uveitis

Non-granulomatous	Granulomatous
Acute	Sarcoidosis
Idiopathic	Syphilis
Ankylosing spondylitis	Tuberculosis
Reiter's syndrome	Systemic lupus erythematosus
Inflammatory bowel disease	Brucellosis
Psoriatic arthritis	Leprosy
Glaucomatocyclitic crisis	Vogt–Koyanagi–Harada syndrome
Herpes simplex or zoster, or varicella zoster	
Lyme disease	
Behçet's disease	
Trauma toxoplasmosis	
Chronic	
Juvenile rheumatoid arthritis	
Chronic iridocyclitis	
Fuchs' heterochromic iridocyclitis	

associated with this are described as large, wet clusters of white cells on the endothelium (mutton-fat) or iris nodules. The non-granulomatous type generally results from an immune or hypersensitivity response. Clinically the KPs are small, dry, discrete white cells on endothelium. Some conditions can present in either way, which sometimes makes this classification unreliable.

The AAO (2003) simplify the classification of causes of intraocular inflammation into that caused by:

- infection
- trauma
- neoplasm
- autoimmune factors.

Symptoms of uveitis depend on the type of inflammation (acute or chronic):

- Pain: may range from mild to severe pain, localized or referred to periorbital region and aggravated by light. This is mainly caused by ciliary spasm and may be referred, so that it feels as though it radiates over a large area served by the trigeminal nerve.
- Photophobia: may range from mild to severe with associated blepharospasm resulting from the irritation of the trigeminal nerve.
- Lacrimation: caused by irritation of the trigeminal nerve by the lacrimal gland.
- Decreased vision: may be moderate or marked according to the level of clouding of the media, compromised tear film, macular involvement or change in lens position.

Uveitis may be found on routine clinical examination in chronic presentations.

Signs

- Conjunctival and perilimbal or circumcorneal injection may be referred to as 'ciliary flush'.
- Distortion of the pupil from reactive miosis of the pupil as a result of dominance of sphincter muscle, iris spasm and/or synechiae.
- Anterior chamber may contain cells and flare and both need to be graded. More severe inflammation may lead to fibrin in the anterior chamber.
- Keratic precipitates are cellular deposits on the corneal endothelium. Distribution and characteristics can indicate the type of uveitis present.

- Hypopyon: layering of inflammatory cells in the inferior angle (Figure 19.2).
- Iris abnormalities in colour; may appear 'muddy'; nodules may be present and are defined as Koeppe or Busacca. Koeppe nodules appear as white fluffy precipitates on the inner surface of the pupillary margin. Busacca nodules are larger and appear on the surface of the iris.
- Heterochromia.
- Posterior synechiae (PSs) are adhesions between the anterior surface of the lens and iris. PSs occur when part or the entire pupillary zone of the iris adheres to the anterior surface of the lens as a result of an inflamed, swollen and slightly 'sticky' iris in close proximity to the lens. This obstructs the flow of aqueous through the pupil, resulting in the build-up of pressure in the posterior chamber. As a result, the iris bulges forward known as iris bombé.
- Peripheral anterior synechiae (PAS) may follow where the peripheral anterior surface of the iris bombé adheres to the peripheral posterior surface of the cornea.
- Increased or decreased intraocular pressure: inflammation of the ciliary process will reduce the production of aqueous, resulting in a low intraocular pressure. Increased pressure will result if secondary glaucoma has occurred.
- Anterior vitreous cells.
- Cystoid macular oedema.
- Neovascularization of choroid or optic nerve.

An inflammatory response to infectious, traumatic, neoplastic or autoimmune processes produces the signs of uveitis as a result of the chemical mediators of the acute stages of inflammation such as serotonin and complement. Other chemicals involved in inflammation include leukotrienes, kinins and prostaglandins. The lymphocyte is the predominant inflammatory cell in uveitis and other cells, including mast cells, also contribute to the inflammatory response. These chemical mediators result in dilatation of blood vessels and ciliary flush, increased vascular permeability resulting in aqueous flare, and the release of inflammatory cells into the eye leading to aqueous or vitreous cells.

Grading of cells

This should be undertaken using a narrow (1 mm) beam of light, about 3 mm high and at maximum intensity and high magnification, and is best observed with the beam of light at a 45–46° angle. Cells are counted and graded as follows:

0	No inflammatory cells
Trace (AAO 2003)	< 5 cells
± (Kanski 2003)	
1+	5–10 cells
2+	11–20 cells
3+	21–30 cells (AAO 2003), 21–50 cells (Kanski 2003)
4+	Cells too numerous to count/hypopyon

Diagnosis

As in other conditions, the diagnosis is based on history and examination; however, a comprehensive history must include an ophthalmic history with current or previous medication usage as well as a detailed systemic health history to determine possible aetiology. There should be a targeted systemic physical examination of the skin and joints.

Not all patients presenting with uveitis should be tested further because at least 25% of presentations are idiopathic and, often, the first episode of uveitis may be the only episode. Generally, then, if there are no significant systemic factors, patients are not investigated further until a second episode (Newell 1996) (Table 19.2).

Table 19.2

Non-tested	Test
Healthy, asymptomatic young to middle age	Recurrent
	Severe
Initial episode of mild-to-moderately severe acute	Bilateral
	Granulomatous
Unilateral	Intermediate, posterior or diffuse uveitis
Non-granulomatous anterior uveitis that responds promptly to treatment	Patients failing to respond promptly to treatment

Once a range of possible causes for the uveitis has been identified, a range of patient specific tests (Table 19.3) may be organized – this is common to all forms of uveitis.

Intermediate uveitis

Chronic inflammation of the pars plana is known as intermediate uveitis and is non-granulomatous with unknown aetiology and insidious onset.

Table 19.3 Special tests

Serology	Syphilis, HIV, Lyme disease, toxoplasmosis, toxocariasis
Chest radiograph, skin tests	TB, sarcoidosis
HLA-B27-positive test	Idiopathic Ankylosing spondylitis Reiter's syndrome Inflammatory bowel disease Psoriasis
Fluorescein angiography/ aqueous and vitreous biopsy	Posterior uveitis

It typically affects people aged between 5 and 40 years and there are two peaks in this age range: from 5 to 15 and then from 20 to 40. Some patients may have self-limiting, short, low-grade episodes. Others may have a lingering chronic bout with sub-acute exacerbation and incomplete remissions. It accounts for up to 15% of all cases of uveitis (AAO 2003).

Cause

The cause is mostly unknown, although it is certainly a feature of sarcoidosis and 10–15% of patients go on to develop multiple sclerosis.

Symptoms

Intermediate uveitis may be painless and the patient may present with an increase in floaters. Macular oedema results in loss of central vision and this may also be a presenting symptom.

Signs

• Minimal anterior chamber cells or flare.
• Cells in the anterior vitreous indicate vitritis: this varies in severity, through individual cells only and including 'snowballs', which are gelatinous exudates and cells, to occasionally a completely opaque vitreous.
• 'Snow-banking': fibrovascular exudates along the inferior pars plana.
• Optic disc swelling.
• Cystoid macular oedema.
• Posterior vitreous detachment.

Complications

- Cystoid macular oedema is the most common cause of visual loss.
- Secondary cataract develops in eyes with severe and prolonged inflammation.
- Tractional detachment may occur.
- Vascularization of exudate behind the posterior lens capsule may cause ciliary detachment, with consequent reduced aqueous secretion, hypotony and, eventually, phthisis bulbi.

Posterior uveitis

This applies to the posterior structures of the eye and may include retinitis, choroiditis, vasculitis and vitritis. These conditions may occur in combination or separately.

Patients with posterior uveitis complain of decreased vision, floaters, metamorphopsia and scotoma, or a combination of these.

Examination shows areas of retinitis or choroiditis as well as cells in the vitreous. There may be posterior vitreous detachment and precipitates on the posterior hyaloid face, which are similar to KPs. Retinitis gives the retina a white, cloudy appearance with obscured vessels and the areas of inflammation tend to have indistinct edges. Vasculitis is seen as fluffy white haziness surrounding blood vessels, and veins are more often affected than arteries.

Causes

Posterior uveitis can be caused by infection or endogenous inflammation or be neoplastic.

- Infection and infestations:
  - viral: herpes zoster, herpes simplex, cytomegalovirus (CMV), HIV
  - bacterial: TB, syphilis, Lyme disease, brucellosis
  - fungi: Candida spp., Aspergillus spp., histoplasmosis
  - parasites: toxocariasis, toxoplasmosis, onchocerciasis
- Systemic disease: sarcoidosis, Behçet's disease, Vogt–Koyanagi–Harada disease, toxoplasmosis
- Multiple sclerosis
- Systemic lupus erythematosus (SLE)
- Inflammatory bowel disease.

Complications include cystoid macular oedema, macular scarring, epiretinal membrane formation, retinal detachment (which may be tractional, rhegmatogenous or exudative), scotomata from chorioretinal scarring or vascular occlusions.

Panuveitis

This may also be referred to as diffuse uveitis, because there is diffuse inflammation of all anterior and posterior structures of the eye. In most case the aetiology is unknown but it is often associated with sarcoidosis, TB and syphilis, and less commonly with sympathetic ophthalmia, Vogt–Koyanagi–Harada syndrome and Behçet's disease.

Treatment of uveitis

Aims

1. To alleviate acute symptoms and suppress inflammation
2. To preserve vision and prevent complications
3. To treat the cause of inflammatory process if known.

Mydriatics and cycloplegics

These are used in anterior uveitis or in intermediate or posterior uveitis when there is overspill of inflammation into the anterior segment.

Mydriatics and cycloplegics dilate the pupil and are used to break down or prevent posterior synechiae. This may include subconjunctival or topical instillation of a combination of drops, such as cyclopentolate 1%, phenylephrine hydrochloride 2.5 or 10%, atropine 1% and homatropine 2%. There may be an initial period of intensive instillation if synechiae are present in order to break down the adhesion between the lens and iris.

These drops also have an analgesic effect via the paralytic effect of cycloplegic eyedrops, which will reduce the iris sphincter spasm. A side effect will be limitation of accommodation affecting close and fairly near work (as with computers).

Practitioner experience shows that application of heat to the eye during intensive dilatation may aid its effectiveness. Heat may be applied in various ways, such as by asking the patient to lean over a bowl or jug of boiling water; a novel method involves filling a surgical glove with hot water, firmly tying a knot in the wrist and asking the patient to apply it, perhaps wrapped in a cover, to the closed eye. Many patients find the application of heat extremely soothing.

If the pupil fails to respond to topical therapy, a subconjunctival drug may be given, often combined with a steroid.

Corticosteroids

The mainstay of management in most cases of uveitis is steroids, which may be delivered as topical, periocular, subconjunctival (useful for severe acute uveitis or cystoid macular oedema), intravitreal and/or systemic treatment. Primarily their action is to suppress the inflammatory response within the eye and they are used only where infection has been ruled out as a possible cause.

Topical treatment can be intensive, initially (1–2 hourly) with a tapering of drops over a prescribed period. Sudden stopping of steroid drops may result in rebound inflammation. Patients need to be aware of the importance of compliance, possible side effects and the importance of completion of prescribed treatment. This may impact on patients' lifestyles if they are working and, if they are unable to self-medicate, frequent assistance may be needed. An ointment may be used at night or if the patient has trouble instilling frequent drops.

Topical steroids are effective for anterior uveitis although they may have useful effects on vitritis or macular oedema if the patient is aphakic. Drugs used include prednisolone acetate, prednisolone sodium phosphate and dexamethasone phosphate.

Periocular or subconjunctival treatment is an option in severe cases of anterior uveitis uncontrolled by drops, intermediate uveitis or in cases where limiting systemic steroids are preferable. Drugs used include methylprednisolone acetate, hydrocortisone sodium succinate and triamcinolone acetonide. Periocular routes include sub-Tenon's or transseptal routes into the orbital floor.

Intravitreal steroids may be given by injection or implantation of a sustained release device. This has been shown to be useful in chronic uveitis and cystoid macular oedema (Antcliff et al. 2001).

Systemic steroids can be used in patients with chronic, vision-threatening uveitis and in severe uveitis not responding to other treatments or when systemic causes must be treated concurrently. They are therefore usually used only for posterior and some intermediate forms of uveitis.

Practitioners and patients need to be aware of the possible complications of steroid use particularly long term. Corneal integrity may be compromised, susceptibility to opportunistic infections increased, or cataracts, usually posterior subcapsular, or glaucoma develops.

Non-steroidal anti-inflammatory drugs

These may be indicated if underlying conditions are present such as arthritis, or juvenile, psoriatic or ankylosing spondylitis.

Immunosuppressants

Although steroids suppress the immune system, the use of immunosuppressants may benefit patients with severe sight-threatening uveitis or those who are resistant to or intolerant of steroids. These drugs are thought to work by killing the lymphocytes that are responsible for inflammation (AAO 2003). They are being used more frequently as a result of the complications of long-term steroid use. Drugs include methotrexate, azothioprine, cyclophosphamide, chlorambucil and ciclosporin. Patients must be monitored closely by practitioners experienced in the use of these agents. Regular blood tests, including blood count, and renal and hepatic tests, should be taken. Serious complications include renal and hepatic toxicity and bone marrow suppression and there is a heightened risk of infection. Some of these drugs are associated with sterility and are all potentially teratogenic, so pregnancy should be avoided.

Antibiotic or antiviral therapy

Topical and/or systemic delivery may be indicated if uveitis is caused by a pathogen.

Anti-glaucoma therapy

This may be necessary to lower the intraocular pressure if secondary glaucoma has occurred. In the acute stage intensive topical treatment and/or systemic acetazolamide is used.

Surgery

Vitrectomy may be useful in vitritis or cystoid macular oedema; other surgery may be needed to deal with the complications of uveitis such as tractional detachment and cataract.

Education

Education about the condition is crucial in aiding compliance with drop regimens. The patient may need to be taught how to instil eyedrops and should understand any possible side effects of treatment. Understanding of the condition will also help to reinforce the importance of attending associated clinics such as for a radiograph or blood tests.

As a result of its dense vascular make-up, the uveal tract mirrors all systemic vascular diseases and uveitis can be an initial presentation of many systemic diseases. Results from diagnostic tests performed in the ophthalmic unit may confirm or discover associated immunological disorders and therefore it commonly falls to the ophthalmic health profession to tell the patients of their diagnosis. The nurse may that find she or he is educating the patients on both their ophthalmic condition and treatment, and associated systemic diseases.

Complications

Secondary glaucoma

This is the most common complication of anterior uveitis. It may be the result of anterior, posterior or peripheral anterior synechiae or a response to steroids. Presence of a hypopyon may cause debris to block the angle and drainage canals, leading to increase in pressure.

Visual impairment

This can take various forms, depending on the cause: inflammation, use of mydriatics, floaters, cataract and glaucoma with visual field loss. If visual impairment is present as a result of cystoid macular oedema, referral to a low-vision assessment clinic may be needed.

Cataract

Formation of a cataract may be secondary to inflammation and steroid use or impairment of metabolism. Corneal band keratopathy may also occur.

Syndromes/conditions and uveitis

Fuchs' heterochromic cyclitis (Fuchs' uveitis syndrome)

This is an uncommon cause of chronic uveitis affecting less than 5% of all patients diagnosed with uveitis. It generally affects those aged over 30 years, is usually unilateral and the common signs and symptoms of uveitis of redness, pain and photophobia are minimal. However, the patient does complain of blurred vision, often from a cataract because cataracts eventually occur in most patients. Often the colour of the iris is affected as a result of stromal atrophy leading to a lighter coloured iris.

On examination changes in the architecture of the iris and a large pupil as a result of iris changes, are seen. Anterior synechiae are sometimes present but posterior synechiae are never seen. Slit-lamp examination reveals KPs, usually present over the entire corneal endothelium, that flare may be present, and there are never more than 2+ cells present. Rubeosis is a common finding.

The two complications of Fuchs' syndrome are cataract and secondary glaucoma as a result of the rubeosis. Cataract surgery is usually successful and the glaucoma is treated with topical medications.

Glaucomatocyclitic crisis (Posner–Schlossman syndrome)

This chronic uveitis is characterized by recurrent episodes of secondary open-angle glaucoma; it generally affects young adults and episodes are unilateral, but 50% of patients will have bilateral episodes at different times. The 'classic' signs and symptoms of uveitis are minimal and the patient usually presents complaining of haloes around lights that are like the colours of the rainbow. These haloes are the result of corneal oedema; however, pain is not a common presenting symptom despite intraocular pressure (IOP) being elevated as high as 40–60 mmHg.

On examination corneal oedema is present but as with open-angle glaucoma the anterior chamber depth is normal. No flare is present, there may be a few cells in the aqueous and KPs are present, but posterior synechiae do not develop.

Treatment during an active episode is to reduce the IOP. Over time some patients may develop a chronic rise in IOP, which can lead to optic disc cupping and visual field loss, as with any glaucoma.

Vogt–Koyanagi–Harada (VKH) syndrome

This syndrome predominantly affects those in populations prone to pigmented skin; it is reasonably common among the Japanese population. It is a multisystem disorder associated with alopecia, poliosis, vitiligo, neurological irritation (headaches, etc.) and auditory disturbances. This syndrome is often divided depending on what the patients present with; if they have mainly skin involvement and anterior uveitis it is described as Vogt–Koyanagi syndrome and if there is neurological and retinal involvement it is described as Harada's disease.

On ocular examination there may be anterior involvement, usually iridocyclitis, or posterior involvement with the presence of posterior synechiae, secondary glaucoma and retina involvement such as retinal detachments or disc oedema.

Sympathetic uveitis (sympathetic ophthalmitis)

This is a very rare presentation of uveitis in the second eye (sympathizing eye) which occurs after a penetrating injury to the other eye (exciting eye), generally as a result of trauma but occasionally after intraocular surgery. In most cases there may have been exposure of some uveal tissue. The patient presents with a mild anterior uveitis in the sympathizing eye from 2–3 weeks to several years after the initial injury, although 65% of cases present within 3 months and 90% within 1 year.

The patient presents with photophobia and blurred vision in the sympathizing eye. On examination the 'classic' signs of uveitis are not present in the sympathizing eye, but there are cells present in the retrolental space, and the exciting eye shows evidence of the original injury and may be injected. However, both eyes eventually develop a severe, chronic inflammation resulting eventually in a panuveitis; in addition posterior synechiae form if not treated early with mydriatics.

Most patients with sympathetic uveitis eventually develop cataract, glaucoma and phthisis bulbi, but in some instances the disease is self-limiting with no long-term effects. Treatment options for patients with sympathetic uveitis are few and often drastic: enucleation of the injured eye within 2 weeks, which seems to have an impact on the incidence, steroid therapy and immunosuppressive therapy.

Systemic disorders and uveitis

HLA-B27

All animals with white blood cells express cell surface glycoproteins (major histocompatibility complex [MHC]) and those in humans are known as human leukocyte antigens (HLAs). HLA-B27 is expressed on the short arm of chromosome 6. Although it is present in only 1–8% of the general population, about 50% of patients with acute anterior uveitis express the HLA-B27 molecule and many of these patients also have other immune disorders such as Reiter's syndrome, inflammatory bowel disease or ankylosing spondylitis (AAO 2003). The mechanism of these immune reactions is still unknown, but it is thought (from animal models) that bacterial gut infection may predispose to arthritis and Reiter's syndrome.

The combination of systemic and ocular disease can be devastating for the patient who not only has to manage a disease process but may also have to align him- or herself to diminishing sight. Here is a brief look at some of the more common systemic diseases; this area is covered more fully in texts dealing with particular systemic diseases.

Ankylosing spondylitis

As previously mentioned there is a strong association between HLA-B27 and this disease. Uveitis almost always occurs at some stage. Ankylosing spondylitis affects men more than women, involves the sacroiliac joints and axial skeleton and ranges in severity from asymptomatic to crippling. Radiographs of the sacroiliac joints show sclerosis and narrowing of joint spaces. HLA-B27 is found in up to 90% of patient with ankylosing spondylitis. Pain, redness and photophobia are the initial complaints and synechiae formation is common. It may be accompanied by iridocyclitis. The iritis is usually recurrent and may lead to permanent damage if not adequately treated.

Reiter's syndrome

This is characterized by a triad of symptoms: non-specific urethritis, polyarteritis and conjunctival inflammation, often with uveitis. It is most common in young adult males. It may be triggered by an episode of diarrhoea caused by a pathogen such as *Chlamydia* spp., *Shigella* spp. or *Salmonella* spp. which acts to trigger inflammation. Arthritis begins within about 30 days of infection in most patients. HLA-B27 is found in up to 95% of these patients.

Crohn's disease and ulcerative colitis

These are both associated with acute uveitis and HLA-B27.

Behçet's disease

Behçet's disease is a generalized occlusive vasculitis of unknown cause and typically affects young men from the eastern Mediterranean region and Japan (Kanski 2003). Its effects include recurrent aphthous ulceration, skin rashes, genital ulceration and uveitis, vitritis or retinitis. Ocular signs with this disease occur in about three-quarters of cases. The uveitis is characterized by the sudden onset of a hypopyon; visual loss is frequent and posterior involvement occurs despite treatment. Combination therapy is often used (steroid plus immunosuppressive) and this can help to reduce visual loss (Kaklamani and Kaklamanis 2001).

Still's disease (juvenile rheumatoid arthritis)

Uveitis presents in about 50% of patients with Still's disease. Low-grade bilateral iridocyclitis may precede or follow joint involvement. Females are more commonly affected and in most cases the onset is insidious. The uveitis may precede the arthritis by 3–10 years; the average age at which the uveitis is detected is 5 years. Corticosteroids and mydriatics are of value in acute episodes but their long-range effect is possibly only to delay the inevitable, which may be severe visual impairment. In 50% of cases, the uveitis is moderate to severe and persists for more than 4 months and in 25% of cases the uveitis is very severe and lasts several years, resulting in cataract, secondary glaucoma and band keratopathy (Kanski 2003).

The treatment of children with uveitis presents some unique problems. There may be a risk of amblyopia in young children, there are different dose requirements for children that may be unique to a particular child, and there are drug-associated risks such as growth retardation with systemic steroids. Gaining cooperation for examination and treatment may also be difficult. Loss of vision in a child will have a greater impact over the lifespan in terms of earning potential and financial burden, and adequate education may also be a problem (Holland and Stiehm 2003).

Sarcoidosis

This is a chronic granulomatous disease of unknown cause characterized by multiple cutaneous and subcutaneous nodules. Thirty per cent of cases are complicated by bilateral anterior uveitis; posterior uveitis is less common. The anterior uveitis is nodular with mutton-fat KPs on the corneal endothelium. This uveitis may lead to severe visual impairment resulting from cataract formation and secondary glaucoma. Corticosteroid therapy given early in the disease may be effective, but recurrences are common and the long-term visual prognosis is poor.

Tuberculosis

Tuberculosis causes a granulomatous type of uveitis and is rare in patients with active pulmonary TB. If the anterior segment is involved iris nodules and mutton-fat KPs are visible on slit-lamp examination. It is the nodules and the localized nature of tuberculous uveitis that help to make a clinical differentiation from sympathetic ophthalmia. After a prolonged course of several months, the disease usually resolves itself. Blurred vision may remain as a result of scarring of the retina.

Infections and uveitis

- Toxoplasmosis and toxocariasis (see Chapter 21)
- Onchocerciasis (see Chapter 13).

Ocular melanoma

Melanoma is a malignancy that develops from cells that produce melanin, the dark-coloured pigment found in skin, hair and the lining of internal organs. The highest incidence of melanoma occurs in the skin and less frequently in other organs of the body such as the eye. The strong link between skin malignant melanoma and exposure to ultraviolet light from the sun is well documented, but the exact cause of ocular melanoma is unknown. The incidence of ocular melanoma is about 28 per million head of population.

Ocular melanoma may involve any part of the eye but the uveal tract is the most common primary intraocular malignant tumour. The tumour can affect any one of the three parts that make up the uveal tract: the iris, ciliary body and choroid. These tumours can also be secondary to primary sites in patients with a history of cancer elsewhere in the body. In particular, in women the breast and lung and in men the genitourinary and gastrointestinal tracts with the liver are the most common primary sites for all secondary ocular melanomas.

The discovery of an ocular melanoma is often an incidental finding from an ophthalmic examination. The patient often has no ocular symptoms unless there is macular involvement and the patient may complain of blurred vision. Sometimes the patient presents with a retinal detachment and will describe the symptoms associated with a retinal detachment.

Iris melanoma

Melanoma of the iris accounts for about 5% of all ocular melanomas. Most are slow-growing tumours and the prognosis is good. The presence of a tumour may discolour the iris or distort the shape of the pupil and so may be noticed by the patient and the family, although they are unlikely to know what the diagnosis is. Often the patient is referred with a differential diagnosis of naevus or melanoma. These tumours are generally observed until growth is noted and then removed by iridectomy.

Ciliary body melanoma

Melanoma of the ciliary body accounts for about 10% of all ocular melanomas. Unlike melanoma of the iris, ciliary body melanoma cannot be visualized without the pupil being dilated and therefore it is difficult to diagnose. Patients may present with a variety of signs and symptoms that on ocular examination may include: secondary astigmatism caused by anterior displacement of the lens from pressure by the tumour, dark mass present on the sclera, dilated episcleral blood vessels, or the anterior chamber invaded by the iris root resulting from erosion, or even retinal detachment, and the patient may present with an anterior uveitis but this is uncommon.

The treatment of choice for ciliary body tumours is enucleation for large melanomas but iridocyclectomy (local resection of the ciliary body) may be undertaken if the tumour does not involve more than one-third of the irido-corneal angle. In selected cases radiotherapy may be the treatment of choice.

Choroidal melanoma

Choroidal melanoma is by far the most frequently diagnosed malignancy of the uveal tract, accounting for about 85% of cases and is the most common primary ocular tumour in adults. The tumour predominantly affects those aged between 50 and 60 years, with only 4% of cases diagnosed in those aged under 30 years.

Patients often have no symptoms until the tumour is quite large and is an incidental finding on ocular examination of the posterior segment, or the patient may present with decreased vision, visual field loss, photopsia or a retinal detachment. The tumour is usually seen as an elevated, oval mass of the choroid which may be pigmented or non-pigmented.

The diagnosis on choroidal melanoma is made only after numerous examinations and investigative tests:

- Ocular examination by slit-lamp with a 60+-D lens, indirect ophthalmoscopy (as long as the ocular media are clear) and transillumination (differentiates between pigmented tumour and dense retinal haemorrhage).
- Fluorescein angiography may assist in diagnosis but does not differentiate between melanoma and other choroidal tumours (haemangiomas).
- Ultrasonography with a 'B scan' is the most helpful tool in detecting ocular tumours.
- Computed tomography has no advantage over a 'B scan' in aiding the diagnosis but does detect any extension of the tumour extraocularly.
- Magnetic resonance imaging.
- Other: colour-coded Doppler imaging and intraocular biopsy.

The treatment of choroidal melanoma remains controversial and each patient should be assessed individually to determine what is the best line of treatment for him or her. The patient's current visual acuity in the affected eye, the size, extent and location of the mass, state of unaffected eye and general health should all be taken into consideration when deciding on a course of treatment/intervention. The aim of any treatment is to retain what vision the patient has, destroy the cancer and prevent recurrence.

There are a variety of treatment options available to patients presenting with choroidal malignant melanoma: enucleation, radioactive plaques, external radiotherapy, photocoagulation, transpupillary thermotherapy and interferon.

Enucleation

This is undertaken if the tumour is extensive, particularly if the patient has lost all sight in the affected eye. It is important during the procedure to avoid any chance of leakage of malignant cells and care must be used by the surgical team during the procedure to prevent this occurring. A prosthesis should be fitted 4–6 weeks after enucleation and the patient must be followed up at regular intervals for possible recurrence of the tumour in the orbit.

Radioactive plaques

These are generally used for treating small- to medium-sized choroidal melanomas and deliver radiotherapy directly to the tumour. There are two types of plaques commonly used – iodine-125 or ruthenium – and it is the ophthalmologist's preference that determines which type of plaque is used. Insertion of the plaque requires a surgical procedure with admission to hospital between usually 1 and 7 days. At the time of surgery the plaque is positioned at the site of the tumour, left in place for a predetermined length of time and then removed during a later surgical procedure. The length of time that a radioactive plaque is left *in situ* is determined by the strength of radiation remaining in the plaque, which defines the required treatment time calculated by an oncology physicist.

Iodine plaques require that more precautions be taken by staff, patients and their families for protection than for the ruthenium plaques; general precautions apply irrespective of what type of 'radiation' is used. The plaques must be stored in the correct lead-lined container, all uses of plaque are logged, and staff providing care for the patient must be provided with radiation monitoring meters and signage warning of radioactive material in use, and have a Geiger counter available. Referral should be made to local hospital policies for specifics.

External radiotherapy

This treatment is undertaken using conventional radiotherapy machines and aims to cause as little damage as possible to surrounding healthy tissue. Therefore, before the radiotherapy a minor surgical procedure is undertaken to attach 'tags' to specific parts of the eye, which act as 'markers' to isolate the area to be treated. The treatment is given over several days in small doses.

Photocoagulation

A laser can be used to seal the blood supply of a tumour but this treatment modality is suitable only for very small melanomas. The patient requires several treatments.

Transpupillary thermotherapy

This is a relatively new laser treatment option for ocular melanomas; it can be used to treat small tumours and may be used together with radiotherapy, but is not readily available in all countries. The transpupillary thermotherapy laser heats the tumour cells, which are more susceptible to heat than normal cells, and destroys them. The patient requires several treatments.

Interferon

Although it is uncertain what interferon may offer in the treatment of ocular melanoma, it is being looked at as a possible future treatment option.

Complications from treatment of ocular melanomas include the following, particularly for treatments involving radioactive material:

- Telangiectasisas: permanent dilatation of superficial capillaries and vessels.
- Keratinization: a process by which the epithelial cells of the cornea are exposed to the external environment, lose moisture and are replaced by horny tissue.
- Corneal vascularization: occurs when corneal tissue becomes vascular and develops proliferating capillaries.
- Radiation retinopathy: changes in retinal vessels resulting from exposure to radiation.
- Radiation cataract: results from exposure to radiation.

Nursing care of patients with ocular melanoma

The role of the nurse in treating patients with ocular melanoma is varied, ranging from providing routine outpatient clinic care to specialist nursing roles within the service to those who provide care to patients throughout the continuum (clinic, ward and sometimes operating rooms). Perhaps the most important role of the nurse is providing support for the patient and the family and ensuring that they are cognisant with all procedures and processes in their care.

As with any patient with a diagnosis of cancer, there are fears experienced by patients and their families that must be dealt with. The nurse is ideally situated to recognize patient concerns, provide support, act as advocate at every decision point for treatment options and refer to appropriate specialist services within oncology if required.

References

American Academy of Ophthalmology (2003) Intraocular Inflammation and Uveitis. San Francisco, CA: AAO.

Antcliff RJ, Spalton DJ, Stanford MR, Graham EM, ffytche TJ, Marshall J (2001) Intravitreal triamcinolone for uveitic cystoid macular edema: an optical coherence tomography study. Ophthalmology 108: 765–72.

Holland GN, Stiehm ER (2003) Special considerations in the evaluation and management of uveitis in children. Am J Ophthalmol 135: 867–78.

Kaklamani VG, Kaklamanis PG (2001) Treatment if Behçet's disease – an update. Semin Arthr Rheum 30: 299–312.

Kanski JJ (2003) Clinical Ophthalmology, 5th edn. London: Butterworth-Heinemann.

Newell FW (1996) Ophthalmology: Principles and concepts, 8th edn. St Louis, MO: Mosby.

CHAPTER TWENTY

The angle and aqueous

AGNES LEE

The drainage system of the eye

To understand glaucoma, it is important first to consider the drainage system of the eye and aqueous dynamics. Abnormalities of the drainage system and the imbalance between the production and drainage of aqueous can lead to glaucoma.

The drainage system includes the anterior and posterior chamber, trabecular meshwork and canal of Schlemm (Figure 20.1).

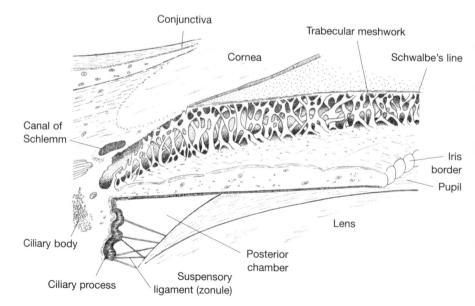

Figure 20.1 The angle and related structures.

420

The anterior chamber

This is a space that is bounded anteriorly by the inner surface of the cornea and posteriorly by the anterior face of the ciliary body, the iris and the lens. The area where the inner cornea meets the iris is known as the angle and is the location for the trabecular meshwork (Snell and Lemp 1998). The depth of the anterior chamber is 2.6–4.4 mm and this decreases by 0.06 mm per year of life. The anterior chamber deepens, in general, by 0.06 mm for each dioptre of myopia and its average volume is 220 µl. It is filled with aqueous humour secreted by the ciliary processes. The blood supply to the anterior segment is shown in Figure 20.2.

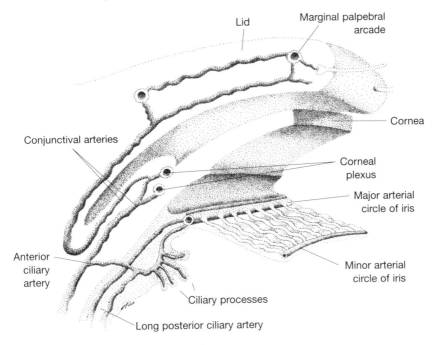

Figure 20.2 Blood supply to the anterior segment.

The posterior chamber

This is bounded anteriorly by the iris peripherally and the ciliary process-es and posteriorly by the lens and the suspensory ligaments (Snell and Lemp 1998). Aqueous first enters the posterior chamber and flows through the pupil into the anterior chamber.

Trabecular meshwork

This is a sponge-like porous network of connective tissue beams arranged as sheets and consisting of three portions: uveal meshwork, corneoscleral and juxtacanalicular. The uveal meshwork portion lies closest to aqueous humour and this portion extends from the ciliary body in the angle recess to Schwalbe's line. The uveal meshwork covers the anterior face of the ciliary body, the scleral spur and the trabecular meshwork. The corneoscleral portion extends from the scleral spur to Schwalbe's line. The endothelial portion (also known as the juxtacanalicular meshwork) is the deepest layer within the trabecular meshwork and is the last layer that the aqueous crosses before entering Schlemm's canal. This canal offers the most resistance to aqueous outflow and consists of endothelial cells, the primary function of which is to digest foreign materials after which the cells migrate away from the trabecular beams into Schlemm's canal. With age and repeated insult, the endothelial cells decrease and so does the flow of aqueous through the trabecular meshwork. Endothelial cells lining the trabecular meshwork have larger and less prominent cells borders than corneal endothelial cells.

Canal of Schlemm

This is a vein-like tube containing septa located at the base of the scleral sulcus. If the intraocular pressure (IOP) is high, the canal can collapse, so subsequently resistance to outflow increases. Its primary function is to collect aqueous from the trabecular meshwork and it drains aqueous into the venous circulation.

Longitudinal muscles situated in the ciliary body open the canal by pulling on the scleral spur (made out of ring of collagen fibres running parallel to the limbus).

Aqueous humour including production

Aqueous humour or 'aqueous' is a clear fluid produced by the non-pigmented portion of the ciliary processes through active secretion, ultra-filtration and diffusion. It is derived from plasma but unlike plasma contains no protein. It contains predominantly water with electrolytes, glucose, amino acids, high concentration of ascorbic acid and dissolved gases and provides nourishment for the posterior cornea and lens as well as maintenance of the shape of the eyeball. The rate of aqueous flow is 2–6 μl/min and turnover in the eye is less than 2 hours.

Aqueous humour drainage

There are two routes of drainage: trabecular and uveoscleral routes. The trabecular route accounts for 90% of aqueous drainage. Aqueous flows from the anterior chamber into the trabecular meshwork and Schlemm's canal and is drained by the episcleral veins. This is a pressure-sensitive route in that increasing the pressure will increase outflow. Trabecular outflow can be increased by drugs such as miotics, sympathomimetics, laser trabeculoplasty and trabeculectomy.

The uveoscleral route accounts for the remaining 10% of aqueous outflow. Aqueous passes across the ciliary body into the suprachoroidal space (space between the sclera and choroid) and is drained away by the venous circulation in the ciliary body, choroid and sclera. Uveoscleral outflow can be decreased by miotics, and increased by atropine sympathomimetics and prostaglandin analogues.

A very small amount of aqueous is also drained away via the corneal endothelium, iris vessels and anterior vitreous surface (Kanski 2003).

Pathological resistance to outflow can be the result of an increase in the thickness of trabecular sheets caused by an accumulation of collagen and basement membrane material, as well as a decrease in the number of trabecular cells.

Understanding intraocular pressure (aqueous dynamics)

Three factors determine the level of IOP:

1. The rate of aqueous secretion by the ciliary processes.
2. The resistance encountered by the drainage of aqueous through the trabecular meshwork.
3. The level of episcleral venous pressure: the episcleral venous pressure is normally relatively stable, except when resulting from alterations in body positions and in certain diseases of the head, neck and orbit. This in turn will obstruct the venous return to the heart or shunt blood from the arterial to the venous system.

According to Alward (2000), a wide range of normal IOPs exists. Pooled data from large epidemiological studies indicate that the mean IOP is about 16 mmHg, with a standard deviation of 3 mmHg (American Academy of Ophthalmology or AAO 2001).

Intraocular pressure can be influenced in the following circumstances:

- time of day (it is higher in the morning and lower in the afternoon and evening – the diurnal curve)
- heartbeat
- respiration
- blood pressure

- age
- sleep
- exercise
- race
- thickness of the cornea (a thicker cornea will give a higher IOP reading and vice versa)
- refractive error
- topical and systemic drugs
- fluid intake
- caffeine
- alcohol
- cannabis.

For these reasons, a single IOP reading is not a sufficient base for a diagnosis of glaucoma.

Glaucoma

The term 'glaucosis' is derived from ancient Greek, meaning cloudy or blue-green hue, and over the years the concept of glaucoma has been extensively refined to the present day.

Glaucoma is a large group of disorders that are characterized by widely diverse clinical and pathological denominators. It is a silent progressive disease and is one of the leading preventable diseases if arrested before significant effects on vision occur. The common denominators of all glaucomas are optic neuropathy, visual field loss and irreversible blindness. One of the risk factors associated with most types of glaucoma is a raised IOP.

Classification of glaucoma

The classification of glaucoma depends on the following factors:

- According to the appearance of the drainage angle (open or closed).
- Presence of any other factors that may contribute to the rise in IOP.
- Primary glaucoma has no other ocular disorders associated with a rise in IOP.
- Secondary glaucoma is associated with another condition such as inflammation, neovascular disease, etc. and accounts for one-third of all glaucoma cases.

Primary open-angle glaucoma

Epidemiology

Primary open-angle glaucoma (POAG) is the most common form of glaucoma in the UK. Glaucoma is also the second leading cause of blindness worldwide. An estimated 13.5 million people may have glaucoma and 5.2 million of those may be blind. It is the leading cause of blindness in African–American individuals in the USA. It is responsible for 12% of blind registration in the UK and the USA. There are a number of risks factors associated with POAG.

Raised IOP
An increase in IOP is a risk factor associated with the development of the disease, and is not the disease in itself. According to Alward (2000), when the IOP is > 21 mmHg, the risk of developing POAG increases 16-fold when compared with eyes in which the IOP is < 16 mmHg.

Ethnicity
Ethnicity affects both the chance of an individual developing glaucoma and the prognosis of his or her disease. The Barbados Eye Study (Leske et al. 1994) highlighted the public health importance of POAG in the African–Caribbean region. The prevalence of POAG by self-reported race was 7.0% in black, 3.3% in mixed-race and 0.8% (1 in 33) in white or other participants. In black and mixed-race participants, the prevalence reached 12% at age 60 years and older and was higher in men (8.3%) than in women, with an age-adjusted male:female ratio of 1.4. Among participants aged 50 years old or older, one in eleven had POAG and prevalence increased to one in six at age 70 years or older.

Age
It affects 1 in 200 of the general population over the age of 40 years and the incidence increases with age. Population-based studies show that the prevalence of POAG ranges from 0.4% to 8.8% in those aged over 40 years. POAG is uncommon before the age of 40. Budde and Jonas (1999) reported that patients with the familial form of glaucoma often have a younger age of disease onset. Both males and females are equally affected.

Inheritance
There is little doubt that familial factors play an important role in POAG. First-degree relatives of POAG patients run a 4–16% risk of developing glaucoma compared with 1–2% for the general population (Alward 2000). The Barbados Family Study (Leske et al. 2001) found a high prevalence of open-angle glaucoma in Barbados and identified family history of glaucoma as a major risk factor. Everyone with a positive family history should undergo an annual IOP check.

In addition to family history, certain genes have been implicated in POAG. Recent studies (Tarwara et al. 2000) reported the discovery of gene *GLC1A* or *MYOC* which produces a protein called myocilin. Myocilin has been detected in several ocular tissues such as the trabecular meshwork, ciliary body and retina. A genetic marker, endothelial leukocyte adhesion molecule 1 (ELAM-1), has also been identified, which could predict the chances of developing glaucoma. The ELAM-1 molecule is found to be the earliest marker for arteriosclerosis.

Myopia

Some studies have demonstrated a correlation between myopia and POAG. It must be acknowledged that some selection bias could have occurred because myopic patients are more likely to attend for their regular optometry examinations than their counterparts who are emmetropic.

Diabetes mellitus

Several older studies have demonstrated a higher prevalence of elevated mean IOP and POAG among patients with diabetes compared with non-diabetic patients. Tielsch et al. (1995), however, found very little link between diabetes and POAG. Klein et al. (1994) found older-onset diabetes (> 30 years of age) was associated with a modest increase in the risk of glaucoma. A more recent study (Ellis et al. 1999) found a strong relationship between patients with diabetes and ocular hypertension. However, they acknowledged that the increased health-care contact in patients with diabetes can lead to an increased detection of glaucoma and ocular hypertension. Gordon et al. (2002) noted that the presence of diabetes seemed to protect patients against developing glaucoma. This finding is controversial because it is thought that patients with diabetes are prone to small vessel involvement; the optic disc of patients with diabetes is therefore more susceptible to pressure-related damage.

Other risk factors

A history of migraine or cold hands and feet (a condition associated with vasospasm), Raynaud's phenomenon, is one of the risk factors and may play a role in the development of POAG. Other risk factors include systemic hypertension, systemic hypotension with nocturnal pressure drops and smoking, which are associated with an increased risk in some studies. Table 20.1 lists the risk factors.

Pathophysiology of POAG

There are multiple theories about how IOP can be one of the factors that initiates glaucomatous damage in a patient's optic nerve. The exact cause of glaucomatous optic nerve damage is unknown and is probably the result of a combination of factors. It is thought that the increase in IOP increases

Table 20.1 Summary – classic risk factors for POAG

Strong association	Intraocular pressure
	Age
	Ethnicity
	Family history
Moderate Association	Diabetes
	Myopia
Weak association	Vasospasm
	Migraine
	Systemic hypertension

From Harvey (1998).

vascular resistance, thereby causing decreased vascular perfusion of the optic nerve and ischaemia. The increased pressure can also cause impaired axoplasmic flow in the ganglion cell axons resulting in aponeurosis and cell dysfunction. As the ganglion cells die, the neuroretinal rim of the optic nerve thins and the optic cup enlarges. This is known as glaucomatous cupping. The increased pressure can also cause mechanical dysfunction by compressing the lamina cribrosa, a sieve-like structure through which the axons pass.

The cause of elevated IOP is generally accepted to be a decreased facility of aqueous outflow through the trabecular meshwork. The increased resistance to the outflow can be associated with the following:

- Age and increased loss of trabecular endothelial cells
- Obstruction of the trabecular meshwork
- Loss of normal phagocytic activity
- Loss of giant vacuoles in the inner wall endothelium and a reduction in the trabecular pore density and size in the inner wall endothelium of Schlemm's canal.

Patients with POAG are usually asymptomatic at presentation; the suspicious features are usually detected by an optometrist and include a rise in IOP measured on several occasions, optic disc changes and visual field defects. Optic disc changes in glaucoma include asymmetry of the neuroretinal rim or cupping and asymmetry of the cup:disc ratio between the two eyes. Other features may include localized thinning or notching of the rim, optic disc haemorrhage and vasculature abnormalities.

A systematic assessment of a patient with POAG

All new patients presenting to the outpatient department as glaucoma suspects should be methodically assessed. Building a good rapport with patients should be the starting point of any assessment because this is crucial in obtaining a complete history with valid information. An ability to be a good listener as well as professional approachability are essential. All new patients with POAG should have:

- a comprehensive medical, surgical and ophthalmic history (including family history)
- social assessment including any disability which might hinder concordance/compliance in treatment
- slit-lamp examination: anterior segment, IOP measurement, gonioscopy and fundal examination, including optic disc and retinal nerve fibre examination
- measurement of anterior chamber by van Herick's or Smith's method
- pupillary examination for relative afferent pupillary defect
- pachymetry
- optic disc assessment
- visual field examination
- optic disc photographs.

Investigations

Slit-lamp examination
This is the same as for any other patient; glaucoma-specific findings might include the following:

- Lids: port wine stain (which may accompany Sturge–Weber syndrome) or naevi
- Cornea: Krukenberg's spindle (a line of deposited pigment on the endothelium, indicative of pigment dispersion syndrome), flecks of extra tissue which may indicate pseudoexfoliation syndrome
- Anterior chamber depth is important and the angle should be assessed
- Iris: transillumination defects may suggest pigment dispersion syndrome, posterior synechiae, new vessels on the iris (rubeosis), deposition of pseudoexfoliative material, heterochromia, iris atrophy, evidence of trauma
- Pupils: differing responses may indicate damage to the optic disc
- Lens: deposition of pigment, pseudoexfoliative material, red blood cells. Anterior capsule opacities may indicate a previous attack of angle-closure glaucoma (*glaukomflecken*).

Pupillary assessment
It is important to evaluate the pupillary reaction between the two eyes because a relative afferent pupillary defect may indicate that there is an inequality in the severity of glaucomatous optic nerve damage between the two eyes of a patient. Careful evaluation and documentation serve as a baseline for future evaluations.

Measuring the IOP

Accurate measurement of the IOP is extremely important in the management of glaucoma patients. In the Collaborative Normal Tension
Glaucoma Study (1998), eyes that had a reduction in IOP of 30% had a
lower rate of visual field progression than those eyes that did not have
their IOP lowered. Grant and Burke, as far back as 1982, made a retrospective study of the long-term interrelationships of IOP, stage of
glaucomatous damage and progressive visual field loss, and commented
that the worse the eye is on first presentation, the lower the pressure needs
to be to prevent further loss or blindness.

The measurement of IOP is based on the Imbert–Fick principle which
states that, in an ideal, dry, thin-walled sphere, the pressure inside the
sphere (P) is equal to the force necessary to flatten the surface (F) divided
by the area (A) of flattening calculated thus: $P = F/A$.

In the eye, a force is applied to the cornea to flatten a specific area of
it and the Imbert–Fick principle is used to calibrate instruments to calculate the pressure inside the globe.

The area of flattening by a prism in Goldmann applanation tonometry
(the gold standard) is 3.06 mm of cornea. The cornea is flattened and the
IOP determined by measuring the applanating force and the area flattened. The force necessary to flatten the cornea is adjusted on a drum
wheel on the instrument and measured in gram force pressure. The gram
force is converted to millimetres of mercury (the international standard
units for pressure measurement) by multiplying the force by 10.

Other methods of intraocular measurements include the following:

- 'Air puff' tonometry which is widely use by community optometrists.
  This non-contact tonometer uses a pulsed jet of air to deform the
  corneal apex. This method carries less risk of cross-infection and is useful in mass screening. It is less accurate than Goldmann tonometry and
  the sudden burst of air can cause the patient to jump and inadvertent-
  ly give a higher IOP reading.
- 'Tonopen': a light portable instrument that applanates a small area of
  cornea. It is useful for immobile or poorly compliant patients. The
  Tonopen has an in-built software that automatically self-calibrates after
  each use and selects the acceptable measurements. It takes the average
  of three 'good' readings and rejects the inappropriate readings. It is
  slightly less accurate than the Goldmann tonometer.
- Schiøtz tonometer: rarely used in developed countries. A preset weight
  is placed on the tonometer which is then placed on the anaesthetized
  cornea. The amount the plunger sinks is measured off the scale and the
  reading is converted to millimetres of mercury from a conversion table.
  This can be used only in a recumbent patient.

- The Perkins' tonometer: a hand-held tonometer that is based on the same principle as the Goldman tonometer. It is useful for bed-bound, anaesthetized patients or patients who are impossible to examine on the slit-lamp. This instrument may be difficult to master initially.
- Digital tonometry: a crude method of measuring how 'hard' the affected eye is in comparison to the normal 'softer' eye by gently palpating the eyeball using the first finger of each hand.

Tonometer readings can be affected by:

- tight collars
- breath holding
- thick or thin corneas
- astigmatism > 3 D
- pressure against the globe from the operator's finger when holding the patient's upper lid
- Valsalva's manoeuvre
- squeezing of the eyelids
- corneal refractive surgery
- inaccurately calibrated tonometer.

Excessive fluorescein results in wide mires, giving an artificially high IOP reading, or insufficient fluorescein with an extremely thin mire, giving an artificially low IOP reading.

Step-by-step guide to measuring IOP using the Goldmann tonometer

This is used together with the slit-lamp. The tonometer consists of two main parts: (1) a small Perspex cylinder that is applied to the eye by (2) a lever attached to a coiled spring, the tension of which is controlled by a calibrated drum at the side of the instrument. Extreme care should be taken when handling the tonometer to avoid damage to the spring-loaded device. It is good practice to calibrate the tonometer before each clinic or at the very least weekly to ensure accurate IOP measurement. Any defective tonometer (> 2 mmHg on calibration) must be sent away for repair.

Method

- A clear, concise explanation is given to the patient to ensure cooperation. Putting the patient at ease also makes measurement much easier.
- Contact lenses should be removed and minims lidocaine (lignocaine)/ fluorescein or proxymetacaine/fluorescein drops instilled into each eye.
- The tonometer prism is sterilized in lens cleaning solution according to local policy. The use of disposable prisms or prism covers is good practice to minimize the spread of infections.
- The prism should be placed in the clip at the end of the tonometer arm. During the attachment of the prism to the tonometer arm, the lever should be supported with a finger to minimize damage to the

spring lever. The prism is placed with the 0 aligned with the white mark on the clip. In patients with astigmatism of 3 D or more, readings should be taken with the bi-prism horizontally and vertically and the two readings averaged. To take the vertical reading, the prism is aligned to the red mark (about 43°) on the tonometer arm.

- The tonometer calibration arm is turned to 1 so that the arm is exerting a slight forward pressure.
- The complete tonometer is placed on the mounting plate on the viewing arm of the slit-lamp and the slit-lamp magnification is set to 10 × with a blue filter in place.
- The illuminating arm of the slit-lamp is placed at an angle of 60° to the slit-lamp.
- The patient should be instructed to look straight ahead and the slit-lamp advanced until a bright blue hue is seen just before touching the apex of the cornea. Up to this point it is best observed by the observer from the side. If the patient is unable to keep the eyes from blinking, the lids can be held open provided that the supporting fingers do not exert any pressure on the eye.
- While looking down the viewing piece of the slit-lamp microscope, the tonometer prism is brought gently into contact with the cornea. As there are two prisms within the tonometer head, on contact with the cornea, two half-circles are seen through the tonometer, adjacent to each other. The two half-circles must be symmetrically placed on the apex of the cornea. It is important that the slit-lamp be pulled slightly away from the cornea should any fine adjustment be needed. This is to minimize any corneal epithelial damage.
- The calibrated wheel is turned until the half-circles just overlap.
- The IOP is read when the inside edges of the half-circles are just touching.

The IOP in the individual varies over the course of a day (diurnal variation) and patients may need a series of readings, taken over the course of a day (phasing or day phasing) to determine the range of pressures particular to their eyes. Figure 20.3 shows the correct placement of mires when undertaking Goldmann applanation tonometry.

Pachymetry
The accurate measurement of IOP is a cornerstone of the diagnosis and management of glaucoma. The influence of corneal thickness on IOP measurements using Goldmann applanation tonometry measurement is well recognized. Research has shown that a thick cornea can cause an elevated IOP reading whereas a thin cornea can give a false reading. Central corneal thickness should be taken into account when assessing the risk for the development of glaucomatous damage among ocular hypertension

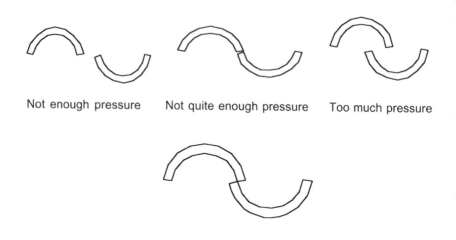

Not enough pressure   Not quite enough pressure   Too much pressure

Perfect amount of pressure exerted on the
cornea by the prism — read off the figure
indicated on the dial

Figure 20.3 Correct placement of mires when undertaking applanation tonometry.

patients. Underestimation of IOP as a result of lower corneal thickness
might led to under-recognition of glaucoma. It has been suggested that a
thin cornea could possibly also have a thin lamina cribrosa or perhaps a
more susceptible optic nerve.

Studies have also shown that patients who have had photorefractive
keratectomy and laser *in situ* keratomileusis have shown significantly lower
IOP measurements. Other pathological corneal variations causing an
alteration in the IOP included corneal oedema, corneal scars, keratoconus, flat anterior chamber, penetrating keratoplasty, bandage contact
lenses, and patients with pituitary adenoma and resultant acromegaly.

Measuring corneal thickness should be a routine procedure to be performed on all patients suspected of having POAG. Pachymetry should be
done before gonioscopy.

Measuring the width of the angle

Van Herick's system is a method of estimating the angle width by making
use of the slit-lamp. This system was devised by van Herick, who felt that
it was too impractical to perform the angle width using direct gonioscopy
and that gonioscopy should be carried out only in cases of extremely narrow angles.

To estimate the angle width, an optic section (narrow slit beam) is placed near the corneal limbus with the light source at 60°. The examiner then compares the depth of the anterior chamber with the thickness of the cornea. If the anterior chamber is thicker than the cornea, the angle is incapable of closure and is thus graded a 4 (wide open angle). The angle is graded a 3 if the anterior chamber depth is between a half and a quarter of the corneal thickness. The angle remains incapable of closure. However, if the thickness of visible aqueous is a quarter (grade 2) or less (grade 1) of the corneal thickness, the angle is probably in danger of closure. A slit (grade 0) indicates that the angle is extremely narrow and that closure is imminent.

Gonioscopy

All patients with suspected glaucoma should undergo gonioscopy examination (Figure 20.4). Gonioscopy is performed to assess and identify the following:

- the drainage angle
- estimation of the width of the chamber angle – open/closed angle
- abnormal angle structures
- the effect of anterior chamber-deepening procedure.

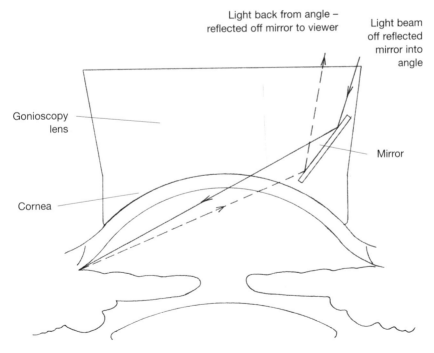

Figure 20.4 Single-mirror gonioscopy lens.

The angle of the anterior chamber cannot be visualized directly so a complex lens is placed onto the cornea, enabling the operator to direct light into the angle and thus see its structures, as a result of the placement of reflecting surfaces in the lens.

This lens is generally called a goniolens and there are a number of different types. The most common ones used are the triple mirror or single mirror Goldmann goniolens or the Zeiss goniolens. The Goldmann lenses require a 'coupling fluid', usually a carbomer gel, which is placed onto the lens before it is placed on the cornea. This forms the interface between the cornea and the lens. Although not painful, this may be an uncomfortable procedure and topical anaesthetic is instilled into the patient's eye to remove corneal sensation. Adequate explanation of the procedure will help the patient to cooperate.

In an ideal world, gonioscopy should be carried out at yearly intervals because it cannot be assumed that the angle configuration will remain constant. When a patient ages, cataracts can develop and cause a pupillary block, and the angle becomes more shallow or even closes in some instances.

The following are the angle structures that can be visualized from a gonioscopy examination:

- Posterior surface of the cornea.
- Schwalbe's line (the point where the cornea and trabecular meshwork meet): a build-up of pigmentation on Schwalbe's line is known as Sampaolesi's line.
- The trabeculum (stretches from Schwalbe's line to scleral spur): divided into two parts – anterior non-pigmented part and posterior pigmented part. Trabecular pigmentation may be visible.
- The scleral spur: most anterior part of the sclera and seen as a shiny band on gonioscopy.
- The ciliary body lies posterior to the scleral spur and appears as a dull brown/slate-grey band.
- Schlemm's canal can occasionally be seen as a darker line deep to the trabeculum.
- Iris processes: thin extensions of the iris that insert into the scleral spur.
- Radial blood vessels are often seen in healthy eyes.

Angle width grading
The angle is graded according to structures seen and grading allows an estimation of the likelihood of angle closure (Kanski 2003):

- Grade 4: ciliary body easily seen and this angle cannot close.
- Grade 3: scleral spur is visible and this angle cannot close.
- Grade 2: trabecular meshwork seen and this angle may close but it is unlikely.

- Grade 1: Schwalbe's line and top of trabecular meshwork are visible and this represents a high angle-closure risk.
- Slit angle: which is in danger of imminent closure.
- Grade 0: a closed angle.

Abnormal angle findings
- Abnormal angle blood vessels which may be rubeotic glaucoma.
- Increased pigmentation of the angle which may indicate pigment dispersion, pseudoexfoliation.
- Peripheral anterior synechiae, which are adhesions of the iris to the angle which prevent aqueous drainage.
- Angle recession as a result of blunt trauma.

Optic disc assessment
Primary angle-closure glaucoma causes damage and loss of ganglion cell axons, leading to changes in the optic nerve head and nerve fibre layer. Significant nerve fibre damage and ganglion cell loss can precede any visual field defect and so the detection of any early pathological signs in the nerve fibre layer and optic nerve head will enable the ophthalmologist to come to an early diagnosis. Documentation of the appearance of the optic disc at the time of the first clinical assessment and subsequent follow-up is as important as coloured optic disc photographs (Figure 20.5).

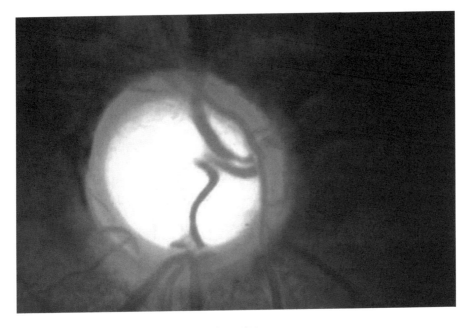

Figure 20.5 Cupped optic disc. (See Plate 47.)

Examination and assessment of the optic nerve head should take into account the following:

- Size
- Symmetry
- Shape/contour
- Colour
- Cup:disc ratio – progressive enlargement or deepening of the cup, asymmetry and vertical elongation all give rise to suspicions of glaucomatous changes
- Thickness of rim-localized nerve rim thinning, known as notching, is significant and this corresponds to visual field changes and nerve fibre layer loss
- Vasculature
- Depth
- Peripapillary atrophy (PPA): caused by poor perfusion from the short posterior ciliary arteries producing visible PPA of the choroid and retinal pigment epithelial layer
- Any haemorrhages, found most commonly temporally and in patients with normal tension glaucoma
- Nerve fibre layer: defects may be visible.

One of the biggest drawbacks when it comes to assessing the optic disc is the huge variation in the appearance of both the normal and the abnormal disc (Alward 2000). The other problem associated with the assessment of the optic disc is that often the early changes in the optic disc are subtle and can also occur within the range of normal diversity and therefore be easily missed even with careful and accurate documentation of the disc. Currently there is no quick, simple, easy, inexpensive, specific and sensitive method of optic nerve head analysis by which glaucoma can be easily and reliably diagnosed and all subtle progression noted.

The assessment of the optic disc routinely employs the direct ophthalmoscope or more commonly the slit-lamp biomicroscopy combined with an indirect lens such as a 90-D, 78-D or 66-D lens. Drawing the optic disc, measuring the vertical height of the disc and estimating the cup:disc ratio will all have to be incorporated in the patient's record.

When the optic disc is being assessed for signs of glaucomatous changes, it must be compared with a presumed previous appearance or prior documented evidence (Pawson and Vernon 1995). Four basic patterns of glaucomatous damage are:

- concentric enlargement of the cup
- notching (focal extension of the cup)

- development of an acquired pit
- development of pallor of the neuroretinal rim.

In addition to these, the examiner must look for other changes in the optic disc such as 'nasal excavation' which is a form of concentric enlargement of the disc. During this excavation process, 'overpass' or 'flyover' vessels may occur. In this scenario, the appearance of a flyover vessel is caused by unsupported neural tissue and the vessels appear suspended over the cup. Normal blood vessels usually follow the contour of the cup as it crosses the disc.

Peripapillary atrophy has also been noted in eyes with maximal excavation of the optic disc. Optic nerve head haemorrhages occurring at the disc margin can predate future excavation, especially in patients with suspected normal tension glaucoma.

It is also important to examine the nerve fibre layers (NFLs) at the same time because the NFL defects may precede visual field defects by as much as 5 years.

Visual field

The visual field is the extent of the area that the eye can see – 'an island of vision surrounded by a sea of darkness' (Kanski 2003). The visual field extends around 50° superiorly, 70° inferiorly, 60° nasally and 90° temporally. Vision is sharpest at the fovea and reduces gradually towards the periphery of the visual field. There is a single area within the visual field where there is no vision. This is the blind spot and represents the optic nerve head. As the size and brightness (luminance) of a point are decreased, the visual field within which it can be seen gets smaller in a series of concentric rings called isopters.

Effects of glaucoma on the visual field One of the features of glaucoma is a reduction in the visual field. There are a number of contributory factors but essentially this is the result of damage to optic nerve fibres caused by a combination of pressure-induced vascular disease of the optic nerve head and direct pressure on the axons passing through the lamina cribrosa, disrupting the axoplasmic flow. Several IOP-independent variables have been found to be associated with glaucomatous field loss, such as disc haemorrhage, altered and disadvantageous blood flow, and haemodynamic characteristics. Nerve fibre bundles passing on to the optic nerve head on the temporal side of the disc, above or below the horizontal, are selectively damaged, resulting in paracentral defects in the nasal visual field (scotomata) which eventually merge to form an arc-shaped area of vision loss (arcuate scotoma). As glaucoma progresses, the cup in the optic nerve head becomes larger with a correspondingly enlarged field defect resulting, eventually, in a small island of central vision and an island of vision on the temporal side that also disappears.

Perimetry

Perimetry can be extremely useful in diagnosing patients with glaucoma as well as determining its progression. Perimetry is a way of evaluating the visual field in a standardized way, attempting to remove all possible variables of patient response and reaction. There is no test that can control for all human variables, however, and the patient should be taken into account when interpreting perimetry results.

Dynamic perimetry involves a moving stimulus of known size and brightness that comes from a non-seeing into a seeing area until it is perceived by the patient. The stimulus is brought into the visual field along straight meridian, often corresponding to clock hours, and the point at which it is perceived by the patient is plotted on a chart. Different sizes and intensities of stimulus can be used for different plots so that the concentric field isopters can be identified. There are a number of ways of undertaking kinetic perimetry, including confrontation where the patient sits opposite the clinician with one eye occluded, fixes the other eye on the eye of the clinician (who can then see any lack of fixation) and tells the clinician when the stimulus comes into view. Other strategies include the tangent screen and the Goldmann perimeter.

Static perimetry forms a three-dimensional assessment of both the visual field and the different light sensitivities of different areas of retina. Static perimetry involves showing the patient static stimuli of varying luminance in the same position. Suprathreshold perimetry (such as Henson's) is often used for screening and presents targets over the normal threshold to the patient. Targets that are noticed indicate areas of grossly normal function; missed targets indicate areas of lowered sensitivity. Threshold perimetry can then be undertaken to quantify the missed areas.

Accurate perimetry takes commitment on behalf of the patient, who needs to fix on a target and remain alert throughout the process, which may be quite difficult. It is for this reason that the patient should always be taken into account along with the printout from any machine. Factors that can affect all visual field testing include patient fatigue or lack of concentration, the spectacle frame, miosis (from pilocarpine drops) and opacities of the ocular media such as cataract.

Goldmann kinetic perimetry The flexible and interactive nature of this form of perimetry makes the test more suitable for those patients unable to cope with automated techniques. Criteria for referring patients include patients with gross visual field loss such as those with extensive retinitis pigmentosa, very extensive glaucoma defects or for the assessment of functional fields in visually impaired individuals. The use of full-threshold fields is probably advisable in the optic neuropathies, provided the central acuity is sufficient, i.e. 6/60 or better. However, Goldmann perimetry is recommended for chiasmal or post-chiasmal field defects or in selected cases of anterior pathway lesions with poorer acuity.

Henson's suprathreshold perimetry Perimetrists will use the extended Henson's 136-point examination, which is an excellent threshold testing for the detection of defects. As this test is much quicker and easier for the patients to comply with (in addition to having a more patient–perimetrist-centred interaction), it may also be a more suitable strategy for those patients in whom concentration may otherwise be a problem. For more serious concentration difficulties, Goldmann perimetry is still recommended. The criteria for referring patients for Henson's suprathreshold perimetry include all new patients in whom visual fields are indicated and follow-up patients who do not manifest a defect or patients at 'low risk' of developing field loss. Suprathreshold perimetry will also be useful for patients in whom static perimetry is desirable, but who have difficulty complying with the lengthy full-threshold testing.

Humphrey: threshold strategies Humphrey's perimeter consists of a white bowl with low background illumination. Target size and luminance of targets on this background can be altered. Only the luminance is altered while the test is in progress. The stimuli are accompanied by sound. The patient must fix on a target for a considerable period of time while stimuli are shown to them. Humphrey's perimeter gives a reliability index for the patient log with the printout, which includes fixation losses and false negatives and positives. A target is presented to where the physiological blind spot should be if the patient were fixating. If they respond, a fixation loss is recorded. A false positive is recoded when a sound is presented without an accompanying visual stimulus and the patient responds; a highly false-positive score indicates an unreliable field. False negatives are indicated when the machine presents a brighter stimulus at an area where a positive has already been indicated and no response is given. This may indicate inattention on behalf of the patient.

Other tests include confocal laser scanning ophthalmoscope, pulsatile ocular blood flow and ultrasound Doppler velocimetry.

Lasers: other diagnostic uses in glaucoma
Retinal nerve fibre layer analysis (RNFLA) can be seen as complementary to IOP measurements, visual field analysis and optic disc photographs. RNFLA can be used as a diagnostic tool to quantify damage to the optic disc and NFL. Three main devices currently available for retinal nerve fibre analysis are optical coherence tomography (OCT), scanning laser ophthalmoscopy such as the Heidelberg retinal tomograph and nerve fibre analysers such as the GDX. The retinal thickness analyser works by projecting a narrow slit (20 µm) of green light on the fundus and the

image is acquired on digital fundus camera. The image thus represents an optical cross-section of the retina and the computer algorithm provided will register the thickness maps of the posterior pole and surrounding peripapillary areas. The RNFLA gives a measurement of macular NFL thickness and the optic nerve (and cup) contour.

The OCT is primarily a retinal tool and uses the principle of index of refraction; the images are produced by detecting differences in the reflectivity of vitreous, e.g. between the vitreous and internal limiting membrane. When used for retinal imaging, 500 points are scanned in a line to form a cross-sectional image. OCT is effective at detecting macular holes, cysts and tumours (surface and retinal pathologies). However, patient dilatation is necessary and OCT is expensive. It is also a large unit and not portable.

Confocal scanning laser ophthalmoscopy uses scanning laser and moving pinhole aperture to acquire multiple image planes and creates a three-dimensional image to determine the optic disc and retinal topography. The edge of the disc is marked by the operator. Subjective marking also determines the cup (area below the retinal surface, red), neuroretinal rim (at the surface, green) and area of slope (blue). The gives information about NFL thickness and quantitative information about the cup is also generated. Retinal topography (contour analysis) indirectly measures the RNFL thickness and requires a reference plane for all measurements.

Making the diagnosis of POAG

When considering the diagnosis of a patient with POAG, the following features may be in evidence:

- Elevated IOP on more than one occasion
- Glaucomatous optic nerve changes
- Typical visual field defects
- May affect only one eye initially.

Some ophthalmologists would wait for evidence of progressive change in disc or field appearance before making the diagnosis. Other options to consider are:

- Glaucoma suspected: only one suspicious feature
- Ocular hypertension: raised IOP but no disc or field changes
- Normal tension glaucoma: normal IOP but optic disc and visual field changes
- Secondary open-angle glaucoma
- Angle-closure glaucoma that may be asymptomatic if it is chronic.

Usually if there are optic disc changes and typical visual field defects are present, treatment for glaucoma is commenced. However, if there is insufficient information to diagnose POAG, repeat assessment for signs of progression will be undertaken. In glaucoma suspects or ocular hypertensive patients, assessments are repeated and the patient is monitored for signs of progression. Measuring IOP throughout a day spent in the ophthalmic unit (phasing) can also provide useful information about the patient's range of IOP.

Informing patients that they have glaucoma

It is never easy to inform patients that they have a condition that requires lifelong management, which involves medication that may cause them to have side effects as well as lifelong visits to the hospital for monitoring their condition. These patients also have to come to terms with their diagnosis and prognosis and to live with the uncertainty of long-term visual loss. The quality of life may be affected if the patient is the main breadwinner and may have to take a lower paid job as a result of further visual field loss at some later stage of the disease. In addition to the financial and social costs, the patients may have the psychological costs. There may be the added burden of coping not only with a physically disabling environment but also with a self-identity involved in learning to be visually impaired in a sighted world, especially if the patient has presented late in the disease (Green et al. 2002).

Before informing patients of their diagnosis, it is important to understand from the patient's perspective the impact that this diagnosis will have. Some patients can feel inhibited and intimidated by health-care professionals. The quality of the patient–health-care professional relationship is an important factor in patient compliance. The quality of the interaction can be improved by showing tact, sensitivity and empathy for the patient in light of the diagnosis. Spending time and talking to the patients may not always be possible in a busy clinic so a contact telephone number of someone to whom they can talk can be very useful. Patients may also have a poor understanding of what is being said to them. Always keep any explanation short and simple and, if necessary, reiterate the information that you have given by using simple words and short sentences. Allow time and opportunity for patients to ask any questions. Important information such as compliance with prescribed medication and regular assessment should be given early in the discussion because research has shown that people tend to remember first those items at the beginning of a conversation or interaction (Robinson 2000). The discussion should include the treatment options available and any side effects of prescribed medication. When patients leave the clinic, they should do so with as much information as possible about their condition. It is also important to check on subsequent visits that the relevant information has been understood and remembered by patients. This is particularly applicable to elderly patients who can be forgetful. So, where possible, any verbal information given should be backed up with appropriate written information in a language appropriate for the patient.

Management of POAG

The goal of glaucoma management is to preserve a patient's vision by reducing IOP to a level safe for the optic nerve by increasing outflow facility while preserving the patient's quality of life. Glaucoma therapy can involve:

- medical therapy
- laser therapy
- surgical therapy.

When making a decision for a chosen therapy, it is important that certain considerations be taken into account. Decision on the best type of treatment option for the individual patient must not be focused on clinical outcomes but on the overall well-being of the patient because glaucoma is a chronic lifelong disease. Ophthalmologists and other health-care workers managing this group of patients must base their assessment on a range of outcomes such as the physical and social functioning and quality-of-life parameters (Robinson 2000).

It is also worth remembering that any treatment regimen selected for patients takes into consideration not only the financial costs but the psychological costs as well. Patients have to live not only with the chronic disease but also with the uncertainty of visual loss and blindness. These patients also face a lifetime of clinic appointments and regular assessments, in addition to the numerous potential side effects associated with treatment. Patients' quality of life will be altered, including lifestyle changes, relationships and loss of independence at a later stage. Sight loss for an individual is clearly dependent on a combination of environmental, social and psychological factors, including physical environment, family circumstances, work roles and adaptive responses to symptoms, rather than medically defined measures of disability (Green et al. 2002).

Target pressure

In recent years, ophthalmologists have come to realize that reducing the IOP to the upper normal range was not sufficient; treatment merely to achieve pressures in the upper normal range has resulted in substantial under-treatment (Palmberg 2001). As a result of the insidious nature of POAG, visual field loss often goes unrecognized as a result of the tendency of comparing only the more recent visual field results with the last few obtained and, over 5–10 years, a proportion, perhaps up to 34% of people, will go blind (King et al. 2000).

Target pressure has been defined by Hitchings (2001) as an IOP level below which further optic nerve damage does not occur. However, in clinical practice, there is a limit on the extent of achievable IOP reduction as a result of the inherent danger of increased ocular morbidity caused by low pressure.

Identification of a target IOP can often be fraught with difficulties and ophthalmologists often have to decide from the mean IOP from a diurnal curve, the peak pressure from day phasing or an isolated pressure reading. Different theories exist, e.g. that IOP-induced damage may be related to peak rather than mean pressure or that it is reasonable to rely on mean IOP and identify it from a diurnal curve and then use that as a baseline from which to calculate the target IOP. When using readings from the diurnal range, it should be borne in mind that the diurnal IOP range does not cover the nocturnal sleep period (about a third of our daily life). It is thought that the nocturnal fall in blood pressure combined with higher IOP (caused by an elevation of episcleral venous pressure at night) may compromise optic nerve circulation at night.

It may be that relying solely on elevated IOP is not a good measure for identifying the potential for conversion to glaucoma. Other risk factors such as family history, race, age, etc. have to be taken into account. Other considerations to take into account in the decision-making process include the risks as well as the benefits of reaching target IOP; this includes the age of the patient (long life expectancy requires lower target IOP) and quality of life; current treatments that would lower the IOP effectively and have the fewest side effects are all important considerations.

Setting a target IOP

Currently lowering the IOP is the only proven treatment for glaucomatous nerve damage. In the Collaborative Normal Tension Glaucoma Study (1998), eyes that showed a reduction of the IOP by 30% had a lower rate of visual field progression than those eyes that did not have their IOP lowered.

Target IOP may be defined as the mean IOP obtained that prevents further damage by glaucoma in the individual under consideration. However, individuals can vary so there is no absolutely safe standard target pressure, although it has been suggested that in order to set a target pressure for patients, the following must be taken into consideration:

- It must be based on the general assessment of each individual patient's disease. No absolute level or percentage change from baseline will be correct for every patient.
- It must be an accurate estimate and the cost of reaching the target IOP should be weighed against the likely benefit.

- It needs to be determined in advance and re-evaluated at regular intervals especially in light of any unacceptable progression.

Other factors to take into consideration when setting target IOP included the following:

- The IOP level before treatment: the higher the IOP at which damage occurred, the higher the target pressure.
- The greater the pre-existing damage, the lower the target IOP should be.
- Rate of progression.
- Age of patient, general condition and expected lifespan of patients.
- Presence of any other risk factors already mentioned.

There are, however, a few limitations to setting target pressures and these are summarized below:

- The frequency at which the IOP is measured. The eye is subjected to IOP all the time yet we have an idea of a patient's IOP only at a given time when the patient attends the clinic. This limits our ability to gauge the level of IOP at which the damage has already occurred.
- The diurnal fluctuation of IOP.
- Patients must get worse in terms of optic nerve damage before the ophthalmologist knows that they did not set the target pressure low enough.

Medical therapy

Medical therapy in the form of eyedrops is still the mainstay of primary therapy in POAG. The new European Glaucoma Society (2003) guidelines suggested that, in order to improve compliance, the number, drug concentration and frequency should be kept to a minimum so that inconvenience caused by the medication can also be kept to a minimum.

There are five classes of topical medications (for further details see Chapter 3):

(1) β-adrenergic antagonists and adrenergic agonists
(2) carbonic anhydrase inhibitors
(3) parasympathomimetics: direct and indirect
(4) prostaglandin analogues
(5) hyperosmotics.

There are number of combined preparations on the market. The greatest advantage of combined preparation is increased patient compliance and reduction in side effects.

General principles of prescribing

- It is important that, when prescribing treatment for the glaucoma patients, all health-care personnel take into consideration not only the clinical parameters of the disease but also the effect of the disease and treatment on the overall well-being of the patient. The main goal in prescribing habit should be aimed at preserving vision for a lifetime with as little inconvenience to the patient as possible (Robinson 2000).

- A target IOP should always be set before starting on treatment.
- If topical medication is ineffective, always consider switching before adding another medication. Only consider adding if there is a reasonable response but target has not achieved. For most patients, the 'maximum medical therapy' should be two bottles of drops.
- Discuss side effects with patient and review any side effects.
- Check on patient's compliance.
- Avoid long-term carbonic anhydrase inhibitors if possible.

Managing compliance/concordance issues with glaucoma patients (see also Chapters 3 and 6)

The term 'non-compliance' is seen by health-care personnel as:

- failure to take medication
- taking too much medication
- taking a drug for the wrong reason
- improper timing of administration
- not filling prescription
- defaulting on the follow-up care.

Various factors that have been associated with non-compliance are:

- dissatisfaction with treatment
- dissatisfaction with the consultation
- health beliefs and attitudes
- lack of understanding of the disease treatment
- little subjective reward for a disease with marginal symptoms
- lack of comprehension/memory
- unexpected side effects
- complex regimen
- visual/physical disability
- lifelong treatment.

The issue of compliance can suggest an underlying authoritarian, dictatorial tone on the part of the health-care personnel and a yielding acquiescent patient who just does as he is told by those who know better. Concordance involves a partnership and negotiation between health-care professional and patient. It takes into account the wishes of patients and respects their beliefs. As a result of concordance, the health professionals and patients to an extent at least determine how and when medicines are to be taken, and this takes into account factors that may reduce 'non-compliance' and involves negotiation and agreement with the patient.

Glaucoma is generally an asymptomatic chronic disease requiring a life-long management and with very little subjective rewards in terms of visual improvement as perceived by the patient. In the face of this, health-care professionals must continuously strive to convince the patients that not taking the prescribed therapy can lead to blindness. The use of fear can be an effective way to alter patients' attitudes and behaviour (Cameron 1996) as long as the suggestions of consequences are realistic. Continuity of care by the same health-care professional can also optimize compliance, although it is acknowledged that this might not always be possible.

To summarize, the various strategies to promote concordance amongst glaucoma patients include the following:

• Patient education about the condition, the treatment, and how to use it
• Minimize treatment regimen
• Minimize inconvenience
• Patient self-help groups may be useful such as the International Glaucoma Association
• Ensure good lines of communication between patients and health-care providers
• Strengthen the quality of interaction between patients and health-care providers.

More glaucoma clinics led by other trained health-care professionals for stable glaucoma patients may enable more contact time between patient and health-care professional and encourage partnership in care (see also Chapter 6).

Surgical treatment

Laser trabeculoplasty

Although the mainstay of glaucoma management is medical, other options have to be considered if medical treatment is insufficient to halt the progression of the disease. Less developed countries may consider laser or surgical intervention as their first choice if patients live in a rural area and are unable to get to a clinic setting or if costs or unavailability of medical treatment is an issue (see Chapter 13). The obvious advantages of surgery compared with medical therapy negate the issue of compliance. Laser trabeculoplasty was first described by Wise and Whiter, in 1979, where discrete burns were applied to the trabecular meshwork to enhance aqueous outflow. It avoids surgery and anaesthesia and is also cost-effective when compared with long-term medical therapy.

Laser trabeculoplasty or surgical trabeculectomy is indicated for the following reasons:

- When target IOP cannot be reached despite maximal medical treatment.
- If there is further progression of the disease such as further optic nerve damage.
- If the patient is unable to tolerate or comply with medication.

Laser is an acronym for light amplification stimulated emission of radiation and is an intense source of coherent monochromatic light. The argon laser produces a therapeutic burn to a pre-selected area of the eye, causing minimal damage to the surrounding tissue, and it emits a blue–green light. The delivery of the argon laser can be done through a slit-lamp via a contact lens, using an indirect laser or endolaser.

Argon laser trabeculoplasty (ALT) involves the application of laser energy (usually argon green) to the trabecular meshwork, by improving the rate of outflow of aqueous humour and thus lowering the IOP. The precise mechanism of ALT is unknown and two main theories have been proposed. It is thought that argon photocoagulation damages the trabecular meshwork, causing collagen shrinkage and scarring of the trabecular meshwork. This tightens the meshwork in the area of each burn and opens up the adjacent, untreated intertrabecular spaces. This is known as the mechanical theory. The second theory put forward is that laser induces coagulative necrosis, causing migration of macrophages, which phagocytose and clear the trabecular meshwork of debris.

Laser trabeculoplasty is contraindicated in the situation where the trabeculum is not visible as a result of narrowing of the angle, in situations where the cornea is cloudy, and in advanced glaucoma where there is a known poor compliance to medical therapy and when there is insufficient time to assess the response to ALT before proceeding to a surgical laser trabeculectomy. It is also contraindicated in paediatric glaucoma and most secondary glaucomas except pigmentary and pseudoexfoliation glaucomas. ALT cannot be repeated if the whole of the trabecular meshwork has been treated. The laser beam is usually applied to the pigmented portion of the trabecular meshwork. Usually 180° of the trabecular meshwork is treated in the first instance. The effects of the ALT may not be obvious for several weeks. Complications include a transient rise in IOP. The IOP is usually reduced by about 25% and 80% of patients show an initial beneficial effect. In at least 50% of these patients, the effect is lost in the first 5 years (Broadway et al. 1994).

The most common complication of ALT is a sudden transient rise in IOP after treatment. The cause is not certain, but increased laser energy has been implicated because greater energy may result in an increased inflammatory response in the anterior chamber. To lessen this risk, topical apraclonidine and oral acetazolamide (Diamox) are prescribed before the laser treatment and immediately afterwards to prevent a spike in IOP. After laser trabeculoplasty, patients should have their IOP checked within the first 6 hours and the next day. Topical steroids may be prescribe four times a day for up to 1 week and patients should continue with all their glaucoma medications until they are seen in the clinic. The optimal effect for ALT is usually seen within 4–6 weeks. The glaucoma medications are withdrawn gradually although complete topical medication withdrawal may not always be possible. The aim of ALT is a safe IOP and not a complete cessation of medication.

Other side effects of ALT included transient iritis and peripheral anterior synechiae, especially if the burns are placed too posteriorly. In addition there is field loss associated with IOP spikes as well as loss of effect and a late rise in IOP.

Another technique used is known as selective laser trabeculoplasty (SLT). SLT requires a specially designed laser with a frequency that doubles the Nd:YAG (neodymium:yttrium–aluminium–garnet) laser which is 532 nm. This laser has specific wavelength that targets only the pigmented cells in the trabecular meshwork, without causing collateral thermal damage to adjacent non-pigmented trabecular meshwork. It causes a biological response in the trabecular meshwork by provoking a release of cytokines, which triggers macrophage recruitment and other changes. SLT has certain advantages over ALT:

- The laser beam bypasses surrounding tissue leaving it undamaged. This is why, unlike ALT, SLT can be repeated several times.
- SLT delivers less than 1% of the energy of ALT, further emphasizing the lack of thermal damage.
- The IOP-reducing effects of SLT and ALT seem to be comparable and there are fewer side effects with SLT.
- SLT can be an additional IOP-lowering treatment in patients who have had previous failed ALT.

In summary, laser trabeculoplasty has been subjected to much investigation and is generally recognized as playing a part in primary glaucoma treatment, especially in patients known to be non-compliant. ALT and its newer counterpart SLT are relatively easy to perform with a low complication rate.

Care and management of patients undergoing laser treatment as outpatients

For patients who have never had any laser treatment, this can be seen as an extremely daunting prospect. Laser trabeculoplasty is usually performed on an outpatient basis.

Patient explanation of the treatment must include a full explanation of the procedure and what to expect during and after it, including the following:

- Purposes, limitations and complications of ALT.
- The procedure, including that a contact lens will be placed on the front of the eye after topical anaesthetic and that flashing lights and clicks will accompany the treatment. Normally the procedure will take 10–15 minutes and it is imperative that the patient remains still during the treatment.
- Ways of communication between the patient and the ophthalmologist must be used so that the patient can attract his or her attention during treatment.
- After treatment, the patient should be warned that vision will be dazzled for about half an hour and the eye may be slightly red and uncomfortable for 2 days.
- The patient should be advised about appropriate pain management afterwards and who and when to contact in cases of complications such as an acute rise in IOP.
- Patients must continue with all anti-glaucoma therapy after ALT, although reduction may subsequently be possible.

Trabeculectomy

The most common surgical procedure for glaucoma is trabeculectomy. In trabeculectomy, an ostium is made in the inner sclera, a fistula covered by a flap fashioned in the outer sclera, thereby providing an alternative drainage site for aqueous humour (Harvey 1998).

Trabeculectomy has been proved to lower the IOP more consistently than anti-glaucoma eyedrops or laser trabeculoplasty, but it can, however, be associated with complications. The trabeculectomy may fail because of either scarring around the scleral flap or closure of the internal ostium (Broadway et al. 1994). Another complication associated with trabeculectomy is cataract, which may progress rapidly.

To increase the success rate of the procedure, topical anti-metabolites such as 5-fluorouracil or mitomycin, can be used intraoperatively or immediately postoperatively to increase the success rate of the trabeculectomy procedure.

Other surgical procedures for glaucoma include the following (Alward 2000):

- Trabeculectomy with filtration devices
- Combined procedure (glaucoma/cataract surgery)
- Goniotomy (paediatric glaucoma)
- Surgical peripheral iridectomy
- YAG laser cyclodestruction
- Cyclodestruction (cyclocryotherapy).

Other glaucomas

Normal tension glaucoma

Patients diagnosed with normal tension glaucoma (NTG) have optic nerve head cupping and visual field loss but with normal document IOP readings. According to Alward (2000), patients who develop glaucomatous changes at normal or low pressures appear to have a more vascular type of damage compared with patients with POAG. NTG patients tend to have notching of the neuroretinal rim and optic disc haemorrhages are also more common. The management of these patients can be challenging because it is more difficult to lower what is already a 'normal' IOP. NTG is treated in the same way as POAG.

Ocular hypertension

Unlike NTG patients, ocular hypertension (OH) patients have IOPs over 21 mmHg but with normal optic nerve head and normal visual field. Some ophthalmologists will advocate treatment only if the IOP has reached a level at which the risk of damage outweighs the costs and side effects of treatment (Alward 2000). If no other risk factors from developing glaucoma are present, the patient should be monitored regularly.

Congenital glaucoma

Congenital glaucoma is present at or near birth and is relatively rare. It can also appear at any time during the first 3 years of life (Figure 20.6). It

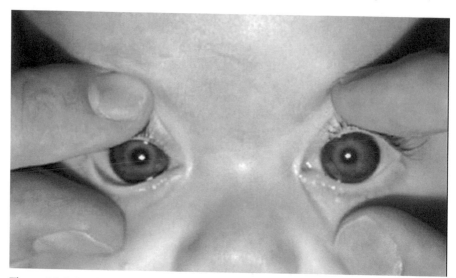

Figure 20.6 Buphthalmos. (See Plate 48.)

occurs in only 1 out of 10 000 babies, and is significant by virtue of the young age of the patients. It occurs as a result of malformation of the angle development or secondary to another eye condition. It is referred to as infantile when it is present within the first 3 years of life and juvenile when it occurs after 3 years of age. According to Alward (2000), 60% of cases are diagnosed by age 6 months and 80% by age 1 year. The disease affects boys more often (65%) than girls and 70% of cases are bilateral.

As there is very little production of aqueous in the first few months of life, most cases are not manifest at birth. The ocular tissues of a baby are quite elastic and stretch easily. As the pressure becomes elevated, the eye becomes enlarged and distended (a condition known as buphthalmos). Sometimes the elevated pressure can cause cracks to appear in Descemet's membrane, known as Haab's striae. In addition, the corneal diameter is also enlarged. The normal newborn corneal diameter is 10.0–10.5 mm and any corneal diameter greater than 12 mm is suggestive of glaucoma. Corneal oedema is another classic sign of glaucoma and the infant cornea can become oedematous at levels of IOP that would be considered only mildly elevated in the adult eye.

Congenital glaucoma can also be associated with many systemic conditions such as neurofibromatosis, congenital rubella and Sturge–Weber syndrome, and related eye problems such as Axenfield, Rieger's and Peter's anomalies, aniridia, nanophthalmos and microcornea.

Presentation
Presentation is often related to the corneal oedema – parents becoming concerned that the child's eye appears 'milky' and often telephoning the unit for advice. Parents often report that the child has very large, blue eyes normally. The child should be seen urgently because, obviously, early intervention is likely to lead to a better outcome. Any parent worried about a child's eyes or vision should be taken extremely seriously – parents see subtle changes that health-care professionals often do not and conditions such as buphthalmos may be overlooked by non-specialist health-care professionals.

Treatment
The normal treatment for congenital glaucoma is a surgical procedure called goniotomy where a goniolens is used to visualize the angle and the anterior portion of the trabecular meshwork is incised (just below Schwalbe's line). Trabeculectomy can also be performed instead of goniotomy. Both give similar IOP control.

Secondary glaucomas

Secondary glaucomas, as the name implies, are secondary to another ophthalmological disease, e.g. inflammation or neovascular disease, and they account for a third of all glaucoma cases (Table 20.2). Patients with secondary glaucomas are typically younger than those with POAG and it is important to rule out secondary glaucoma in patients with POAG and NTG. The angle in patients with secondary glaucoma may be closed or open.

Table 20.2 Secondary glaucoma: features of the angle

Secondary glaucomas	Angle
Pigmentary	Open
Pseudoexfoliation	Open
Steroid induced	Open
Neovascular	Closed
Lens induced	Open or closed
Inflammatory	Open or closed
Early or late traumatic	Open or closed
Miscellaneous causes	

Pigment dispersion syndrome

Pigment dispersion syndrome (PDS) is an aggressive form of glaucoma typically affecting myopic men in their mid-20s. It is usually bilateral but may be asymmetrical. During blinking, aqueous is driven from the posterior to the anterior chamber The aqueous from the anterior chamber causes an increase in iridozonular contact, liberating pigment from the posterior surface of the iris and depositing it in the anterior and posterior chambers. The pigment epithelium may be abnormally prone to shedding and exercise may precipitate acute episodes. One of the key findings is deposition of pigment on the corneal endothelium in a spindle shape (Krukenberg's spindle), along with iris atrophy and transillumination.

IOP rise is a result of obstruction of intertrabecular spaces and up to 50% of people with PDS will go on to develop ocular hypertension or pigmentary glaucoma (Kanski 2003). This is often quite an 'aggressive' disease and management and treatment are as for POAG.

Pseudoexfoliation glaucoma

Pseudoexfoliation (PEX) syndrome involves the deposition of a greywhite, fibrogranular material on all structures in the anterior segment as well as the anterior vitreous face and conjunctiva. Systemic changes may also be found with deposition elsewhere in the body. The material is produced by ageing abnormal epithelial cells and may have a genetic component. The trabecular meshwork is blocked by deposits, resulting in secondary glaucoma. The risk of glaucoma in people with PEX increases with time and a yearly ocular examination should be part of the management of the condition. Medical treatment is as for POAG but, often, surgery is needed.

Steroid-induced glaucoma

Steroids are thought to change the trabecular meshwork ability to process aqueous and both topical and oral steroids can cause a rise in IOP. About two-thirds of populations are thought to be steroid responders and response is dependent on frequency and dose of application. Patients with myopia and POAG are at increased risk. Treatment is by stopping steroids if possible or by using drop therapy or surgery to lower the IOP. Patients with uveitis who are steroid responders will need therapy to control the IOP along with their treatment for uveitis.

Neovascular glaucoma

This is relatively common and potentially devastating. Retinal hypoxia leads to neovascularization of the iris and the new vessels will proliferate on to the iris, known as iris rubeosis (open angle), with contraction of the fibrovascular membrane (closed angle). It may follow central retinal vein occlusion (36%), diabetic retinopathy (32%) and other carotid disease (13%), central retinal artery occlusion, chronic uveitis and intraocular tumours. Prompt panretinal photocoagulation (PRP) is required if the media are clear or cryotherapy if the view is poor. Atropine and steroids will reduce flare and improve the vascular component. Surgery may be needed to control IOP and eventually, if the eye becomes blind and painful, enucleation may be discussed with the patient.

Lens-induced glaucoma

Phakolytic glaucoma is caused by lens protein leaking through the intact lens capsule into the aqueous and then obstructing the trabecular meshwork. It is more common in less developed countries where people with cataract may often present late or not be able to access treatment. Treatment involves control of IOP and surgery to remove the cataract and lens material.

Phakomorphic glaucoma is acute, secondary angle closure caused by a large, swollen, cataractous lens. The lens moves anteriorly as a result of slackened suspensory ligaments and the size of the lens precipitates pupillary block. Treatment is by control of the IOP, laser iridotomy when IOP is controlled and cataract surgery when the eye has settled.

Inflammatory glaucoma: uveitic glaucoma

Glaucoma may occur secondary to intraocular inflammation and may be transient or persistent and damaging. Secondary glaucoma is the most common cause of blindness in children and young people with chronic anterior uveitis (Kanski 2003). Uveitis can result in posterior synechiae. If 360° of posterior synechiae occur, aqueous outflow into the anterior chamber is obstructed, the angle will close as the iris moves forward and the IOP will rise rapidly. Treatment is with topical therapy and laser iridotomy.

Posner–Schlossman syndrome (glaucomatocyclitic crisis)

Unilateral, acute, secondary open-angle glaucoma occurs in association with mild anterior uveitis. The rise in the IOP is presumed to be a result of trabeculitis. It is most common in young people and more common in men. Patients who have repeat episodes are often a good source of information about their condition. Treatment combines uveitis therapy with topical therapy to suppress the production of aqueous.

Traumatic glaucoma

Glaucoma can result from blunt trauma, immediately or months to years later, and in late presentations is the result of angle recession. Patients with blunt trauma should be encouraged to have follow-up assessments, perhaps in the form of regular eye tests with an optometrist to ensure that any IOP rise is identified promptly.

Primary angle-closure glaucoma

Primary angle-closure glaucoma (PACG) is a condition in which the iris is apposed to the trabecular meshwork at the angle of the anterior chamber of the eye. Angle closure may occur by two mechanisms: pupillary block or plateau iris, which is rare and not considered here.

There are three interrelated factors that predispose to pupillary block:

1. Lens size: the lens continues to grow in all dimensions throughout life. Growth in diameter allows the suspensory ligaments to slacken and the lens may then move forward, nearer to the iris; along with this, it also becomes 'fatter' and this, again, leaves its anterior surface nearer to the front of the eye. Both these factors lead to a more shallow anterior chamber.
2. A smaller corneal diameter ensures a smaller anterior chamber.
3. A short eye, one with a smaller than average axial length, ensures that there is a smaller corneal diameter and more crowded structure within the eye.

Therefore, primary pupillary block glaucoma is most prevalent in elderly individuals with hypermetropic eyes. Races with anatomically narrower angle, such as Asians and Eskimos, have a higher incidence of angle closure than white people. Among the latter, the incidence of angle-closure glaucoma is three times higher in women. Women have a slightly smaller mean axial length than men, but the calculated ocular volume of the average female eye is 10% less than that of men (Quigley et al. 2003). In other races, men and women are affected equally (Noecker 2001) and PACG is uncommon in black people. Several studies have found a bimodal peak, with the first peak at age 53–58 years and the second at 63–70 years.

Aqueous is normally produced by ciliary, non-pigmented, epithelial cells in the posterior chamber and flows through the pupil to the anterior segment, where it drains out of the eye through the trabecular meshwork and Schlemm's canal. If contact occurs between the lens and iris, aqueous accumulates behind the pupil, increasing posterior chamber pressure and forcing the peripheral iris to shift forward and block the anterior chamber angle. The anterior surface of the iris may be apposed to the posterior surface of the cornea, as with total posterior synechiae, or to the trabecular meshwork as in relative pupillary block. Newer theories seem to suggest that expansion of choroidal volume, leading to increased vitreous cavity pressure and poor vitreous fluid conductivity, may also be responsible for the occlusion. Each of these features can appear as an isolated dominant cause in a single condition (nanophthalmos and malignant glaucoma, respectively) or they may be contributory features in acute primary angle closure. The full pathogenesis of PACG is not yet fully understood.

Recent literature on PACG has highlighted the importance of this disease as a worldwide cause of blindness. According to Foster et al. (2002), in a population-based survey people with PACG are three times more likely to be blind than those with POAG; they concluded that PACG may be the leading cause of glaucoma blindness in the world today. There is a need to develop screening tests that will identify both people with occludable angles and those likely to develop frank angle closure and angle-closure glaucoma.

Signs and symptoms of PACG

- Haloes around lights as a result of corneal oedema
- Rapidly progressive visual loss caused by corneal oedema
- Severe pain, in and around the eye, and headache as a result of the acute rise in IOP
- Nausea, vomiting and abdominal pain caused by vagal stimulation
- Lacrimation.

In general settings, acute glaucoma (Figure 20.7) may be missed or the patient's systemic symptoms of nausea, abdominal pain, vomiting or headache may lead to clinicians overlooking eye signs and symptoms. On examination the following are found:

- A 'red eye'.
- Corneal oedema caused by the acutely raised IOP overcoming the pumping action of the corneal endothelium and forcing fluid into the corneal tissue.
- Shallow or flat anterior chamber with peripheral contact between iris and cornea.
- The iris may be bowing forwards (iris bombé).
- Flare and cells in the aqueous (once oedema has settled) as a result of breakdown of the blood–aqueous barrier.
- An oval (vertically) fixed, unreactive and semi-dilated pupil.
- Dilated iris vessels.
- Raised IOP (50–100 mmHg).

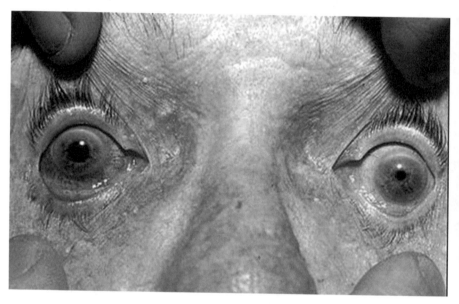

Figure 20.7 Acute glaucoma. (See Plate 49.)

Gonioscopy and optic disc evaluation

Once the pressure is controlled and corneal oedema has resolved, gonioscopy should be undertaken to assess the angle in both eyes. It is also important to evaluate and assess the optic disc for any glaucomatous damage. Even a short elevation of acute IOP can result in a posterior displacement of the lamina cribrosa. The most likely explanation for the IOP-dependent changes of the topography of the optic disc is a mechanical displacement of the optic nerve head tissues. An elevation of IOP could compress, rearrange and/or displace the tissues of the optic nerve head, resulting in a larger cupping.

Immediate medical and nursing management

Acute angle-closure glaucoma is a common ophthalmic emergency that requires early recognition followed by appropriate treatment to minimize visual loss. There is considerable variation in the details of treatment among the various ophthalmologists, but it is generally accepted that treatments should be aimed at reducing any acute IOP (thereby limiting any ischaemic sequelae) (Seang-Mei et al. 2003) and removing any element of pupil block (to minimize further iris–trabecular meshwork apposition) through use of IOP-lowering medications, followed by laser peripheral iridotomy or in some cases filtration surgery to relieve pupillary block.

Immediate medical treatment

- Intravenous acetazolamide (Diamox) 500 mg followed by an oral dose of 500 mg, provided that the patient is not vomiting.
- Prednisolone forte 1% or dexamethasone four times a day to both eyes to reduce anterior chamber activity.
- Pilocarpine 2% drops: the use of pilocarpine to induce pupillary constriction, which leads to the opening of the narrow angle and thus facilitates aqueous outflow, can also cause shallowing of the anterior chamber by increasing axial lens thickness, and induce anterior lens movement, particularly if a 4% concentration is used. Cholinergic agonists must be used only after the IOP has decreased sufficiently to allow perfusion of the iris (< 40 mmHg). The few cases of cholinergic toxicity reported from pilocarpine are typically the result of over-administration of this drug during attacks of acute angle-closure glaucoma.
- There is no place in the treatment of acute glaucoma for intensive miotic therapy (Kanski 2003).
- Analgesics and antiemetics as required.
- Lying down for a period of time not only will be more comfortable for the patient, but will aid pressure reduction.
- Intravenous fluid if dehydrated.
- Reassurance and explanation must be paramount to alleviate anxiety and fears.
- Oral 50% glycerol 1 g/kg may be administered if the IOP does not fall quickly and 20% mannitol 1–2 g/kg i.v. may be used subsequently or if the patient is unable to tolerate glycerol.

Apraclonidine is a relatively new α_2-agonist that acts primarily by decreasing aqueous production. Its effects are additive to topically administered β blockers. It has been reported to be effective in treating acute angle-closure glaucoma.

Subsequent nursing management

Patients with an acute attack of angle closure are usually admitted to the eye unit (although not in all cases) for further monitoring. These patients are often elderly and may be in a great deal of pain in addition to feeling nauseous. They may have been feeling unwell for a few days before seeking treatment. They may be dehydrated which further adds to their confusional state. On admission to the ward, a full nursing assessment must be carried out. The assessment and care should include issues such as:

- maintaining a safe environment, taking into account the mental, visual and mobility state of the patient
- controlling pain and nausea
- communication issues – hearing, language barriers, speech
- ensuring understanding of condition and treatment
- nutrition, including the care of any intravenous fluids (input and output chart)
- care of intravenous infusion
- observations as necessary – pulse, blood pressure, temperature
- investigations as necessary, such as bloods for urea and electrolytes, especially if the patient has had nausea and vomiting for some time
- skin integrity assessment using a Waterlow score
- care of any other relevant medical problems – diabetes, cardiovascular, respiratory
- identification of relevant previous ophthalmic problems
- medications
- allergies
- social assessment and communication with relatives, carers and others who need to know about the patient's admission.

Subsequent medical treatment

When the IOP has been brought under control, a laser (peripheral) iridotomy (LPI) is normally carried out to both the affected and unaffected eye because the fellow eyes of acute angle-closure patients have been found to have very high risks of developing PACG. Acute angle closure in the fellow eye occurs most frequently during the period between the initial onset of symptoms in the acute eye and the end of the first month of outpatient follow-up. Contralateral eyes of patients with acute ACG are at significant risk of an acute attack and iridotomy virtually eliminates this risk.

Laser iridotomy creates an opening in the iris through which aqueous humour trapped in the posterior chamber can reach the anterior chamber and trabecular meshwork. As aqueous flows into the anterior chamber through the iris defect, pressure behind the iris falls, allowing the iris to recede towards its normal position. The procedure opens the anterior chamber angle and relieves the blockage of the trabecular meshwork.

A number of laser burns are delivered to the mid-peripheral iris until a hole is seen and aqueous flows through.

An evidence-based update on interventions for ACG concluded that LPI has been recommended as an effective and safe treatment for acute angle closure and acute ACG. It found that LPI was less expensive, less invasive, more convenient and safer than surgical peripheral iridectomy, although it was also found that it could be associated with an increased rate of cataract formation (Seang-Mei et al. 2003). Other possible adverse side effects included development of posterior synechiae and, in theory, endothelial changes in the cornea. Many eyes treated with peripheral iridectomy will eventually require medication to control chronic pressure elevation and some will need filtering surgery.

The use of argon laser peripheral iridoplasty (ALPI), where a ring of contraction burns is placed on the peripheral iris to contract the iris stroma near the angle, has been reported to be an efficient and effective option in opening up the angle. This mechanically pulls open the angle, thus lowering the IOP and thereby allowing the eye to become quiet before definite treatment is performed (Ritch 2001). ALPI is most useful when LPI cannot be performed because of corneal oedema or a very shallow anterior chamber. The usual practice is to perform ALPI 3–6 hours after maximal medications fail to control IOP (Lim et al. 1993).

References

Alward W (2000) Glaucoma: The requisites in ophthalmology. New York: Mosby.

American Academy of Ophthalmology (2001) Preferred Practice Patterns: Primary Open Angle Glaucoma Suspect and POAG. San Francisco, CA: AAO, pp. 1–36.

Broadway DC, Grierson I, O'Brien C, Hitchings RA (1994) Adverse effects of topical antiglaucoma medication 11. The outcome of filtration surgery. Arch Ophthalmol 112: 1446–54.

Budde WM, Jonas JB (1999) Family history of glaucoma in the primary and secondary open-angle glaucomas. Graefes Arch Clin Exp Ophthalmol 237: 554–7.

Cameron C (1996) Patient compliance: recognition of factors involved and suggestions for promoting compliance with therapeutic regimens. J Adv Nursing 24: 244–50.

Collaborative Normal Tension Glaucoma Study Group (1998) Comparison between glaucomatous progression between untreated patients with normal tension glaucoma and patients with therapeutically reduced intraocular pressures. Am J Ophthalmol 126: 498–505.

Ellis JD, Morris AD, MacEwen CJ (1999) Should diabetic patients be screened for glaucoma? Br J Ophthalmol 83: 369–72.

European Glaucoma Society (2003) Key issues for nurses from the European Glaucoma Society Guidelines (www.eugs.org).

Foster PJ, Buhrmann R, Quigley HA, Johnson GJ (2002) The definition and classification of glaucoma in prevalence surveys. Br J Ophthalmol 86: 238–42.

Gordon MO, Beiser J, Arandt JD (2002) The Ocular Hypertension Treatment Study: baseline factors that predict the onset of primary open angle glaucoma. Arch Ophthalmol 120: 714–20.

Grant W, Burke P (1982) Why do some people go blind from glaucoma? Ophthalmology 100: 991–8.

Green J, Siddall H, Murdoch I (2002) Learning to live with glaucoma: a qualitative study of the diagnosis and the impact of sight loss. Soc Sci Med 55: 257–67.

Harvey RB (1998) Practical Ophthalmology – CD-ROM. Birmingham: Palmtrees Publishing.

Hitchings R (2001) Target pressure. J Glaucoma 10(5, suppl 1): 68–70.

Kanski JJ (2003) Clinical Ophthalmology, 5th edn. London: Butterworth Heinemann.

King AJ, Reddy A, Thompson JR (2000) The rates of blindness and of partial sight registration in glaucoma patients. Eye 14: 613–19.

Klein BE, Klein R, Jensen SC (1994) Open-angle glaucoma and older-onset diabetes. The Beaver Dam Study. Ophthalmology 101: 1173–7.

Leske MC, Connell AMS, Schachat AP, Hyman L (1994) The Barbados Eye Study: prevalence of open angle glaucoma. Arch Ophthalmol 112: 821–9.

Leske MC, Nemesure B, He Q (2001) Patterns of open angle glaucoma in the Barbados Family Study. Ophthalmology 108: 1015–22.

Lim A, Tan A, Chew P (1993) Laser iridoplasty in the treatment of severe acute angle closure glaucoma. Int Ophthalmol 17: 33–6.

Palmberg P (2001) Risk factors for glaucoma progression. Where does intraocular pressure fit in? Arch Ophthalmol 119: 897–8.

Pawson P, Vernon SA (1995). The optic disc in glaucoma. Optom Today 6: 20–6.

Quigley H, Friedman D, Congdon M, Nathan G (2003) Possible mechanisms of primary angle closure and malignant glaucoma. J Glaucoma 12: 167–80.

Ritch R (2001) Angle closure glaucoma: current thoughts. Glaucoma – Perspectives in Practice, Issue 3.4.

Robinson R (2000) How to inform patient about glaucoma. Glaucoma World 21 December: 17–18.

Seang-Meis, Gazzard G, Friedman D (2003) Interventions for angle closure glaucoma. An evidence-based update. Ophthalmology 110: 1869–78.

Snell R, Lemp M (1998) Clinical Anatomy of the Eye, 2nd edn. Oxford: Blackwell Science.

Tarwara A, Okada Y, Kubota T (2000) Immunohistochemical localisation of MYCO/TIGR protein in the trabecular tissue of normal and glaucomatous eyes. Curr Eye Res 21: 934–43.

Tielsch JM, Katz J, Quigley HA (1995) Diabetes, intraocular pressure and primary open angle glaucoma in the Baltimore Eye Survey. Ophthalmology 102: 48–53.

Wise JB, Whiter SAL (1979) Argon laser therapy for open-angle glaucoma. Arch Ophthalmol 97: 319–22.

CHAPTER TWENTY-ONE

The retina and vitreous

SUSANNE RAYNEL AND OLGA BROCHNER

The posterior segment contains the retina, vitreous, optic disc and macula/fovea. These structures are not visible to the naked eye because they are situated behind the lens and iris at the 'fundus' of the globe and consequently are perhaps the least understood of the structures of the eye. It is imperative that the retina and associated structures can be identified and understood in order to understand associated diseases, particularly as retinal conditions often impact on patients' vision and/or visual outcome (Batterbury and Bowling 1999).

The retina

The retina is the most complex ocular tissue (Figure 21.1). It lines the inner two-thirds of the wall of the globe, extending from the ora serrata

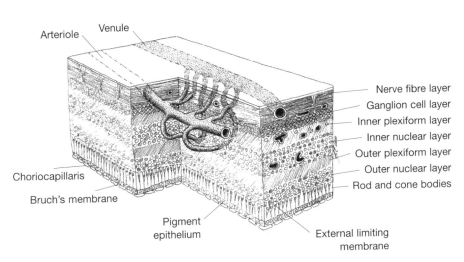

Figure 21.1 Photoreceptors and the retinal pigment epithelium (RPE).

to the optic nerve head, with the choroid and sclera posteriorly and vitreous humour anteriorly occupying the cavity of the posterior segment. It is in the retina where sight begins; the neurosensory segments are responsible for receiving the light stimulus and transmitting the visual information to the brain's occipital cortex for interpretation.

It is only relatively recently that technology has enabled us actually to 'see' and 'explore' the posterior segment. To begin to understand the retina it is necessary to have an understanding of its anatomy and physiology.

Anatomy and physiology

Embryology

The optic cup develops from the optic vesicle in the first 6–7 weeks of gestation. This consists of two layers of neuroectoderm separated by a space. The outer layers form the retinal pigment epithelium (RPE) whereas the inner layers form the neurosensory retina, with a potential space between them. This is an important factor in the development of retinal detachments.

The retina consists of a semi-transparent, multi-layered sheet of neural tissue with the RPE at the 'bottom' and nine neural layers on top. It is important to know how the layers interact because a healthy retina is essential to the formation of vision and any disruption in retinal layers can lead to visual disturbances.

There are two functional layers in the retina: the RPE and the neural retina (Table 21.1). Figure 21.3 shows a normal retina.

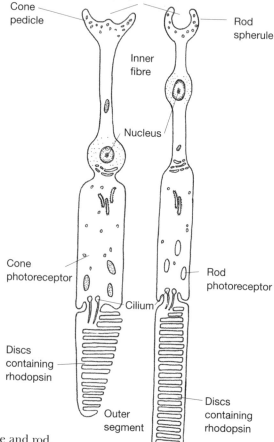

Figure 21.2 Photoreceptors: cone and rod.

Table 21.1 Function of the layers of the retina

Functional layer	Function/Purpose
Retinal pigment epithelium (RPE)	RPE is a single layer of cells that provides the metabolic support for the neurosensory retina, recycles vitamin A (essential for the rods and cones) and reduces photoreceptor damage by absorbing scattered light
Neural retina consisting of several identified layers: photoreceptors, external limiting membrane, outer nuclear, outer plexiform, inner nuclear, inner plexiform, ganglion cell, nerve fibre layers and internal limiting membrane	The retina is transparent as light must pass through all the neural layers before reaching the photoreceptor cells. Light (photons) interacts with the photoreceptor molecules causing a chemical and then a neural response (nerve impulse) that is transferred to the occipital lobe of the brain
	The neural layers include the photoreceptor cells (rods and cones), bipolar cells and ganglion cells. These cells are connected though the different neural layers, e.g. the bipolar cells transmit signals from the photoreceptor cells to the ganglion cells from the outer plexiform layer, through the inner nuclear and inner plexiform layer to the ganglion cell layer itself
	Cones are sensitive to colours and function best with light. There are 6–7 million cones which are mainly situated in the macula, and the fovea comprises only cones. The cones are also responsible for visual acuity, i.e. when you are reading, watching TV or looking at a person, the eyes will move so that the object that you are watching is fixed on the fovea for the best visual acuity. This is a result of the way that they are 'wired' to the rest of the neural cells. Cones have a direct one-to-one connection with the ganglion cells, which are large neurons responsible for conducting impulses from the retina to the brain
	Rods are mainly situated in the periphery of the retina. They are more numerous than cones because there are 120 million rods, and they function in dim light. Rods contain the photoreceptor protein molecule rhodopsin, which is very light sensitive. But it takes the rods about 20 minutes to become properly dark adapted, because rhodopsin is 'bleached' by bright light, hence that dazzled feeling when you go from darkness into a lightened room (Figure 21.2)

Blood supply

The retinal arteries, veins and capillaries are located primarily within the superficial nerve fibre layer of the central retinal artery, which enters the

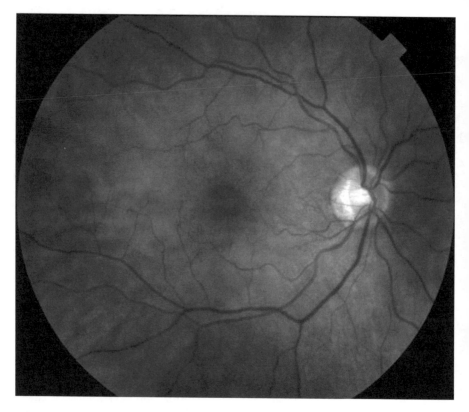

Figure 21.3 Normal retina. (Courtesy of Ophthalmic Imaging Department, Manchester Royal Eye Hospital.) (See Plate 50.)

eye at the optic nerve. The inner retina receives its blood supply from retinal branches whereas the choroid supplies inner areas of the retina and the macular region.

The vitreous

Embryologically the vitreous develops in two stages: primary and secondary. The primary vitreous is forming at the same time as the retina, at 6–7 weeks, between the neural ectoderm and the lens vesicle. The hyaloid vascular system (hyaloid canal) runs through the primary vitreous nourishing the developing lens. In months 6–7 the hyaloid system begins to atrophy; at the same time the primary vitreous is replaced by the transparent secondary vitreous. If the primary vitreous is not replaced the patient is diagnosed with persistent hyperplastic primary vitreous.

The vitreous occupies the posterior segment cavity and is the largest structure within the globe, occupying about 80%. It is a clear, avascular, gelatinous body made up of 99% water and 1% collagen and hyaluronic acid molecules, which are necessary to bind this large volume of water. Vitreous has an outer surface, the hyaloid membrane, which is firmly attached to the retina, the posterior capsule of the lens, the posterior surface of the zonules and the optic disc. If the vitreous attachment to these structures is disrupted holes may form, which can result in retinal detachment. It is a normal part of ageing for the vitreous to shrink, collapse in on itself and separate posteriorly from the retina, and this is known as a posterior vitreous detachment (PVD). The spaces formed are filled by aqueous.

Optic disc

The optic disc is a relatively pale, almost circular area at the posterior pole where retinal nerve fibres leave and retinal blood vessels enter and leave the interior of the eye. The optic disc is 1.5 mm in diameter and this is often used as a unit of measurement within the eye.

Macula and fovea

The macula is situated in the central part of the retina and measures about 5–6 mm in diameter. The macula differs structurally and functionally from the rest of the retina and has a high concentration of cones, whereas the peripheral retina has a high concentration of rods. The fovea is situated at the centre of the macula.

Ora serrata

This is the junction between the retina and pars plana (posterior to the ciliary processes). The ora comprises a series of crescent-shaped indentations making it look like a scallop shell.

Pars plana

This is a landmark at the posterior region of the ciliary body, situated behind the lens and above the retina.

Vitreous base

This is a firm attachment of vitreous to the retina and pars plana, which straddles the ora serrata. It is about 3.2 mm wide.

Assessment of retinal disorders

The retina reacts in a limited way to disorder and disruption and can exhibit only a limited range of physical signs, so similar fundus appearances may be produced by a number of different 'disease' processes. As a result of the position of the retina in the globe, it is difficult to view and so again there are limited ways in which conditions/disease assessment can be undertaken.

Generic signs and symptoms of retinal disorders

Patients presenting with retinal conditions may provide a similar description of their symptoms, although there are some descriptions that patients articulate that are indicative of specific retinal conditions. When the eye is being examined it can appear 'normal' but there are signs in the anterior segment that can be observed and documented initially before the posterior segment is examined.

The visual acuity is often normal unless there is macular involvement or vitreous opacity resulting from a haemorrhage or an inflammatory process in the posterior segment.

A careful patient history should be taken because retinal disorders, unless associated with trauma, are painless. In particular, the patient should be asked about any metamorphopsia (distortion in vision), photopsia (flashing lights), sudden increase in floaters, curtain-like appearance in visual field and a sudden loss of vision as such symptoms are associated with specific retinal disorders.

Anterior segment examination should include:

- Presence of red reflex
- Relative afferent pupillary defect (RAPD).

Posterior segment examination

- The use of either an indirect ophthalmoscope using a 20-D lens with indentation of the sclera to view the peripheral retina or a slit-lamp with a 90-D lens is required. The view through a direct ophthalmoscope is too limited to assist in the diagnosis and does not provide a stereoscopic view.

Vitreous opacities

As with any ocular opacity, floaters interfere with the passage of light and cast a shadow on the retina, which in turn is seen in that area of the visual field. Floaters may present in one or more 'shapes' and patients usually describe them as cobwebs, threads, spots or blobs in the visual field. They are more commonly seen against a uniform background, such as looking up at the sky. Floaters can be the sign of something innocuous or more sinister; however, floaters that move do not normally indicate any serious underlying condition.

Floaters are usually the result of the clumping of collagen and hyaluronic acid molecules in the vitreous as one ages, i.e. vitreous degeneration. Syneresis, resulting in a PVD, may also cause floaters as can vitreous haemorrhages. In turn, these haemorrhages can be secondary to a rupture of retinal vessels caused by trauma, retinal traction or the bleeding of abnormal vessels as occurs in proliferative diabetic retinopathy (PDR). The disruption to the visual acuity depends on the cause of the floater or size of the haemorrhage. A large retinal bleed into the vitreous may cause a reduced red reflex (Chawla 1999).

There is no associated pain with floaters, unless they are the result of trauma; however, the underlying cause of floaters should be identified particularly if the patient notices a sudden increase in number or if they are associated with 'flashing lights'. Usually no treatment is required for floaters. Small haemorrhages are left to clear unless the pathology (as in PDR) signifies the need for a vitrectomy to preserve sight.

Diagnostic tools and investigations in retinal disorders

Amsler grid

This is grid of black on white lines used to assess macular function. If macular changes are present lines in the central grid are distorted; patients with age-related macular degeneration (AMD) are often given a grid to take home and advised to return if they notice deterioration. To use the grid, one eye must be occluded and the patient should look only at the central spot on the grid and describe or draw areas of the grid that are distorted. Patients with macular disease should be encouraged to undertake this on a regular basis and attend the eye unit for review should changes occur.

Two-dimensional ultrasound (B scan)

If no view of the retina is possible a B scan may be undertaken to aid diagnosis. This is the ophthalmic equivalent of an ultrasound scan used in other specialities. Sound waves are projected through the globe, providing a two-dimensional image of the interior of the globe. The two dimensions appear as white or black, with white being known structures and abnormalities such as haemorrhage and black being the vitreous cavity and anterior segment.

Retinal colour photography

Photographs of the retina are used for screening in conditions such as diabetes but their main function is for serial assessment of retinal disorders such as naevi or stereoscopic images to assess maculopathy.

Fundus fluorescein angiography (FFA)

This is currently the gold standard for imaging of ocular circulation. Fluorescein, a mineral-based dye, is injected intravenously and quickly reaches the retinal circulation. The dye will not leak from healthy vessels but where damaged or new vessels are situated the fluorescein will leak out and show up as hyperfluorescent areas. Fluorescein is used extensively in ophthalmic practice to aid in the diagnosis of maculopathy and retinal circulation abnormalities caused by a number of conditions such as diabetes or Age-Related Macular Degeneration (AMD). It is not without risk, and it should be treated as any medication or allergy status discussed before administration. Dosages vary, but a common prescription is 2.5 ml of 20% fluorescein given intravenously in the antecubital fossa while the patient is positioned at a posterior segment camera. Patients should be told that their skin may appear yellow and their urine will be bright yellow/green until all of the fluorescein has been excreted. Patients should be encouraged to drink copious amounts of fluid to aid in excretion.

Electroretinography

This is commonly referred to as electrophysiology testing used for the diagnosis of hereditary dystrophies. Electroretinography (ERG) is to the eye what an electrocardiogram (ECG) is to the heart. When the retina is stimulated by a light source the resultant action potential is recorded between two electrodes; rod and/or cone responses are then analysed to determine the visual potential.

Electro-oculography

Electro-oculography (EOG) measures the activity of the RPE and photo-receptors.

Indocyanine green (ICG)

This is a relatively new diagnostic aid; it highlights the choroidal circulation and is used as an adjunct in the diagnosis of macular disorders such as exudative AMD. Patients who have an iodine or shellfish allergy may have an allergic reaction to indocyanine green (ICG). It is administered in a similar way to fluorescein.

Ocular coherence tomography

Ocular coherence tomography (OCT) is similar to a B scan but uses infrared waves rather than sound waves. It is useful in providing a topographical map of the retinal thickness. It is non-invasive.

Heidelberg retinal tomography

This is a laser scanning system that ultimately provides a three-dimensional image. It has become an important tool for disc and nerve fibre layer evaluation in glaucoma. It is also used to assess conditions such as macular oedema.

Retinal thickness analyser

This is a laser scan used to calculate retinal thickness.

Watzke–Allen test

A narrow slit beam of light is projected onto the macula and can be used to detect macular pathology. It is considered to be a crude method for detection of abnormality and, with the current diagnostic aids available, is obsolete.

Retinal detachment

Retinal detachment refers to the separation of the neural retina from the RPE. Retinal detachments are generally divided into two main types: rhegmatogenous and non- rhegmatogenous. Rhegmatogenous is derived from the Greek *rhegma* meaning 'break' or 'tear'.

This detachment recreates a potential space between the two layers of the original embryonic cup briefly discussed earlier in this chapter.

Rhegmatogenous retinal detachments (Figure 21.4)

This means simply that the detachment is caused by a full-thickness break (hole or tear) in the continuity of the retina, allowing fluid to collect between the neural retina and RPE as a result of the tension between the vitreous and the retina, and so the break cannot close without intervention. This is the most common type of detachment with an incidence of 1 in 10 000 in western populations, with about 10% being bilateral. The retinal break most often described is a horseshoe-shaped tear.

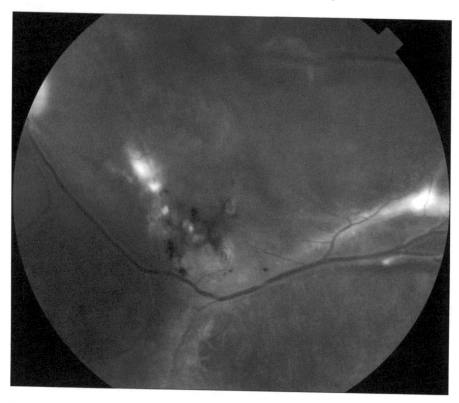

Figure 21.4 Retinal detachment. (Courtesy of Ophthalmic Imaging Department, Manchester Royal Eye Hospital.) (See Plate 51.)

This break can occur spontaneously as a consequence of PVD, or as a result of trauma to the globe allowing fluid through the break; fluid then accumulates, precipitating separation of the neural retina and RPE. The cause of spontaneous retinal detachments is often not found, and not all patients presenting with PVD will progress to retinal detachment because, if the vitreous detaches evenly, there is no traction on the retina to produce a hole. These breaks most frequently occur in the periphery of the retina, making viewing difficult. People with myopia have 42% of all retinal detachments but make up only 10% of the population as a result of increased incidence of lattice degeneration in this group of patients and a high frequency of PVD at a younger age (Taylor et al. 1995). Another common cause of retinal breaks is degeneration of the retina. Lattice degeneration is present in about 7% of the population and about 40% of eyes with a retinal detachment have lattice degeneration.

There are also several other ophthalmic conditions that may contribute to the development of rhegmatogenous detachments: cataract extraction (resulting from movement of the vitreous, in around 1% of patients), peripheral cystic retinal tufts and senile retinoschisis. Blunt trauma may result in detachment because the retina may become detached at the ora serrata (retinal dialysis), or in retinal holes which may occur at the time of injury or months later (Newell 1996). Penetrating trauma may damage the retina directly or result in tears and lead to detachment at a later date.

Timing of surgery is important. If the macular area is not affected, or has only recently become involved, detachment surgery is likely to be undertaken as a matter of urgency in order to preserve macular function. If the macular area has been detached for some time, there is less chance of recovering macular function and surgery may be delayed (Ross and Kozy 1998).

Non-rhegmatogenous retinal detachments

There are two types of non-rhegmatogenous retinal detachments: traction and exudative.

Traction detachments

These occur when there is a proliferation of vitreoretinal membranes creating a localized traction on the retina pulling the neural retina away from the RPE. This type of detachment is associated with proliferative diabetic retinopathy (PDR), proliferative vitreoretinopathy (PVR) and retinopathy of prematurity (ROP). Traction membranes grow on the surface of the retina and can even grow into the vitreous cavity using the vitreous as a type of scaffolding. Membranes, such as in PVR, can create traction, which causes new retinal breaks or results in the recurrence of retinal detachments. PVR is often the cause of failed detachment procedures.

To restore vision, the traction needs to be removed and to gain access to the membranes the vitreous must be removed. Vitreoretinal surgery is currently the only treatment option.

Exudative detachments

Exudative detachments occur when there is damage to the RPE by choroidal or retinal disorders. The conditions associated with this type of detachment are AMD, tumours of the choroid, choroidal haemorrhage, inflammation and retinopathies. These have a poor prognosis and there are few treatment options; those that are available are not necessarily recognized as conventional treatment as a result of the guarded outcome and because the variables contributing to success or failure are still not fully understood.

Signs and symptoms

Patients presenting with retinal detachments provide a similar description of their symptoms, irrespective of what type of detachment. Symptoms that patients complain about are photopsia (flashing lights), floaters, distorted vision or straight lines appearing wavy (metamorphopsia), loss of some the visual field (peripheral or central), with no associated pain.

As vitreous separates from the retina and moves within the eye, floaters may be seen by the individual. They appear as spots, curly lines or rings, and may be dark or clear. They move with the eye and may be especially troublesome when looking at a pale surface or the sky. Vitreous tugging on the retina stimulates it and the only way that this can be interpreted by the brain is as a flashing light. The appearance of flashing lights may, therefore, be an indication of traction on the retina, and a possible retinal hole. If a retinal blood vessel may be damaged, blood may emerge into the vitreous (vitreous haemorrhage). A small amount of blood may be seen as a shower of spots and larger amounts of blood can cause darker patches in the field of vision. A retinal detachment may appear as a patch of vision that is missing or as something moving around in the periphery of vision. Another common visual symptom described by patients is to feel that they can see a spider's web, or be trying to brush away stray hairs that seem to be over their vision.

Examination

Anterior segment

- There may be an absence of the red reflex.
- Relative afferent pupillary defect may be noted with extensive retinal detachment.
- Intraocular pressure (IOP) difference between the affected and normal eye of up to 5 mmHg.
- A mild anterior uveitis may be present.

If major, the pupil may appear white (leukocoria) as a result of the detached retinal tissue floating behind the lens.

Posterior segment

- The detached retina has the appearance of a tissue waving in the breeze, whereas a retina that remains attached appears red from the posterior choroidal circulation.
- Tobacco dust, pigment from the RPE, may be seen.
- Haemorrhage may be present if there is trauma or the detachment has occurred directly over a vessel.
- If no view of the retina is possible, a three-dimensional ultrasound scan (B scan) may be undertaken to aid diagnosis.

Treatment options

These are dependent on the type and severity and fall into two categories: surgical and non-surgical. Before the 1920s there was no recognized successful treatment option available for any type of retinal detachment; people eventually lost their sight. The goal of any intervention is the preservation of vision, and to restore pre-detachment vision when possible. The aim of treatment is to close the retinal break and realign the neural retinal epithelium and the RPE.

Retinopexy

This is the least complex method of repairing, i.e. closing, a retinal break. It is least invasive option and is used only when the break is small.

Patient
- Pre-procedure: explain procedure including feeling of an uncomfortable pressure when indenting and need for positioning/posturing post-procedure, probable visual disturbance from the introduced gas.
- The pupil of affected eye is dilated, the patient is positioned supine, local anaesthetic eye drops instilled, sometimes local infiltrate required.
- Post-procedure: patient requires positioning or posturing; this allows the gas bubble to provide an internal tamponade to the break. Positioning is vital to the successful outcome of this procedure. Regular IOP checks are required and the patient must be warned about visual disturbance from the injection of gas (Shelswell 2002).

Procedure – sometimes staged
- An expandable gas is injected into the posterior segment through a 30-gauge needle at the pars plana (pneumatic retinopexy). Two commonly

used gases are perfluoropropane (C_3F_8) and sulphur hexafluoride (SF_6). This bubble of gas acts as a tamponade to prevent more fluid entering the retinal break and therefore allows the RPE and choroid to reabsorb the subretinal fluid.

- A paracentesis is frequently required to reduce IOP because the gas goes into a cavity that has a finite capacity. The gas introduced is absorbed over a few weeks.

- Indirect laser (photocoagulation) or cryotherapy is applied around the retinal break to create a chorioretinal scar and permanently seal the break.

- The use of cryotherapy is not influenced by the presence of excessive subretinal fluid and may be used if a laser is not available, but the patient usually experiences more pain as a result of postoperative conjunctival oedema.

- If laser is the preferred treatment option, this may be a staged procedure because, if there is excessive subretinal fluid present, this prevents sufficient uptake of laser. However, after positioning following insertion of a gas bubble, subretinal fluid is reduced as a result of the pump action of the RPE, and laser can be effectively applied to create scarring and seal the retinal break.

Scleral explants

Scleral explant surgery is often referred to as a conventional retinal detachment repair and used when there is a peripheral retinal break(s). This procedure not only closes the retinal break, but also reduces the vitreous tension on the retinal surface caused by the indentation created by an external tamponade. The external tamponade may be a scleral buckle, tyre, band or 'plomb'. It is essential that there is a good view of the break(s) if this option is to be successful. The explants are generally made out of silicone because of the material's properties. Before the advent of vitreoretinal surgery, this was the treatment of choice for most retinal detachments.

Patient
- Pre-procedure: preparation as for retinopexy.
- Post-procedure: positioning required only if air or gas has been inserted in the posterior segment.
- Adequate analgesia.

Procedure
- The break is closed with cryo- or indirect laser therapy. The application of an external tamponade (explant) aims to bring the RPE, choroid and sclera into contact with the retinal break. Although the vitreous may

still be causing a traction-like force on the retina, this inward force will be decreased as the wall of the eye is indented by the explant. There are many different shapes and sizes of scleral explants, and use depends on the size of the break and often the surgeon's preference.

- Subretinal fluid may be drained to aid the contact of the retinal break to the underlying RPE.
- Air or expandable gas may also be inserted into the posterior segment, acting as an internal tamponade.

Vitreoretinal surgery

This is more commonly known as a three-port pars plana vitrectomy or just 'vitrectomy'. The vitrectomy has revolutionized the treatment of complicated retinal detachment repairs. A vitrectomy may also be performed in combination with a scleral buckling procedure, especially in complicated retinal detachment repairs such as giant retinal tears (where the retinal edge has rolled in on itself).

Patient
- Pre-procedure: prepare as for retinopexy.
- Post-procedure: positioning or posturing will always be required.

Procedure
- A vitrectomy involves making three incisions (sclerotomies) at the pars plana; this is the safest method to gain access to the posterior segment. As the word suggests, 'vitrectomy' is the removal of the vitreous. However, as vitreous is a gel, it cannot simply be sucked out of the eye; instead a special device that cuts as well as sucks the vitreous is required to remove vitreous safely. As a result of the shape of the eye and the presence of the lens, it is physically impossible to remove all the vitreous, but careful attention ensures that the posterior hyaloid and as much vitreous as necessary are removed, thereby releasing the traction on the retina and enabling it to be reapposed to the RPE.
- Subretinal fluid can be drained via the retinal break or another retinotomy (retinal hole made by the operator/surgeon).
- Heavy liquid (perfluorocarbon liquid) is injected into the vitreous cavity to reappose the neural epithelium to the RPE to assist in the repair of the retinal detachment, but this substance is toxic to the retina and so is used only as a temporary tamponade. The retinal break(s) is then closed with the formation of a chorioretinal scar by laser, which may be either endo (internal) or indirect, or cryotherapy.
- The vitreous does not regenerate, so something is needed to replace it. During the operation an ocular compatible solution (such as balanced salt solution or BSS) is used to maintain IOP, but postoperatively BSS

would not create the required internal tamponade to ensure a successful detachment repair. For this reason an expandable gas or silicone oil is inserted into the vitreous cavity, thus providing an intraocular tamponade. The substance used depends on the retinal break and the ability of the patient to position postoperatively.

- If an expandable gas is used, it will naturally be a much larger volume than that used for a pneumatic retinopexy or during a scleral buckle retinal detachment procedure, where the vitreous has not been removed. To reduce the risk of central retinal artery occlusion, the gases are mixed with non-expandable air to create an appropriate mix. Expandable gases are absorbed after a few weeks (and aqueous fills the remaining space). A large break may require a longer-acting tamponade, in which case silicone oil may be a better option than a gas replacement for the removed vitreous.
- A further surgical procedure is required to remove the oil, if this is used during the procedure to repair the detachment.

Retinal tamponades

Unlike other organs in the body it is impossible to apply direct pressure to the eye without potential damage to the ocular structure and so tamponades are used. These tamponades can be external (scleral explants) or internal. The internal tamponades consist of air, expandable gases e.g. SF_6 or C_3F_8, silicone oil or heavy liquid (perfluorocarbon liquids), and it is essential that the implications of these substances are understood when providing care to patients, particularly for discharge information. Complications of tamponade use include increased IOP and cataract formation. If an internal tamponade is likely to be required during a surgical procedure the nurse should highlight to the medical staff the need for a preoperative A scan, as a result of the potential for cataract development.

Patients are required to posture postoperatively to ensure that the tamponade is effective irrespective of which substance is used. Positioning is also dependent on where the tamponade needs to be applied. Macular hole repair requires face-down posturing, whereas a superior temporal hole may require patient to posture 'cheek to pillow'.

Air
This is seldom used as a tamponade because it is absorbed too readily from the vitreous cavity.

Gases
As discussed, there are a number of expandable gases available for use. However, with all gases, atmospheric pressure and nitrogen and oxygen pressure affect the rate of expansion and activities such as diving or flying

could adversely affect the gas, causing further expansion, resulting in occlusion of the central retinal artery. For this reason, education must be given to the patient, particularly if they intend to fly immediately after surgery because alternative arrangements may need to be made either to transport or to treatment. Nitrous oxide is a commonly used general anaesthetic agent, but when there is an expandable gas in the vitreous cavity the use of nitrous oxide will adversely affect the rate of the gas's expansion as described above.

An application of a 'gas bracelet' is recommended to remind the patient of the potential complications of the gas and to highlight to other medical staff the presence of the gas in the eye. An example could be one that states: 'No nitrous oxide, expandable gas in eye.' This bracelet would be removed by the ophthalmologist when there is no further viable presence of gas in the vitreous cavity.

Silicone oil

Unlike gas, silicone oil cannot be absorbed; it requires a surgical procedure for removal. Silicone oil is a transparent substance that is lighter than water. It is indicated for use in giant retinal tears, diabetic retinopathy, post-traumatic retinal detachments, if the patient has to travel by air postoperatively or if the patient may not be compliant with positioning.

The removal of the oil is undertaken 3–6 months postoperatively but the timeframe is dependent on the stability of the retina and may be left *in situ* in some cases. A cataract extraction and insertion of an intraocular lens (IOL) is often performed when removing the silicone oil, if required.

Heavy liquids

These have a low viscosity that makes then easily injected and aspirated during vitreoretinal surgery. They are a useful tool for repairing retinal detachments such as unfolding the edge of a giant retinal tear, but are never left *in situ* long term because of ocular toxicity.

Other potential vitreous substitutes are under development.

Retinoschisis

In retinoschisis the neural retina splits and separates, generally in the outer plexiform layer. There are three major types of retinoschisis: congenital, acquired/degenerative or secondary to other retinal trauma or disease. It affects a small number of the population and is more common in hypermetropic individuals. For most people it is asymptomatic with no visual impairment.

Congenital retinoschisis is uncommon and always bilateral and causes a vitreoretinal degeneration; the patient has an impaired visual acuity as a result of maculopathy. Congenital retinoschisis is found almost exclusively in males.

No treatment is necessary for most patients with retinoschisis, except when there are complications such as retinal detachment.

Diabetic retinopathy

Diabetes mellitus is classified as type 1 (no insulin produced) or type 2 (decreased insulin production or insulin resistance) diabetes and is reaching epidemic proportions in many countries. Type 1 and 2 diabetes can affect a variety of ocular structures, but one of the most universal complications of diabetes is diabetic retinopathy (DR). Diabetic retinopathy, microangiopathy where the retinal vasculature is pathologically altered, is a microvascular complication that is similar to changes found in other regions of the body as a result of diabetes. The result is DR. Studies have shown that a person with diabetes is 10–20 times more likely to go blind than a non-diabetic person and diabetes is the most common cause of blindness in those aged 30–60 years in the western world.

The likelihood of having a degree of DR increases with the duration of diabetes with almost all type 1 and 60% of those with type 2 diabetes developing some form of retinopathy after 20 years. The development and progression of DR is also influenced by several factors, including chronic hyperglycaemia, pregnancy and hypertension, and, if untreated, the retinopathy will progress causing loss of vision. To date there is no cure for DR.

The dense network of capillary vessels in the retina is vulnerable to microvascular disease and diabetes affects retinal blood vessels, resulting initially in features of microvascular occlusion and leakage. The exact mechanisms causing the development of DR are not yet completely understood; however, thickening of the capillary basement membrane and endothelial damage are believed to contribute to retinal microvascular occlusion which may begin the cascade of DR changes that can result in blindness. The development of DR is progressive and the clinical manifestations of different stages are related to the changes occurring in the retinal vasculature. However, different stages may exist together. The classification or stages and clinical features observed as retinopathy develops are outlined in Table 21.2.

Non-proliferative diabetic retinopathy

In this early (mild) stage, changes are limited to the surface of the retina, there is no growth of new vessels (neovascularization) and this stage lasts many years and does not interfere with vision. It is also known as

Table 21.2 Classification and visible clinical features of diabetic retinopathy

Classification	Clinical features	Visual symptoms
Non-proliferative diabetic retinopathy (NPDR) Mild to moderate	Microaneurysms Small intraretinal haemorrhages Hard exudates Retinal oedema	→ asymptomatic
Pre-proliferative diabetic retinopathy Moderate-to-severe NPDR	Cotton-wool spots Changes to venous vessels – 'beading' or 'looping' Intraretinal microvascular abnormalities	→ asymptomatic
Proliferative diabetic retinopathy (PDR)	Neovascularization: new vessels at optic disc, elsewhere in retina or on iris Fibrous traction bands Vitreous haemorrhage	→ asymptomatic → sudden ↓ in vision
Diabetic maculopathy	Macular oedema Clinically significant macular oedema (CSMO)	→↓ in visual acuity →↓ central vision

Adapted from Hamilton et al. (1996).

'background retinopathy' and/or mild non-proliferative DR (NPDR). This stage is characterized by microaneurysms, which are outpouchings from the walls of the capillaries (Figure 21.5).

As retinopathy progresses, microaneurysms from the basement membranes of the capillaries thicken, resulting in impaired cell integrity. Pericytes are responsible for structural integrity in the retinal capillary walls and chronic hyperglycaemia may lead to pericyte and capillary wall damage. Advanced glycation end-products (AGEs) have also been indicated in the development of basement membrane abnormalities. The affected retinal capillary basement membranes thicken and may become entirely blocked, thus cutting off the blood supply to the cells served by that capillary. The vessels also become more permeable, resulting in vascular leakage of blood, protein and lipid.

Moderate NPDR is characterized by dot-and-blot haemorrhages as the distended vessels burst, resulting in small haemorrhages, and the presence of hard exudates resulting from diminished permeability of the capillary walls. Hard exudates are yellow in appearance, composed of lipoproteins and deposit in the outer plexiform area/layer of the retina.

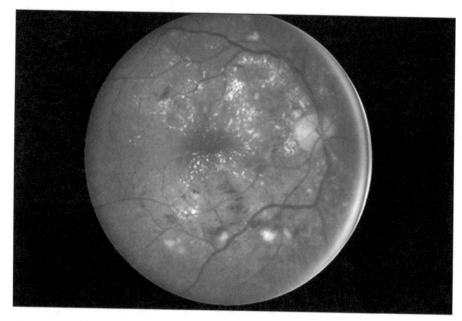

Figure 21.5 Non-proliferative diabetic retinopathy. (See Plate 52.)

Flame-shaped haemorrhages occur in the nerve fibre layer; these are also seen in hypertensive retinopathy.

Diabetic maculopathy

If the diabetic damage results in increased blood vessel permeability with fluid accumulating at the macula, oedema, hard exudates, or both, accumulate at the macula and are associated with macular thickening and the development of maculopathy. Vision is initially blurred, but long-term clinically significant macular oedema (CSMO) will cause permanent loss of central vision as a result of the separation of neurosensory retina from the RPE. CSMO is the principal mechanism of visual loss in NPDR, but it can occur at any time during the progression of retinopathy.

Severe or pre-proliferative NPDR

The microvasculature changes and resulting capillary non-perfusion lead to the progression of DR and the development of retinal ischaemia. The severe stage is characterized by signs of retinal ischaemia, including cotton-wool spots, intraretinal microvascular abnormalities (IRMAs) and beaded or looped blood vessels.

Cotton-wool spots overlie the retinal vessels and lie in the nerve fibre layer of the retina. They are white fluffy patches that imply retinal ischaemia, but do not interfere with vision and are transient. Chronic capillary changes, defects in the red blood cells and increased platelet stickiness also contribute to this.

Proliferative diabetic retinopathy

Proliferative diabetic retinopathy (Figure 21.6) is defined as 'the presence of new vessels on the surface of the retina or optic disc' (Ferris et al. 1999, p. 669). This is advanced retinal vessel disease associated with advanced diabetes and other blood vessel disease; it always impedes vision. Ischaemia is the major influencing factor in the progression to PDR. In an attempt to correct ischaemia, the body tries to improve the circulation and angiogenic factors are released, stimulating the proliferation of new blood vessels (neovascularization). The vessels can grow from the remaining vessels at the edge of the non-perfused areas (new vessels elsewhere or NVE) or at the optic disc (new vessels at disc or NVD). These vessels do not resolve the ischaemia but can instead 'grow upwards' off the retina's surface and up into the vitreous using it as scaffolding. As the vitreous shrinks forward, the vessels are pulled forward and bleed, resulting in a haemorrhage known as a vitreous or intragel haemorrhage.

The new vessels are fragile and tend to bleed, which can result in haemorrhages between the posterior hyaloid membrane and the retinal surface:

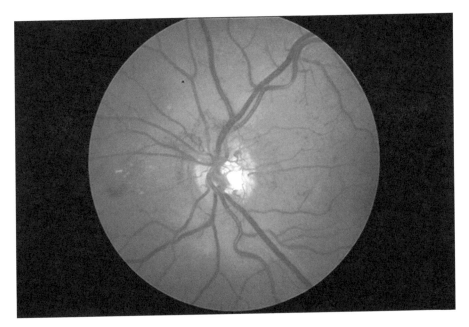

Figure 21.6 Proliferative diabetic retinopathy. (See Plate 53.)

preretinal, subhyloid or retrogel haemorrhage. They also have an accompanying fibrotic glial tissue or scar-like component; this tissue is white and non-transparent so it interferes with visual acuity, plus it behaves like scar tissue and contracts. As this occurs, the tissue pulls on retinal vessels leading to breaks and/or haemorrhages. The vessels also pull on the retina, causing distortion and retinal breaks leading to vitreous haemorrhage, retinal detachment and severe visual loss.

In PDR, bleeding from the new vessels results in sudden loss of vision as a result of a vitreous haemorrhage. In the contraction stage vision loss may occur secondary to tractional complications of the neovascular fibrotic membrane on the retinal surface, causing neurosensory retinal separation from RPE. The detachment may be localized, causing loss of vision if it involves the macula, or it may be a combined local – rhegmatogenous – retinal detachment secondary to tractional forces from the PDR.

Diagnosis

Diabetic retinopathy often does not cause any visual loss symptoms until a vitreous haemorrhage occurs; by then, the retinopathy can be quite advanced. The diagnosis of DR is made by either visual examination or retinal photography. Hence the need for regular and accurate checks of all those with diagnosed diabetes to assess the state of the retina in relation to diabetes. Early diagnosis and treatment are always more effective and give better results in the long term. Failing this, the aim is to diagnose and treat before permanent vision loss occurs.

Treatment options

The rate of development of diabetes-related complications, such as DR, can be affected by diabetic control. Management of diabetes is the only viable option to reduce the occurrence of blinding DR. This involves education about factors that effect diabetes, including glucose control, blood pressure control, diet, physical activity and pharmacological agents. Patient education should begin early in the patient's disease process, and diabetic liaison nurses, GP nurses and diabetic clinics have an important role to aid patients by empowering them to gain the knowledge and skills required to facilitate the prevention of complications.

Patients with diabetes need to understand the importance of regular eye examinations for the management of DR. A health intervention plan for a patient with diabetes must include education about the importance of regular ophthalmic assessment because the rate and development of retinopathy progression in an individual cannot be predicted. Patients with DR may remain asymptomatic, unaware of their condition and the potential for loss of vision, and retinopathy can be well advanced before visual symptoms occur and the patient presents for assessment and treatment.

Diabetic retinopathy screening consists of retinal photography, ophthalmoscope examination (fundoscopy) or a combination of both. Once screened, patients with retinopathy changes can receive appropriate follow-up or photocoagulation treatment (Hamilton et al. 1996).

Retinal photography

There are two ways in which the retina is photographed to aid in the diagnosis and treatment options: retinal photoscreening or fluorescein angiography.

Retinal photoscreening

This is a process whereby patients with diabetes are screened primarily and then on a regular basis using retinal photography for those who have minimal or no DR. In some countries this is undertaken annually; in others the expectation is every 2 years if no DR is present, but the frequency of subsequent retinal photoscreening depends on the presence of the retinal disease. Photographs of the retina are taken and reviewed; primary and secondary screening are increasingly undertaken by nurses and other trained personnel with tertiary screening by consultant ophthalmologists for photographs identified as abnormal (Shah and Brown 2000).

Digital cameras are increasingly being used for retinal photoscreening because the images can be transmitted electronically which has several advantages over celluloid images. The image can be viewed by ophthalmologists as needed in the clinical setting and, for tertiary screening, the screener can be offsite and the images can be used for the teaching purposes of health-care personnel (Ryder 1995). However, perhaps most importantly, the image can be used as a teaching tool for the patient and the family to assist them in understanding the degree of retinopathy and the possible outcome or treatment required. The photographs are a hard record of the presence or absence of DR and offer a safer alternative to a retinal drawing, which could be misinterpreted. Digital cameras also allow flexibility in the provision of screening services with outreach facilities closer to the patients, making attendance easier than to a large hospital.

Patient preparation is dependent on whether the camera is non-mydriatic or mydriatic. Non-mydriatic cameras do not require the patient to have the pupil dilated whereas pupil dilatation is required for a mydriatic camera.

Fluorescein angiography

Fluorescein angiography (FFA) may be used for diagnosis of maculopathy and to aid in decisions about photocoagulation.

Photocoagulation

Two ground-breaking trials, the Diabetic Retinopathy Study (DRS Group 1978) and the Early Treatment of Diabetic Retinopathy Study (ETDRS Research Group 1985), demonstrated the risk of severe visual loss from PDR and that maculopathy can be reduced by retinal photocoagulation (laser). Laser was developed in the 1970s. Before this, there was no established form of treatment for DR. The rationale behind laser treatment is as follows:

1. To destroy abnormal new vessels by treating where the capillaries are not perfused; consequently the stimulation for neovascularization is reduced. Panretinal, or scatter, photocoagulation (PRP) laser for PDR treatment involves the application of thermal energy to the peripheral retina in order to ablate the ischaemic retina, causing a reduction in its oxygen need and therefore in the stimulation of vasogenic factors, leading to regression of neovascularization (Figure 21.7). Although the peripheral retina is 'burnt' by the laser, central vision should be maintained. Destruction of the ischaemic areas in the peripheral areas may even lead to shrinkage of new vessels at the optic disc.
2. Focal or grid macular photocoagulation consists of precise focal points of laser burns to blood vessels leaking into the macular area. Laser treatment destroys or occludes leaking vessels near the macula, thereby reducing the leakage of fatty deposits and fluid accumulation. This is the treatment of choice for diabetic maculopathy. If nerve cells are

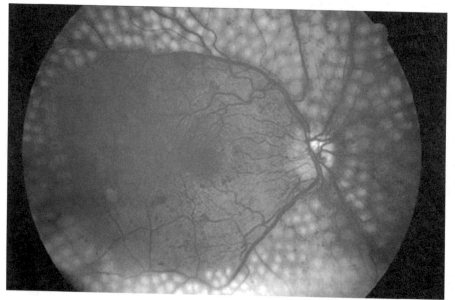

Figure 21.7 Panretinal photocoagulation for retinopathy. (By courtesy of the National Eye Institute, National Institutes of Health, USA.) (See Plate 54.)

already destroyed treatment cannot heal them or improve the visual acuity, but instead aims to maintain vision at the current level.

There are a number of lasers currently suitable for use in treating DR, yet, despite the proven effectiveness of photocoagulation treatment, it does not improve or restore any lost vision. Photocoagulation can only delay the progression of retinopathy and reduce loss of vision if it is instigated in the early stages of DR. The most effective method of preventing loss of vision is to prevent NPDR from progressing.

Patient preparation for laser

- Dilate pupil
- Information about the procedure: bright flashes are occasionally uncomfortable; laser burns for PRP may be uncomfortable and they will often require more than one treatment.

Side effects may include headache, choroidal detachment and macular oedema.

Vitreoretinal surgery

In the early 1960s, the concept of a controlled removal of vitreous was realized when Kasner performed a planned 'open sky vitrectomy'. Machemer went on to develop the pars plana vitrectomy which has successfully allowed visual rehabilitation, for many patients, of eyes that were previously untreatable. Vitrectomy for the complications of proliferative changes has resulted in the preservation of vision for many patients with PDR and traction detachments. Indications for a vitrectomy in diabetic eye disease include:

- Severe non-clearing vitreous haemorrhage
- Traction retinal detachment especially when involving the macula
- Combined traction and rhegmatogenous retinal detachment
- Severe progressive fibrovascular proliferation.

Surgical steps are similar to vitreoretinal surgery for other reasons but include a membranectomy to dissect off and remove the proliferating tissue and relieve the traction. PRP is always performed via indirect laser at the time of surgery. If there is a combined tractional–rhegmatogenous detachment, the surgical procedure will also involve the identification of retinal breaks, removal of subretinal fluid, photocoagulation to seal the breaks, insertion of an internal tamponade and possible explant, and postoperative posturing for the patient. In cases of severe persistent retinal traction, a retinectomy (planned incision of the scleral surface of the retina) may need to be performed in order to salvage the macula and central vision.

Postoperative complications
- Infection
- Cataract formation
- Recurrent vitreous haemorrhage
- Rhegmatogenous retinal detachment
- Fibrin clot formation
- Neovascular glaucoma
- Flat anterior chamber
- Transient rise in IOP.

Pharmacological control of diabetic retinopathy

Research into the possibility of pharmacological control includes the pharmacological control of angiogenesis to reduce proliferative diabetic neovascularization and a drug to dissolve the vitreous, thereby reducing vitreoretinal traction. However, at present these are not viable options (Ferris et al. 1999). The prevalence of diabetes is predicted to increase, reflecting changing demographic factors (including increased population size and changes in population age structure) and epidemiological factors (such as obesity and physical inactivity). The increasing incidence of diabetes will inevitably mean that diabetes-related complications, such as DR, will have an increasing impact on society, health care and economics.

Retinopathy of prematurity

Retinopathy of prematurity (ROP) is a relatively new ophthalmic diagnosis. It was first described in 1942 by Terry as retrolental fibroplasia (RLF). It was initially thought that the tissue developed postnatally and the white retrolental mass might be a congenital cataract. However, the cause was unknown with different aetiologies proposed, including infection transmitted by either the mother or the primary source, vitamin E deficiency and/or anoxia.

History of ROP

In 1948 Owens and Owens ophthalmoscopically observed normal fundi in pre-term infants undergo a transformation over several weeks, but it was not until the early 1950s that hyperoxia was implicated in the incidence of RLF. The judicious use of inspired oxygen for pre-term infants reduced the amount of RLF but the incidence of death and brain damage among pre-term infants was increased. However, with the technological developments of the 1960s, low-birthweight pre-term infants who would have previously died survived, but required the use of oxygen to do so and the incidence of RLF continued to increase in the 1960s and 1970s despite sophisticated oxygen-measuring techniques. In the 1980s ROP replaced RLF as the accepted terminology to describe this condition.

Incidence of ROP

Small infants are increasingly susceptible to ROP despite meticulous monitoring of oxygen therapy and this continues to be the case today; there has been no safe mean discovered to dates to prevent ROP. It is now thought that prematurity and associated low birthweight (< 1000 g) are the primary contributors to ROP as opposed to overzealous use of oxygen, as suggested in the past.

Cause of ROP

Although it is not fully understood how or why ROP develops, the retinal vasculature is not completely developed in a very pre-term infant. The nasal ora is reached by the inner retina vasculature at about 8 months' gestation, although the temporal ora is not reached until 9 months' gestation and once vascularization is complete, oxygen does not affect the retina. Currently it is thought that the pre-term baby is at higher risk as a result of ischaemic areas of the retina. Since 1984 the International Classification of Retinopathy of Prematurity (ICROP) has been used. The classification defined the location of disease and the extent of developing vasculature. The location is divided into three zones and the abnormal vascularization is divided up into five progressive stages.

The most common outcome is regression for most babies who develop ROP; this occurs spontaneously and does not require intervention. However, a small minority progress to advanced ROP requiring intervention.

Treatment for ROP

- All pre-term babies must be monitored, particularly those at or below 26 weeks' gestation, because they have an increased risk of developing ROP.
- It is necessary to dilate pupils to examine these babies with an indirect ophthalmoscope and indenting of the retina as a result of retinal pathology in ROP begins at the periphery.
- Advanced ROP requires cryotherapy or laser treatment to ablate the ischaemic areas, resulting in regression of the abnormal vasculature. Rarely, babies with ROP develop retinal detachments and these require surgical intervention.

Nursing care

It is essential that the parents be supported and provided with education and given time to absorb information and encouraged to ask questions, irrespective of the extent of the disease.

Hypertensive retinopathy

Hypertensive retinopathy occurs secondary to an elevated systemic blood pressure, resulting in changes in the vasculature of the retina and choroid. The elevated systemic blood pressure can cause either primary hypertension or secondary hypertension as a result of renal disease or toxaemia of pregnancy. Sustained hypertension causes disruption of the blood–retina barrier with the resultant increase in vascular permeability. Specific ocular manifestations associated with systemic hypertension are retinal vein occlusion, retinal artery occlusion, exudative retinal detachment and ischaemic optic neuropathy.

The incidence of hypertensive retinopathy is dependent on the control of the patient's systemic hypertension. The initial response is narrowing of the retinal arterioles; however, if there is a lot of involutional sclerosis in older patients, the same degree of narrowing does not occur despite the presence of hypertensive retinopathy.

Signs and symptoms

Patient symptoms

- Symptoms depend on the severity of the retinopathy present.
- It is generally asymptomatic with minimal retinopathy.
- The patient will complain of blurred or distorted vision with moderate-to-severe hypertensive retinopathy caused by haemorrhages and exudates affecting the macula, and consequently affecting central vision.
- If moderate-to-severe hypertensive retinopathy is present, the patient may also complain of headaches.

Signs

- The retinal image is characterized by vasoconstriction and leakage of vessels.
- Hypertensive retinopathy has four distinct gradings (Table 21.3).

Treatment

Control of hypertension is the key to controlling the retinopathy.

Table 21.3 The grading and visible clinical features of hypertensive retinopathy

Grading of hypertensive retinopathy	Clinical features	Visual symptoms
Grade 1: mild retinopathy	Arteriolar narrowing Broadening of arteriolar light reflex	→ asymptomatic
Grade 2: moderate	Arteriovenous crossing changes. Cotton-wool spots	→ asymptomatic
Grade 3: severe	Flame-shaped haemorrhages, mainly in nerve fibre layer Microaneurysms Hard exudates 'Copper wiring' of arterioles Marked arteriolar constriction Secondary telangiectasias Serous detachment	→generally asymptomatic →symptomatic if retinal involvement
Grade 4: malignant	Signs as for grade 3 Disc swelling/ischaemic papillopathy Macular star from hard exudates around fovea	→symptomatic only if macular involvement

Retinal vein occlusion

Retinal vein occlusion is the second most common retinal vascular disease after diabetic retinopathy; the occlusions can be central (central retinal vein occlusion or CRVO) or branch (branch retinal vein occlusion or BRVO). Factors that predispose to retinal vein occlusions can be systemic or ocular (Table 21.4).

Table 21.4 Causes of retinal vein occlusion

Cause	Contributing factors
Systemic	Age Hypertension Blood abnormalities (dyscrasias), e.g. sickle-cell disease
Ocular	Raised intraocular pressure Hypermetropia Congenital anomalies Periphlebitis, e.g. Behçet's disease

From Recchia and Brown (2000).

Branch retinal vein occlusion

Occlusion of a vein draining any section of the retina results in stagnation of blood flow and hypoxia of the corresponding retinal area, and increased vessel permeability. The occlusion can occur in the periphery or the macular region. The latter may result in macular oedema with a noticeable decrease in the patient's visual acuity.

At the acute stage features seen include tortuous veins, flame-shaped haemorrhages and retinal oedema, which may resolve in 6–12 months, but which may be replaced by vascular sheathing, chronic macular oedema and RPE degeneration at the macula. The larger the area affected by the BRVO, the poorer the visual recovery prognosis. With a main BRVO, vitreous haemorrhage may be present; this will usually clear over a number of months. Complications of BRVO include secondary neovascularization and chronic macular oedema.

Management

It is important that the patient be aware that, in 5% of cases, both eyes can be affected by a BRVO, and control of systemic hypertension is paramount. The following are alternatives for the management of secondary complications:

- If an FFA shows macular oedema as opposed to macular ischaemia, laser photocoagulation may be useful.
- Laser photocoagulation is indicated for neovascularization.
- Persistent or recurring vitreous haemorrhage requires a vitrectomy.
- Vitrectomy and sheathotomy, by opening the sheath surrounding the retinal vessels, provide a release of the arteriovenous (AV) pressure and enable the occlusion to resolve.

Prognosis

If the underlying cause, systemic hypertension, is controlled visual prognosis is reasonably good unless the macula is involved. In about 50% of patients, collateral vessels develop and take over the role of the occluded vein but, if the perifoveal capillary network is too badly affected, the visual prognosis is poor.

Central retinal vein occlusion

Central retinal vein occlusion can be divided into three specific groups; the treatment and prognosis vary according to which group the vein occlusion falls into (Table 21.5).

Table 21.5 Central retinal vein occlusion (CRVO)

Groups	Clinical features	Symptoms	Prognosis	Treatment
Non-ischaemic	Tortuous and dilated branches of CRV Retinal haemorrhages Disc oedema Macular oedema	Loss of VA Slight Marcus–Gunn pupil	50% regain near normal VA Loss of VA is the result of chronic cystoid macular oedema	Inconclusive if laser beneficial for macular oedema
Ischaemic	Tortuous and engorged veins Retinal haemorrhages Cotton-wool spots Disc oedema Macula Haemorrhages and cystoid changes	Loss of VA (6/60) Marcus–Gunn pupil	Poor Potential development of neovascular glaucoma and vitreous haemorrhage	Laser photo-coagulation to prevent neovascul-arization
Young individuals (rare)	Optic disc vasculitis and oedema Retinal haemorrhages	Mild decrease in VA, worse in the morning	Good as little retinal ischaemia	Observe

A recent development in the treatment of CRVO is vitrectomy and optic neurotomy. After the vitreous is removed, the surgeon will 'stab' an outer area of the disc to widen the lamina cribrosa, allowing more room for the central retinal vein and thus decreasing the pressure on the vein, thereby decreasing the amount of the occlusion.

Retinal artery occlusion

This can be central retinal artery occlusion (CRAO) or branch retinal artery occlusion (BRAO); they are commonly associated with an embolic blockage from heart or carotid artery disease such as cholesterol plaques. They may also be caused by systemic conditions that result in arteritis and secondary occlusion of the artery, e.g. giant cell arteritis. A severe rise in IOP may also cause an RAO but this is rare and tends to be a complication associated with pressure on the globe or secondary to a gas tamponade.

Central retinal artery occlusion

This is an ophthalmic emergency and is most often the result of an atheroma or embolus. The patient presents with sudden, complete, painless loss of vision. Externally the eye will look quiet. The fundal image is of a pale, swollen retina with an absence of red reflex. As the fovea does not have the thick nerve fibre layers present in the rest of the retina, the reflex from choroidal vessels is still evident so the fovea stands out as a 'cherry-red spot'; this spot will disappear after a few weeks. Although retinal veins appear normal, the arteries are narrowed.

Treatment needs to be prompt and is aimed at increasing retinal perfusion. Medically, intravenous acetazolamide can help lower the IOP as can intermittent ocular massage, with the added aims of increasing blood flow and dislodging the arterial blockage. Re-breathing (into a paper bag) as a strategy to increase CO_2 levels and cause vessel dilatation, which may allow the embolus to move to a branch artery, may also be used. Other options are: an anterior chamber paracentesis to reduce IOP (again, to take pressure off the central retinal artery and allow the embolus to travel to a branch artery) or a gas exchange if the raised IOP is caused by a gas tamponade. However, the visual prognosis for patients with CRAO is usually poor.

Branch retinal artery occlusion

These occlusions are commonly the result of emboli and patients present with a painless sudden defect noticed in their visual field. On examination, a pale ischaemic area of the retina is seen. Over time the inner retinal layers atrophy and the patient is left with a permanent visual field defect.

In both CRAO and BRAO, retinal emboli suggest carotid artery disease and the patient should be investigated for cardiovascular disease to prevent a stroke.

Age-related macular degeneration

Age-related macular degeneration (AMD), until recently known as ARMD, is the most common cause of irreversible loss of central vision in people aged over 65 years in the western world, and with the ageing population it is expected that the incidence will continue to increase. AMD is divided into two main types: non-neovascular and neovascular. Non-neovascular AMD, the more common form, affects roughly 10% of people aged over 60, and is characterized by drusen and abnormalities of the RPE, including atrophy of the RPE. Non-neovascular AMD normally has little impact on vision unless significant atrophy develops and is slowly progressive.

Severe and rapidly progressing vision loss is characteristic of the neo-vascular form of AMD, which affects roughly 2% of people over 60. Although non-neovascular AMD is the most common form of the disease (80%), loss of vision results most often from neovascular AMD (90%) and, in general, central vision loss associated with AMD occurs after the development of serous and haemorrhagic detachment of the neurosensory retina and/or RPE as a result of choroidal neovascularization (CNV) (80–90%), and geographic atrophy of the RPE without exudation or haemorrhage (< 5%). Almost half of patients with bilateral neovascular AMD are likely to be legally blind within 5 years of diagnosis because 42% of patients with neovascular AMD will develop it in the other eye within 5 years (Macular Photocoagulation Study Group 1997). Late diagnosis may be partly responsible for the poor prognosis: as loss of vision can go unnoticed if one eye is unaffected, many patients may not present with AMD until the condition has developed bilaterally, and is already relatively advanced in the first eye.

Age-related macular degeneration affects central vision although peripheral vision is maintained, which allows the retention of 'navigational' vision. However, the loss of central vision severely restricts the ability of elderly people to live completely independently, because they are unable to recognize faces, read, sign documents, watch television, drive cars or see bus numbers, leading to frustration and for some depression from loss of independence. People with AMD require constant reassurance and assistance to retain some independence but there will always be a reliance on the assistance of others for every activity. There is also the fear of blindness if both eyes are affected.

Risk factors for AMD

The prevalence of AMD increases with age and several risk factors have been identified, including cigarette smoking and a family history (Arnold and Sarks 2000).

Other factors that may be associated with AMD include gender (female), ethnicity (white), hypertension and cardiovascular disease, ultraviolet light exposure, and aphakia as well as nutritional status. Findings from the Age-Related Eye Disease Study (AREDS Research Group 2001) show that high levels of antioxidants and zinc reduce the risk of advanced AMD by 25%.

AMD development

Age-related macular degeneration specifically affects the outer layers of the retina and portions of the choroid. The areas involved include the photoreceptors, the RPE, Bruch's membrane and the choroidal circulation.

The exact cause of AMD is unknown. It is thought that a combination of genetic and environmental factors, which may involve free radicals, disrupts the normal metabolic activity of the RPE. This leads to an accumulation of debris, with thickening of Bruch's membrane, which forms the barrier between the RPE and the choroid. Ophthalmoscopically, these deposits are visible because they accumulate in Bruch's membrane as drusen. Drusen are a common retinal lesion but are also the earliest clinical sign of AMD and vary in size.

Non-neovascular AMD

In non-neovascular AMD, diffuse drusen may predispose an individual, for unknown reasons, to develop localized areas of atrophy in the RPE. Disappearance of the RPE layer causes progressive damage to the photoreceptors and a gradual failure of central vision if the centre of the fovea is involved. On examination, in non-exudative AMD the retina will appear patchy from RPE atrophy. The RPE cells atrophy, leaving areas of depigmentation in the macula which is seen as 'geographic atrophy'. Geographic atrophy simply relates the appearance of the non-functioning retina affected by AMD.

Neovascular AMD

In neovascular AMD, breaks in Bruch's membrane provide sites through which CNV may grow and proliferate. This process causes rapid, widespread and progressive damage to photoreceptors and is accompanied by a build-up of fibrous tissue. The RPE can detach from the outer aspect of Bruch's membrane and this can damage the RPE and photoreceptors, leading to significant loss of vision. Damaged RPE may produce angiogenic growth factors, which stimulate growth of new blood vessels from the choroid. If left untreated, fibrocytes build up between and within the RPE and photoreceptors; disc-like fibrovascular structures called disciform scars are formed, which replace the RPE, photoreceptors and inner choroid in the central macula and are associated with vision loss.

Signs and symptoms

The patient often presents with normal visual acuity with distortion (metamorphopsia) of central vision being the most common presenting symptom. Patients generally notice this distortion only when for some reason they close one eye; they see distortion of normally straight lines such as doorframes. This metamorphopsia is indicative of foveal pathology. There is also a decrease in contrast sensitivity. As severe loss of vision is often a consequence of CNV, strategies for early detection of this condition's effect on vision are extremely important. Recognition of changes in visual acuity as early as possible could limit vision loss. Patients with recognized AMD should monitor their own sight by noting their ability to carry out daily activities. Patients should be encouraged to use an Amsler grid, one eye at a time, to recognize when their sight is deteriorating and should report any changes promptly for subsequent diagnosis and, possibly, treatment.

Diagnostic tests

Retinal, or fundal, fluorescein angiography allows accurate visualization of the CNV necessary for treatment options (Figure 21.8). Areas of CNV appear as hyperfluorescence and leakage. The terms 'classic' and 'occult' are used to describe the CNV leakage. Classic refers to leakage that occurs early in the angiogram, whereas occult leakage is a later occurrence. ICG angiography is used to investigate the choroidal circulation and often used as an adjunct to the FFA. Stereoscopic FFA is becoming the standard for evaluating CNV, on which treatment decisions are based. If part or all of the lesion is under the centre of the foveal avascular zone, the lesion is defined as subfoveal; lesions within 200 μm of the foveal centre, but not beneath it, are defined as juxtafoveal and extrafoveal lesions are those where lesions are at least 200 μm from the foveal centre.

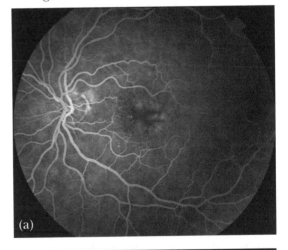

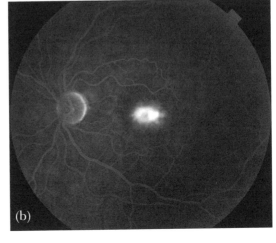

Figure 21.8 Fluorescein angiography of (a) early and (b) late, wet macular degeneration. (By courtesy of Ophthalmic Imaging Department, Manchester Royal Eye Hospital.)

Treatment options

For most patients with AMD, there are no treatment options at present for non-exudative AMD and very limited options for exudative AMD. For patients identified with bilateral age-related macular changes with normal central vision, a diet rich in fruit and green vegetables and the cessation of smoking, are recommended, but this does not necessarily halt progression of the disease. For a minority of patients affected by exudative (or wet) AMD, laser photocoagulation may be applied to 'seal' off, or cauterize, the leaking vessels. This is effective, however, only if the CNV is located outside the foveal area, otherwise the laser burns can damage the fovea as well as all other normal tissue. Well-demarcated extrafoveal and juxtafoveal lesions have been successfully treated with photocoagulation for several years and maintenance of vision has been achieved for an extended interval, but CNV does recur frequently.

Laser photocoagulation is used to limit the spread of neovascularization across the fovea in extrafoveal and juxtafoveal lesions and, in subfoveal cases, may confine damage, thereby limiting the size of the central scotoma and further vision loss.

Recent innovations in treatment of AMD

Photodynamic therapy
Non-thermal laser treatment, known as photodynamic therapy (PDT), has been developed as a treatment option for exudative AMD. This combines a photosensitizing drug (verteporfin is the drug currently available) with non-thermal laser therapy in an attempt to close the leaking vessels. Multiple treatments are required and studies have indicated that PDT is useful only for some patients. To restrict the loss of vision patients must be referred early. However, many patients feel that distorted vision is 'normal' and a result of 'old age' and may not present until they have already lost central vision in one eye. PDT does not restore vision and in some countries, such as New Zealand, it is available only through the private sector, so that the expense of the multiple treatments puts it out of the range of many elderly, retired individuals. The UK's National Institute for Clinical Excellence (NICE 2004), after considering a number of large studies, has recommended PDT for patients with classic and predominantly classic AMD, and it should be available to all eligible patients. Occult lesions may be treated within the NHS as part of a clinical trial.

Verteporfin is rapidly and selectively taken up and retained by neovascular endothelial cells and malignant cells. The timing of photoactivation is critical to the selectivity of PDT with verteporfin. The optimal timing of non-thermal laser delivery is exactly 15 minutes after the start of a

10-minute intravenous infusion (via an infusion pump) of verteporfin 6 mg/m^2. The procedure is time critical and the patient must be well prepared for it. Verteporfin is metabolized mainly in the liver and cleared primarily via the bile and faeces, with less than 1% cleared via the kidneys and urine.

Verteporfin is taken up slowly by the skin, and can be activated in the peripheral vasculature by light. Precautions must therefore be taken against skin photosensitivity after a verteporfin infusion, and patients should avoid direct sunlight and bright lights for 48 hours after treatment and wear a brimmed hat, sunglasses and be fully covered with clothes when out of doors after treatment. The use of a bracelet to inform the patient and other health-care professionals about the needs of the patient after verteporfin therapy is recommended. Some patients report severe back pain following infusion of the drug and the mechanisms for this are not fully understood.

Anti-angiogenic drugs
Research is also underway on anti-angiogenic drugs as a means of stopping the neovascularization. The CNV is attributed to vascular endothelial growth factor (VEGF), a substance that stimulates angiogenesis. Without the stimulation for the CNV there will be a reduction in disease progression and loss of functional vision. Such medications are administered intravitreally or via a sub-Tenon's approach, and they may offer a therapy with the potential to stabilize or even improve vision in patients with exudative macular degeneration.

Surgery
Vitreoretinal surgical intervention with macular translocation, or rotation, has been investigated to offer such patients some chance of regaining central vision. This involves a three-port pars plana vitrectomy, after which there is a planned retinectomy and then a retinal detachment is created, allowing the retina to be 'spun' around. This means that the macula/fovea is translocated to a site away from the underlying CNV. Laser photocoagulation is used to seal the retinectomy. Further surgery is then required to correct the resultant strabismus, and there is a high risk of postoperative complications, including PVD, retinal detachment and macular folds. Translocation surgery is not undertaken lightly.

Dietary supplements
Daily high-dose supplements, including vitamins A, C and E, zinc oxide, lutein and β-carotene may be prescribed as preventive medication for those at risk of developing exudative AMD. However, it has recently been suggested that smokers and ex-smokers should not take the β-carotene component because of the risk of lung cancer.

Ultraviolet light avoidance
Protection against ultraviolet (UV) light has also been recommended, although there are no data yet to support this (Murphy and Nesbitt 2001, Mittra and Singerman 2002).

The end-result of AMD can be a central scotoma (blind spot) and loss of vision, but the progression of AMD is variable among different patients. Some patients with AMD may experience a phenomenon known as Charles–Bonnet syndrome, where the person with visual impairment/central scotoma may have hallucinations that are well defined, organized, clear images (Menkhaus et al. 2003). The precise mechanism is unknown but is believed to originate from the visual association areas of the cerebral cortex. Charles–Bonnet syndrome has been described as phantom vision and likened to phantom limb phenomenon.

Age-related macular degeneration has far-reaching implications not only on an affected patient's quality of life, but also on social and health costs. In an attempt to offer some support to affected patients, it has often been stressed that they will not become totally blind because 'only central vision is lost', although they will be classified as legally blind. This view is, however, likely to be of little comfort to anyone (which must include nearly everyone) who is reliant on their central vision for a normal life. The search for a curative therapy continues. When CNV has developed in both eyes, it is important to maximize existing vision. Good lighting can improve visual function significantly, as can low-vision aids, if some central vision remains. Referral to support agencies and low-visual aid assessors is paramount so that the patient has the option to use low-visual aids to buttress the remaining vision. Disturbances such as metamorphopsia, however, make visual rehabilitation more challenging.

Retinoblastoma

Retinoblastoma is a rare ocular malignant tumour of the retina. It is the most common childhood intraocular malignancy and retinoblastoma can be life threatening if undiagnosed and untreated, although with the current treatment modalities available the survival rate is over 90%. An accurate diagnosis and prompt initiation of treatment interventions that are ongoing for several years are necessary to save the child's life and where possible, to maintain vision. The development of retinoblastoma can occur in the embryo *in utero* and up to 7 years of age, with 18 months as the average age of diagnosis. Retinoblastoma affects about 1 in 20 000 live births (Kanski 2003) and is generally diagnosed within 3 years of birth although it can be diagnosed at any age.

Retinoblastoma is a complex ocular 'disease' process that can be unilateral, bilateral or even trilateral (involving the pineal gland); it can also be familial or sporadic in origin. Familial retinoblastoma occurs from an autosomal dominant gene mutation to chromosome 13 and accounts for only about 6% of cases (Kanski 2003). Children with familial retinoblastoma tend to have an early onset of the disease, are generally bilateral and are at risk of developing other tumours late in life. Sporadic retinoblastoma cases can be either unilateral or bilateral and the cause is unknown. However, if the child with a sporadic presentation has bilateral retinoblastoma, he or she is considered to have a gene mutation, the same as familial cases, and therefore is a carrier of the disease.

Presentation and diagnosis

Occasionally retinoblastoma is 'picked' up as an incidental finding on a regular ultrasound scan during pregnancy. The child commonly presents with leukocoria and/or strabismus with about 60% of cases presenting with leukocoria. Parents may notice 'something strange' about their child's eye, and report a cat's eye appearance, a twinkling easily seen in photographs or even an absence of the normal red reflex from photographs. All such signs require prompt investigation and referral to an ophthalmologist. Although not all of these children will have retinoblastoma, any strabismus or leukocoric eye requires investigations.

A suspicion of retinoblastoma requires an ophthalmic examination of all ocular media, in particular the retina, and this is generally done under general anaesthesia. At the same time the child may undergo ultrasonography, computed tomography (CT) or magnetic resonance imaging (MRI) and bone marrow biopsy depending on the facility in which the ophthalmic examination takes place.

Bilateral indirect ophthalmoscopy, with both pupils fully dilated, is the most important ophthalmic examination undertaken. The examination must include scleral indentation to ensure that tumours located anteriorly in the retina are seen and documented. Documentation of the tumour may be recorded in a variety of ways: hand-drawn sites of the tumour or retinal photographs (conventional celluloid or digital 'retcam'). The tumour appears nodular and from there it can seed out to form a multitude of small retinoblastoma intraocular tumours; there may be a retinal detachment present. It is essential to determine the location of the tumour in relation to the optic nerve because malignant cells can track back to the brain via the optic nerve.

Adjunctive investigations are generally undertaken in collaboration with a paediatric oncology service and include radiological investigation such as CT and MRI which highlight involvement of other organs, e.g. the optic nerve and pineal gland. Bone marrow biopsies are also taken at this time to exclude any metastasis.

Treatment

As retinoblastoma typically occurs in pre-school children, the treatment involves not only the patient, but also the family and significant others. A large part of the care involves education and support, not only concerning the initial diagnosis, but also during the ongoing monitoring necessary for the child.

There are a variety of options depending on the size and location of the tumour. An examination under anaesthetic is performed in order to assess the tumour; this may also involve obtaining retinal photographs (commonly digital) of the tumour. The major contributors to the current survival rate in children with retinoblastoma are the treatment modalities available. The treatment modality may differ from one child to the next because these are often tailored to the individual patient.

Previous to the development of other therapies, enucleation was the treatment of choice. Today this may still be required if the tumour does not respond to other treatment modalities or if it is encroaching on the optic nerve. Postoperatively, the socket will be assessed and the child will require fitting for a prosthesis.

Photocoagulation and/or cryotherapy to the cancer destroys the tumour and prevents it seeding. These treatments are used for treating small tumours and also in combination with chemotherapy agents. Photocoagulation (laser) applies burns to the tissue surrounding the tumour, destroying its blood supply without direct treatment. During cryotherapy, the cryo-probe is placed on the sclera as in a retinal detachment repair. As with all cryo-treatments, the eye may appear oedematous after the procedure.

Chemotherapy has been the major advance and over the last few decades has had the most impact on saving sight and the long-term survival rate for children with retinoblastoma. Chemotherapy works by preventing cell division and replication; it interferes with the DNA and is used to treat retinoblastoma that has become metastatic, and in cases of bilateral disease and advanced unilateral disease to decrease the size of the tumour, in combination with focal treatment to the lesions with laser therapy or cryotherapy to destroy the tumour. There are a number of side effects associated with chemotherapy, and the child's family will also require support and education about these.

External beam radiotherapy or radiotherapy is also used in some cases; however, side effects include cataract formation and disruption to the structure of the bony orbit, resulting in deformity, so it is not often a treatment option pursued today. Radiotherapy is also used in some cases, but is rarely a treatment of choice today.

New treatments continue to be explored; transpupillary thermotherapy laser is currently being explored as an option with what appear to be positive results (Abramson and Schefler 2003) if used alone and also in combination with focal treatment (Lumbroso et al. 2003). Advances in gene technology have enabled some centres to offer retinoblastoma identification markers, so parents are aware of the potential risk to their offspring.

All children born to parents with retinoblastoma or who have siblings diagnosed with retinoblastoma are routinely examined and followed up to ensure early detection of the development of a tumour. This is a type of screening where the children are followed regularly, initially with retinal examinations under anaesthetic but, as the child grows older, retinal examinations can occur in an outpatient setting and generally cease when the child is about 5 years old.

It is common for families to be offered genetic counselling and screening, particularly if their child with retinoblastoma is the first, to determine whether there is a genetic cause of the tumour. Although counselling can be undertaken in any ophthalmic unit, the screening will generally have to be undertaken at a major centre and it will take time to get the results, during which time the family will require support.

Nursing care

A diagnosis of retinoblastoma is devastating for the parents of the child and it is essential that education and support be provided, particularly as there are frequent ocular examinations and treatments required, often for several years. Perhaps the most important role for the nurse is providing support for the patient and the family, and ensuring that they are cognisant with all procedures and processes in their care. Nurses in units that provide care for retinoblastoma patients come to know the children and their parents very well. The parents meet each other frequently and offer support to each other that health-care personnel cannot; the children also often form friendships.

Many ophthalmic units have nurses who are pivotal to coordinating the care of these children with retinblastoma: they organize follow-up visits, liaise with oncology departments, liaise with cancer societies, liaise with ophthalmologists, etc. Some units also have the services of a play therapist, which assists the children in understanding what is happening to them and making their frequent visits for ocular examinations 'fun' to do rather than a 'dread', which in turn helps the parents. Most ophthalmic care for children with retinoblastoma is undertaken on a day-stay basis and so there is little specific nursing care for these children other than what has already been outlined and the routine preparation of any patient having a retinal examination through dilated pupils.

To manage retinoblastoma successfully, early detection is vital. A test as simple as checking for a red reflex could be incorporated into the newborn health assessment checks as an early assessment for retinoblastoma.

Other retinal conditions

Asteroid hyalosis

This is a form of vitreous gel degeneration where calcium 'soaps' aggregate on the vitreous. They are asymptomatic and rarely impair vision. On examination, however, they appear like stars in the vitreous and a B scan shows bright 'spots' in the vitreous body.

Retinitis pigmentosa (RP)

This a hereditary degenerative ocular disease causing a photoreceptor dystrophy with resultant progressive loss of RPE and photoreceptor function. There is also an atypical retinitis pigmentosa which may be associated with a variety of systemic disorders including Usher's syndrome. Usher's syndrome is characterized by profound deafness and blindness.

RP is a bilateral condition with more males affected than females. Although both rods and cones are affected, the damage to the rods is predominant so the patients present with problems with dark adaptation, often described as night blindness (nyctalopia) because the rods are predominantly at the periphery of the retina. Patients frequently present in their teenage years with nyctalopia and by age 30 over 75% are symptomatic with progressive loss of peripheral vision, and often tunnel vision, occurring by the time the patient is in his or her 50s for most.

In patients with retinitis pigmentosa there are few signs in the early stages, but with progression of the disease coarser pigmentary changes occur, seen as clumping of retinal pigment on ocular examination. There is no known treatment for this condition and generally patients are referred to supportive organizations. Genetic counselling may be offered to patients who carry the gene.

Sickle-cell disease

Sickle-cell disease is the most common haemoglobinopathy affecting humans; it is caused by the presence of abnormal haemoglobins in the red blood cells. In conditions such as hypoxia and acidosis, the abnormal haemoglobin cells become sickle shaped and more rigid than normal. These sickle cells obstruct small blood vessels, resulting in tissue ischaemia locally. Once ischaemia is present a cycle is commenced where more sickling occurs. It is predominantly found in people of African or Afro-Caribbean background, affecting about 8% of that population in the US. There are varying degrees of sickle-cell disease and the severity depends on the amount of normal versus abnormal haemoglobins present.

A proliferative retinopathy can develop secondary to a sickle-cell disease and has five distinct stages from arteriolar occlusion to ischaemia and neovascularization and finally vitreous traction and retinal detachment. Treatment, as for other retinopathies, is laser photocoagulation to stop neovascularization.

Macular dystrophies

Family history, electrophysiological tests and the retinal appearance are all important for the diagnosis of these inherited macular dystrophies. There are no current treatment options, so ongoing support is vital along with prompt referral to low-vision agencies.

Cone dystrophy

This is a progressive deterioration of the cones and most cases are sporadic rather than inherited; however, it is linked to an autosomal dominant gene and has a poor visual prognosis. As discussed previously, the cone photoreceptors are responsible for colour vision and central vision, so a cone dystrophy results in a decreased visual acuity, a decrease in colour sensitivity and photophobia. On examination the retina may appear normal until late in the disease progression when RPE changes and an atrophic macula may be seen. A 'bull's-eye' pattern of depigmentation, with a surrounding zone of hyperfluorescence and a central spot of non-fluorescence, is indicative of a cone–rod dystrophy on FFA. Electrophysiological tests assist in the diagnosis as ERG shows a decreased cone function with some loss of rod function. There is currently no treatment for cone–rod dystrophy.

Best's dystrophy

Best's dystrophy is also know as vitelliform dystrophy and is linked to an autosomal dominant trait, with the onset of the disease process affecting those aged between 4 and 20 years. Presenting symptoms vary from none to decreased visual acuity and, for some, strabismus. On ophthalmoscopic examination, the retinal appearance varies from a mild pigmentary disturbance in the fovea to a yellow material resembling 'egg yolk'. Degeneration of the macula may lead to subretinal neovascularization, extensive macular scarring and subretinal haemorrhage.

Stargardt's disease

Stargardt's disease is caused by an autosomal recessive gene and is bilateral. Children will often present with a loss of central vision but at whatever age the patient presents, it generally results in an untreatable loss of central vision. Early symptoms include a decrease in vision followed by a decrease in night vision as a result of poor dark adaptation. The retina usually has the appearance of creamy-white flecks that change with time. Initially the macula appears normal but then develops changes that ultimately result in the macula appearing like 'beaten bronze'. The visual prognosis is poor.

Retinopathies

Diabetic retinopathy and hypertensive retinopathy are the most common presentations, but the other retinopathies that patients may present with include the following.

Valsalva's retinopathy

This can follow a rise in intrathoracic or intra-abdominal pressure against a closed glottis/Valsalva's manoeuvre. The result is a rupture in superficial retinal veins causing small inter-retinal haemorrhages without any leakage. These are asymptomatic and there is no loss of vision or permanent retinal damage.

Solar retinopathy

This is caused by intense exposure to visible light in the blue and near UV wavelengths (250–441 mm). This can be a result of observing the sun or a solar eclipse without using the correct safety filters. There are also case reports of people using hallucinatory drugs and staring at the sun or unconsciously exposing their eyes to the sun with a resultant macular burn. A larger pupil size will naturally result in more damage. Initially the retina may appear normal, but the retinal burn will result in RPE depigmentation and may even cause a macular cyst or hole. In mild cases the photoreceptors and RPE will regenerate in time.

Inflammation in the posterior segment

There are a number of conditions that can cause severe posterior segment inflammations. Some are systemic, such as the human immunodeficiency virus (HIV), which allows opportunistic retinal infections resulting in retinal necrosis and loss of vision. Other infections, such as herpes infections, toxoplasmosis and tuberculosis, can cause posterior uveitis, chorioretinal inflammation and lesions, and vitritis.

As with management of any infection, a range of interventions from topical and systemic medication regimens to surgical procedures may be indicated.

Vitreous inflammation

Known as 'vitritis' this is a sign of inflammatory cells in the vitreous. Vitritis can be a result of posterior uveitis or lesions in the retina or choroid, such as toxoplasmosis, or tumours such as lymphoma. The inflammation can be localized and small causing only a few cells that appear as floaters. However, if there is a larger amount of infiltrate, the resulting opaque vitreous will cause a decrease in visual acuity. In such cases, a vitrectomy may be indicated to clear the media. Vitritis of unknown origin may be an indication for a vitrectomy or a vitreous biopsy to identify the underlying pathology.

Human immunodeficiency virus

HIV is associated with a range of ocular diseases and in the retina it can present within a spectrum from minimal ocular symptoms and signs to those infections secondary to the patient's immunodeficiency, with consequences including loss of vision.

HIV microvasculopathy is a non-sight-threatening, non-infective condition with cotton-wool spots and is the most common ocular sign seen in patients with HIV. These are transient and, although retinal microaneurysms may also be seen, no treatment is indicated. These signs are also seen with other retinal conditions, including hypertension and diabetic retinopathy, highlighting the need to obtain an accurate, detailed health and social history from the patient.

Cytomegalovirus

This is an opportunistic infection associated with the common herpes virus but was rarely seen in ophthalmology departments until the advent of AIDS. Retinal cytomegalovirus (CMV) causes a severe retinal infection known as CMV retinitis, causing in turn an inflammation that results in a necrotic, thinned retina that has a high risk of developing retinal breaks and a corresponding retinal detachment. CMV retinitis can occur in any immunocompromised patient, but it is most commonly seen to affect a large percentage of patients with advanced AIDS.

Initial presentation may be when the patient complains of painless blurred vision, but on examination the retinal picture provides the diagnosis. CMV retinitis causes a 'pizza' appearance of the retina as a result of flame-shaped haemorrhages along the retinal vessels and large areas of yellow–white exudates. It may be when a patient presents with CMV retinitis that a diagnosis of AIDS is made, which can be devastating for the patient and the family.

The CMV infection is treated with antiviral medications including ganciclovir and foscarnet. Any retinal detachments occurring secondary to CMV are difficult to repair because of retinal necrosis. For this reason CMV retinitis is commonly sight threatening.

Toxoplasmosis

This is caused by the *Toxoplasma gondii*, a protozoon with the domestic cat as the primary host although other felines also carry the disease. Toxoplasmosis is a common cause of posterior segment inflammation worldwide and may even be acquired *in utero*. Oocysts are excreted in cat faeces with infection occurring directly or indirectly through ingestion of undercooked meat or even transplacentally. This acquired infection tends to result in a subclinical illness and often detection is the incidental finding of chorioretinal scars. These lesions may be reactivated and cause symptoms varying from nil to floaters and blurred vision and, in severe cases, pain and photophobia.

On ocular examination a vitritis, an inflammatory process in the vitreous, can be seen which may be mild or dense enough to obscure the retina from view. The retina itself may have focal areas of necrotic tissue.

Testing for the presence of toxoplasma antibodies is not routine, because large numbers of the population may be positive without the presence of active disease. Therefore, diagnosis is usually based on clinical observations. Treatment is not normally required, because most cases of reactivation resolve spontaneously. However, if the patient's vision is threatened or affected, antimicrobial treatment is necessary. Steroids may be indicated to help reduce the inflammation.

Toxocariasis

This is caused by roundworms passed from dogs and cats to humans. Ocular manifestations of toxocariasis may appear without systemic involvement and usually affect children from 7 years of age, because they tend to have a close association with family pets and may also eat dirt that harbours the toxocara ova.

This disease tends to be unilateral and the child may present with a red eye, complain of blurred vision or have leukocoria. On examination the patient may have a vitritis and choroidal granuloma or possibly chronic endophthalmitis.

These patients are treated with systemic or periocular corticosteroid injections and sometimes a vitrectomy is undertaken to obtain a vitreous sample for biopsy, or if there is a vitreous opacity or retinal traction.

Nursing care of retinal patients

Although the retina has numerous diseases and conditions that affect its function and ultimately impacts on the patient's vision, there are many similarities when providing care that apply to this group of patients. Rather than provide advice for specific diseases and conditions, it is more appropriate to provide guidelines because the care of retinal patients differs from one country to the next and the doctor's preference. It is the new frontier for advances in ophthalmic care and preservation of vision, surgically and non-surgically, so how care is provided is changing all the time. There are some specific differences between the provision of care for some retinal patients, namely those who require surgical intervention.

As with any other ophthalmic disorder, one of the most important strategies in care is adequate, comprehensive and timely information presented in a way that is understandable for the patient.

Nurses are generally the first health professional that the patients and their family will see, whether they present to a hospital service, private clinic or the GP's office. It is essential to establish a rapport with the patients and family from the outset, because this will assist not only the individual nurse but also the team in dealing with the patient and family in the future. For most patients who have a retinal problem the interaction with health professionals is likely to be lifelong and so it is essential to achieve a good relationship for the best outcome for the patient.

Many retinal patients will not regain their vision once it is lost and often require referral to and input from specialized services such as low-vision clinics and charities associated with low vision or specific disease entities. Nurses should ensure that this occurs in a timely manner for the patient and the family.

Posturing after surgery

Patients are often required to position or posture postoperatively and this is the greatest challenge not only for the patient but also for nursing staff. The patient is required to lie in specified positions such as head down, and the sensory deprivation and physical deprivation experienced by the patient are often not appreciated. Make sure that you tell the patient who you are when you enter the room, explain what you are going to do, position anything they need within easy reach and answer call bells promptly. Positioning and posturing are important for a successful visual outcome from surgical intervention when internal tamponades are used (refer to 'Retinal detachment'). Patients required to posture often find this difficult to maintain for any length of time and again, depending on the doctor, the patient may be permitted to stop posturing for periods of time throughout the day. There are several aids that can assist patients to maintain the required position but these may vary from one country to another. Positioning aids that have an area that allows the patient to position correctly, but also to continue to read or work, such as massage-type chairs which have a head support with an opening, are sometimes used.

Analgesia after surgery

Analgesia is generally required and, if prescribed analgesia does not relieve pain postoperatively, the IOP should be checked. Some patients may have their IOP monitored at regular intervals after surgery, again dependent on the hospital and doctor. A raised IOP requires urgent intervention to preserve vision. Some surgeons at the end of the surgical procedure give the patient a sub-Tenon's block which provides excellent postoperative analgesia without the use of opiates, which reduces the incidence of postoperative nausea and vomiting.

References

Abramson DH, Schefler AC (2004) Update on retinoblastoma. Retina 24: 828–48.
Abramson DH, Frank CM, Susman M, Whalen MP, Dunkel IJ, Boyd NW (1998) Presenting signs of retinoblastoma. J Paediatr 132: 505–8.
Age-Related Eye Disease Study Research Group (2001) A randomised, placebo controlled, clinical trail of high-dose supplementation with vitamins C and E, beta-carotene, and zinc for age-related macular degeneration and vision loss. Arch Ophthalmol 119: 1417–36.
Arnold JJ, Sarks SH (2000) Age related macular degeneration. BMJ 321: 741–4.
Batterbury M, Bowling B (1999). Ophthalmology: An illustrated colour text. London: Churchill Livingstone.
Chawla HB (1999) Ophthalmology – A symptom-based approach, 3rd edn. London: Reed Educational and Professional Publishing Ltd.
Diabetic Retinopathy Study Research Group (1978) Photocoagulation treatment of proliferative diabetic retinopathy: the second report of Diabetic Retinopathy Study findings. Ophthalmology 85: 82–106.
Early Treatment Diabetic Retinopathy Study Research Group (1985) Photocoagulation for diabetic macular edema. Early Treatment Diabetic Retinopathy Study report number 1. Arch Ophthalmol 103: 1796–806.
Ferris FL, Davis MD, Aiello LM (1999) Drug therapy: treatment of diabetic retinopathy. N Engl J Med 341: 667–78.
Hamilton AMP, Ulbig MW, Polkinghorne P (1996) Management of Diabetic Retinopathy. London: BMJ Publishing Group.
Kanski JJ (2003) Clinical Ophthalmology, 5th edn. London: Butterworth-Heinemann.

Lumbroso L, Doz F, Levy C et al. (2003) Diode laser theromotherapy and chemotherapy in the treatment of retinoblastoma. J Fr Ophtalmol 26: 154–9.

Macular Photocoagulation Study Group (1997) Risk factors for choroidal neovascularisation in the second eye of patients with juxtafoveal or subfoveal neovascularisation secondary to age related macular degeneration. Arch Ophthalmol 115: 741–7.

Menkhaus S, Wallesch CW, Behrens-Baumann W (2003) Charles-Bonnet syndrome. Ophthalmology 100: 738–9.

Mittra R, Singerman LJ (2002) Recent advances in the management of age-related macular degeneration. J Am Acad Optometr 79: 218–24.

Murphy S, Nesbitt P (2001) Advances in management of age-related macular degeneration. Ophthal Nursing 5(3): 20–3.

National Institute for Clinical Excellence (2004) Guidance on the use of photodynamic therapy for age-related macular degeneration: www.nice.org.uk

Newell FW (1996) Ophthalmology: Principles and concepts. St Louis, MO: Mosby.

Recchia F, Brown GC (2000) Systemic disorders associated with retinal vascular occlusion. Curr Opin Ophthalmol 11: 462–7.

Ross WH, Kozy DW (1998) Visual recovery in macula-off rhegmatogenous retinal detachments. Ophthalmology 105: 2149–50.

Ryder B (1995). Screening for diabetic retinopathy. BMJ 311: 207–8.

Shah GK, Brown GC (2000) Photography, angiography, and ultrasonography in diabetic retinopathy. In: Flynn HW, Smiddy WE (eds), Diabetes and Ocular Disease: Past, present and future therapies. San Francisco, CA: Foundation of the American Academy of Ophthalmology, pp. 101–13.

Shelswell N (2002) Perioperative patient education for retinal surgery. AORN J 75: 801–7.

Taylor RH, Shah P, Murray PI (1995) Key Topics in Ophthalmology. Oxford: BIOS Scientific.

CHAPTER TWENTY-TWO

The orbit and extraocular muscles

ALLYSON RYDER

This chapter examines the anatomy of the orbit and discusses some orbital problems, including thyroid eye disease (TED), orbital infection, orbital inflammatory disease and orbital tumours. It then looks at the extraocular muscles and ocular movements, and strabismus (squint) and its management, as well as giving an overview of a basic orthoptic assessment.

Anatomy of the orbit

The bony orbits are pyramid-shaped cavities composed of four walls (roof, floor, medial and lateral), converging on the apex posteriorly (Figure 22.1). The medial walls are parallel and the lateral walls make an angle of about

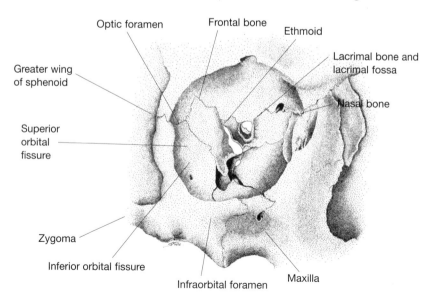

Figure 22.1 The bones of the orbit.

90° with each other. The widest part of the orbit is about 15 mm behind the orbital margin, or rim, and this overhang protects the globe from injury.

The average height of an adult orbit is 35 mm and the average width 40 mm. In an adult the average volume of the orbit is 30 ml (Bron et al. 1997).

Seven bones form the four walls of the orbit: frontal, maxilla, zygoma, sphenoid, ethmoid, lacrimal and palatine (Snell and Lemp 1998). There are several openings within and adjacent to the orbits, through which nerves and blood vessels supply the globe, extraocular muscles and nearby structures (see box).

Superior orbital fissure } Inferior orbital fissure	Motor nerves to ocular muscles and ophthalmic nerve and vein
Optic foramen	Optic nerve
Supraorbital notch	Supraorbital nerves and vessels
Infraorbital foramen	Infraorbital nerve and artery

Roof

The very thin orbital plate of the frontal bone primarily forms the roof. The lesser wing of the sphenoid lies posteriorly at the apex, perforated by the optic canal.

Relationships

• Above, the roof is indented by the convolutions of the frontal lobe and the frontal sinus lies anteriorly.
• Anteromedially, 4 mm behind the orbital rim, lies the fovea, or small depression, for the pulley of the superior oblique. The supraorbital notch lies on the supraorbital margin, approximately a third of the way along from the medial wall.
• Anterolaterally in the frontal bone lies the fossa for the lacrimal gland; this is bounded below by the suture between the frontal and zygomatic bones.
• Immediately below the roof lie the frontal nerve, supraorbital artery and levator palpebrae superioris, with the superior oblique between the roof and the medial wall.

Medial wall

From front to back the medial wall is made up of the frontal process of the maxilla, the lacrimal bone, the very thin lamina papyracea of the ethmoid, which forms the major part of the wall, and then a small part of the body of the sphenoid.

Relationships

- Anteriorly the lacrimal sac lies in the lacrimal fossa, which leads down into the lacrimal canal.
- Medially lie the ethmoidal air cells and posteriorly the sphenoidal air cells.
- The medial rectus runs along the medial wall, and the superior oblique runs along the angle between the medial wall and the roof. The nasociliary nerve and the anterior part of the ophthalmic artery lie between the two muscles.

Floor

The floor is formed mainly by the orbital plate of the maxilla. The orbital surface of the zygoma forms the anterolateral part, with the apex formed by the orbital process of the palate.

Relationships

- Below the floor lies the maxillary antrum and above lies the inferior rectus. Posteriorly the inferior rectus is in contact with the floor, whereas anteriorly it is separated from the floor by the inferior oblique and orbital fat. The inferior oblique rises from an area lateral to the opening of the nasolacrimal canal. It then crosses the floor outwards and backwards.
- Posteriorly the inferior orbital fissure separates the floor from the lateral wall and the infraorbital sulcus runs forwards from the middle of this fissure. Anteriorly the sulcus becomes a canal, emerging in the infraorbital foramen, about 4 mm from the orbital rim.

Lateral wall

This is formed by the orbital surface of the zygoma anteriorly and the orbital surface of the greater wing of the sphenoid posteriorly. The superior and inferior orbital fissures separate the sphenoidal part of the wall from the roof and floor, respectively.

Relationships

- The lateral rectus originates from a small bony spur on the lower margin of the superior orbital fissure, at the junction of the narrow and wide parts. The muscle then runs forward in contact with the wall. The lacrimal nerve and artery run above the muscle.
- The zygomatic nerve runs within the zygomatic groove, from the anterior end of the inferior orbital fissure to the zygomatic foramen.

Superior orbital fissure

The superior orbital fissure is the largest opening between the middle cranial fossa and the orbit. It is a gap about 22 mm long, lying between the lesser wing of the sphenoid in the roof and the greater wing of the sphenoid in the lateral wall. It is closed anteriorly by the frontal bone. Medially it lies below the optic foramen, separated from it by the posterior root of the lesser wing of the sphenoid; from here it runs up and laterally.

The superior orbital fissure consists of two parts – a wider medial portion and a narrow lateral portion – and these are separated by the spine of the lateral rectus muscle. There is an oval tendinous ring, the annulus of Zinn, which divides the wide portion into two and also encloses the optic foramen. This ring is the common origin of the four rectus extraocular muscles.

Passing through the fissure above the annulus are, from above down, the lacrimal, frontal and fourth (trochlear) nerves, with the superior ophthalmic vein below and lateral. Passing through within the annulus, from above downwards, are the superior division of the third (oculomotor) nerve, the nasociliary and sympathetic root of the ciliary ganglion, the inferior division of the third nerve and then the sixth (abducens) nerve. Occasionally the inferior ophthalmic vein passes through the fissure below the annulus.

Inferior orbital fissure

The inferior orbital fissure lies between the greater wing of the sphenoid on the lateral wall and the maxilla on the floor of the orbit. It starts below and lateral to the optic foramen, close to the medial end of the superior orbital fissure, and then runs forwards and laterally to about 20 mm from the inferior orbital margin.

It forms a communication between the orbit and the pterygopalatine fossa and transmits the infraorbital nerve, the zygomatic nerve, branches from the pterygopalatine ganglion to the orbital periosteum and a communication between the inferior ophthalmic vein and the pterygoid plexus.

Optic canal

Within the optic canal, and adherent to its roof, runs the optic nerve, with its covering of dura, arachnoid and pia mater. The ophthalmic artery runs alongside, first below and then lateral to the nerve.

The canal runs forwards, laterally and slightly downwards from the optic groove of the sphenoid bone in the middle cranial fossa, between the two roots of the lesser wing of the sphenoid, and opens into the apex of the orbit at the optic foramen.

Orbital disorders

As a result of the rigid bony structure of the orbit, with only an anterior opening for expansion, anything that causes an increase in the orbital contents will displace the eyeball. Pressure behind the globe will push it forward (proptosis), whereas pressure to one side will push it to the opposite side. Displacement of the globe will result in diplopia (double vision). Pressure, which affects the blood supply to the optic nerve and retina, will result in reduced vision (Stephenson 1966).

Thyroid eye disease

Thyroid eye disease (TED) is also referred to as dysthyroid ophthalmopathy or Graves' ophthalmopathy. The thyroid gland is the largest endocrine gland in the body, situated just below the cricoid cartilage in the neck. It has numerous small follicles, which secrete thyroxine (T_4) and triiodothyronine (T_3). Secretion of thyroid hormones is initiated by the hypothalamus, which secretes thyrotrophin-releasing hormone (TRH). This stimulates the pituitary gland to release thyroid-stimulating hormone (TSH), which binds to receptors on the thyroid gland. This new protein, thyroid-stimulating hormone receptor protein (TSH-R), activates a complex system that regulates the functions of the thyroid gland and results in secretion of the two thyroid hormones (Newell 1996). Thyrotoxicosis (Graves' disease) is a systemic disease secondary to excessive secretion of thyroid hormones. Women are predominantly affected with the incidence peaking in the mid-40s (Newell 1996). It is suggested that this is caused by an autoimmune abnormality in which IgG antibodies bind to TSH receptors in the thyroid gland and stimulate secretion of thyroid hormones (Kanski 2003).

Thyroid eye disease commonly occurs in patients with a history of thyroid dysfunction, specifically Graves' disease. Eye problems may precede, coincide with or follow the hyperthyroidism. In fact 25% of patients present to an ophthalmologist with eye signs and symptoms before the discovery of hyperthyroidism. Patients who are euthyroid but exhibit eye signs and symptoms may be referred to as having ophthalmic Graves' disease. About 1% of patients with Graves' ophthalmopathy are hypothyroid, with thyroid hormone levels depressed but the TSH level increased (Newell 1996).

Thyroid eye disease is believed to be an organ-specific autoimmune disorder in which an antibody is responsible for hypertrophy of the extraocular muscles (caused by round cell infiltration), lymphocyte infiltration of the interstitial tissue and proliferation of orbital fat, connective tissue and lacrimal glands.

Environmental factors play a part in the development and severity of autoimmune disease and severe TED has recently been linked with smoking, which is known to affect the immune system.

Signs of TED

- Upper eyelid retraction (Dalrymple's sign)
- Lid lag (von Graefe's sign)
- Staring, frightened appearance (Kocher's sign)
- Periorbital and lid swelling
- Chemosis: oedema of the conjunctiva
- Conjunctival hyperaemia
- Superior limbic keratoconjunctivitis
- Proptosis – axial
- Mechanical restriction of ocular movements
- Increased intraocular pressure
- Compressive optic neuropathy.

These signs may be unilateral or bilateral, but if unilateral it is likely that the other eye will be affected at a later stage. In about 30% of cases of unilateral proptosis the aetiology is TED (Char 1997).

Symptoms of TED

- Pain/discomfort from soft tissue involvement
- Photophobia
- Lacrimation
- Grittiness/discomfort from corneal exposure
- Diplopia
- Progressive impairment of central vision
- Defective red–green colour vision.

Classification of ocular changes (Char 1997)

The acronym NO SPECS is one that can be used to classify the severity of TED into seven classes – 0 to 6:

Class 0 – **n**o signs or symptoms
Class 1 – **o**nly signs, no symptoms
Class 2 – **s**oft tissue involvement
Class 3 – **p**roptosis
Class 4 – **e**xtraocular muscle involvement
Class 5 – **c**orneal involvement
Class 6 – **s**ight loss – optic nerve involvement.

Natural history of TED

Thyroid eye disease has two identifiable phases: the active inflammatory phase, in which the eyes are red and painful, and the cicatricial phase.

The inflammatory phase

The inflammatory process that affects the extraocular muscles and eyelids gives rise to most of the characteristic features of TED. There is round cell infiltration of the muscles, causing oedema, and deposition of mucopolysaccharides between the muscle fibres. The muscles enlarge and can increase in volume up to 10 times more than normal. This, combined with the proliferation of orbital fat and connective tissue, increases the orbital volume and causes proptosis, which can lead to corneal exposure. Intraorbital pressure can rise and the blood supply to the optic nerve may be embarrassed. This risk of optic neuropathy has been found to be directly linked to the size of the extraocular muscles. These swollen muscles become inelastic and cause mechanical restriction of ocular movements. Botulinum toxin (BT) injection of the muscles during this phase has been found to be successful in reversing the mechanical restriction.

The upper lid retraction and lid lag in this phase are thought to be the result of sympathetic over-stimulation, secondary to high levels of thyroid hormone, resulting in overaction of Müller's muscle.

The cicatricial phase

The inflammatory phase is followed by fibrosis of the extraocular muscles and secondary muscle contracture. The muscle swelling subsides, the proptosis gradually reduces and hence the risk of optic neuropathy also reduces. Ocular movement restriction becomes more symmetrical and there is a gradual development of a large, vertical, fusional amplitude, which means that diplopia may be less troublesome.

Eyelid retraction normally persists and may be caused by contraction of the levator and fibrosis between it and the overlying orbital tissues, or by secondary increased innervation to the superior rectus, in order to try to elevate the eye after the fibrosis of the inferior rectus.

Management of TED

For the purposes of management TED can be categorized into:

• soft tissue involvement
• lid retraction
• proptosis
• optic nerve involvement
• extraocular muscle involvement.

Soft tissue involvement

This includes periorbital and lid swelling, chemosis, conjunctival hyper-aemia, especially over the insertion sites of the horizontal recti, keratoconjunctivitis sicca and superior limbic keratoconjunctivitis.

Management is often unsuccessful but the following may benefit the patient to some extent:

- Topical therapy: lubricants, such as artificial tears during the day and ointment at night, may help if there is ocular irritation resulting from corneal exposure, conjunctival inflammation and keratoconjunctivitis sicca. Patients with superior limbic keratoconjunctivitis may need 1% topical adrenaline (epinephrine) and 5% acetylcysteine.
- Head elevation: increasing pillows during sleep may help to reduce periorbital oedema.
- Taping lids: during sleep may aid patients with exposure keratopathy.
- Diuretics: at night may reduce periorbital oedema in the morning.

Eyelid retraction

Fifty per cent of patients with Graves' disease have lid retraction, which may be mild, moderate or marked. Patients with mild lid retraction do not normally need treatment and it may improve spontaneously or after treat-ment of associated hyperthyroidism.

Surgical treatment is indicated in cases of marked, but stable, lid retrac-tion with exposure keratopathy and poor cosmesis. The following are the main surgical procedures:

- Inferior rectus recession: if the fibrotic inferior rectus is thought to be causing the lid retraction.
- Disinsertion of an overactive Müller's muscle.
- Lengthening a contracted levator with donor sclera.
- Lateral tarsorrhaphy: sewing the upper and lower lids together at the lateral canthus. This is rarely used because it is unsightly and does not benefit corneal exposure.

Proptosis

Thyroid eye disease is the most common cause of proptosis in adults. It may be unilateral or bilateral and is permanent in about 70% of patients. It is uninfluenced by any hyperthyroidism treatment and if severe will prevent adequate lid closure, leading to exposure keratopa-thy, corneal ulceration and endophthalmitis.

Management of proptosis can involve:

- Systemic steroids: these are used during the early stages of the disease where there is rapidly progressing and painful proptosis. Oral pred-nisolone 80–100 mg/day is prescribed, with relief of symptoms expected within 48 hours. Ciclosporin can be used in addition and this permits a reduction in the dosage of prednisolone. Steroids should be discontinued after 3 months.

- Radiotherapy: can be considered in patients who are unresponsive to steroids or where steroid therapy is contraindicated.
- Surgical decompression: can be considered when medical treatment has failed or is contraindicated. Some authorities favour this as a primary treatment. The aim of orbital decompression is to create space for the orbital contents and reduce proptosis by removing one or more of the orbital walls. The most common procedure is to remove part of the floor and the posterior portion of the medial wall, allowing the orbital contents to prolapse into the maxillary and ethmoidal sinuses. This achieves 3–6 mm retroplacement of the globe.

Optic nerve involvement

About 5% of patients have optic neuropathy, caused by direct compression of the optic nerve or its blood supply (Char 1997). Patients present with decreasing visual acuity, defective red–green colour vision and central or paracentral field defects. Optic atrophy will develop if treatment is delayed.

Management is the same as for severe proptosis and the threat to vision is classed as a medical emergency:

- Systemic steroids
- Radiotherapy
- Surgical decompression.

Extraocular muscle involvement

Between 30% and 50% of patients develop ophthalmoplegia and diplopia can be a persistent problem. Diplopia may be vertical, horizontal or a combination of both.

As mentioned previously, the muscles become enlarged during the inflammatory stage, followed by a mechanical restriction of movements; this is caused by oedema in the infiltrative stage and fibrosis in the cicatricial stage. A single muscle in one eye may be affected or a number of muscles in both eyes. In order of frequency the affected muscles are:

- Inferior rectus: restricting elevation (most common)
- Medial rectus: restricting abduction (lateral gaze)
- Superior rectus: restricting depression
- Lateral rectus: restricting adduction (medial gaze).

Management may be conservative or surgical.

Conservative management

The following are the aims:

- To monitor the process of the disease, record and measure changes in the condition.

- To overcome symptoms and maintain binocular single vision (BSV). This can be achieved by:
  - prism therapy: using prisms to join the diplopia and restore BSV
  - botulinum toxin (BT): injection of BT into an affected muscle in the inflammatory stage can be successful in helping to regain BSV
  - occlusion: this is used as a last resort to eliminate diplopia when other conservative methods have failed.

Surgical management
Extraocular muscle surgery should be carried out only when the patient is euthyroid, the ocular muscle imbalance has been stable for between 3 and 6 months and there is no evidence of congestive ophthalmology. The aim of surgical management is to achieve a field of BSV in the primary position and the reading position, i.e. down-gaze. The patient should be aware that binocularity in all positions of gaze is difficult to achieve and further surgery may be necessary.

Surgery is tailored to the affected individual muscle, but the most commonly performed surgery is an inferior rectus recession and/or medial rectus recession, using adjustable sutures.

Orbital infections

Preseptal cellulitis

This is an infection of the subcutaneous tissues anterior to the orbital septum. It is not strictly an orbital disease but must be differentiated from orbital cellulitis which is less common, although much more serious. Rapid progression to orbital cellulitis can occur in some patients. Preseptal cellulitis can be a result of trauma to the skin or from infected insect bites. Local infection such as infected chalazion or dacryocystitis may spread to become preseptal cellulitis, or a more remote infraction such as a middle-ear infection may be transmitted via the blood supply to the lids.

Presentation will be as a unilateral, tender and red periorbital area with some lid oedema. Treatment is with a course of oral antibiotics such as flucloxacillin or amoxicillin.

Orbital cellulitis

Orbital cellulitis is a bacterial infection of the soft tissue behind the orbital septum and is caused by the same organisms that cause acute sinusitis, i.e. pneumococci, streptococci or staphylococci (Figure 22.2). These enter the orbit from the infected frontal, maxillary, ethmoidal or sphenoidal sinuses via the vascular channels or by direct extension. It may also be post-traumatic or postoperative, following retinal, lacrimal or orbital surgery. It may also result from an extension of preseptal cellulitis through the orbital septum or from local spread from, for example, dacryocystitis. If not treated successfully, infection can spread to the cavernous sinus or meninges, resulting in cavernous sinus thrombosis, meningitis or abscess of the brain. It is therefore potentially life threatening and, although it can occur at any age, it is more common in children (Kanski 2003). Orbital abscess can occur in post-traumatic or postoperative cases.

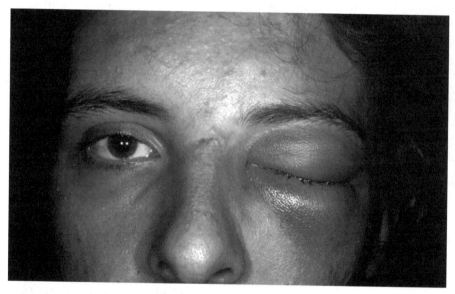

Figure 22.2 Orbital cellulitis. (See Plate 55.)

Signs and symptoms

Orbital cellulitis is almost always unilateral, with a sudden onset. Mild cases involve swelling and redness of the eyelids, chemosis, proptosis and dull pain. In more severe cases the pain is more intense and there is pain on eye movements, which will be restricted. In advanced cases there may be signs of optic nerve dysfunction, with optic neuritis after severe inflammatory reactions. Other symptoms can range from mild fever and malaise to high fever and marked debility.

Differential diagnosis

- Tendonitis
- Orbital periostitis

- Cavernous sinus thrombosis
- Rhabdomyosarcoma in children.

Treatment

The patient should be admitted to hospital and assessed frequently because orbital cellulitis can be vision threatening or even life threatening. However, almost all cases respond well to large doses of systemic antibiotics, and visual prognosis is good in the absence of complications. Investigations include white cell count, blood culture and computed tomography (CT) of the orbit and brain. Antibiotic regimens differ but often include intravenous antibiotics and therapy should be continued until the patient has been fever free for 4 days. Optic nerve function should be monitored every 4 hours while the orbital cellulitis is in its acute phase. Pupil reactions, visual acuity, colour vision and brightness appreciation should form part of this monitoring and patients must have sufficient information and awareness of their condition to recognize the importance of these investigations at a time when they may well be feeling very ill. Monitoring may be more of a problem in children with orbital cellulitis because it is likely that they will be nursed in a specialist paediatric area where, although the nursing staff will have a wealth of knowledge about the care of the sick child, they may know little about ophthalmic care and will therefore be unaware of both the tests that should take place and their importance and significance. Ophthalmic clinicians must be very clear therefore in their handover of the child to a paediatric setting, and may have to take responsibility for the ophthalmic care of the child by enquiring regularly about the progress of the child in the paediatric setting and by physically attending to ensure that investigations are carried out.

Cavernous sinus thrombosis

Cavernous sinus thrombosis is normally caused by infection spreading along the venous channels draining the orbit, central face, throat and nasal cavities.

Signs and symptoms

It is normally bilateral, with proptosis, orbital oedema, swelling of the eyelids, diminished or absent pupillary reflexes, papilloedema and reduced vision. There may be involvement of the cranial nerves that traverse the cavernous sinus, i.e. nerves III and IV, and the ophthalmic division of nerves V and VI. There will be severe headache, fever, nausea and vomiting.

Differential diagnosis

This is orbital cellulitis, which is unilateral, with normal pupillary reflexes, no papilloedema and less severe pain.

Treatment

High doses of systemic antibiotics will normally ensure good visual recovery.

Orbital inflammatory disease

Idiopathic orbital inflammatory disease (pseudotumour)

This is an uncommon inflammatory disorder characterized by non-infectious and non-neoplastic space-occupying orbital lesions. Its cause is unknown.

Signs and symptoms

It is normally unilateral in adults but in 30% of children it is bilateral. There is a gradual onset of proptosis, sometimes with lateral displacement of the globe and restriction of ocular movements, causing diplopia. There will be periorbital swelling, chemosis and conjunctival injection. There may be optic nerve dysfunction if the inflammation involves the posterior part of the orbit.

Differential diagnosis

- Orbital cellulitis
- Thyroid eye disease
- Orbital tumours
- Ruptured dermoid cyst.

Treatment

- Observation in mild cases, because there may be a remission.
- Systemic steroids (usually prednisone) are successful in over 50% of moderate-to-severe cases.
- Radiotherapy is carried out if there is no improvement after 2 weeks of steroid therapy.
- Cytotoxic drugs (usually cyclophosphamide) are used if there is no improvement with steroids or radiotherapy.

Orbital tumours

Kanski (2003) classifies orbital tumours into:

- Vascular
- Lacrimal gland
- Neural
- Miscellaneous.

Vascular tumours

Capillary haemangioma

This is the most common childhood orbital and periorbital tumour. It may present as a small isolated lesion or a large disfiguring mass, causing impairment of vision and associated with visual complications.

Signs
- The tumour presents at birth and may be superficial, subcutaneous or deep. If superficial there will be the classic strawberry naevus on the eyelids.
- If subcutaneous, the skin on the eyelids will appear dark blue or purple and there may be displacement of the globe.
- A deep tumour will cause unilateral proptosis with no skin discoloration.
- About 25% of cases have coexisting capillary haemangiomas on other parts of the body and large tumours may be associated with high-output cardiac failure.

Treatment
- Of patients 40% spontaneously resolve by the age of 4 years and this increases to 70% by age 7 years.
- Early treatment is indicated if there is a threat to visual acuity, poor cosmesis, necrosis or infection, or high-output cardiac failure.
- The methods of choice are steroid injections, effective in the early stages of subcutaneous tumours, or systemic steroids, which are used if there is a large orbital component.

Cavernous haemangioma

This is the most common benign orbital tumour in adults, normally presenting in the fourth to fifth decades. It consists of large dilated veins with an endothelial lining and normally occurs in the fat space behind the globe.

Signs
There is slow progressive unilateral axial proptosis, which may be associated with disc oedema and chorioretinal folds.

Treatment

Surgical excision is required in most cases as the tumour enlarges. It is usually well encapsulated and relatively easy to remove.

Lymphangiomas

These are rare benign vascular malformations, normally presenting in early childhood.

Signs

If anterior there will be soft bluish masses in the upper nasal quadrant, with conjunctival cysts.

If posterior there may be slow progressive proptosis or, if the tumour initially lies dormant, there may be a sudden onset of painful proptosis, following a spontaneous haemorrhage.

Treatment

These are difficult to treat, as a result of the fact that they are not encapsulated. There is a tendency to haemorrhage easily and they may infiltrate normal orbital tissue. They may be treated by drainage or by controlled vaporization using a carbon dioxide laser.

Lacrimal tumours

Pleomorphic lacrimal gland adenoma

This is a benign mixed-cell tumour and is the most common epithelial tumour affecting the lacrimal gland (about 50% of cases).

Signs and symptoms

It presents normally in the fifth decade as a slowly progressive, firm, painless swelling in the superotemporal orbit.

There may be proptosis and downward and medial displacement of the globe with diplopia, especially in the field of action of the superior rectus.

Treatment

This is by surgical excision.

Lacrimal gland carcinoma

This is a very rare tumour, presenting in the fourth to sixth decades, with a high morbidity and mortality.

Signs and symptoms

There will be a fast growing, often painful, lacrimal gland mass, causing downward and medial displacement of the globe, with associated diplopia.

Twenty-five per cent of cases have swelling of the optic disc and 25% have hypoaesthesia in the region supplied by the trigeminal nerve.

Treatment
Prognosis for life is poor. Radical surgery involving orbital exenteration or mid-facial resection is normally unsuccessful because the tumour is past surgical excision. Radiotherapy may reduce pain and prolong life.

Neural tumours

Optic nerve glioma (juvenile pilocystic astrocytoma)

This is a primary tumour of the glial cells of the optic nerve, which presents in the first decade, normally before age 5 years. Kanski (2003) reports that 25–50% of cases have associated neurofibromatosis, whereas Levine and Larson (1993) increase this figure to 60%.

Signs and symptoms
There is slow, painless, progressive loss of vision and axial proptosis. As a result of the contours of the orbital walls, the globe is eventually displaced outwards and downwards. The optic nerve is initially swollen and then becomes pale. CT scan will show a smooth fusiform enlargement of the optic nerve.

Treatment
- Observation only if vision is good and the tumour is confined to the orbit.
- Surgical excision, with preservation of the globe, is carried out if the tumour is growing towards the optic foramen, vision is reducing and cosmesis is poor.
- Radiotherapy, combined with chemotherapy, is indicated in cases where the tumour has extended into the cranium.

Neurofibroma

Diffuse or plexiform neurofibroma is the most common peripheral nerve tumour of the orbit. It presents in early childhood and occurs in patients with neurofibromatosis 1.

Signs
There is diffuse orbital involvement, with overgrowth and hypertrophy of periorbital tissues and a mechanical ptosis following eyelid involvement. Kanski (2003) reports that on palpation the tissues 'feel like a bag of worms'.

Treatment
This is difficult because of the close involvement of the extraocular muscles and lacrimal gland.

Miscellaneous tumours

Rhabdomyosarcoma

This is the most common primary malignant orbital tumour of childhood, presenting in the first decade of life.

Signs
There is rapid progressive proptosis with displacement of the globe. It can involve any part of the orbit but the most common location is retrobulbar followed by superior. Thirty-three per cent of cases have ptosis, with a palpable mass. Swelling and injection of skin develop later. CT scan will show a poorly defined, irregular orbital mass, which may extend into adjacent bones or sinuses.

There may be metastatic spread to the lungs, bone or, rarely, the lymphatic system.

Treatment
• Radiotherapy combined with chemotherapy.
• If the tumour is resistant to radiotherapy, exenteration may be carried out.

Metastatic tumours

In adults orbital involvement is the presenting sign in 25% of cases of carcinoma, with breast, bronchus, prostate and skin being the most common primary sites (Levine and Larson 1993).

Signs and symptoms
These depend on the exact position of the tumour. There will be displacement of the globe, diplopia and inflammation, similar to orbital pseudotumour. If the orbital apex is affected, there will be involvement of the cranial nerves (II, III, IV, V, VI) and mild proptosis.

Treatment
Most patients die within 1 year so treatment is aimed at relieving pain and preserving vision. Radiotherapy, chemotherapy and hormonal therapy in breast metastases are the options of choice.

Eye removal

Enucleation

This is the surgical removal of the globe and a portion of the optic nerve from the orbit. The indications for enucleation are primary intraocular malignant tumours, irreparable trauma, where there is a possibility of sympathetic ophthalmia and blind painful eyes. The patient is likely to need a great deal of support both pre- and postoperatively. One of the greatest concerns for the patient is often that the incorrect eye might be removed. Marking of the forehead preoperatively helps to reassure the patient that this will not happen and this can be confirmed by the usual preoperative checks at the theatre door and, later, in the theatre.

Procedure

A 360° limbal periotomy is performed, preserving as much of the conjunctiva as possible. The conjunctiva is then undermined back to the four rectus muscles, which are isolated, tagged and severed from their insertions. The two obliques are identified, severed and allowed to retract. Fascial bands, nerves and vessels are cut to allow exposure of the optic nerve, which is identified and transected 5 mm from the globe. This can then be removed.

Donor sclera, which has been soaked for 10 minutes in antibiotic solution, is placed around a spherical implant (e.g. hydroxyapatite) and this is inserted into the muscle cone. The sutures used to tag the rectus muscles are attached to the anterior lip of windows cut in the donor sclera, so that the muscle is in direct contact with the implant. This will aid in vascularization of the implant. Tenon's capsule and then the conjunctiva are sutured closed.

The patient is likely to return to the ward with a pressure dressing *in situ* and nurses must be aware of possible complications of surgery (haemorrhage particularly) and should check the dressing very frequently. Pressure on the dressing may be maximized by nursing the patient on his or her operated side.

A shaped conformer or shell is placed in the socket at surgery in order to maintain the shape of the socket. The patient must know how to remove, clean and reinsert the shell, before discharge to avoid discomfort and infection, and become adept at manipulating the shell and later the prosthesis. This is obviously a very upsetting time for both the patient and his or her relatives or carers and they may find the whole process extremely distasteful. Enough time must be allowed so that the patient can be supported adequately through this period.

Socket implants may be integrated or non-integrated. Integrated implants are more commonly used now because of the potential for a much better cosmetic effect. Hydroxyapatite is a substance that was initially manufactured from coral but now more often consists of a synthetic substitute that can bio-integrate – it is porous and allows fibrovascular ingrowth, thus becoming integrated into the orbit. This reduces the incidence of migration and extrusion. The position of the implant and the fibrovascular ingrowth allow it to be drilled, and a peg is introduced for direct coupling of a prosthesis. The peg fits into the back of the prosthesis and, in this way, movement of the artificial eye is equal to that of the other eye. The peg also supports the weight of the prosthesis, taking the pressure off the lower lid (Leatherbarrow 2003).

A prosthesis can be fitted in 4–6 weeks and, later, when the implant has vascularized, the implant can be drilled and a peg placed.

Evisceration

This is the removal of the contents of the globe while leaving the sclera and the optic nerve intact. The advantages over enucleation are that there is less disruption of orbital anatomy, reduced socket deformity, better mobility of a prosthesis and better cosmesis. The disadvantages are that it does not remove any unsuspected intraocular tumour, does not stop the development of sympathetic ophthalmia and, as a result of continued ciliary innervation to the globe, there may be persistent pain. However, it may be the procedure of choice when endophthalmitis is present, to reduce the spread of infection via the cut dura.

Exenteration

Exenteration is the removal of the entire contents of the orbit and is usually performed to remove life-threatening malignancy. Exenteration may be total, subtotal or extended. Subtotal exenteration spares the eyelids and is performed when the disease is behind the globe. Extended exenteration removes surrounding bone. There is a considerable loss of tissue during exenteration and, often, a skin graft is needed which may be taken at the time of surgery. A split skin graft lining the cavity will heal faster than a cavity that is left to granulate. The patient must be aware of the need for skin grafting and that there will be a second painful site postoperatively. The donor site must be prepared preoperatively and must be an area where there is minimal growth of hair, such as the inner thigh or arm. When the exenteration site has healed, osseo-integrative techniques can help to achieve a good cosmetic effect for the patient.

Extraocular muscles (Table 22.1 and Figures 22.3 and 22.4)

There are six extraocular muscles, which allow the eye to move into different positions: four recti (medial, lateral, superior and inferior) and two obliques (superior and inferior).

Table 22.1 Summary of the nerve supply and actions of the extraocular muscles

Muscle	Nerve supply	Primary action	Secondary action	Tertiary action
Lateral rectus (LR)	VI	Abduction		
Medial rectus (MR)	Inferior division III	Adduction		
Superior rectus (SR)	Superior division III	Elevation in adduction	Adduction	Intorsion
Inferior rectus (IR)	Inferior division III	Depression in abduction	Adduction	Extorsion
Superior oblique (SO)	IV	Depression in adduction	Abduction	Intorsion
Inferior oblique (IO)	Inferior division III	Elevation in adduction	Abduction	Extorsion

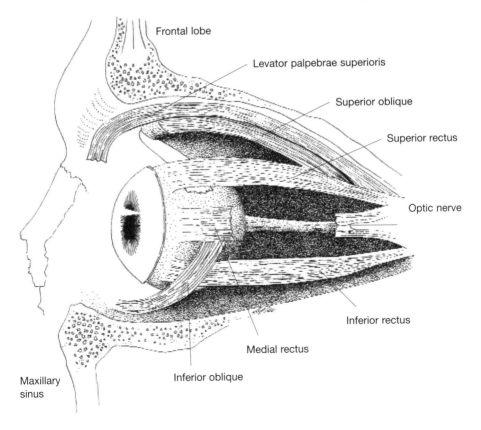

Figure 22.3 Extraocular muscles.

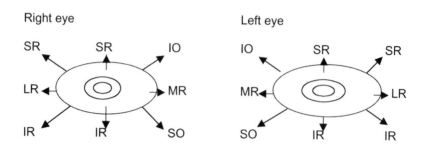

Figure 22.4 Actions of the extraocular muscles.

Lateral rectus

Action

- Abducts, i.e. pulls the eye laterally.

Origin

The lateral rectus originates from the lateral part of the tendinous annulus of Zinn, where it bridges the superior orbital fissure. Lateral to this tendinous ring is a small spine rising from the surface of the greater wing of the sphenoid, to which the lateral rectus is also attached.

Insertion

The lateral rectus passes forward along the lateral wall, pierces Tenon's capsule and is inserted into the sclera 6.9 mm from the limbus by a tendon 8.8 mm long. The line of insertion is almost vertical.

Relationships

- Above lie the lacrimal nerve and artery and then the superior rectus
- Below is the orbital floor
- Laterally is the lateral wall and anteriorly lies the lacrimal gland
- Medially lie nerve VI, the ophthalmic artery, the ciliary ganglion and then further forward the tendon of the inferior oblique.

Nerve supply

- Nerve VI (abducens).

Blood supply

- Lacrimal artery
- Lateral muscular branch of the ophthalmic artery.

Medial rectus

Action

- Adducts, i.e. pulls the eye medially.

Origin

The medial rectus originates from the medial part of the annulus of Zinn and is attached to the dural sheath of the optic nerve. It is the largest of the extraocular muscles.

Insertion

It passes forwards along the medial wall, pierces Tenon's capsule and is inserted into the sclera 5.5 mm from the limbus by a tendon 3.7 mm long. The line of insertion is almost vertical.

Relationships

- Above lie the superior oblique, the ophthalmic artery, with its anterior and posterior ethmoidal branches, and the nasociliary nerve
- Below is the orbital floor
- Laterally is the optic nerve and orbital fat
- Medially is the orbital plate of the ethmoid bone and the ethmoidal air cells.

Nerve supply

- Inferior division nerve III (oculomotor).

Blood supply

- Medial muscular branch of the ophthalmic artery.

Superior rectus

Action

- Elevates, i.e. pulls the eye up
- Adducts
- Intorts, i.e. rotates the eye medially.

Origin

The superior rectus originates from the superior part of the annulus of Zinn, above the optic foramen, and, like the medial rectus, is attached to the dural sheath of the optic nerve.

Insertion

It passes forwards and laterally, making an angle of 25° with the median plane, pierces Tenon's capsule and is inserted into the sclera 7.7 mm from the limbus by a tendon 5.8 mm long. The line of insertion is oblique and slightly curved.

Relationships

- Above lie the levator palpebrae superioris, the frontal nerve and the orbital roof
- Below are the optic nerve, the ophthalmic artery, the nasociliary nerve and orbital fat
- Laterally lie the lacrimal artery and nerve and then the lateral rectus
- Medially lie the ophthalmic artery, the nasociliary nerve, the medial rectus and the superior oblique.

Nerve supply

- Superior division nerve III (oculomotor).

Blood supply

- Lateral muscular branch of the ophthalmic artery.

Inferior rectus

Action

- Depresses, i.e. pulls the eye down
- Adducts
- Extorts, i.e. rotates the eye laterally.

Origin

The inferior rectus is the shortest of the recti, originating from the inferior part of the annulus of Zinn, below the optic foramen.

Insertion

It passes forwards and laterally, making an angle of 25° with the median plane, pierces Tenon's capsule and is inserted into the sclera 6.5 mm from the limbus by a tendon 5.5 mm long. The line of insertion is oblique and slightly curved.

Relationships

- Above lie the inferior division of nerve III, the optic nerve and orbital fat, and then the globe
- Below is the orbital floor, the infraorbital vessels and nerve, in their canal, and the maxillary sinus; the inferior oblique crosses below, between the inferior rectus and the orbital plate of the maxilla, and here the two muscle sheaths are united
- Laterally lies the nerve to the inferior oblique.

Nerve supply

- Inferior division nerve III (oculomotor).

Blood supply

- Medial muscular branch of the ophthalmic artery.

Superior oblique

Action

- Depresses
- Abducts
- Intorts.

Origin

The superior oblique is the longest and thinnest of the extraocular muscles. It originates outside the annulus of Zinn, above and medial to the optic canal. The muscle runs forward between the roof and the medial wall of the orbit, giving rise to a rounded tendon, about 10 mm behind the trochlea.

Trochlea

This is a U-shaped pulley of fibrocartilage, attached to the trochlear fossa on the frontal bone, a few millimetres behind the orbital margin. It is lined by a synovial sheet, which surrounds the tendon as it runs through the pulley and then continues with it until its insertion.

Insertion

As the tendon emerges from the trochlea it bends downwards, backwards and laterally, at an angle of about 55°. It pierces Tenon's capsule, passes beneath the superior rectus, fans out and is inserted into the sclera, posterior to the equator of the globe.

Relationships

- Above are the orbital roof and the supratrochlear nerve
- Below lie the nasociliary nerve, the ophthalmic artery and its posterior and anterior ethmoidal branches.

Nerve supply

- Nerve IV (trochlear).

Blood supply

- Superior muscular branch of the ophthalmic artery.

Inferior oblique

Action

- Elevates
- Abducts
- Extorts.

Origin

The inferior oblique is the only muscle that has its origin at the front of the orbit. It arises from a small depression in the orbital floor, just behind the orbital margin and lateral to the nasolacrimal canal.

Insertion

The inferior oblique passes backwards and laterally, parallel with the reflected tendon of the superior oblique, making an angle of 50° to the median plane. It follows the curve of the lower surface of the globe, running between the inferior rectus and the orbital floor. It is inserted into the sclera at the posterolateral part of the globe, under the lateral rectus. The line of insertion is oblique and convex above.

Relationships

- Above lie the inferior rectus and the globe
- Below are the orbital floor and then laterally the lateral rectus.

Nerve supply

• Inferior division III nerve (oculomotor).

Blood supply

• Infraorbital artery
• Medial muscular branch of the ophthalmic artery.

An easy way to remember the secondary and tertiary actions of the muscles is: RADSIN

    Recti – **AD**duct   Superior – **IN**tort

Therefore:

• obliques abduct
• inferior extorts.

Ocular movements

Normal ocular movements are dependent on the integrity of the ocular muscles, the infra- and internuclear pathways and the oculomotor nuclei. Ocular movements take place around three axes of Fick:

• X: the horizontal axis around which vertical movements are made
• Y: the sagittal or anteroposterior axis around which torsional movements are made
• Z: the vertical axis around which horizontal movements are made.

Ocular movement terminology

Ductions

These are uniocular movements around the axes of Fick from the primary position. They are:

• adduction – moving the eye medially
• abduction – moving the eye laterally
• elevation
• depression
• intorsion
• extortion.

Versions

These are binocular conjugate movements of the eyes, i.e. the eyes move in the same direction:

- dextroversion: right gaze
- laevoversion: left gaze
- dextroelevation: up and right
- laevoelevation: up and left
- dextrodepression: down and right
- laevodepression: down and left.

Vergences

These are binocular disjugate movements of the eyes, i.e. in opposite directions. They are:

- convergence: both eyes moving in
- divergence: both eyes moving out.

Positions of gaze

There are six cardinal positions of gaze:

1. Dextroversion: right gaze
2. Laevoversion: left gaze
3. Dextroelevation: up and right
4. Laevoelevation: up and left
5. Dextrodepression: down and right
6. Laevodepression: down and left.

Ocular movements are assessed in nine positions of gaze. These are the six cardinal positions plus:

7. Primary position: straight ahead
8. Elevation
9. Depression.

Laws of ocular movements

Sherrington's law of reciprocal innervation

This states that when there is increased innervation to one muscle to contract there is decreased innervation to its direct antagonist, which is therefore relaxed, i.e. when the right lateral rectus contracts the right medial rectus relaxes. This is a uniocular law.

Hering's law of equal innervation

This states that when an impulse to contract is sent to one muscle, a simultaneous and equal impulse is sent to its contralateral synergist or yoke muscle, i.e. to look to the right, the right lateral rectus and the left medial rectus receive equal innervation to contract. This is a binocular law, aiding the maintenance of binocular single vision.

Antagonists are pairs of muscles in the same eye, which move the eye in opposite directions, i.e. right superior oblique and right inferior oblique.

Synergists are pairs of muscles in opposite eyes, which move both eyes in the same direction, i.e. right superior oblique and left inferior rectus (Table 22.2).

Table 22.2 Synergists and antagonists

Muscle	Contralateral synergist	Ipsilateral antagonist	Contralateral antagonist
RMR	LLR	RLR	LMR
LMR	RLR	LLR	RMR
RLR	LMR	RMR	LLR
LLR	RMR	LMR	RLR
RSR	LIO	RIR	LSO
LSR	RIO	LIR	RSO
RIR	LSO	RSR	LIO
LIR	RSO	LSR	RIO
RSO	LIR	RIO	LSR
LSO	RIR	LIO	RSR
RIO	LSR	RSO	LIR
LIO	RSR	LSO	RIR

See Addendum for abbreviations. R and L at the beginning of each abbreviation here signify right and left.

Muscle sequelae

These are the series of changes that take place affecting the muscle pairings after an ocular motility defect:

1. Primary underaction
2. Overaction of contralateral synergist (Hering's law)
3. Contracture of ipsilateral antagonist (Sherrington's law)
4. Secondary inhibition of contralateral antagonist (Hering's law).

The overaction of the contralateral synergist will occur at the onset of the defect but the other sequelae take time to develop.

Testing ocular movements

1. The patient sits straight but comfortably, with a straight head and without spectacles.
2. A light fixation target is used at a distance of 50 cm.
3. The light is initially held in the primary position, the corneal reflections observed and a cover test performed.

4. The light is slowly moved into each of the positions of gaze in turn, where a cover test is carried out, and then back into the centre.
5. The patient must not move the head to look, only the eyes.
6. The patient is asked to report any diplopia or pain/discomfort in any positions of gaze.
7. Any anomalous movements are noted.
8. Changes in palpebral fissures, lids and globe position should be noted, e.g. ptosis, lid retraction, lid lag, globe retraction.
9. Any nystagmus should be noted.

Recording ocular movements

Ocular movements can be recorded in various ways, written, graphic, photographically or Hess charts (Figure 22.5).

When recording it is important to note:

- what happened, i.e. over-/underaction or restriction
- which eye
- which position
- size of defect, i.e. slight, small, moderate, marked.

Underaction

This is where the eye does not move fully on a vergence movement (both eyes open), but on duction (where the other eye is covered) the eye moves fully, e.g. on dextroelevation the right eye does not move fully up but when the left eye is covered the movement is completed. This is recorded as:

small underaction of the right eye on dextroelevation.

Overaction

This is where the eye moves past the position that it should be in and moves back to fixate when an alternate cover test is performed, e.g. on dextroelevation when the right eye fixates the light the left eye moves upwards. When the right eye is covered the left eye moves down to fix. This is recorded as:

small overaction of the left eye on dextroelevation.

As mentioned previously, the development of muscle sequelae means that underaction of a muscle of one eye in a particular position of gaze is accompanied by overaction of its contralateral synergist. In the above example, the underacting muscle is the right superior rectus and the overacting muscle is the left inferior oblique.

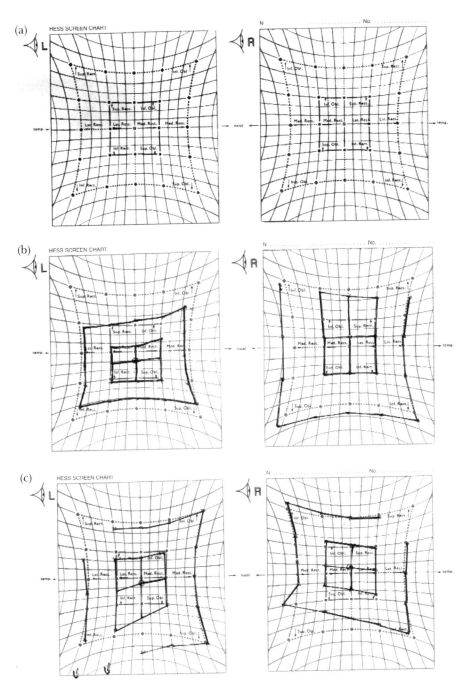

Figure 22.5 Hess charts: (a) the chart; (b) mechanical limitation of elevation in the left eye; (c) right fourth nerve palsy.

Restriction/Limitation

This is where the eye does not move fully on either version or duction.

Written notation

As seen in the above example, this indicates the size (small), action (underaction), eye (right) and direction of gaze (dextroelevation).

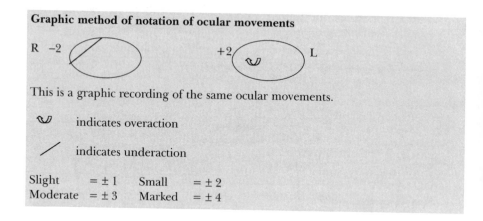

Graphic method of notation of ocular movements

R −2   +2   L

This is a graphic recording of the same ocular movements.

     indicates overaction

     indicates underaction

| Slight | = ± 1 | Small | = ± 2 |
| Moderate | = ± 3 | Marked | = ± 4 |

Hess/Lees screen

This test plots the function of the extraocular muscles and is used in cases of incomitant squint, paralytic squint and to provide a baseline in cases such as TED where defective ocular movements change during the course of the disease. It also provides a record of improving eye movements in a recovering muscle palsy.

The test is based on foveal projection, Hering's and Sherrington's laws of innervation and dissociation of the eyes.

Method

The patient sits in front of a screen, which is a large version of the grid on the chart (see Figure 22.5). Their eyes are dissociated either by red and green goggles (Hess screen) or by a double-sided plane mirror (Lees screen). Each eye is tested in turn as the patient fixes on the different points on the grid and indicates with a pointer where they see the points projected. The position of the points is then recorded on the chart.

Interpretation

- The position of the central dot in each field indicates the deviation in the primary position.
- Each small square on the grid subtends 5° so the measurement of the deviation can be calculated in the different positions of gaze.

- As it is based on foveal projection, patients must have normal retinal correspondence, otherwise the field plotted will not be an accurate representation of the eye position. On the chart the position of the field reflects the position of the eye; the higher field is the higher eye, as opposed to diplopia where the higher image belongs to the lower eye.
- As a result of Hering's law the smaller field belongs to the eye with limitation of movement; underactions are noted by the inward displacement of the dots. There will be maximum displacement in the direction of action of the affected muscle. Overactions have an outward displacement of dots, with the maximum displacement occurring in the field of action of the contralateral synergist.
- A squashed or narrow field indicates a mechanical restriction of ocular movements (see Figure 22.5c).

Orthoptics

Orthoptists investigate, diagnose and treat disorders of binocular vision, ocular motility and visual development. The work includes patients of all ages, especially children (Rowe 1997).

Up to the age of 7 years about 8% of children have impaired vision as a result of a need for spectacles and 5% have a squint. Visual development can be monitored from birth and abnormalities diagnosed at an early stage; no child or baby is too young to be assessed by the orthoptist. Vision develops quickly during the first year of life and finishes developing at about 7 years so early detection and treatment lead to a more successful outcome.

The orthoptist normally sees adults if they complain of diplopia. This could be of sudden onset or a more long-standing problem. It is the orthoptist's role to detect which muscles are causing the problem and which cranial nerves may be affected and deduce where the lesion may be. Diplopia has many causes, e.g. trauma, cerebrovascular accident (CVA), tumour, hypertension, diabetes or thyroid disorders; it may be the first sign of multiple sclerosis (MS) or myasthenia, so an inaccurate diagnosis by the orthoptist can have serious consequences for the patient (McNamara 1995).

Squint (strabismus)

Strabismus or squint (turn, cross eyed, wall eyed) is a condition where the eyes are not parallel, so only one of the visual axes is directed towards the fixation object, whereas the other deviates horizontally, vertically or a combination of both. A squint can be manifest (heterotropia) or latent (heterophoria). It may be concomitant, the same in all positions of gaze or incomitant (paralytic), varying according to the position of gaze and the affected muscle (Ansons and Davis 2001).

Heterotropia

This is the term for a manifest deviation where one of the visual axes is not directed towards the fixation point. It may be constant (present all the time) or intermittent (present only at certain distances or under certain circumstances, e.g. when tired or unwell):

- Esotropia: convergent squint – one eye deviates nasally, i.e. turns in.
- Exotropia: divergent squint – one eye deviates temporally, i.e. turns out.
- Hypertropia: one eye deviates up.
- Hypotropia: one eye deviates down.

Heterophoria

This is the term for a latent deviation where both eyes are directed towards the fixation point when both eyes are open, but deviate on dissociation, i.e. when one eye is covered.

- Esophoria: latent convergent squint.
- Exophoria: latent divergent squint.
- Hyperphoria: latent upwards deviation.
- Hypophoria: latent downwards deviation.

Concomitant squint

Concomitant squints are predominantly horizontal and the size of the deviation is the same whichever eye is fixing in the primary position. The onset is in childhood, usually before the age of 6 years, with infantile strabismus developing between 2 and 4 months of age.

Aetiology

Anything that disrupts the development of binocular vision during the developmental period will result in squint and there are a number of factors that may contribute to this.

Heredity

Sixty per cent of children with squint have a close relative with a squint and a child with a parent who has a squint is four times more likely to develop one.

Refractive error

Uncorrected refractive error can influence the development of squint; specifically moderate hypermetropia is associated with accommodative esotropia. Children who develop microtropia often have anisometropia, which has affected visual development, resulting in central suppression and amblyopia.

Neurological defects
Pre-term, low-birthweight and brain-damaged babies (especially cerebral palsy) have a higher incidence of squint.

Febrile illness
Squint is often reported after chickenpox or measles but often these children have a predisposition for squint and the illness precipitated it rather than caused it.

Incomitant (paralytic) squint

In incomitant squints the size of deviation differs depending on the position of gaze and according to which eye is fixing, with the size of squint increasing in one or more positions of gaze depending on the underlying cause of the limitation of movement. The aetiology may be:

- neurogenic, as a result of a cranial nerve palsy of nerve III, IV or VI
- mechanical, e.g. caused by a blow-out fracture
- myogenic, e.g. caused by myasthenia gravis or TED.

Detection of squint

The methods of detection are observation of appearance, observation of corneal reflections and the cover test.

Observation of appearance

Any obvious deviation, abnormal head posture, abnormal lid position or other anomaly, which may indicate an oculomotor defect, should be noted.

Corneal reflections

The patient is asked to look at a pen light held at a distance of 33 cm and the positions of the corneal reflections in each eye are noted. If the corneal reflections are central and symmetrical the eyes are straight but if the reflections are asymmetrical there is a manifest deviation present.

The reflection will be central in the fixing eye and displaced in the deviating eye. Temporal displacement indicates a convergent squint, medial displacement a divergent squint and vertical displacement a vertical squint.

The amount of displacement also indicates the size of squint: 1 mm of displacement represents about 7° of deviation so if the corneal reflection is on the border of the pupil the deviation is about 15°.

Pseudostrabismus

The corneal reflection test is also useful for detecting a pseudostrabismus or pseudosquint. Often children have flat noses with the presence of skin folds on the inner canthi, called epicanthic folds. This results from the fact that their facial features are not fully formed. Many babies and young children may appear to have a convergent squint as a result of their facial appearance but the corneal reflections will be central and symmetrical in either eye, showing that the eyes are straight. Epicanthus normally resolves as the facial skeleton develops.

Cover test

This is the most accurate assessment of a deviation and, as Ansons and Davis (2001) state, the cornerstone of the investigation of squint. It is an objective dissociative test, which elicits the presence of a latent or manifest squint, relying on the observation of the behaviour of the eyes while either eye is covered and uncovered in turn.

The cover test is performed for near (33 cm), distance (6 m) and far distance (in the case of divergent deviations) and with and without spectacles. The test is carried out first with a pen light for near and then with an accommodative target. There are two types of cover test:

1. The cover–uncover test
2. The alternate cover test.

Performing the cover–uncover test

The test consists of two parts: cover then uncover.

Part 1 – cover

1. The patient sits comfortably facing the examiner.
2. The patient fixes a pen light held in the primary position (straight ahead) at 33 cm while the examiner observes the corneal reflections.
3. One eye is covered and any movement of the **uncovered** eye to take up fixation is noted.
4. If there is no movement to fix, the test is repeated, covering the other eye and any movement of the **uncovered** eye is noted.
5. A movement out to fix indicates esotropia and a movement in to fix indicates exotropia. A movement down to fix indicates hypertropia, whereas a movement up to fix indicates hypotropia.

Part 2 – uncover

1. The test is repeated but now the eye behind the occluder is observed.
2. The right eye is occluded for a few seconds and then the covering removed with the examiner noting any movement of the right eye.

3. If the eye moves out as the cover is removed, the eye has been deviated inwardly, indicating an esophoria or latent convergent squint.
4. If the eye moves in when the cover is removed, it has been deviated outwards, indicating an exophoria or latent divergent squint.
5. Downward movement indicates a hyperphoria, whereas upward movement indicates a hypophoria.
6. The test is repeated for the other eye.
7. No movement indicates orthophoria.

The cover–uncover test is repeated using an accommodative target for near, suitable for the vision and age of the patient, then at 6 m and, if required, at the far distance.

Performing the alternate cover test
This is the repeated alternate covering of each eye in turn so that binocular vision is prevented and fusional stimuli are eliminated. It reveals the total deviation: tropia + phoria. It should be performed only after the cover–uncover test, otherwise it will be impossible to differentiate between the manifest and latent components of the squint:

1. The patient fixes the light or accommodative target while the examiner covers the right eye for about 2 seconds.
2. The occluder is quickly transferred to cover the left eye completely, ensuring that there is no chance of binocular interaction between the two eyes.
3. The left eye is covered for a couple of seconds and then the occluder is moved back to the right eye.
4. As the occluder is moved alternately between the two eyes for a few more times, the eye movements are noted. The eyes will be completely dissociated and so the maximum deviation will be elicited.
5. When the cover is removed the eyes will return to their pre-dissociated state and the examiner notes the speed and smoothness of recovery.

Information gained from the cover test
1. Direction of deviation: eso-/exo-/hyper-/hypo-/torsional
2. Type of deviation: manifest or latent
3. Size: small/slight/moderate/marked
4. Variations between near and distance: this aids in the classification of squint
5. Comitance or incomitance: if the size of the deviation differs according to which eye is fixing
6. The effect of spectacles on the deviation
7. The effect of accommodation on the deviation
8. In a latent squint the rate and speed of recovery to binocular single vision (BSV) indicates the ability to control the deviation.

Management of squint

Concomitant squint

The aims of management of a concomitant squint are to:

- attain and then maintain the best possible vision by correction of any refractive error and treatment of amblyopia
- achieve BSV where there is the potential for it
- restore a good cosmetic appearance.
  The methods of achieving these aims are:
- conservative
- surgical
- a combination of the two.

Conservative treatment

Optical/spectacles All children attending an orthoptic clinic will have a cycloplegic refraction carried out by the ophthalmologist. If there is a refractive error spectacles will be prescribed:

- To correct vision
- To correct the squint – certain lenses can reduce the angle of a squint and possibly restore BSV, e.g. a hypermetropic correction in an esotropia will reduce the angle of squint and may allow it to be controlled to an esophoria. Prisms may also be used to correct a deviation to restore BSV.

Occlusion (patching) This is the most effective way to treat amblyopia (lazy eye). The aim of occlusion is to achieve the best possible vision in the amblyopic or lazy eye by occluding or covering the good eye. A patch is used, preferably on the face (to avoid peeping) either full time (FTTO), i.e. all day, or part time (PTTO), i.e. for a specific period and prescribed activities, depending on the level of vision and the age of the child.
The optimum results are achieved from occlusion therapy if:

- the treatment is commenced as soon as possible
- the child is in the critical period of visual development, i.e. up to the age of about 7 years
- spectacles if needed are worn with the patch
- most importantly of all, compliance is good, the patch is worn as prescribed and the child attends regularly.

Occlusion is continued until equal, or the best possible, vision has been achieved.

Orthoptic exercises Exercises are used in a number of different ways and in different types of squint. They are most frequently used to help a patient control a latent squint, which may be causing asthenopic symptoms, i.e. headache, blurred vision or diplopia, or to teach control of an intermittent squint.

Surgical treatment
Surgery is performed to:

• restore BSV
• improve a cosmetically poor appearance.

The following are the two main methods of surgical procedure used in squint surgery:

1. Recession – weakening: where the muscle is detached from its insertion and reattached further back.
2. Resection – strengthening: where the muscle is detached from the globe, a piece is cut out, thereby shortening the muscle, and it is then reattached in the original position.

The choice and amount of surgery depend on the type and size of the squint. In the case of a left esotropia, where the left eye turns in and therefore needs to be pulled laterally into a straight ahead position, the left medial rectus will be recessed or weakened and the left lateral rectus will be resected or strengthened.

Incomitant squint

The aims of management of an incomitant squint are to:

• diagnose which muscles are under- and overacting
• establish the type of limitation, i.e. neurogenic, mechanical or myogenic
• differentiate between a long-standing and a recently acquired palsy
• diagnose and treat the cause of the palsy
• monitor the progress of the condition by maintaining an accurate and repeatable record of the condition
• alleviate symptoms until there is spontaneous recovery, or squint surgery can be carried out if full recovery does not take place.

Orthoptic assessment

An orthoptic assessment uses different methods to assess and measure visual acuity, detect the presence of squint or abnormal ocular movements, to measure any deviation present and to assess binocular functions.

There follows an overview of a basic orthoptic assessment, giving examples of orthoptic terminology that may be seen in an orthoptic report.

History

A detailed history will always be taken eliciting the reason for attendance, what has been noticed, what the symptoms are, when it first occurred and how often it is noticed now, if there were any precipitating factors and if there has been any previous ophthalmic treatment.

Vision

This is always assessed monocularly to ascertain the level of vision in each eye. The test used depends on the age and ability of the patient.

Cover test

This is carried out as above to establish the type of deviation.

Ocular movements

These are assessed as above to determine if there is an ocular motility problem and which muscles are involved.

Binocular functions

The aim of the assessment of binocular functions is to determine if the patient has binocular vision or the potential for binocular vision because this will affect the course of treatment undertaken. Tests used to assess binocular functions are:

- Bagolini glasses
- Prism fusion range (PFR) or prism reflex test in young children
- Stereoscopic tests, e.g. Wirt, TNO, Frisby.

Measurement

A squint can be measured using the following methods:

1. By approximation using the corneal reflections (see above), recorded in degrees.
2. By the prism cover test (PCT), recorded in prism dioptres (Δ), $2\Delta = 1°$. Prisms are used in conjunction with the cover test to neutralize the movement of the eyes and so determine the size of the squint.
3. By the synoptophore, recorded in degrees.

Examples of orthoptic reports are given in the box.

Examples of orthoptic reports

Case 1: Child aged 3

VA	c gls R 6/60 L 6/6 SG	Vision with spectacles using Sheridan–Gardiner test
CT	c gls n & d sl/mod RCS c poor fix	Right convergent squint
	s gls n & d mod RCS	Increasing without spectacles
OM	sl lim RE on ABD	
Conv	c dev to nose	
PCT	c gls n 20ΔBO	Measurement with prisms
	d 18ΔBO	
	s gls n 40ΔBO	
	d 35ΔBO	
Synop	c gls obj + 10°	Measurement with synoptophore
	subj R supp	
	s gls obj +20°	

Diagnosis: partially accommodative R esotropia with amblyopia

Treatment: PTTO LE – 6 hours a day (part-time total occlusion left eye)

To see again 4/52 (4 weeks)

Case 2: Adult aged 60

VA	s gls R 6/6	L 6/6
CT	n sl R hypertropia c diplopia	
	d sl latent R/L c fair rec – diplopia before rec	
OM	mod elev RE on ADD	
	mod limit RE on laevodep c o/a LE	
	mod o/a RE c u/a LE on laevoelev	
	R/L in all pos > on laevo versions	

Diplopia: vertical for near in all pos > on laevo versions

Saccades: horiz + vert – normal resp

Conv	c dev to approx. 8 cm	
PFR	n nil	Prism fusion range
	d 8ΔBO – 2ΔBI	
PCT	n 10ΔR/L	Prism cover test
	D 4ΔR/L	

Diplopia joined for near c 8Δ BD RE

Bagolini Gls	n vertical diplopia	Test for binocular vision
	d BSV resp	
	n c 8Δ BD RE BSV resp	

Frisby	c 8Δ BD RE 120"	Stereopsis
Lees no. 1	RSO palsy	

Diagnosis: recently acquired R VI nerve palsy

Diplopia: joined with 8Δ prism BD RE

For further investigations

Addendum

Orthoptic abbreviations

ACS	alternating convergent squint
ADS	alternating divergent squint
AHP	abnormal head posture
ARC	abnormal retinal correspondence
BD	base down
BE	both eyes
BEO	both eyes open
BI	base in
BO	base out
BSV	binocular single vision
BT or BTXA	botulinum toxin
BU	base up
BV	binocular vision
BVA	binocular visual acuity
CC or CAC	Cardiff acuity cards (vision test for babies)
CI	convergence insufficiency
c/o	complains of
Conv	convergence/convergent
CPEO	chronic progressive external ophthalmoplegia
CT	cover test
D	dioptre
Dep	depression
Dist	distance
Div	divergence/divergent
DVD	dissociated vertical deviation
DVM	delayed visual maturation
EE	either eye
EF	eccentric fixation
Elev	elevation
Eso	esotropia/-phoria
Exo	exotropia/-phoria
FCPL	forced choice preferential looking (vision test for babies)

FEE	fixing either eye
FLE	fixing left eye
FRE	fixing right eye
FTTO	full-time total occlusion
H/A	headaches
HES(1)	hospital eye service prescription
HM	hand movements
INO	internuclear ophthalmoplegia
IO	inferior oblique
IR	inferior rectus
Kay Pics	Kay pictures (vision test for children)
LCS	left convergent squint
LDS	left divergent squint
LE	left eye
LPS	levator palpebrae superioris
LR	lateral rectus
L/R	left over right (left hypertropia/-phoria or right hypotropia/-phoria)
LVA	low visual aid or left visual acuity
MR	medial rectus
N	nerve
NAD	no apparent deviation
NPA	near point of accommodation
NPC	near point of convergence
NRC	normal retinal correspondence
NPL	no perception of light
NVA	near visual acuity
o/a	over action
OKN	optokinetic nystagmus
OM	ocular movements
PBD	prism base down
PBI	prism base in
PBO	prism base out
PBU	prism base up
PCT	prism cover test
PFR	prism fusion range
PH	pin hole
PL	perception of light
PMT	post-mydriatic test
PRT	prism reflection test
PTTO	part-time total occlusion
RAF	Royal Air Force rule measurement of convergence and accommodation
RAPD	relative afferent pupillary defect
RCS	right convergent squint
RDS	right divergent squint
Recess	recession

Resect	resection
R/L	right over left (right hypertropia/-phoria or left hypotropia/-phoria)
ROP	retinopathy of prematurity
rr	rapid recovery (as in latent deviations)
RVA	right visual acuity
SG or SSG	single Sheridan–Gardiner (vision test for children)
Sl rec	slow recovery (as in latent deviations)
Sn	Snellen's
SO	superior oblique
SP	simultaneous perception
SR	superior rectus
u/a	underaction
VA	visual acuity
VEP	visual evoked potential
VER	visual evoked response
VF	visual field
VOR	vestibulo-ocular reflex

Acknowledgements

Orthoptic Department, Wrightington, Wigan and Leigh NHS Trust, for use of information in their teaching pack.

References

Ansons A, Davis H (2001) Diagnosis and Management of Ocular Motility Disorders, 3rd edn. Oxford: Blackwell Science.

Bron A, Tripathi R, Tripathi B (1997) Wolff's Anatomy of the Eye and Orbit, 8th edn. London: Chapman & Hall Medical.

Char D (1997) Thyroid Eye Disease, 3rd edn. Oxford: Butterworth-Heinemann.

Kanski JJ (2003) Clinical Ophthalmology, 5th edn. Oxford: Butterworth-Heinemann.

Leatherbarrow B (2003) Oculoplastic Surgery. London: Taylor & Freeman.

Levine M, Larson D (1993) Orbital tumours. In: Tenzel R (ed.), Orbit and Oculoplastics. Textbook of ophthalmology, Vol. 4. London: Mosby-Wolfe.

McNamara R (1995) Orthoptics. In: Parry JP, Tullo AB (eds), Care of the Ophthalmic Patient, 2nd edn. London: Chapman & Hall.

Newell FW (1996) Ophthalmology: Principles and concepts, 8th edn. St Louis, MO: Mosby.

Rowe F (1997) Clinical Orthoptics. Oxford: Blackwell Science.

Snell RS, Lemp MA (1998) Clinical Anatomy of the Eye and Orbit, 2nd edn. Oxford: Blackwell Science.

Stephenson RW (1966) Anatomy, Physiology and Optics of the Eye. London: Kimpton.

CHAPTER TWENTY-THREE

Visual and pupillary pathways and neuro-ophthalmology

YVONNE NEEDHAM

The complexity of the visual system though the brain's hemispheres often leads to confusion, but knowledge of the primary pathways and their progress will assist the ophthalmic nurse in supporting patients with visual, pupillary and neurological problems. The anatomy and physiology of the visual pathway must be understood in order to put it into perspective for patients, to explain and help them deal with the issues that they face with a variety of conditions. This chapter provides an overview and a basis for further study and initially identifies the relevant anatomy and physiology of the visual pathway from the optic nerve to the visual cortex and goes on to discuss how damage to the pathway affects the patient's vision and in some cases movement and balance. In some conditions interventions using medication or surgery may be advised but in all cases patients and their relatives will need advice and support in managing their condition and maintaining a healthy lifestyle. Visual disturbances that patients face can often lead to isolation and loss of confidence.

Components of the visual pathway

The primary visual pathway in humans consists of the retina (see Chapter 21), optic nerves, optic chiasma, optic tracts, lateral geniculate bodies, optic radiations and the visual cortex (Glaser 1990, Perry and Tullo 1993) (Figure 23.1). The visual pathways travel horizontally though the brain using parallel systems in each hemisphere from the retina to the cortex. The whole pathway is regarded as part of the 'central nervous system', growing forward from the brain into the orbital cavities.

Optic nerve

The second cranial nerve is known as the optic nerve. Each is about 51 mm in length commencing at the optic nerve head in the globe and ending as

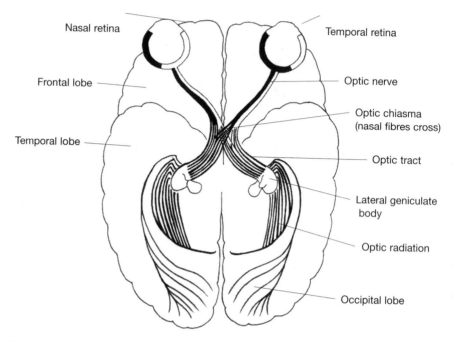

Nasal retina

Temporal retina

Frontal lobe

Optic nerve

Optic chiasma
(nasal fibres cross)

Temporal lobe

Optic tract

Lateral geniculate
body

Optic radiation

Occipital lobe

Figure 23.1 Visual pathways.

the two optic nerves joined at the chiasma situated in the third ventricle. It is surrounded by cerebrospinal fluid contained within the meninges. The optic nerve contains oligodendrocytes, astrocytes and microglia rather than the Schwann cells, fibroblasts and macrophages of peripheral nerves. It has the same structure as the brain's white matter and therefore has no powers of regeneration. It is not myelinated in the same way as peripheral nerves (by oligodendrocytes rather than Schwann cells) and is covered by the meninges (pia, arachnoid and dura mater). It is the only cranial nerve that is visible and can be seen though the eye at the optic disc.

Visual development commences with the optic stalk identified at day 27 of fetal gestation (Forrester et al. 1996); by week 8 the ganglion cells of the optic nerve and the optic nerve sheath can be identified clearly. The optic nerve can be split into four distinct sections: intraocular, orbital, intracanalicular and intracranial (Forrester et al. 1996).

The intraocular portion of the optic nerve is about 1 mm in length. The optic disc is the commencement of the optic nerve, and is visible when the eye is viewed internally though the pupil. The optic disc is pale in comparison to the retina and on examination may appear yellowish and vertically ovoid, about 1.5 mm in diameter; it contains 1.2 million ganglion cell axons in the nerve fibre layer which converge to form a raised area known as the papilla. The protrusion of the optic disc through the retina creates an area with no visual receptors and hence the blind spot (Forrester et al. 1996).

The optic nerve exits the eye though the choroid and sclera. At the exit point the nerve fibres thicken, causing a doubling in size of the optic nerve. In some individuals the optic nerve exits the sclera at less than a 90° angle which would make the disc margin elevated, giving it a tilted appearance known as tilted disc. Tilted discs are usually small and bilateral and often associated with astigmatism (Ragge and Easty 1999). When viewing the optic disc this should be considered as a common normal variant (Acheson and Riordan-Eva 1999). The blood supply to this part of the optic nerve is by branches from four sources: central retinal vessels, scleral vessels (circle of Zinn–Haller), choroidal vessels and pial vessels. The first three are derived from the central retinal artery, with the pial vessels from the internal carotid artery.

The orbital portion of the optic nerve is about 30 mm long and extends backwards medially from the sclera to the optic canal at the apex of the orbit. It is covered by the meninges and surrounded by the four rectus muscles. The dura and arachnoid blend with the sclera. The orbital portion of the optic nerve has an S-shaped bend which enables the full range of eye movement and up to 8 mm of proptosis without the optic nerve being stretched. The central retinal vessels travel though this space before entering the optic nerve 1 cm behind the globe. The central retinal vessels must cross the subarachnoid space, making them vulnerable to compression when raised intercranial pressure occurs.

The intracanalicular portion of the optic nerve is about 10 mm in length and passes though the optic canal accompanied by the optic artery and the sympathetic nerves. The optic canal is formed by the two roots of the lesser wing of the sphenoid bone.

The intracranial portion of the optic nerve is 10 mm in length and travels from the optic canal medially backwards and slightly upwards, coming together with the other nerve to form the optic chiasma in the fold of the third ventricle. The olfactory tract, frontal lobe and anterior cerebral arteries lie above the optic nerve with the internal carotid arteries laterally.

Optic chiasma

The optic chiasma is situated at the junction of the floor and the anterior wall of the third ventricle. It is quadrangular in shape and approximately 12 × 8 mm in size, consisting of a flattened bundle of nerve fibres. The posterior angles form the optic tract. In the chiasma, the fibres from the nasal half of each retina (those that collect light from the temporal side), including the nasal half of the macula, cross over and enter the optic tract on the opposite side. The fibres from the temporal retina pass backwards along the optic tract on the same side. This partial crossing of the nerve fibres is essential for binocular vision (Snell and Lemp 1998).

Optochiasmal glioma may have its origins in the differentiation of cells during month 4 of fetal development.

The optic tracts

The optic tracts extend as cylindrical bands of fibres from the chiasma backward towards the midbrain. Most of the fibres terminate in the lateral geniculate body and are concerned with conscious vision. Ten per cent pass the lateral geniculate body and enter the pre-tectal nucleus; these are concerned with visual body and light reflexes. The nerve fibres conducting these reflexes synapse in the pre-tectal nuclei with neurons connecting to the Edinger–Westphal nuclei (Perry and Tullo 1993).

Lateral geniculate bodies

The lateral geniculate bodies are oval in shape and are highly differentiated structures lying in the thalamus (Acheson and Riordan-Eva 1999). The function of these bodies is to transmit the visual information from the eye, via the lateral root of the optic tract, to the cortex. As a result of the crossing of fibres in the chiasma, each of the lateral geniculate bodies receives information from both retinas (Forrester et al. 1996).

Optic radiations

Optic radiations consist of nerve fibre bundles, the bodies of which lie in the lateral geniculate bodies with their axons terminating in the visual cortex of the occipital lobe. As a result of their path though the temporal lobe along the lateral aspect of the lateral ventricle, they are of major clinical significance because they are frequently disturbed during cerebrovascular disturbances or tumour growth. The optic radiations stimulate the whole of the visual cortex. Those stimulating the lower visual cortex carry information from the peripheral retina and those supplying the upper visual cortex carry information from the macular area of the retina.

The visual cortex

The visual cortex is found in the occipital lobe of the brain. Very simplistically, the cortex differentiates between impulses sent from the peripheral and those sent from the central retina. Damage to any part of the visual pathway will result in characteristic field loss.

Malformation of the optic nerve head

Failure of the posterior optic fissure to close leads to the formation of an optic nerve head coloboma with bulging of the sclera. The coloboma may be seen as a small recess on the rim of the disc. This will be associated with visual loss resulting from the leakage of fluid from the optic pit and formation of exudates beneath the macula (Forrester et al. 1996).

Axial coloboma or morning glory syndrome

This presents with a symmetrically enlarged and excavated optic disc, which may be unilateral or bilateral (Forrester et al. 1996). This malformation of the optic nerve causes a displacement into the optic meninges of the optic nerve; the meninges contain fat and smooth muscle. This distortion of the normal optic nerve structure results in severe visual loss and the nerve impulses cannot be transmitted for interpretation in the visual cortex.

Congenital optic disc abnormalities

Optic disc colobomas prevent visual development in babies and children. It is essential that from an early stage children's visual development and stimulation be maximized. Parents will need information about this condition and the effects that this will have on the sight of their child. Often parents who have children with congenital abnormalities feel responsible for the child's problems. It is important to allow the parents time to come to terms with their child's condition and it would not be unexpected for the parents to go through the stages of grieving. Parents need to know that their reaction to the news that they have been given is normal and what to expect in terms of the rollercoaster of emotion that they will go though during the years to follow. It is essential that parents are made aware of services to support them with their child's visual impairment and how to access that support. Referrals need to be made promptly so parents are not left for a long period without support after the initial diagnosis.

As ophthalmic nurses may rarely see these children and parents when they visit outpatients, it is important that the parents know that they can still access support from the outpatient clinics. It is thus valuable to have available information about the locations of local child development centres and educational development centres and their telephone numbers. Specialist child development teams will assist parents in caring for their child pre-school and educational development teams will support the child and parents though the school years. These services, along with mobility officers and local, national and international organizations for people with visual disability, will assist the parents in enabling the child to maximize the vision that they have. Parents will need ongoing support from social workers, counsellors and health visitors because having a child with such a condition requires adjustments to be made to family life and the potential for isolation is great in families with children with disabilities (Goffman 1990, Daniels 2001).

Optic disc hypoplasia

This may be accompanied by other ocular or forebrain abnormalities and visual function may be good or poor. Where optic disc hypoplasia is bilateral, there is poor vision and nystagmus. As a rule, the smaller the disc the poorer the visual acuity. Although the cause is unknown maternal diabetes has been linked to optic disc hypoplasia (Burde et al. 1992), as has intake of toxic substances such as alcohol, quinine, phenytoin and lysergic acid diethylamide (LSD) (Glaser 1990). Care of the child and parents will follow similar routes to those identified above for optic nerve coloboma. However, if the condition is identified as being caused by maternal diabetes or ingestion of toxic substances, additional support will be needed for both parents, because of their feelings of guilt and blame, in coming to terms with their child's condition.

Nystagmus

Nystagmus is an involuntary to-and-fro movement of the eyes and may be a consequence of optic nerve problems because it tends to develop in children where central vision is lost before the age of 2 years – movements may be right, left, up, down or rotary.

There are many causes of nystagmus; in this case it is caused by sensory deprivation. There are three types (Kanski 2003) known as:

• pendular movements of equal velocity in each direction (similar to a pendulum)
• jerk nystagmus: slow movement in one direction and fast in the other
• mixed nystagmus where pendular movements occur in the primary position and jerk movements when the eyes deviate laterally.

As a result of the constant eye movement accommodation is very difficult and objects appear blurred.

Visual development may be restricted in children by nystagmus, and accurate assessment of vision will assist in planning the use of the vision that they have for mobility and education.

Acquired optic nerve problems

Optic neuritis

Optic neuritis in children presents with bilateral visual loss with disc swelling associated with viral illness such as measles, mumps and chicken-pox (Glaser 1990, Wormald et al. 2004).

Optic neuritis normally presents in adults between the ages of 20 and 50 (Burde et al. 1992) with an acute unilateral loss of vision and with pain behind the eye and on movement (Maclean 2002), and possibly brow ache (Glaser 1990). This pain may precede or accompany the visual loss. The optic disc may appear swollen (optic neuritis) but is usually normal in appearance because the nerve is swollen behind the globe and is then known as retrobulbar optic neuritis (Wormald et al. 2004). Decreased colour vision is often obvious because objects appear drab and 'washed out'. Contrast sensitivity, central scotoma and a relative afferent pupillary defect are also seen on examination (Burde et al. 1992). Visual loss is rapid and progressive, reaching its lowest level after around a week. Visual loss may be partial or total but normally begins to improve in the second or third week and is back to normal by the fourth week. In the optic neuritis treatment trial the mean visual acuity was 6/5 with only 7% having a visual acuity of 6/12 after 1 year (Beck and Cleary 1993).

Causes in adults

Optic or retrobulbar neuritis is the first presentation of multiple sclerosis (MS) in a large number of patients with about 70% of women and 35% of men going on to develop other neurological problems associated with MS later (Maclean 2002). These figures do vary between different authors but the risk is very significant.

Optic neuritis may also develop secondary to inflammation of sinuses, orbit or meninges (Acheson and Riordan-Eva 1999). Syphilis, sarcoidosis, tuberculosis and cytomegalovirus infection have also been implicated (Burde et al. 1992), although many cases are idiopathic.

Management of the patient involves full blood count (FBC), erythrocyte sedimentation rate (ESR) of plasma viscosity, and a VDRL (Venereal Disease Reference Laboratory) test should be done to exclude vasculitic and other diseases (Ragge and Easty 1990). High-dose corticosteroids may be used in severe cases but studies (Wormald et al. 2004) have found that this may speed up visual recovery although it does not affect long-term outcome or lessen the frequency of recurrence. Their use may have side effects such as insomnia, mild mood changes, stomach upsets, oedema and weight gain.

With the loss of vision patients need to be assured that in 75% of cases vision is restored to normal within a few weeks, although it is likely to worsen initially. Timescales for visual recovery and colour sensitivity need to be conveyed accurately. In this way, as the patient's vision recovers, he or she will be reassured. Where visual recovery is not within the time scales identified patients need to be kept informed of their progress and improvements from the initial loss identified. Time should be taken to listen to patients' concerns and support and advice given about the difficulties that they may be encountering. Each patient is an individual and recovery of vision will vary. Discussion relating to how the visual loss is affecting the patient must include home and work, and advice and assistance should be offered. Loss of binocular vision and how this will affect the patient will need identifying. Patients may be more prone to tripping or misjudging depth and generally appearing clumsy, thus increasing their anxiety, especially if the cause for the optic neuritis has been linked to MS.

Where other systemic disease is identified as the cause, additional support will be necessary. Information about the need to treat the underlying cause will assist the patient with dealing with the uncertainty during the tests required. When MS is suspected referral to a neurologist is indicated, and it could be argued that the possibility of MS should be discussed only by a neurologist, or an ophthalmologist together with a neurologist, so that the patient gains the best possible advice from someone who will be able to discuss all the disease possibilities. Tests to diagnose MS involve magnetic resonance imaging (MRI) to show demyelination, lumbar puncture and evoked potentials (Kanski and Nischal 1999). A number of these patients are likely to be followed up in the ophthalmic department and, after being informed of the possibility that the cause of the visual loss may be MS, they are likely to be extremely shocked because a confirmed diagnosis will have a profound effect on their future health and life. During this time it is vital that the patient has help from a friend or family member who will be able to offer support and retain information that can be discussed at a later time.

It is common for patients not to hear important information or focus on the negative when receiving bad news. Although MS has the potential to be life altering, patients can experience long periods of remission and as with all disease progression varies. It is important that patients are aware of support from social workers, counselling services and support groups. Family support should not be overlooked because, if the diagnosis of MS is confirmed, this may require changes. Although it is not likely that the nurse in the ophthalmic clinic will be required to provide all this information, it is useful to know what the patient will experience in terms of the referral and possible tests needed to confirm the diagnosis. Fear of the unknown in terms of the next stage in the process can often cause distress and it may be that referral to the neurologist takes several weeks, during which time the patient and family may feel very isolated, so providing a contact number for the clinic or social worker may be valuable.

Optic neuropathies

Anterior ischaemic optic neuropathy

This is caused by an acute infarction of the optic nerve head and may be divided into non-arteritic and arteritic ischaemic optic neuropathy.

Non-arteritic ischaemic optic neuropathy

This affects individuals aged 45 years and over (Burde et al. 1992), with the average age of onset being around 60 years of age (Wormald et al. 2004). Visual loss is sudden and painless and mostly irreversible but non-progressive. Various vascular risk factors have been associated with non-arteritic ischaemic optic neuropathy (NAION), such as hypertension, diabetes mellitus and cigarette use (Wormald et al. 2004). Tests will include an ESR to exclude giant cell arteritis; blood pressure and blood sugar tests to check for risk factors will need to be recorded.

Although there is no evidence to suggest that the use of aspirin may prevent the recurrence of NAION, retrospective studies have found an increased risk of these patients dying from vascular-related diseases such as myocardial infarction and stroke (Wormald et al. 2004), so the treatment of NAION patients with aspirin may reduce this risk. Burde et al. (1992) and Maclean (2002) both advocate the use of aspirin. The NAION patient should, however, have the risk of vascular disease assessed initially by his or her GP. Patients are now more aware that aspirin is prescribed to help prevent the risk of myocardial infarctions and strokes, and once vascular diseases such as these are mentioned they may question the use of aspirin if is not advised. Nurses must be ready to support patients with information in such cases and advise them to ensure that they get the vascular risk assessment done. If patients smoke they may need to be advised of the possible links between smoking and their NAION. Information such as national and local helpline numbers and other information about the assistance that they can receive to help them to stop smoking may be useful.

Arteritic ischaemic optic neuropathy

The most common cause of arteritic ischaemic optic neuropathy (AION) is giant cell/temporal arteritis. Giant cell arteritis is considered to be a severe variant of polymyalgia rheumatica, with a combination of genetic and environmental factors thought to play a role in its aetiology (Huang et al. 2001). Adults over the age of 50 years are affected, with the mean age of onset being 70 (Wormald et al. 2004). Loss of vision is initially in one eye and may be profound, reducing vision to perhaps 'count fingers', but may be followed rapidly by loss of vision in the other eye if treatment is not started (Burde et al. 1992, Wormald et al. 2004). In 30% of patients visual acuity may improve over 2 years (Wormald et al. 2004). Loss of vision may be accompanied by headache, which is temporal over the scalp; patients may complain of pain when brushing their hair. Jaw claudication will be present in giant cell arteritis; it occurs on chewing and is relieved by rest (Kanski 2003). Morning muscle stiffness, anorexia, anaemia, fever and fatigue may also be present (Burde et al. 1992).

Tests to confirm giant cell arteritis are ESR and temporal artery biopsy. The presence of jaw claudication, anaemia and European origin have been significantly correlated with biopsy results that are positive for giant cell arteritis (Burde et al. 1992).

Treatment involves initial intravenous hydrocortisone followed by 60–80 mg orally daily as a starting dose. This will be tapered as the ESR is reduced (Wormald et al. 2004). Patients may be required to continue treatment for up to 2 years and will require frequent visits to outpatients during this time. Information in relation to giant cell arteritis and the risk of the other eye being affected must be discussed with patients because, in 40% of patients, the other eye was subsequently found to be affected (Kanski 2003).

Patients will need referral for treatment of anaemia and any underlying rheumatic disease, and this may involve referral to the GP and/or a rheumatologist. Explanation of steroid use and the possible side effects must be explored with patients, which may include osteoporosis, peptic ulcer, diabetes, hypertension, immunosuppression, weight gain, psychiatric disturbances, and ocular complications such as cataract and glaucoma.

Patients may need to adapt to field loss and can, with hemianopia, learn to move their eyes or head in the direction of field loss. In older adults, until these skills are acquired there is a greater risk of falls. Both patients and family members need to be aware of these risks. It is important that the team caring for the patient and family – nurse, orthoptist, low-visual aid optician and/or social worker – spend time discussing how the treatment and visual loss may impact on daily life. Taking a team approach in this way will provide the best support to the patient and the family. Nurses can give information and advice on the use of steroids, and the orthoptist will advise on prisms to combat any diplopia and using the visual field that the patient has. Some patients may not be able to tolerate prisms for walking and this should be assessed before dispensing. Patients may be able to have prisms for reading, watching television or computer work (Melore 1997). Social workers will be able to advise on services available to assist at home, in mobility and with work if this is relevant. The low-visual aid optician will dispense and advise on the use of low-visual aids and lighting (Melore 1997). Throughout the patient's care nurses in the outpatient department will be able to assess the patient and discuss how he or she is coping with treatment and managing at home. These interactions will be crucial because there is the potential for the patient to become depressed and isolated. Clear documentation of the patient's appearance, mobility and concerns will enable continuity of care.

Other optic neuropathies

Leber's optic neuropathy

This is a rare hereditary disorder and is transmitted by mitochondrial DNA, most of which comes from the mother, rather than by nuclear DNA. It normally affects healthy young men but there is no transmission down the male line. Women transmit the disease to sons and the carrier state to their daughters, although some carrier females are also affected (Kanski 2003). Burde et al. (1992) indicate that these cases are so rarely seen in clinical practice that they are often misdiagnosed. Visual loss is initially monocular, painless and progresses to bilateral over weeks or months. These young people will need extensive support because their visual impairment may have a profound effect on their lives. It will be important that family members be examined (Glaser 1990, Burde et al. 1992) and counselling about the hereditary aspect of this condition will be necessary. Depending on the visual acuity, the patient will need different types of support and advice about mobility, and life and work options. The process of acceptance and rehabilitation may be lengthy and patients may be at risk of becoming depressed and isolated. Friends and family will play a large part in rehabilitation, but will need advice and support and, with the patient's permission, must be included in discussions.

Toxic optic neuropathies

Toxic amblyopia typically affects heavy drinkers and pipe smokers who have a diet deficient in B vitamins (Burde et al. 1992, Kanski 2003). Visual loss is gradual, progressive and bilateral. Vision will improve with treatment of hydroxycobalamin for 10 weeks. The classic field defect is bilateral central or caecocentral scotomata. Patients need advice on reduction of alcohol and/or smoking cessation, and may need social work involvement to enable them to access a treatment programme. Without reduction of the cause the condition will recur.

Drug induced

Ethambutol can cause optic neuropathy but doses of up to 25 mg/kg per day are rarely toxic (Burde et al. 1992). Patients who become toxic often have concurrent alcoholism or diabetes. Onset is sudden and associated with loss of red–green colour vision (Kanski 2003). Visual recovery is normally complete but may take up to 12 months. As ethambutol is part of the treatment for tuberculosis, it is vital that the treatment be continued. These requirements will need full explanation to the patients to ensure compliance. Patients may need help with daily life, mobility and any associated underlying condition treated.

Papilloedema

This is swelling of the optic nerve head produced by raised intracranial pressure. Finding the cause and treating the pressure will relieve the papilloedema and prevent long-term visual loss. Visual loss initially may be in the form of diplopia and an enlarged blind spot. Other signs may be loss of consciousness, headache worsened by coughing or straining, and vomiting without nausea (Kanski 2003). Papilloedema is invariably bilateral unless there is previous disease of the optic nerve (Burde et al. 1992). There are three stages of papilloedema:

1. Early papilloedema where there is minimal hyperaemia of the disc and oedema.
2. Acute papilloedema includes haemorrhages and exudates which are present in addition to the early symptoms. Visual acuity is normal unless there is macular oedema. The disc margins become indistinct and the central cup is obliterated.
3. Vintage: the acute haemorrhagic and exudative components resolve. Once oedema resolves the optic disc is pale and nerve fibre visual field defects are seen on field testing (Burde et al. 1992, Kanski 2003).

Initial referral to an ophthalmologist will be at an ophthalmic clinic and may come via an optician or GP. Patients will require detailed explanations of the possible causes and what will be required to identify the underlying cause. The main causes of papilloedema are tumours in the cranium and urgent referral to a neurologist or neurosurgeon will be required.

Optic nerve tumours

Gliomas

Gliomas present in two different forms. Benign tumours are found in children between the ages of 4 and 8 years with unilateral proptosis and visual impairment (Acheson and Riordan-Eva 1999, Kanski 2003). Investigations include radiographs, computed tomography and ultrasonography and will be able to identify the size and extent of the tumour. Kanski (2003) identifies that about 55% of patients will also have neurofibromatosis. If proptosis becomes aesthetically unacceptable and the eye is blind from optic atrophy, a local resection is the treatment of choice. Intracranial extensions to the tumour may need the assistance of a neurosurgeon and radiation is used for tumours too big for surgical excision. Parents and children will require support and information about the condition and treatments. Loss of vision will require additional support for the child in terms of education.

In adults, normally men aged 40–60, the presence of the tumour may mimic optic neuritis with rapid monocular visual loss, retrobulbar pain and disc oedema. Even with steroid treatment complete blindness ensues in several weeks. Radiotherapy and/or chemotherapy may be of some value but death usually occurs within months.

Meningiomas

These are invasive tumours that typically affect middle-aged women (Kanski 2003). The meningiomas spread along the lines of least resistance, along the subarachnoid space, and are usually encapsulated by intact dura (Acheson and Riordan-Eva 1999). Visual loss is slow but progressive with loss of acuity and central scotoma, and loss of colour vision. Treatment for intracranial tumours is surgical but prognosis is poor (Acheson and Riordan-Eva 1999). By contrast primary optic nerve sheath meningiomas, when removed by stripping the optic nerve sheath with its blood supply, are not normally fatal although they do have a profound effect on visual acuity.

Pituitary tumours

These tumours affect the chiasma as they grow so visual field loss is normally bitemporal. Headaches may initially accompany the blurring of vision and diplopia would indicate that the third, fourth or sixth nerve may be involved. As the pituitary gland is responsible for producing hormones, depending on which tumour is present, different features may present (Kanski 2003).

Care for patients with tumours varies depending on the treatment but nurses must ensure that the patient and family are fully informed throughout all the investigations and treatments. Coming to terms with a potentially life-threatening illness requires skilled support and may need the intervention of specialist nurses in this field and referral to local hospice services. For those patients who survive, the loss of vision will require a significant amount of adjustment.

Aneurysms

The proximity of the carotid artery to the chiasma when a carotid aneurysm occurs initially causes a unilateral nasal hemianopia. As the aneurysm becomes larger, it may press against the opposite carotid artery (Kanski 2003).

Supranuclear disorders of eye movement

In these conditions patients may be unaware of visual disturbance, such as the inability to see food on their plate, and may attribute problems that they are experiencing to simple solutions such as inappropriate spectacles (Burde et al. 1992). Differentiation between problems with fixation and the location of objects will determine which area of the visual pathway is affected and determine the underlying cause, such as sixth nerve palsy, Huntington's disease, Parinaud's syndrome or internuclear ophthalmoplegia (Kanski 2003). Patients may adopt varying head postures to accommodate visual disturbances. Given that the patient may not attribute problems to visual disturbances, initially after diagnosis nurses may need to spend time listening to the patient determining to what extent the visual loss is affecting their life.

Nerve palsies (see also Chapter 22)

About 25% of third, fourth or sixth nerve palsies have no known cause and 50% of these will resolve spontaneously (Kanski 2003). Nerve palsies may be the first sign of patients developing complications of systemic disease and conditions such as diabetes, hypertension and atherosclerosis are the most common causes. Other causes may include herpes zoster, tuberculosis, basal meningitis, syphilis, otitis media and Guillain–Barré syndrome. The nerves are susceptible to trauma as a result of their pathways and this is a common cause of palsy. Aneurysms may cause third nerve palsies (Kanski 2003).

Generally, in nerve palsy, surgical intervention will be carried out only after symptoms have been present for about 6 months. This is to allow time for spontaneous resolution. During this time, depending on the visual disturbances, patients may benefit (apart from in fourth nerve palsy) from the use of prisms applied to spectacles, or even occlusion of the affected eye. Support and advice on how to manage at home and work may require referral to a specialist social worker.

Third nerve (oculomotor)

The third nerve is situated in the midbrain (Kanski 2003) and supplies the medial, inferior and superior rectus, superior oblique and lid levator muscles (Acheson and Riordan-Eva 1999). Paralysis of the nerve may be compete or partial leading to a variety of different symptoms. Complete third nerve palsy will lead to ptosis, which may mask diplopia. Paralysis and unopposed action of extraocular muscles will cause diplopia, and loss of pupillary function as a result of interruption of the parasympathetic pathway to the sphincter pupillae causes a fixed, dilated pupil non-reactive to direct or consensual light (Kanski 2003). Vascular disease often causes pupil-sparing third nerve palsy. A painful palsy may be associated with diabetes but should be investigated thoroughly because it may be a sign of a more sinister causation. Posterior communicating artery aneurysm is an important cause of a painful third nerve palsy with pupil involvement.

Fourth nerve palsy (trochlear)

The fourth cranial nerve lies in the midbrain at the caudal aspect of the oculomotor nuclear complex and exits the brain stem dorsally (Acheson and Riordan-Eva 1999). It innervates the superior oblique muscle. Bilateral palsy is common and is characterized by hyperdeviation in gaze. There is limitation in adduction as a result of superior oblique weakness; diplopia is vertical, torsional and worse on looking down. Diplopia may be reduced by abnormal head posture. Frequent causes of fourth nerve palsies are congenital lesions that may manifest later in life. Trauma is also an important cause, as are vascular lesions.

Sixth nerve (abducens)

This nerve lies in the midportion of the pons inferior to the floor of the fourth ventricle. There is frequently a facial nerve palsy and weakness of the lateral rectus prevents abduction. If palsy is complete, there will be no abduction beyond the midline and patients may adopt face turning in order to reduce diplopia. Acoustic neuroma is an important cause of sixth nerve palsy and hearing and corneal sensitivity should be tested because these are the first signs and symptoms of acoustic neuroma. Other causes include nasopharyngeal tumours, raised intracranial pressure and basal skull fractures as well as vascular causes.

Pupillary pathways

The pupil changes size as a result of the actions of two opposing muscles in the iris: the constrictor and dilator pupillae. The size of the pupil at any given time is the result of balance of the innervations of the two (Perry and Tullo 1993) (Figure 23.2).

(a)

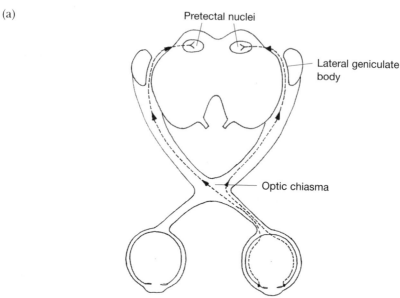

(b)

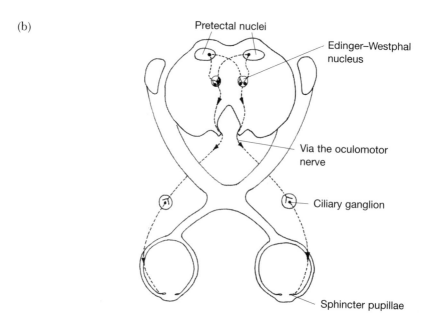

Figure 23.2 The pupillary light reflex: (a) to the pretectal nuclei – the afferent pathway; (b) from the pretectal nuclei to the Edinger-Westphal nuclei – the pretecto oculomotor pathway, and from there to the sphincter pupillae – the efferent pathway.

As photoreceptors in the retina are stimulated by light, impulses travel through the optic nerve to the lateral geniculate body as described earlier. Those fibres that bypass the lateral geniculate body synapse on nerve cells in the pretectal nucleus. The impulse travels via axons of the pretectal nerve cells to the Edinger–Westphal nuclei of the oculomotor nerve (parasympathetic nuclei) on each side (which accounts for the consensual response). This forms the afferent pathway. From here, the fibres synapse and travel through the oculomotor nerve to the ciliary ganglion within the orbit. The short ciliary nerves take the impulses to the constrictor pupillae muscle – the efferent pathway.

The pupil also constricts in response to accommodation, which consists of a triad of convergence, accommodation and miosis. The three light reflexes are therefore:

1. The **direct** light reflex occurs when light is focused on the eye.
2. At the same time, the pupil of the other eye constricts as well – the **consensual** reflex.
3. The **near** reflex in accommodation.

The dilator pupillae is under sympathetic nerve control from the hypothalamus via the spinal cord and superior cervical ganglion and then in the sympathetic fibres that run alongside the carotid artery and ciliary nerves to the eye. Stimulation of these nerve pathways causes the pupil to dilate, in low intensity light and during excitement or fear.

The size of the pupil is in a constant state of movement (hippus) adjusting to changes in illumination, fixation distance and psychosensory stimuli. Pupillary sizes tend to be smaller in children and older adults than young adults and smaller in brown eyes than blue (Burde et al. 1992).

Examining the pupils

To examine the pupil the light should be dim and preferably directed onto the face from below so that both pupils are seen simultaneously; the size should be measured with a millimetre rule (Kanski 2003). Anisocoria, a difference in pupillary size between the two eyes, may normally be found in 41% of people examined (Burde et al. 1992). To determine whether this is normal the pupillary dimensions of the individual should be reassessed, varying the amount of illumination in the room; anisocoria that varies with the degree of illumination is pathological (Kanski 2003).

Reaction to light should be brisk and full and should be tested when the patient is fixating at distance to prevent constriction caused by the near response.

Pupillary pathway defects

Afferent pupil defect

If the afferent pathway is completely compromised, no light impulse will reach the Edinger–Westphal nucleus and therefore no direct response is possible. The pupil will still show a consensual response if light is shone into the other eye because the efferent pathway is susceptible to impulses directed to it from the fellow eye. Complete afferent pupillary defects are uncommon but relative afferent pupillary defects (RAPDs) are a sensitive measure of optic nerve damage or disease.

The test for this is commonly known as the swinging flashlight test and should take place in a dimly lit room. Both pupils must be observed at once so complete darkness is unhelpful. A bright light is shone on to the un-affected eye and the pupil's direct response and the consensual response of the other eye are noted. The light is swung to the affected eye and, if a defect of the afferent pathway is present, the pupil appears to dilate to a greater or lesser degree. Both pupils are larger at this phase of the test as a result not of not dilating, as such, but of a lesser degree of constriction because of a compromised afferent pathway of the affected eye, and therefore a lesser impulse reaching the unaffected eye through its efferent pathway. (In simplistic terms, if only 50% of the optic nerve is working on the affected eye, then only 50% of the 'signal' can reach the Edinger–Westphal nucleus and only 50% return down each of the efferent routes.) As the flashlight is swung back to the unaffected eye, the pupil constricts further and the pupil of the affected eye does the same (100% of impulse reaching the Edinger–Westphal nucleus means 100% down each efferent pathway). RAPDs should be recorded according to an agreed taxonomy such as 'mild', moderate' or 'severe'.

Although RAPDs are felt to be characteristic of optic nerve disease, they can also be present in some retinal lesions, including detachment, age-related macular degeneration and retinal vein occlusion. RAPDs may also be seen in some people with amblyopia, although the mechanism is not clear and the severity of the RAPDs is not related to the degree of amblyopia.

Efferent pupil defect

If there is damage to the nerve parasympathetic pathway controlling the action of the constrictor pupillae, the pupil will respond poorly to both direct and consensual stimulation. Abnormalities of the efferent pathway may be caused by lesions anywhere from the midbrain to the pupillary sphincter muscle. The cause and site of the nerve damage will need to be determined for a diagnosis to be made.

Light–near dissociation

The light reflex is absent or sluggish and the near response is normal. Compression of the dorsal midbrain can selectively damage the dorsally located light reflex fibres while leaving the more ventrally located near reflex fibres intact. The most commonly seen bilateral light/near dissociation is an Argyll Robertson pupil whereas a common cause of unilateral near–light dissociation is Adie pupil (or Adie's tonic pupil).

Argyll Robertson pupil

Argyll Robertson pupils are small (> 2 mm), irregular and react to near but not to light. They are the result of tertiary syphilis involving the central nervous system. Iris atrophy is frequent and dilatation is poor after mydriatic instillation. It is important to assess visual acuity accurately in these patients because optic atrophy, which may also cause light–near dissociation, is also a consequence of syphilis. Argyll Robertson (-like) pupils are also seen in diabetes, chronic alcoholism and some degenerative disorders as well as encephalitis.

Adie pupil/Adie's tonic pupil/Adie syndrome

Adie pupil is a common cause of anisocoria and is commonly seen in young adults (Kanski 2003). This pupillary abnormality is caused by damage to the postganglionic supply to the sphincter pupillae and the ciliary muscle. The cause is not understood but it is a benign condition and does not indicate any underlying pathology.

The affected pupil is larger and does not react to light, although it reacts slowly to near stimuli. A tonic near response is one where the pupil remains constricted after accommodative effort has ceased. Accommodation may also be tonic giving the person blurred vision for some time after he or she has stopped accommodating. Deep tendon reflexes are diminished in many patients but the reasons for this are unclear (Holmes–Adie syndrome). The palsy of the sphincter pupillae is almost always segmental. Slit-lamp examination reveals bunching of the iris stroma in those areas where the sphincter pupillae is intact. The segmental response may be described as vermiform or worm-like. A test for Adie pupil is the instillation of 0.05–0.125% pilocarpine. Many of these patients have a hypersensitivity to this strength of pilocarpine.

A change in anisocoria of more than 1 mm after 45 minutes is considered to be a positive result. The test should not be carried out within 24 hours of any other test that changes the corneal permeability (because this will affect the results – perhaps giving a false positive as a result of increased uptake of the pilocarpine), such as instillation of topical anaesthetic, applanation tonometry, etc., so the patient may have to come back to the department to have this carried out. Patients with Adie pupil may have photophobia or accommodative symptoms but, often, they have no symptoms and state that the anisocoria was noted by a friend or relative. Accommodative problems tend to resolve within months. About half of Adie pupils will resolve within 2 years but involvement of the second eye is common.

Lesions at any point along the sympathetic pathway results in Horner's syndrome.

Horner's syndrome

Here one pupil is smaller as a result of paralysis of the dilator muscle along with a moderate degree of ptosis. Anisocoria is more apparent in dim light and there is delayed or absent dilatation. Reactions to light and near are normal. The lesion may be congenital (associated with birth injury to the brachial plexus) or associated with acquired lesions of the pathway. These will result in a degree of anhidrosis (lack of sweating) in the areas of the body innervated by the pathway in which the lesion occurs – the entire side of the body, the same side of the face or just the forehead. Causes involving first-order neurons include central nervous system lesions such as vascular occlusion, tumours and cervical disc problems. Second-order neuron lesions may be caused by lung tumours and thoracic surgery, carotid or aortic aneurysm, and trauma to the brachial plexus. Third-order neuron lesions include tumours in the neck, cluster headaches and carotid artery surgery. Location of the lesion is important so patients may undergo a battery of investigations that they feel are irrelevant to their eye problem.

Instillation of cocaine 4% into both eyes confirms the diagnosis. The normal pupil will dilate as a result of the cocaine blocking the reuptake of noradrenaline (norepinephrine) which terminates its action. There is therefore an accumulation of adrenaline (epinephrine) at the postganglionic sympathetic nerve endings and the pupil dilates. There is no noradrenaline released in the pupillary pathway of the eye with Horner's syndrome and therefore cocaine has no effect.

Support from ophthalmic clinicians will be needed at this time so that the person understands the relevance of the tests and investigations.

References

Acheson J, Riordan-Eva P (1999) Neuro-ophthalmology. Fundamentals of Clinical Ophthalmology. London: BMJ Publications.

Beck RW, Cleary PA (1993) The Optic Neuritis Study Group: Optic Neuritis Treatment Trial one year follow up results. Arch Ophthalmol 111: 773–5.

Burde RM, Savino PJ, Trobe JD (1992) Clinical Decisions in Neuro-Ophthalmology, 2nd edn. St Louis, MO: Mosby.

Daniels E (2001) Losing Your Sight. London: Robinson.

Forrester JK, Dick AJ, McMenamin P, Lee RW (1996) The Eye: Basic sciences in practice. London: WB Saunders.

Glaser JS (1990) Neuro-Ophthalmology, 2nd edn. Philadelphia, PA: JB Lippincott.

Goffman E (1990) Stigma Notes on Management of Spoilt Identity. Harmondsworth: Penguin Books.

Huang D, Zhou Y, Hoffman GS (2001) Pathogenesis immunogenetic factors. Best Pract Res Clin Rheumatol 15: 239–58.

Kanski JJ (2003) Clinical Ophthalmology, 5th edn. London: Butterworth-Heinemann.

Kanski JJ, Nischal KK (1999) Ophthalmology: Clinical signs and differential diagnosis. London: Mosby.

Maclean H (2002) The Eye in Primary Care. Oxford: Butterworth-Heinemann.

Melore GG (1997) Treating Vision Problems in the Older Adult. St Louis, MO: Mosby.

Perry JP, Tullo AB (1993) Care of the Ophthalmic Patient. London: Chapman & Hall.

Ragge NK, Easty DL (1999) Immediate Eye Care. London: Wolf Publications Ltd.

Snell RS, Lemp MA (1998) Clinical Anatomy of the Eye, 2nd edn. Oxford: Blackwell Science.

Wormald R, Smeeth L, Henshaw K (2004) Evidence Based Ophthalmology. London: BMJ Books.

CHAPTER TWENTY-FOUR
The eye and systemic disease

DOROTHY E FIELD

The eye is said to be 'the window of the human body', a phrase attributed to Leonardo Da Vinci (1452–1519). For the physician, or the expert ophthalmic nurse, it may also provide a window into the general health of the body, because examination through a dilated pupil will provide a view of retinal blood vessels and the relative health of the retina, and the optic disc may provide evidence of raised intracranial pressure. It is therefore true to say that distinctive changes in the eye may be pointers to many general health problems. With this in mind, the ophthalmic clinician should be aware of these possible eye changes, because they may be relevant to an ophthalmic diagnosis or form the basis for giving further, more general health advice. As general health may affect the eye, producing a 'new' condition, a careful general history in terms of family eye problems, the patient's general health and any current medications being taken should always be noted.

Only an overview can be taken here, regarding systemic health and the eye, and it is proposed therefore to discuss the eye and systemic disease under the following headings:

- Congenital problems, because these will be particularly within the remit of those working in paediatric areas
- Problems acquired throughout life
- Problems that may require health advice.

Congenital problems

The list that follows provides only a brief indication of some of the problems with each syndrome. Ophthalmic clinic nurses who are likely to come across these, or other unlisted, problems are advised to make separate, detailed studies to heighten their awareness of systemic disease and its ocular consequences. Similarly, nurses working in paediatric areas, particularly those who deal with children who are likely to require anaesthesia, are advised to develop information folders for the purposes of providing safe, informed care to children and their families. This having been said, children become adults, so this information is also necessary for every ophthalmic clinician. Helpful information regarding anaesthesia for children with congenital syndromes may be found in Bevan (1998) and Mitchell et al. (1995).

Sight problems in people with a learning disability

The Royal National Institute for the Blind (RNIB 2003) remarks that the prevalence of visual problems in people with learning difficulties is higher than in the general population. The more profoundly disabled a person appears, the more likely he or she is to have sensory disabilities. About 40% of learning-disabled people have a hearing problem and about 35% have a significant sight problem. In addition to the higher incidence of eye problems within this group, many of these difficulties, both of eye problems and of focusing (refractive) errors, may go unrecognized and, even if easily managed, may go untreated. The RNIB additionally cautions that people who have difficulties communicating their needs to others may, out of frustration, develop self-injuring behaviour that can result in eye injury, e.g. detached retinas. This, too, may go unrecognized.

Bourneville's disease (tuberous sclerosis)

* Systemic problems: epilepsy, particularly infantile spasms, learning difficulties, adenoma sebaceum, consisting of numerous pink or red–brown papules on the face, mostly around the nose. Renal or cardiac tumours occur in about 50% of cases.
* Eye problems: slowly maturing retinal tumours in 50% of cases.

Coats' disease (exudative retinitis)

* Systemic problems: may be associated with other systemic disorders (Robitaille et al. 1996).
* Eye problems: this progressive disease of the retinal capillaries affects mainly males. Problems start in the first 10 years of life, with the chronic progressive inflammation that may threaten to cause retinal detachment. Treatment may be with argon laser, photocoagulation and cryotherapy. Secondary cataract, uveitis and rubeosis have also been linked to Coats' disease.

Cerebral palsy

- Systemic problems: specific to the individual and may result in only mild or very severe disability.
- Eye problems: people with cerebral palsy are likely to have difficulties with processing visual information (cortical visual impairment).

Down's syndrome

- Systemic problems: degrees of learning disability, congenital cardiac anomalies, recurrent chest infections.
- Eye problems: upslanting, narrow palpebral fissures, hyperplasia of the iris, congenital blue-dot lens opacities, tendency to high myopia (33% of people with Down's syndrome – Vaughan et al. 1999). In addition, children with Down's syndrome are likely to have decreased corneal thickness, which may give an artificially low intraocular pressure measurement by applanation tonometry (Evereklioglu et al. 2002). They are more likely than the general population to require penetrating keratoplasty for keratoconus (Kuchle and Naumann 1992).

Edward's syndrome

- Systemic problems: learning disability and developmental problems, congenital heart defects and renal problems. Of these children 90% die in the first year of life, but a small proportion survive into their teens and twenties (Holmes and Coates 1994).
- Eye problems: corneal and lens opacities, unilateral ptosis and optic atrophy. Although many do not have associated ocular abnormalities that might affect vision, visual acuity is difficult to measure as a result of the profound developmental delay (Holmes and Coates 1994).

Galactosaemia

- Systemic problems: impairment of galactose metabolism causing failure to thrive, lethargy, vomiting and diarrhoea, which untreated would lead to enlarged liver, renal disease, anaemia, deafness and learning disability. Treatment of galactosaemia requires a galactose-restricted diet. Weese et al. (2003) suggested that, based on current recommendations, most baby food meals should be acceptable for infants with galactosaemia.
- Eye problems: development of an early, central cataract, which may regress if the systemic condition is recognized and treated early. In addition to cataracts, Levy et al. (1996), alerted by ophthalmological examination, initiated the observation of clouding of a child's eye, or on

routine examination noted that infants with severe neonatal manifestations of galactosaemia were more likely to have vitreous haemorrhages. Long-term follow-up of patients with this disorder, by Bosch et al. (2002), showed that, in spite of a severely galactose-restricted diet, most patients still develop abnormalities such as a disturbed mental and/or motor development, dyspraxia and hypergonadotrophic hypogonadism.

Laurence–Moon–Bardet–Biedl syndrome

- Systemic problems: obesity, learning disability, additional fingers or toes, and impaired sexual development. Beales et al. (1999) found the average age at diagnosis to be 9 years, late for such a debilitating condition, but the slow development of the clinical features of this syndrome probably accounts for this. Their study identified some novel clinical features, including neurological, speech and language deficits, behavioural traits, facial dysmorphism and dental anomalies, which may facilitate earlier diagnosis of this disorder. Their findings have important implications for the care of these patients and their unaffected relatives.
- Eye problems: retinitis pigmentosa may develop in infancy or early teens.

Lowe's syndrome

- Systemic problems: Lowe's syndrome, a rare genetic condition, which affects only males, causes medical problems and physical and mental disability. As Lowe's syndrome involves the eyes, brain and kidney, it is also known as OCRL (oculocerebrorenal) syndrome.
- Many boys with Lowe's syndrome go on to develop kidney problems, namely Fanconi-type renal tubular dysfunction at about a year. In Lowe's syndrome, the Fanconi-type renal dysfunction may be mild or severe.
- Eye problems: affected males are born with bilateral cataracts, and about 50% of these children also go on to develop glaucoma.

Marchesani's syndrome

- Systemic problems: slight maxillary underdevelopment, narrow palate, malformed and malaligned teeth, and cardiac defects. Late ossification of the ends of the long bones is a consistent feature of this condition. Children may have squat, stiff fingers and may be short in stature.
- Eye problems: small shallow orbits, small lenses and myopia, with or without glaucoma, frequent lens dislocation and occasional blindness.

Marfan's syndrome

- Systemic problems: unusually long limbs and fingers, scoliosis, heart problems, muscular underdevelopment.
- Eye problems: dislocated lenses, megalocornea, keratoconus, severe refractive problems, glaucoma resulting from angle anomaly, lattice degeneration and retinal detachment.

Patau's syndrome

- Systemic problems: cerebral defects, cleft palate, heart problems, additional fingers or toes and haemangiomas. Vaughan et al. (1999) suggest that death by age 6 months is common.
- Eye problems: anophthalmos (congenital failure of the eye to develop), microphthalmos, cataracts and retinal problems.

Refsum's syndrome

- Systemic problems: this is a metabolic disease, which may cause peripheral neuropathy, ataxia, deafness, ichthyosis or cardiac arrhythmias.
- Eye problems: pigmentary retinopathy, causing night blindness; cataracts.

Rubella

If a fetus *in utero* is infected by the mother via the transplacental route, during the first 24 weeks of pregnancy, a number of physical malformations may occur, depending on when organogenesis is complete:

- Systemic problems: congenital heart problems, deafness, mental handicap, enlarged liver and many others.
- Eye problems: retinopathy, microphthalmos and glaucoma. Vaughan et al. (1999) suggest that maternal rubella is responsible for 75% of congenital cataracts.

Stickler's syndrome

- Systemic problems: deafness, cleft palate, skeletal abnormalities and mitral valve prolapse. Stickler et al. (2001) found wide variations of symptoms and signs among affected people, even within the same family. They highlighted delays in diagnosis, lack of understanding among family members and denial about the risk of serious eye problems.
- Eye problems: high myopia, presenile cataract, dislocation of the lens (caused by dysfunction of the lens zonule fibres) and early retinal

detachment. Leiba et al. (1996) studied the ocular manifestations in a family of 42 people with Stickler's syndrome, and the results of laser photocoagulation as preventive treatment for retinal detachment are described. They demonstrated that retinal detachment was significantly higher in non-lasered than in lasered eyes.

Sturge–Weber syndrome

- Systemic problems: this condition involves one side of the face with naevus flammeus ('port wine stain'), which may also affect the meninges and eyes. As a result of a same-sided brain lesion, it may be associated with epilepsy, hemiparesis and learning disability.
- Eye problems: involvement of the eyelid and conjunctiva nearly always indicates eye involvement, in particular glaucoma, possible diffuse choroidal haemangioma, and haemangioma of the iris and ciliary body. Possible hemianopia may result from brain involvement. Awad et al. (1999) highlight the fact that medical treatment often fails to control intraocular pressure and, in their study of 18 patients, note that late postoperative complications resulted in loss of vision in three eyes that underwent surgical procedures.

Turner syndrome

- Systemic problems: affects girls, and causes growth retardation and impaired sexual development. Lawrence et al. (2003) have discovered a hitherto hidden aspect of Turner syndrome. People with the condition show an impairment in remembering faces and classifying 'fear' in face images. Lesniak-Karpiak et al. (2003), using parental reports, documented social skills impairment in children with Turner syndrome. Anxiety, shyness and difficulty understanding social cues have been reported for girls with Turner syndrome. Self-report and parental ratings did not suggest higher levels of anxiety in females with Turner syndrome, but did reflect higher levels of social difficulty.
- Eye problems: 8% of people with Turner syndrome have impaired colour vision (Vaughan et al. 1999). Other potential eye problems include ptosis, pterygia and keratoconus, blue sclera.

Usher's syndrome

- Systemic problems: Kanski (2001) says that Usher's syndrome is responsible for about 5% of all congenital, severe deafness, and about half of all cases of deaf blindness.
- Eye problems: progressive pigmentary retinopathy.

Problems acquired throughout life

Amaurosis fugax

Amaurosis fugax is a transient, often complete, loss of vision experienced in one or both eyes.

The most likely mechanism of retinal ischaemia and embolism in patients with amaurosis fugax was identified by Babikian et al. (2001) as extracranial internal carotid artery occlusion or stenosis – 22% of cases, in a study of 77 patients, making it the largest aetiological subgroup. Uncommon but treatable conditions were identified in 10% of patients, and no causative diagnosis could be made in 45% of patients. Significant to all ophthalmic personnel who deal with this condition was that further adverse health events followed in 18% of patients, within 1 month, and in 8% of patients at the 3-month follow-ups. This included two myocardial infarcts and two deaths.

Behçet's syndrome

This is described by Kanski (2001) as a multisystem disease, associated with an increased incidence of HLA-B51. Among a range of other symptoms, patients may exhibit stomatitis, skin lesions, recurrent genital ulceration, and arthritis of knees and ankles. Eye manifestations include recurrent iridocyclitis, frequently accompanied by hypopyon and occlusive vasculitis of the retinal vessels.

Diabetes and the eye

Diabetic retinopathy

Aiello (2003) describes diabetic retinopathy as a microvascular complication of diabetes mellitus that is a significant cause of blindness, and describes laser photocoagulation as treatment for proliferative diabetic retinopathy and diabetic macular oedema. He promotes the value of intensive glycaemic control in reducing the risk of onset and progression of diabetic eye disease and other microvascular complications of diabetes, believing that severe and moderate visual loss from diabetes is essentially preventable with early detection, treatments and effective long-term follow-up. Nurses, however, should note that, as with patients with open-angle glaucoma, eye diseases appear to have a more aggressive course in some individuals than in others, and should always avoid 'victim blaming'.

However, nurses should note their role in preventing and alleviating the complications of disease. Leslie and Pozzilli (2002) note that the

Diabetes Control and Complications Trial and the UK Prospective Diabetes Study found that improved control of blood glucose reduced the risk of major diabetic eye disease by 25%, serious deterioration of vision by nearly 50%, and early kidney damage by 33%. They state that studies have demonstrated the importance of blood pressure control and reduced cholesterol, in addition to the use of aspirin in limiting the progression of macrovascular disease. Diabetic retinopathy is discussed further in Chapter 21.

Cataract formation

Cataract formation in people with diabetes is thought to result from an increase in glucose in the lens that is subsequently reduced to sorbitol. The lens capsule is relatively impermeable to sorbitol, which remains within the lens where it attracts water, causing an osmotic imbalance that eventually leads to cataract formation. People with type 2 diabetes do not develop true diabetic cataracts but tend to develop age-related cataracts on average 10 years earlier than people who do not have diabetes. Fluctuating vision and rapid-onset myopia caused by shifts in the glucose, electrolyte and water balance within the lens are early symptoms of diabetes (Vaughan et al. 1999).

Macular oedema after cataract surgery in people with diabetes

Nurses managing postoperative cataract clinics should be aware that swelling of the central retina (macular oedema) is fairly common among patients with diabetes after cataract surgery. It causes reduced central visual acuity and is an important risk consideration for patients with diabetes according to Dowler et al. (1999), who carried out a study of 32 people to examine the frequency of macular oedema postoperatively in patients with diabetes. During the first year after surgery, only 6% of patients had no change in their macular oedema (retinal swelling), whereas the other 94% had worsening. However, by the end of the first postoperative year, 43% of the patients' macular oedema had returned to the preoperative state. A more severe degree of swelling of the macula, known as clinically significant macular oedema, occurred in 56% of patients during the first year after surgery. However, of these patients, 69% had resolution of the condition by the end of the first postoperative year, without laser therapy. For nurses who are involved with obtaining patients' written consent, it is noteworthy that Dowler et al. (1999) recommend that patients with diabetes who are considering cataract surgery should understand that macular oedema may worsen during the first year after surgery, reducing visual acuity. The good news is that the condition frequently resolves spontaneously.

Pupil dilatation

Experienced ophthalmic nurses are aware of the difficulties in dilating the pupils of people with diabetes, particularly on clinic visits. Worryingly, according to Pittasch et al. (2002), pupillary autonomic neuropathy is considered to be an early sign of the development of systemic autonomic neuropathy, and is related to the duration of diabetes and the development of systemic dysfunction, e.g. trouble with circulation to the feet, development of silent cardiac ischaemia, etc. Clearly smoking should be discouraged in this group of patients, and good foot care and frequent health monitoring should be encouraged.

Drug misuse and the eye

Augsten et al. (1998) suggest that *Aspergillus* spp. are a rare cause of endophthalmitis, but note that aspergillus ocular manifestations have mostly been reported in connection with immunosuppression, severe diseases or drug misuse. Weishaar et al. (1998) note that aspergillus endophthalmitis usually has an acute onset of intraocular inflammation and often has a characteristic chorioretinal lesion located in the macula. They noted that treatment with pars plana vitrectomy and intravitreous amphotericin B may eliminate the ocular infection, but the visual outcome is poor, especially when there is direct macular involvement. Augsten et al. (1998) also note the case of a kidney transplant recipient, on immunosuppressive drugs, who developed an endogenous aspergillus endophthalmitis.

Lyme disease

Lyme disease, although not actively affecting the eye, impacts on the eye unit in relation to tick removal. Lyme disease is carried by ticks in the UK, and is common in children, who frequently present with ticks in their eyelids and eyebrows. In addition to frequently recognized manifestations, such as erythema migrans, a characteristic rash spreading from the site of a tick bite, which typically starts about 2–30 days after the tick bite, may often affect the skin, heart, joints and nervous system. Clinical diagnosis of Lyme disease is supported by blood tests. It is not considered necessary to provide routine prophylactic antibiotics after the removal of a tick, but it is advisable to remove the tick very carefully to avoid it regurgitating its stomach contents into the host. Ophthalmic departments should carefully consider their policies in respect of safe tick removal and the provision of information leaflets for these patients. The chances of developing Lyme disease after tick bites are very small, but patients/parents should be warned to watch for a red spot or rash developing close to the original bite, which may be accompanied by a headache and fever within 3–30 days of the bite and, in this event, are advised to seek medical consultation urgently.

Sarcoidosis

Kanski (2001) describes sarcoidosis as a common, multisystem, idiopathic, granulomatous disease that involves the lungs in 90% of patients. It may also cause neurological symptoms, a variety of skin problems and affect kidneys, liver, bones and heart. Ophthalmic presentations include conjunctival granulomas, dry eyes, acute and chronic uveitis, and retinal problems. Bradley et al. (2002) have demonstrated that 25–50% of patients with sarcoidosis will have ocular manifestations that are likely to cause significant sight-threatening problems for these patients. They go on to state that the frequency with which eye disease is seen, and the course that it takes, will vary with the person's age and race.

Shaken baby syndrome

Vaughan et al. (1999) recommend that unexplained retinal haemorrhages in children under 3 years without external evidence of head injury should be investigated as possible child abuse. All ophthalmic professionals should be conversant with the child protection procedures in their units.

Stevens–Johnson syndrome (toxic epidermal necrolysis)

Views on the causation of Stevens–Johnson syndrome vary. Kanski (2001) suggests that hypersensitivity to some drugs, and to infections caused by *Mycoplasma pneumoniae* and herpes simplex, may be implicated. Vaughan et al. (1999) also suggest that it may occur as a hypersensitivity reaction to food, noting that children are most susceptible. It is characterized by painful blistering of the skin and mucous membrane involvement. In many cases it is preceded by flu-like symptoms and a high fever. As the condition develops, skin from the lesions may literally slough off. Ocular involvement includes severe conjunctivitis, iritis, lid oedema, conjunctival and corneal blisters and erosions, and corneal perforation. Prins et al. (2003) describe the use of high-dose intravenous immunoglobulin therapy, which is being examined as a means of blocking the progression of Stevens–Johnson syndrome and reducing the time taken to effect skin healing.

Temporal arteritis (giant cell arteritis)

This is a disease of older people, and any history of recent 'new' headaches, combined with recent visual loss, jaw or tongue pain in a patient older than

50 years, should prompt the ophthalmic clinician to consider this diagnosis. Temporal arteritis is a symptom of a generalized inflammation of the tunica intima (inner lining) of the medium and large arteries of the body. Early recognition and treatment are critical to prevent monocular or binocular blindness. Prompt treatment with corticosteroids will relieve the condition, which will be monitored with regular ESR checks. A temporal artery biopsy often gives a conclusive diagnosis.

Thyroid eye disease

Thyroid eye disease (TED) is, in many patients, mild and non-progressive, but Bartalena et al. (2002) state that in 3–5% of cases it is severe. They suggest that non-severe TED requires only supportive measures, such as eye ointments, sunglasses and prisms, but comment that severe TED requires aggressive treatment, either medical (high-dose glucocorticoids, orbital radiotherapy) or surgical (orbital decompression). Most ophthalmic nurses, however, would counter Bartalena et al.'s (2002) trivializing view that non-severe TED requires only supportive measures. The change in cosmetic appearance is very emotionally upsetting for most patients, as evidenced by the publications of the TED patients' organization.

Metcalfe and Weetman (1994) suggest that treatment for TED involves persuading patients to discontinue smoking because it is a risk factor in thyroid-associated ophthalmopathy, an inflammatory process primarily affecting the fibroblasts in extraocular muscles. Wiersinga and Prummel (2002) state that hypoxia stimulates these fibroblasts, and this could contribute, as an enhancing factor, to the adverse effects of smoking on TED. For patients with severe TED, corticosteroids, radiation and orbital decompression may be necessary. Stable patients may require surgery to correct lid retraction and strabismus surgery with adjustable sutures to relieve diplopia.

Uveitis and systemic disease

A number of systemic diseases are associated with the pathogenesis of uveitis. Work by Berthelot et al. (2002) discusses new theories and suggests that the chiefly 'immunological' theory of spondyloarthropathies, which blamed a cross-reaction between self-proteins and bacterial peptides for the disease process, is giving way to a more 'microbiological' concept in which latent bacteria residing within macrophagic or dendritic cells undergo reactivation through a process facilitated by HLA-B27 (human leukocyte antigen). Berthelot et al. (2002) suggest that improved understanding of the mechanisms that give some bacterial strains the potential for persisting within cells, including macrophages, may point the way towards new treatment approaches capable of suspending the disease process, and towards antibiotic therapy to kill dormant bacteria located within cells.

DiLorenzo (2001) states that, within ophthalmology, HLA associations are strongest in diseases of the uvea and in patients with uveitis. She says that 19–88% have the HLA-B27 characteristics, depending on the population studied. HLA-B27 appears in 80–90% of patients with ankylosing spondylitis, thus illustrating the link.

Lyons and Rosenbaum (1997), in a study of inflammatory bowel disease and spondyloarthropathies such as Reiter's syndrome, noted that they were also characterized by diarrhoea, arthritis, stomatitis and uveitis. They set out to investigate whether the characteristics of the uveitis in the eyes of this group of patients could help distinguish these two diagnoses. Their research revealed that uveitis with spondyloarthropathies was predominantly anterior, unilateral, sudden in onset and limited in duration, in contrast to patients with inflammatory bowel disease who frequently had uveitis that was bilateral, posterior, insidious in onset and/or chronic in duration. Episcleritis, scleritis and glaucoma were also more common among patients with inflammatory bowel disease. In 59% of the patients with inflammatory bowel disease in the Lyons and Rosenbaum's (1997) study, the diagnosis of uveitis preceded that of the bowel disorder.

Sexually transmitted infections and AIDS

Acquired immune deficiency syndrome

This is caused by infection with the human immunodeficiency virus (HIV), transmitted by sexual intercourse or accidental inoculation with infected blood. Vaughan et al. (1999) suggest that 30% of people with HIV who develop full-blown AIDS symptoms may present at a hospital's eye department. Ophthalmic manifestations of AIDS may include (Kanski 2001): Kaposi's sarcoma of the eyelid or conjunctiva, multiple molluscum lesions of the lids, severe herpes zoster ophthalmicus, orbital cellulitis, herpes simplex keratitis, anterior uveitis, HIV retinopathy, cytomegalovirus retinopathy and other eye conditions caused by opportunistic infection.

Chlamydial genital infection

Kanski (2001, p. 145) suggests that chlamydial genital infection only infrequently presents as an eye infection. It will present as a follicular conjunctivitis with a mucopurulent discharge that has failed to respond to conventional antibacterial treatments. A diagnostic feature is the presence of a superior micropannus (infiltration of the cornea with blood vessels). Bacterial, viral and chlamydial swabs will be required to confirm the diagnosis. A positive finding will necessitate referral to a genitourinary clinic for treatment, advice and identification of contacts (see also Chapter 15).

Ophthalmia neonatorum

Neonates may present with gonococcal infection (2–3 days after delivery), chlamydial eye infections (5–12 days) or herpes simplex virus 2 (HSV-2) keratoconjunctivitis (2–3 days), having become contaminated during the birth process.

Gonococcal infections, which may rapidly lead to corneal ulceration and even perforation, need to be treated most urgently. Following the results of an urgent Gram stain, which demonstrates the broad type of bacteria involved, and pending actual identification of the organism, the eyes may be treated with topical penicillin, chloramphenicol, gentamicin or tetracycline and systemic antibiotics. In the UK, this is a notifiable illness (see also Chapter 15) and parents will need treatment and advice.

Problems that may require health advice

Sexually transmitted infections

For details of this see above.

Xanthelasma

These are fatty lesions that characteristically present around the eye. Baumgartner et al. (1992) state that xanthelasmas occur more frequently in people with diabetes than in the rest of the population. Surprisingly, according to Baumgartner et al. (1992), only about 5% of patients with xanthelasma have hyperlipidaemia. However, as they may be symptomatic for congenital hyperlipidaemia, or arise in people with raised serum lipids, people who develop these should be advised to have their blood cholesterol checked.

Hypertension

A routine blood pressure check on a person who has attended an ophthalmic emergency department with a subconjunctival haemorrhage may reveal hypertension as a possible causative factor. Further blood pressure checks by the practice nurse should be advised before the GP will be able to make a firm diagnosis of hypertension.

Hypotension

Although not actively treated in the UK, hypotension is increasingly being scrutinized as a possible factor in low-tension glaucoma. Gherghel et al. (2001), in a study to evaluate the relationship between the circadian blood pressure rhythm and the retrobulbar blood flow in glaucoma patients, concluded that glaucoma patients with a marked drop in their nocturnal systemic blood pressure seem to have altered retrobulbar blood flow parameters, suggesting that an abnormal systemic blood pressure profile may be the manifestation of some kind of systemic vascular dysregulation relevant to the ocular circulation. Marcus et al. (2001) suggested that 'sleep-disturbed breathing' may be a risk factor for normal tension glaucoma and, although unable to provide evidence for a cause-and-effect relationship, suggested that various physiological factors produced by sleep-disturbed breathing might play a significant role in its development. They recommended obtaining a sleep history from these patients and possible referral to a sleep apnoea clinic.

Migraine

Migraine accounts for many visits to ophthalmic accident and emergency departments. The practice by some departments of encouraging the public to telephone before attendance has helped to reassure patients and reduce these attendances. One of the key questions that the ophthalmic nurse needs to ask the patient who is complaining about flashing lights is whether the phenomenon is affecting both eyes. If it is, and the visual aura lasts for about 30 minutes, and clears, the symptom that the patient is reporting is most likely to be caused by migraine.

However, Comoglu et al. (2003) have demonstrated a possible interrelationship of the pathophysiology of migraine, visual field defects and glaucomatous optic neuropathy, and do suggest visual field screening for normal tension glaucoma in patients who have regular migraine attacks.

References

Aiello L (2003) Perspectives on diabetic retinopathy. Am J Ophthalmol 136: 122–35.
Augsten R, Konigsdorffer E, Oehme A, Strobel J (1998) Bilateral endogenous endophthalmitis. Klin Monatsbl Augenheilkd 212: 120–2.
Awad A, Mullaney P, Al-Mesfer S, Zwaan J (1999) Glaucoma in Sturge–Weber syndrome. J Am Assoc Pediatr Ophthalmol Strabismus 3: 40–5.
Babikian V, Wijman C, Koleini B, Malik S, Goyal N, Matjucha I (2001) Retinal ischemia and embolism – etiologies and outcomes based on a prospective study. Cerebrovas Dis 12: 108–13.

Bartalena L, Marcocci C, Tanda ML, Pinchera A (2002) Management of thyroid eye disease. Eur J Nuclear Med Mol Imaging 29(suppl 2): S458–65.

Baumgartner R, Spina G, Senn B (1992) Lid tumors in systemic illness. Klin Monatsbl Augenheilkd 200: 543–4.

Beales P, Elcioglu N, Woolf A, Parker D, Flinter F (1999) New criteria for improved diagnosis of Bardet-Biedl syndrome: results of a population survey. J Med Genet 36: 437–46.

Berthelot JM, Glemarec J, Guillot P, Laborie Y, Maugars Y (2002) New pathogenic hypotheses for spondyloarthropathies. Joint Bone Spine 69: 114–22.

Bevan J (1998) Congenital syndromes in paediatric anaesthesia: what is important to know. Part 2. Can J Anaesth 45(5 suppl): R3–9.

Bosch A, Bakker H, van Gennip A, van Kempen J, Wanders R, Wijburg F (2002) Clinical features of galactokinase deficiency: a review of the literature. J Inherited Metab Dis 25: 629–34.

Bradley D, Baughman R, Raymond L, Kaufman A (2002) Ocular manifestations of sarcoidosis. Semin Respir Crit Care Med 23: 543–8.

Comoglu S, Yarangumeli A, Koz O, Elhan A, Kural G (2003) Glaucomatous visual field defects in patients with migraine. J Neurol 250: 201–6.

DiLorenzo AL (2001) HLA-B27 syndromes: www.emedicine.com/oph/topic721.htm (accessed 4/04/05).

Dowler J, Sehmi K, Hykin P (1999) The natural history of macular oedema after cataract surgery in diabetes. Ophthalmology 106: 663–8.

Evereklioglu C, Yilmaz K, Bekir NA (2002) Decreased central corneal thickness in children with Down syndrome. J Pediatr Ophthalmol Strabismus 39: 274–7.

Gherghel D, Orgul S, Gugleta K, Flammer J (2001) Retrobulbar blood flow in glaucoma patients with nocturnal over-dipping in systemic blood pressure. Am J Ophthalmol 132: 641–7.

Holmes J, Coates C (1994) Assessment of visual acuity in children with trisomy 18. Ophthal Genet 15(3–4): 115–20.

Kanski J (2001) Systemic Diseases and the Eye. London: Mosby.

Kuchle M, Naumann G (1992) Penetrating keratoplasty for keratoconus in patients with Down's syndrome. Klin Monatsbl Augenheilkd 200: 228–30.

Lawrence K, Campbell R, Swettenham J et al. (2003) Interpreting gaze in Turner syndrome: impaired sensitivity to intention and emotion, but preservation of social cueing. Neuropsychologia 41: 894–905.

Leiba H, Oliver M, Pollack A (1996) Prophylactic laser photocoagulation in Stickler syndrome. Eye 10: 701–8.

Leslie RD, Pozzilli P (2002) An introduction to new advances in diabetes. Diabetes/Metabolism Res Rev 18(suppl 1): S1–6.

Lesniak-Karpiak K, Mazzocco M, Ross J (2003) Behavioral assessment of social anxiety in females with Turner or fragile X syndrome. J Autism Dev Dis 33: 55–67.

Levy HL, Brown AE, Williams SE, deJuan E (1996) Vitreous hemorrhage as an ophthalmic complication of galactosemia. J Pediatr 129: 922–5.

Lyons JL, Rosenbaum JT (1997) Uveitis associated with inflammatory bowel disease compared with uveitis associated with spondyloarthropathy. Arch Ophthalmol 115: 61–4.

Marcus D, Costarides A, Gokhale P et al. (2001) Sleep disorders: a risk factor for normal-tension glaucoma? J Glaucoma 10: 177–83.

Metcalfe R, Weetman A (1994) Stimulation of extraocular-muscle fibroblasts by cytokines and hypoxia – possible role in thyroid-associated ophthalmopathy. Clin Endocrinol 40: 67–72.

Mitchell V, Howard R, Facer E (1995) Down's syndrome and anesthesia. Pediatr Anesth 5: 379–84.

Pittasch D, Lobmann R, Berens-Baumann W, Lehrent H (2002) Pupil signs of autonomic neuropathy in patients with type 1 diabetes. Diabetes Care 25: 1545–50.

Prins C, Vittorio C, Padilla RS et al. (2003) Effect of high-dose intravenous immunoglobulin therapy in Stevens–Johnson syndrome: a retrospective, multicenter study. Dermatology 207: 96–9.

Robitaille JM, Monsein L, Traboulsi EI (1996) Coats' disease and central nervous system venous malformation. Ophthal Genet 17: 215–18.

Royal National Institute for the Blind (2003) www.rnib.org.uk (accessed 28/8/03).

Stickler G, Hughes W, Houchin P (2001) Clinical features of hereditary progressive arthroophthalmopathy (Stickler syndrome): a survey. Genet Med 3: 192–6.

Vaughan D, Asbury T, Riordan-Eva P (1999) General Ophthalmology. Norwalk, CT: Appleton & Lange.

Weese S, Gosnell K, West P, Gropper S (2003) Galactose content of baby food meats: considerations for infants with galactosemia. J Am Diet Assoc 103: 373–5.

Weishaar P, Flynn H, Murray T et al. (1998) Endogenous aspergillus endophthalmitis – clinical features and treatment outcomes. Ophthalmology 105: 57–65.

Wiersinga W, Prummel F (2002) Graves' ophthalmopathy: a rational approach to treatment. Trends Endocrinol Metab 13: 280–7.

Plates 2, 4, 17, 18 and 24–43
by courtesy of Angela Chappell, Ophthalmic
Imaging Department, Flinders Medical
Centre, Adelaide, South Australia.

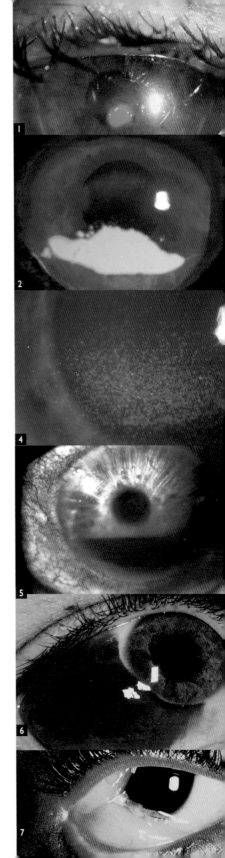

Plate 1 Corneal abrasion.

Plate 2 Exposure keratitis.

Plate 3 Foreign body.

Plate 4 Punctate epithelial erosions.

Plate 5 Hyphaema.

Plate 6 Subconjunctival haemorrhage.

Plate 7 Chemosis.

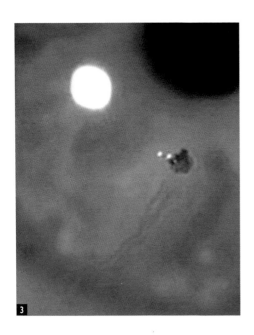

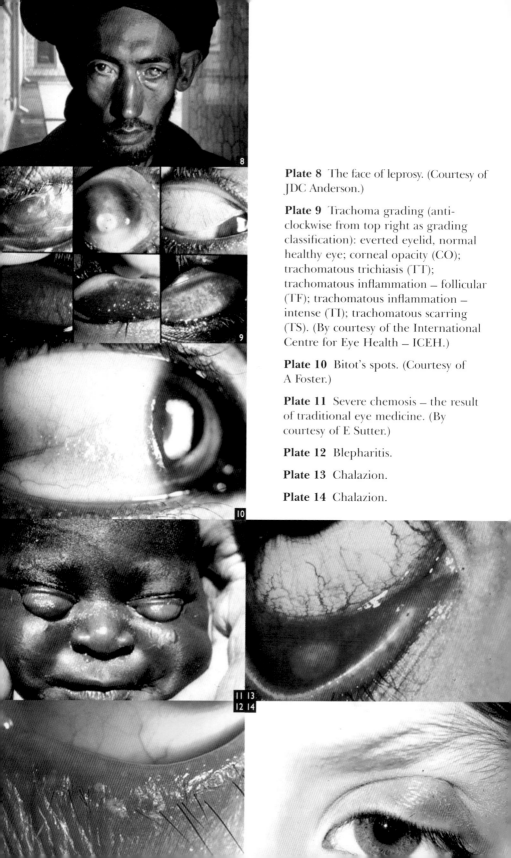

Plate 8 The face of leprosy. (Courtesy of JDC Anderson.)

Plate 9 Trachoma grading (anti-clockwise from top right as grading classification): everted eyelid, normal healthy eye; corneal opacity (CO); trachomatous trichiasis (TT); trachomatous inflammation – follicular (TF); trachomatous inflammation – intense (TI); trachomatous scarring (TS). (By courtesy of the International Centre for Eye Health – ICEH.)

Plate 10 Bitot's spots. (Courtesy of A Foster.)

Plate 11 Severe chemosis – the result of traditional eye medicine. (By courtesy of E Sutter.)

Plate 12 Blepharitis.

Plate 13 Chalazion.

Plate 14 Chalazion.

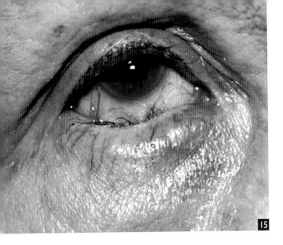

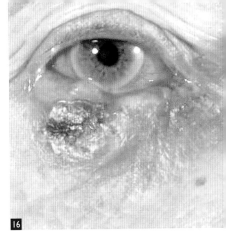

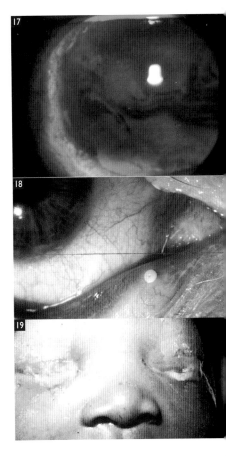

Plate 15 Entropion.

Plate 16 Basal cell carcinoma. (By courtesy of the Ophthalmic Imaging Department, Manchester Royal Eye Hospital.)

Plate 17 Tear film break-up time.

Plate 18 Punctal plugs.

Plate 19 Gonococcal conjunctivitis (baby).

Plate 20 Viral conjunctivitis.

Plate 21 Follicles.

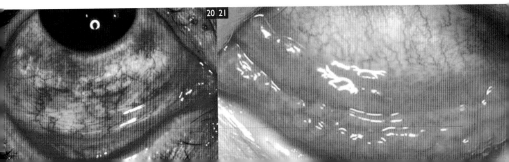

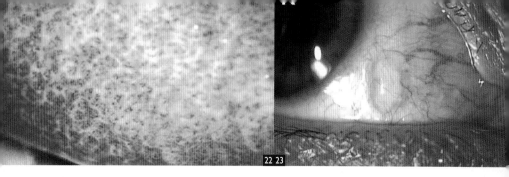

Plate 22 Papillae.

Plate 23 Conjunctival cyst.

Plate 24 Corneal topography of astigmatism.

Plate 25 Specular micrograph of a normal endothelium.

Plate 26 Filamentary keratitis.

Plate 27 Bacterial keratitis.

Plate 28 Dendrite. Dentritic ulcer caused by herpes simplex virus.

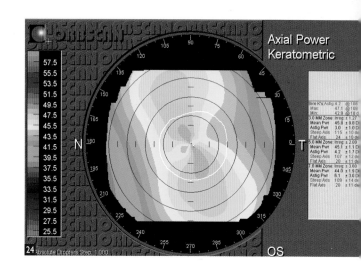

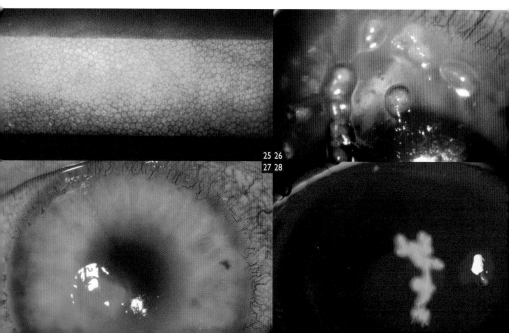

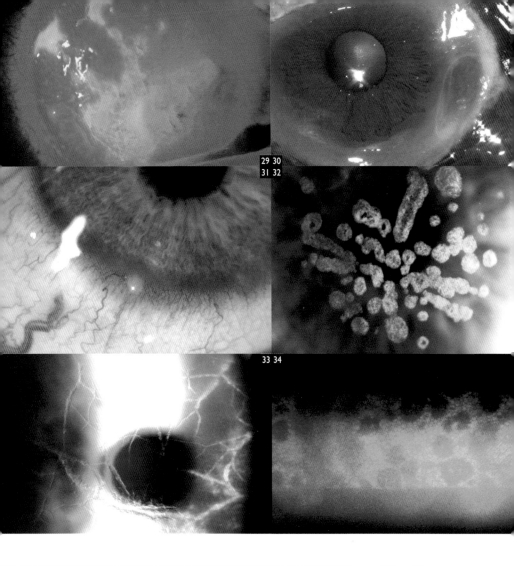

29 30
31 32
33 34

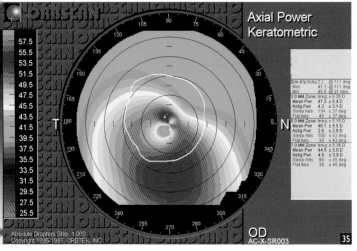

Axial Power Keratometric

57.5
55.5
53.5
51.5
49.5
47.5
45.5
43.5
41.5
39.5
37.5
35.5
33.5
31.5
29.5
27.5
25.5

T 180

N

OD
AC-X-SR003

35

Absolute Diopters Step: 1.000
Copyright 1995-1997, ORBTEK, INC

Plate 29 Geographic ulcer. Caused by herpes simplex virus.

Plate 30 Corneal dellen.

Plate 31 Phlycten.

Plate 32 Granular dystrophy.

Plate 33 Lattice dystrophy.

Plate 34 Fuchs' endothelial dystrophy.

Plate 35 Orbscan of keratoconus.

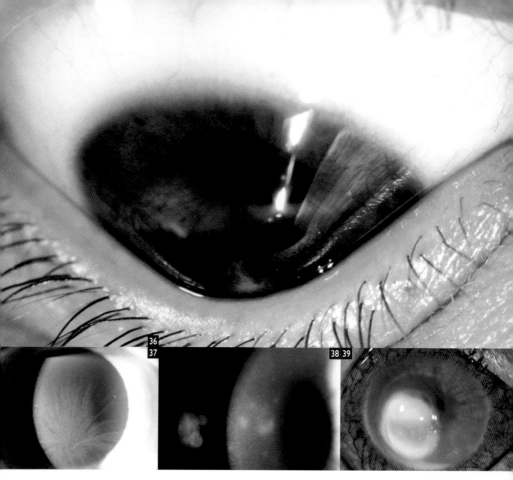

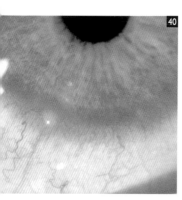

Plate 36 Munson's sign.

Plate 37 Vortex keratopathy.

Plate 38 Contact lens induced hypoxia.

Plate 39 Bacterial keratitis caused by pseudomonas aeroginosa.

Plate 40 Loose corneal suture in penetrating keratoplasty.

Plate 41 Radial keratotomy.

Plate 42 Episcleritis.

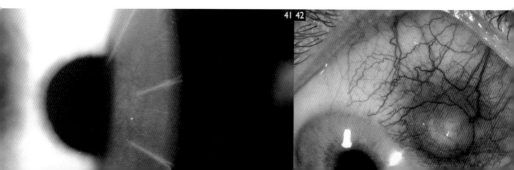

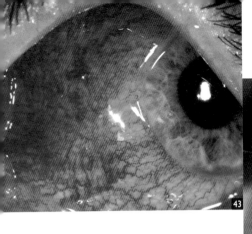

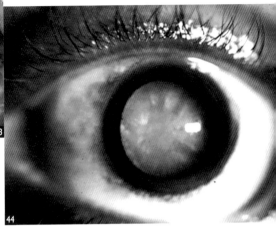

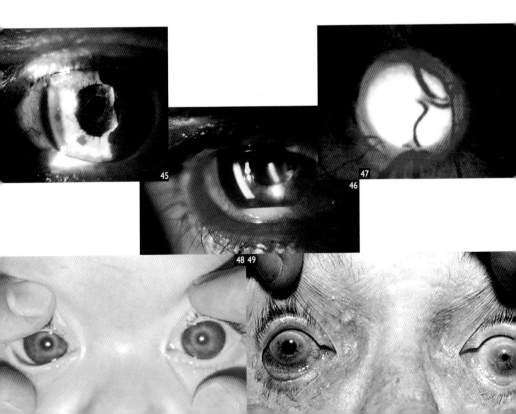

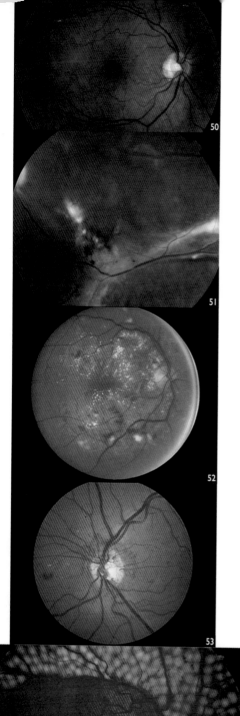

Plate 50 Normal retina. (By courtesy of Ophthalmic Imaging Department, Manchester Royal Eye Hospital.)

Plate 51 Retinal detachment. (By courtesy of Ophthalmic Imaging Department, Manchester Royal Eye Hospital.)

Plate 52 Non-proliferative diabetic retinopathy.

Plate 53 Proliferative diabetic retinopathy.

Plate 54 Panretinal photocoagulation for retinopathy. (By courtesy of the National Eye Institute, National Institutes of Health, USA.)

Plate 55 Orbital cellulitis.

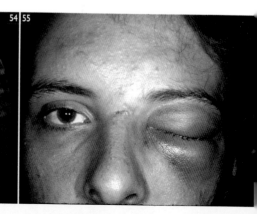

Appendix

Addresses

Christian Blind Mission International (CBMI)
Nibelungenstrasse 124
64625 Bensheim, Germany
Website: www.cbmi.org

Healthlink Worldwide
Cityside
40 Adler Street
London E1 1EE, UK
Website: www.healthlink.org.uk

International Agency for the Prevention of Blindness (IAPB)
VISION 2020 – Central Office/IAPB Secretariat
L.V. Prasad Eye Institute
L.V. Prasad Marg
Banjara Hills
Hyderabad, India
Website: www.iapb.org

International Resource Centre (IRC)
International Centre for Eye Health (ICEH)
London School of Hygiene and Tropical Medicine
Keppel Street
London WC1E 7HT, UK
Website: www.iceh.org.uk

National Radiological Protection Board (NRPB)
Chilton
Didcot
Oxford OX11 0RQ, UK
Website: www.nrpb.org.uk

ORBIS International Inc.
520 Eighth Avenue
11th Floor
New York, NY 10080, USA
Website: www.orbis.org
ORBIS exists to preserve and restore sight worldwide. They work in partnership with local health professionals to improve the quality of eye care available for people in countries where the need is great.

Royal College of Ophthalmologists
17 Cornwall Terrace,
London NW1 4QW, UK
Tel: +44 (0) 20 7935 0702
Fax: +44 (0) 20 7935 9838
Website: www.rcophth.ac.uk

St John Eye Hospital
Nablus Road
Sheikh Jarrah
Jerusalem 97200, Israel
Website: www.stjohneyehospital.org

Sight Savers International
Grosvenor Hall
Bolnore Road
Haywards Heath
West Sussex RH16 4BX, UK
Website: www.sightsavers.org.uk

Teaching-aids At Low Cost (TALC)
PO Box 49
St Albans
Hertfordshire, AL1 5TX, UK
Website: www.talcuk.org

VISION 2020 – London Office
London School of Hygiene and Tropical Medicine
Keppel Street
London WC1E 7HT, UK
Website: www.v2020.org

Vision Aid Overseas (VAO)
12 The Bell Centre
Newton Road
Manor Royal
Crawley RH10 2FZ, UK
Website: www.vao.org.uk

World Health Organization (WHO)
Prevention of Blindness and Deafness (PBD)
1211 Geneva 27, Switzerland
Website: www.who.int/pbd

Websites

Action for Blind People
www.afbp.org
Enables blind and partially sighted people to transform their lives through work, housing, leisure and support. Offers a wide range of services to visually impaired people, their families, advocates, professionals and the general public.

Anaesthesia for ENT, Ophthalmic, Dental and Facial Surgery
www.virtual-anaesthesia-textbook.com/vat/ent.html
The Virtual Anaesthesia Textbook, Anaesthesia for ENT, Ophthalmic, Dental and Facial Surgery

British Blind Sport
www.britishblindsport.org.uk

Diabetes UK
www.diabetes.org.uk
Diabetes UK is the leading charity working for people with diabetes.

English Blind Golf Association
www.blindgolf.co.uk/index.php
The EBGA is a voluntarily run organization, which provides quality competition and training in golf for registered blind people throughout England and Wales.

EQUIP – Electronic Quality Information for Patients
www.equip.nhs.uk/topics/eye.html
A gateway to quality-checked websites of information for patients.

Eye Cancer Network
www.eyecancer.com
Provides education and services to patients and professionals.

The Eyecare Trust
www.eyecare-trust.org.uk
The Eyecare Trust is a registered charity that exists to raise awareness of all aspects of ocular health, the importance of regular eye care and good eye wear. They do this by providing accurate, unbiased eye care information to the public and the media.

Eyesite
www.nurseseyesite.nhs.uk
An on-line community for ophthalmic nurses.

Eyetext
www.eyetext.net
Eyetext is an interactive ophthalmology site.

EyeUK
www.eyeuk.com/
Links to and reviews of UK WWW sites related to the eye, vision and ophthalmology.

Global Vision
www.global-vision.org.uk
"A charitable organisation dedicated to the relief of blindness in developing countries"

The Guide Dogs for the Blind Association
www.guidedogs.org.uk/

International Council of Ophthalmology
www.icoph.org
The International Council of Ophthalmology's Eye Site is a guide to finding information, resources and connections related to ophthalmology and vision around the world. It offers information on ophthalmological organizations, ophthalmic education, preservation and restoration of vision, and prevention of blindness. The Eye Site is also the internet home for the International Federation of Ophthalmological Societies (IFOS) and the International Council of Ophthalmology (ICO).

Ophthalmic Hyperguide
www.ophthalmic.hyperguides.com
Educational resource for eye care specialists.

Positive Vision
www.positivevision.co.uk
Positive vision charity that aims to help people with sight loss and to help their families and carers.

Sense
www.sense.org.uk
A voluntary organization working with people of all ages who are deaf-blind or have associated disabilities.

SPECS
www.eyeconditions.org.uk
A not-for-profit organisation. Contains a list of other eye organisations and their websites of use to professionals and their patients and acts as an umbrella group for specific eye condition support groups.

Glossary

Accommodation	The adjustment of the eye for seeing at near distances. The shape of the lens is changed through action of the ciliary muscle, focusing a clear image on the retina.
Achromatopsia	Colour blindness.
Agnosia	The inability to recognize common objects despite an intact visual apparatus, e.g. prosopagnosia – the inability to recognize faces.
Amaurosis fugax	Transient loss of vision, often caused by carotid artery disease.
Amblyopia	Reduced visual acuity (uncorrectable) in the absence of detectable anatomical defects in the eye or visual pathways.
Ammetropia	An optical defect preventing light rays from being brought to a focus on the retina.
Amsler grid	A chart with vertical and horizontal lines and a central spot, used in the assessment of macular disease.
Angiography	A diagnostic test in which the retinal vascular system is examined. Intravenous injection of fluorescein demonstrates the retinal circulation, whilst that of indocyanine green demonstrates the choroidal circulation.
Aniridia	Congenital absence of the iris.
Anisocoria	Unequal pupillary size.
Anisometropia	Difference in refractive error of the eyes.
Anophthalmos	Absence of a true eyeball.
Aphakia	Absence of the lens.
Asthenopia	Eye fatigue from muscular, environmental or psychological causes.
Astigmatism	Refractive error preventing the light rays from coming to a focus on the retina because of different curvatures of the meridians of the cornea (or lens).

596

Binocular vision	Ability of the eyes to focus on one object and then to fuse the two images into one.
Bitot's spots	Keratinization of the conjunctiva near the limbus, resulting in raised spots – caused by vitamin A deficiency.
Blepharitis	Inflammation of the lid margins.
Blepharoptosis	Drooping of the eyelid, usually known as ptosis.
Blepharospasm	Involuntary spasm of the eyelids.
Blind spot	Missing area of the visual field, corresponding to where light falls on the optic nerve head.
Botulinum toxin	Neurotoxin A of the bacterium *Clostridium botulinum* used in very small doses to produce temporary paralysis of the extraocular muscles.
Buphthalmos	Large eyeball in congenital glaucoma resulting from raised pressure.
Canthotomy	Usually a lateral canthotomy – cutting of the lateral canthal tendon in order to widen the palpebral fissure. Usually after trauma because of haematoma in the orbit.
Canthus	The angle formed at the junction of the upper and lower lids, inner (medial) and outer (lateral).
Capsulorrhexis	Removal of the anterior capsule of the lens before phakoemulsification, using a single circular tear.
Capsulotomy (posterior)	Laser treatment after extracapsular cataract extraction involving the making of a hole in the posterior capsule of a lens that has become opaque.
Cartella	Protective eye shield.
Chalazion	Swelling of a meibomian gland resulting from infection or granuloma post-infection.
Chemosis	Conjunctival oedema.
Coloboma	Congenital cleft in ocular tissue resulting from the failure of a part of the eye or adnexae to form completely.
Concave lens	Lens having the power to diverge rays of light; also known as a diverging or minus (–) lens.
Cones	Retinal receptor cells, concerned with visual acuity and colour discrimination.
Convex lens	Lens having the power to converge rays of light; also known as converging or plus (+) lens.
Cyclodestructive procedures	Surgical techniques to reduce aqueous production by destroying part of the ciliary body using cryotherapy (cyclocryotherapy), laser (cyclophotocoagulation) or diathermy.

Cycloplegic	A drug that temporarily paralyses the ciliary muscle.
Cyclitis	Inflammation of the ciliary body.
Cylindrical lens	A segment of a cylinder (the refractive power of which varies in different meridians) used to correct astigmatism.
Dacryoadenitis	Infection of the lacrimal gland.
Dacryocystitis	Infection of the lacrimal sac.
Dacryocystorhinostomy	A procedure by which a channel is made between the nasolacrimal duct and the nasal cavity to bypass an obstruction in the nasolacrimal duct or sac.
Dark adaptation	The ability to adjust to decreased illumination.
Dellen	An area of epithelial loss on the cornea caused by drying because of shadowing by conjunctiva swollen as a result of chemosis or subconjunctival haemorrhage.
Dendritic ulcer	A corneal ulcer caused by the herpes simplex virus – named thus because of the characteristic pattern of the ulcer on the cornea.
Diopter	Unit of measurement of the refractive power of lenses.
Diplopia	Double vision – the eyes' inability to fuse two images into one – disappears when one eye is covered.
Discission	Operation for congenital cataract or certain types of traumatic cataract in which the anterior capsule is ruptured and the lens substance left to absorb or, later, be evacuated.
Echymosis	'Black eye'.
Ectropion	Turning out of the eyelid (eversion).
Emmetropia	An eye with no refractive error.
Endolaser	Application of laser from a probe inside the globe.
Endophthalmitis	Intraocular infection.
Enophthalmos	Abnormal retrodisplacement of the eyeball.
Entropion	A condition where the eyelid turns inwards (inversion).
Enucleation	Surgical removal of the eyeball.
Epicanthus	Congenital skin fold that overlies the inner canthus.
Epiphora	Watering eye – tearing.
Evisceration	Removal of the contents of the globe.
Exenteration	Removal of the entire contents of the orbit, including the globe and lids. Can be more or less radical.

Exophthalmos	Abnormal protrusion of the eyeball (proptosis).
Field of vision	The entire area that can be seen without moving the point of gaze.
Floaters	Moving images in the visual field as a result of vitreous opacities.
Fornix	The junction of the bulbar and palpebral conjunctivae.
Fovea	Depression in the macula adapted for most acute vision.
Fundus	The posterior portion of the eye visible through an ophthalmoscope.
Glaukomflecken	Opacities on the anterior lens capsule indicative of a previous episode of acute, angle-closure glaucoma.
Gonioscopy	An examination technique for the anterior chamber angle, using a corneal contact lens containing a mirror and a light source.
Hemianopia	Blindness in one-half of the field of vision of one or both eyes (bitemporal where both temporal fields are missing or homonymous where the defect is on the same side).
Hippus	Spontaneous rhythmic movements of the iris.
Hordeolum, external (stye)	Infection of the glands of Moll or Zeiss.
Hordeolum, internal	Meibomian gland infection – chalazion.
Hypermetropia (far-sightedness)	A refractive error in which the focus of light from a distant object is behind the retina.
Hyphaema	Blood in the anterior chamber.
Hypopyon	Pus in the anterior chamber.
Hypotony	Abnormally soft eye from any cause.
Injection	Congestion of blood vessels.
Iridodialysis	Detachment of the iris from the ciliary body, usually caused by blunt trauma.
Iridodonesis	Trembling of the iris after cataract extraction.
Ishihara colour plates	A test for colour vision based on the ability to see patterns in a series of multicoloured charts.
Isopter	A device for testing visual fields. Isopters can be of different colours and sizes and form concentric rings on field testing (perimetry).
Keratic precipitate (KP)	Accumulation of inflammatory cells on the corneal endothelium in uveitis.
Keratitis	Corneal inflammation.
Keratoconus	Cone-shaped deformity of the cornea.
Keratomalacia	Corneal softening, usually associated with vitamin A deficiency.
Keratometer	An instrument for measuring the curvature of the cornea.

Keratoplasty	Corneal graft – may be lamellar or full thickness. An area of opaque cornea is replaced in order to achieve corneal clarity.
Keratotomy	An incision in the cornea. Radial keratotomy is a procedure in which radial incisions are made in the cornea to change the curvature of the cornea and correct refractive error.
Leukocoria	White pupil.
Limbus	Junction of the cornea and sclera.
Macula lutea	The small avascular area of the retina surrounding the fovea, containing yellow xanthophyll pigment.
Megalocornea	Abnormally large cornea.
Metamorphopsia	Distortion of vision.
Microphthalmos	Abnormally small eye with abnormal function.
Miotic	A drug causing pupillary constriction.
Mydriatic	A drug causing pupillary dilatation.
Myopia (near-sightedness)	A refractive error in which the focus for light rays from a distant object is in front of the retina, so images from a distance appear blurred.
Nanophthalmos	Abnormally small eye with normal function near point – the point at which the eye is focused when accommodation is fully active.
Nystagmus	An involuntary movement of the globe that may be horizontal, vertical, torsional or mixed.
Ophthalmia neonatorum	Conjunctivitis in the newborn.
Optic disc	Ophthalmoscopically visible portion of the optic nerve.
Pannus	Infiltration of the cornea with blood vessels.
Panophthalmitis	Inflammation of the entire globe.
Papillitis	Optic nerve head inflammation.
Perimeter	An instrument for measuring the visual field.
Peripheral vision	Ability to perceive the presence or motion of objects outside the direct line of vision.
Phacoemulsification	Technique of extracapsular cataract extraction in which the nucleus of the lens is disrupted into small fragments by ultrasonic vibrations, allowing aspiration of lens matter through a small wound, leading to faster visual recovery.
Phlycten	Localized lymphocytic infiltration of the conjunctiva or corneal margin resulting in a small, raised, staining area.
Photocoagulation	Thermal damage to tissues, in ophthalmology, usually as a result of laser energy.
Photophobia	Abnormal sensitivity to light.

Photopsia	Appearance of flashes of light within the eye as a result of traction on the retina.
Phthisis bulbi	Atrophy of the globe with blindness and decreased intraocular pressure, caused by end-stage ophthalmic disease.
Pinguecula	A thickening of the conjunctiva, usually medial to the cornea, bilateral and a normal finding.
Placido's disc	A disc with concentric black and white rings used to determine the regularity of the cornea by observing the ring's reflection on the corneal surface.
Presbyopia	Physiologically blurred near vision, caused by a reduction in the ability of the eye to accommodate, because of increasing size and rigidity of the lens, with age.
Pseudophakia	Presence of an artificial intraocular lens after cataract extraction.
Pterygium	A triangular growth of tissue that extends from the conjunctiva over the cornea.
Ptosis	Drooping of the eyelid.
Puncta	External orifices of the upper and lower canaliculi.
Refraction	(1) Deviation in the course of light rays passing from one transparent medium into another of different density. (2) Determination of refractive errors of the eye.
Retinal detachment	A separation of the neurosensory retina from the pigment epithelium.
Retinitis pigmentosa	A hereditary degeneration of the retina.
Retinoscope	An instrument designed for objective refraction of the eye.
Rods	Retinal receptor cells concerned with peripheral vision and vision in decreased illumination.
Rubeosis	Aberrant blood vessels, often on the iris (rubeosis iridis).
Scleral spur	The protrusion of sclera into the anterior chamber angle.
Scotoma	A blind or partially blind area in the visual field.
Subconjunctival haemorrhage	Haemorrhage, generally idiopathic, underneath the conjunctiva.
Staphyloma	A thinned part of the coat of the eye resulting in protrusion of ocular contents.
Strabismus	Misalignment of the eyes – a squint.
Symblepharon	Adhesions between the bulbar and palpebral conjunctivae.

Sympathetic ophthalmia	Inflammation in a normal eye resulting from inflammation in the fellow eye.
Synechiae	Adhesion of the iris to the cornea (anterior synechiae) or lens (posterior synechiae).
Syneresis	A degenerative process within the vitreous involving a drawing together of particles within the gel, separation and shrinkage of the gel.
Tarsorrhaphy	A surgical procedure by which the upper and lower lid margins are joined.
Tonometer	An instrument for measuring intraocular pressure.
Trabeculectomy	Surgical procedure for creating a channel for additional aqueous drainage in glaucoma.
Trabeculoplasty	Laser photocoagulation of the trabecular meshwork to aid aqueous outflow.
Trachoma	A serious form of infectious keratoconjunctivitis.
Trichiasis	Inversion and rubbing of the eyelashes against the globe.
Uveal tract	The iris, ciliary body and choroid.
Uveitis	Inflammation of one or all portions of the uveal tract.
Visual acuity	Measure of central vision.
Visual axis	A theoretical line connecting a fixation point with the fovea centralis.
Vitritis	Inflammation of vitreous.
Xerosis	Drying of tissues lining the anterior surface of the eye.
Zonule	The suspensory ligaments that stretch from the ciliary processes to the lens equator and hold it in place.

Index